WHAT'S A SERVING SIZE?

FRUITS

1 serving of fruit looks like:

1 medium peach

or

1 mango

1 medium apple

or

1 cup chopped apples

or

1 8-inch banana

1 cup (8 fl. oz) 100% fruit juice

compare with

VEGETABLES

1 serving of vegetables looks like:

2 cups lettuce

or

1 cup cooked broccoli

or

1

7 baby carrots

1 large bell pepper

DAIRY

1 serving of dairy looks like:

8 oz yogurt

1 cup (8 fl. oz) milk

compare with

How Much Do I Eat?

When you're creating a healthful diet for yourself, or doing a diet assessment project, it's important to keep in mind not only the types of foods you eat, but also how much. However, it can be difficult to know what a particular number of cups, ounces, or ounce-equivalents looks like. Here is a visual tip sheet that will help you translate the food on your plate into common serving sizes. Tear it out and bring it with you to the dining hall, the café, or the kitchen table.

A "Hand-y" Way to Estimate Serving Size

The following photos show how to judge serving sizes with something you always have with you—your hand.

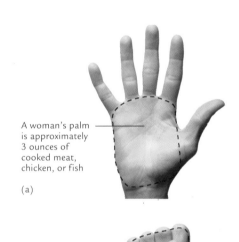

A woman's palm is approximately 3 ounces of cooked meat, chicken, or fish

(a)

A woman's fist is about 1 cup of pasta or vegetables (a man's fist is the size of about 2 cups)

(b)

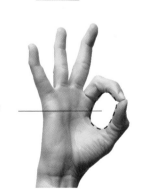

About 1 tbsp. of vegetable oil

(c)

GRAINS

1 serving of grains looks like:

| 1/2 cup rice | or | 1/2 cup pasta | or | 1/2 cup oatmeal | = | 1/2 baseball |

| 1 slice bread | 1 cup cereal | 1 piece cornbread | one 6-inch tortilla | one 3-inch (mini) bagel |

MEAT & BEANS

1 serving of meat or beans looks like:

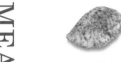 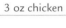

| 3 oz chicken | or | 5 oz steak | or | 4 oz pork | or | 6 oz tofu | = | mouse |

| 3 oz fish | = | checkbook |

| 1/2 cup garbanzo beans | or | 1/2 cup pinto beans | = | light bulb |

| 1 oz peanuts | or | 1 oz almonds | or | 2 T. peanut butter | = | ping pong ball |

FATS

1 serving of fats looks like:

| 1 t. butter | 1 oz potato chips | 1 T. salad dressing | 2 T. cream cheese | or | 2 T. olive oil | = | ping pong ball |

ALCOHOL

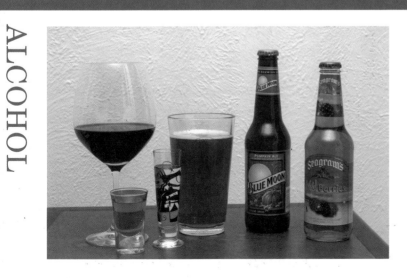

One "drink" of alcohol is defined as the amount of a beverage that provides 1/2 fl. oz of alcohol, which normally equals 1-1/2 oz of distilled spirits, 5 oz of wine, or 12 oz of beer or wine cooler.

NUTRITION
FOR LIFE

SECOND EDITION

Janice Thompson, PhD, FACSM

University of Bristol
University of New Mexico

Melinda Manore, PhD, RD, FACSM

Oregon State University

Benjamin Cummings

San Francisco   Boston   New York
Cape Town   Hong Kong   London   Madrid   Mexico City
Montreal   Munich   Paris   Singapore   Sydney   Tokyo   Toronto

Senior Acquisitions Editor: Sandra Lindelof
Senior Project Editor: Marie Beaugureau
Development Manager: Barbara Yien
Development Editor: Laura Bonazzoli
Assistant Editors: Jacob Evans and Shannon Cutt
Assistant Media Producer: Lee Ann Doctor
Supplements Editor: Jennifer Cassidento
Managing Editor: Deborah Cogan
Production Supervisor: Beth Masse
Production Management and Composition: S4Carlisle Publishing Services
Interior and Cover Designer: Riezebos Holzbaur Design Group
Illustrators: Precision Graphics
Senior Art Editor: Donna Kalal
Photo Researcher: Kristin Piljay
Image Rights and Permissions Manager: Zina Arabia
Manufacturing Buyer: Jeffrey Sargent
Senior Marketing Manager: Neena Bali
Text Printer: Quebecor World Dubuque
Cover Printer: Phoenix Color
Cover Design: Riezebos Holzbaur Design Group
Cover Photo Credit: Paul Conrath/Getty Images

Credits can be found on page CR-1.

Library of Congress Cataloging-in-Publication Data

Thompson, Janice, 1962–
    Nutrition for life / Janice Thompson, Melinda Manore.—
    2nd ed. p. cm.
Includes bibliographical references and index.
ISBN 978-0-321-57084-0
1. Nutrition—Textbooks.   I. Manore, Melinda, 1951–
    II. Title.

TX354.T46 2010
613.2—dc22   2008044432

1 2 3 4 5 6 7 8 9 10—**QWD**—11 12 10 09 08
Manufactured in the United States of America.

ISBN-10: 0-321-57084-7 (Student edition)
ISBN-13: 978-0-321-57084-0 (Student edition)

ISBN-10: 0-321-57166-5 (Professional copy)
ISBN-13: 978-0-321-57166-3 (Professional copy)

Benjamin Cummings
is an imprint of

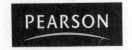

www.pearsonhighered.com

"To our moms—your consistent love and support are the keys to our happiness and success. You have been incredible role models.

"To our dads—you raised us to be independent, intelligent, and resourceful. We miss you and wish you were here to be proud of, and to brag about, our accomplishments.

ABOUT THE AUTHORS

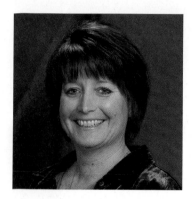

Janice Thompson, PhD, FACSM

University of Bristol
University of New Mexico

Janice Thompson earned a PhD from Arizona State University in exercise physiology and nutrition. She is currently a Professor of Public Health Nutrition at the University of Bristol in the Department of Exercise, Nutrition and Health Sciences, and is also an Adjunct Faculty member at the University of New Mexico Health Sciences Center. Her research focuses on designing nutrition and physical activity interventions to reduce the risks for cardiovascular disease and type 2 diabetes in high-risk populations. She also teaches nutrition courses and mentors graduate research students.

Janice is a Fellow of the American College of Sports Medicine (ACSM), and member of the American Society of Nutrition (ASN), the American Diabetes Association (ADA), the British Association of Sport and Exercise Science (BASES), and The Nutrition Society (UK). Janice won an undergraduate teaching award while at the University of North Carolina, Charlotte. In addition to *Nutrition for Life*, Janice coauthored the Benjamin Cummings textbooks *Nutrition: An Applied Approach* with Melinda Manore and *The Science of Nutrition* with Melinda Manore and Linda Vaughan. Janice loves cats, yoga, and hiking. She likes almost every vegetable except fennel and believes chocolate should be listed as a food group.

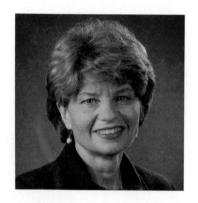

Melinda Manore, PhD, RD, FACSM

Oregon State University

Melinda Manore earned a PhD in human nutrition with a minor in exercise physiology at Oregon State University (OSU). She is the past chair of the Department of Nutrition and Food Management at OSU, and is currently a professor in the Department of Nutrition and Exercise Sciences. Prior to her tenure at OSU, she taught at Arizona State University for 17 years. Melinda's areas of specialization include the role that nutrition and exercise play in health, energy balance, obesity, and disordered eating, especially in active women.

Melinda is an active member of the American Dietetic Association (ADA) with advanced credentialing as a Certified Specialist in Sport Dietetics (CSSD), and the American College of Sports Medicine (ACSM). She is the past chair of the ADA Research Committee and the Research Dietetic Practice Group, and served on the ADA Obesity Steering Committee. She is a Fellow of ACSM and is a member of the Board of Trustees. Melinda is also a member of the American Society of Nutrition (ASN) and the North American Association for the Study of Obesity. Melinda has been an associate editor for Medicine and Science in Sports and Exercise and ACSM's *Health and Fitness Journal*. She also serves on the editorial boards of numerous research journals, and has won awards for excellence in research and teaching. In addition to *Nutrition for Life,* Melinda coauthored the Benjamin Cummings textbook *Nutrition: An Applied Approach* with Janice Thompson, and *The Science of Nutrition* with Janice Thompson and Linda Vaughan. Melinda is an avid walker, hiker, and former runner who loves to garden, cook, and eat great food. She is now trying her hand at birding.

WELCOME TO NUTRITION FOR LIFE!

Why We Wrote the Book

You stop at the convenience store for a snack. Blaring across the front of a bag of chips is a banner *No Trans Fats!* while a bag of pretzels claims *Now With Whole Grains!* What does this stuff really mean, you wonder, and should you care? You buy the chips and take them to a party, where the game is on TV. It's half-time and an athlete is pushing some new protein supplement. A friend comes up and offers you a can of something called *Action!* "It's this new high-energy drink," he explains. But then your roommate snickers, "Yeah, and the caffeine in it disintegrates your bones! You know, they've banned that stuff in France!"

No doubt about it, nutrition is a hot topic, but do you ever wind up with information overload? Everybody claims to be an expert, but what's their advice based on? Is it reliable? How do you navigate through the endless recommendations and come up with a way of eating that's right for you—one that energizes you, allows you to maintain a healthful weight, and helps you avoid disease?

We Wrote This Book to Help You Answer These Questions

Nutrition for Life began with the conviction that students would benefit from an accurate and clear textbook that links nutrition to their health and encourages them to make nutrition part of their everyday lives. As authors and instructors, we know that students have a natural interest in their bodies, their health, their weight, and their success in sports and other activities. By demonstrating how nutrition relates to these interests, *Nutrition for Life* empowers students to reach their personal health and fitness goals. We use several strategies to capture students' interest, from highlighting how nutrients are critical to health, to discussing the vitamins and minerals based upon their functions within the body, to a variety of special features and activities that bring nutrition to life. In addition, throughout the chapters, material is presented in a lively narrative that continually links the facts to students' lifestyles and goals. Information on current events and research keeps the inquisitive spark alive, illustrating that nutrition is not a "dead" science, but rather the source of considerable debate. We present nutrition in an easy-to-read, friendly narrative and with engaging features that reduce students' fears and encourage them to apply the material to their lives. Also, we made sure the organization and flow of the information and the art come together to provide a learning experience that is enjoyable for both instructors and students.

As teachers, we are both familiar with the myriad challenges of presenting nutrition information in the classroom, and we have included tools in the book and ancillary package to assist instructors in successfully meeting these challenges. Through broad instructor and student support with print and media supplements, we hope to contribute to the excitement of teaching and learning about nutrition: a subject that affects every one of us, a subject so important and relevant that correct and timely information can make the difference between health and disease.

Features of *Nutrition for Life*

The following features are integrated into every chapter of *Nutrition for Life,* to help you learn, study, and apply all the fascinating concepts of nutrition to your own life. As you read through each chapter, be sure to look at the feature boxes and work through their activities, complete the margin journaling features, and test your knowledge with the Review Questions. You can also find more information, resources, and self-quizzing activities on the book's Companion Website, available at www.pearsonhighered.com/nutritionplace.

- *New feature!* **Where I'm Starting From . . . and Where I'm At Now . . .** margin journaling features help you assess how your real-life practices relate to the nutrition information provided in the chapter. Fill out Where I'm Starting From. . . before you read the chapter, and complete Where I'm At Now. . . once you've read it.

- **Test Yourself questions** are found at the beginning of each chapter. These questions will help you dispel common myths about nutrition. The answers can be found at the end of each chapter.

- **What About You?** feature boxes are another feature that will help you figure out where you stand with regard to important nutrition issues. These boxes provide self-assessments that allow you to determine whether your diet and lifestyle are as healthful as they could be, or whether you should be concerned about a particular nutrition-related issue.

- **Game Plan** feature boxes offer you detailed strategies for adopting healthful eating and lifestyle changes. New for this edition, they have been updated into a checklist format, making it even easier to follow the recommended tips and guidelines.

- **Nutrition Label Activities** will teach you how to evaluate the labels from real food products so you can make educated decisions about the foods you eat and purchase. New for this edition, these activities have been made even more interactive so you have hands-on practice that you can apply when you do your own food shopping. Answers to Nutrition Label Activities, when applicable, can be found at the end of the chapter.

- **Nutrition Myth or Fact?** feature boxes provide the facts behind the hype on many current nutrition and dietary issues. They dispel common misconceptions and teach you how to critically evaluate information you hear from the Internet, the mass media, and your peers.

- **Highlight** feature boxes give further insight into topics that you will recognize from the mass media and popular culture, such as sports beverages, alternative sweeteners, and fad diets. Highlight boxes discuss the facts and theories that attempt to explain these interesting topics.

- **Nutri-Case** case studies follow the stories of five recurring characters with various nutritional needs. Two Nutri-Cases appear in each chapter, and through them we discuss the implications of nutrition on these characters. By prompting you to help the characters choose the most sensible option, these cases help you apply the material you've just learned to real life. The full background for each Nutri-Case character is provided on pages viii–ix.

- **Healthwatch** sections are designed to highlight the health effects of various nutrients and foods, illuminating the real consequences of diet on health.

- **Recaps** are placed consistently throughout the text and rephrase what you have just learned in the preceding sections, using new wording, so you understand the concepts and don't just memorize the words.

- **Organization of vitamins and minerals** is unique in this book. Traditionally students have learned the vitamins and minerals by memorizing each one along with its deficiency and toxicity symptoms. We found that with that approach, students quickly forget the information and don't really understand why these nutrients are important. In *Nutrition for Life,* we organize the vitamins and minerals based on what they do inside your body, giving you a framework for understanding why they're important, what they do, and what happens when you don't get enough—or get too much!—of each one.

- **Art, photos, and tables** have been specially designed to walk you through your body's processing of nutrients. Figures were developed to show you step-by-step what happens to the food you eat, as well as to show you what foods are good sources of each nutrient. We chose photos that illustrate conditions created by deficiency and toxicity, as well as to show you foods that you may not immediately think of as good sources for specific nutrients.

- **Review Questions** at the end of each chapter help you assess your retention and understanding of the material you have covered in the chapter. Answers to Review Questions appear at the end of the book.

- **Web Links and References** provide students with references to all of the research used in the chapter as well as related Web Links for further information and study.

Additional Features Available on the Companion Website, www.pearsonhighered.com/nutritionplace

- *New feature!* **Full Student Study Guide** Word files available in a password-protected section. To gain access, use the password provided in the front of your new textbook. This study guide will help you get the best grade possible with its large variety of review questions for each chapter. Great for preparing for a test or just making sure you understand the content!

- *New feature!* **Find the Quack** scenarios for each chapter help promote critical thinking and encourage you to become a better consumer of nutrition information.

- **Chapter Summaries** for each chapter provide quick reviews of the major points covered in each chapter. By going through the chapter summaries you can determine whether you've understood information about each point.

- **Critical Thinking Questions** allow you to test your understanding of the content and think critically. Offered in an essay-style format that you can email to your instructor.

- **And More!** The Companion Website also includes features such as answers to each Nutri-case, self-quizzing, web links, flashcards, an interactive glossary, and instructor resources.

NUTRI-CASE   YOU PLAY THE EXPERT!

Our Nutri-Case feature will give you lots of chances to evaluate the nutrition-related beliefs and behaviors of five individuals who represent a wide range of backgrounds and nutritional challenges. Throughout this text, you will read about these five characters as they deal with nutrition concerns in their lives. As you do, you might find that they remind you of people you know, and you may also discover you have something in common with one or more of them. Our hope is that by applying the information you learn in this course to their situations, you will deepen your understanding of the importance of nutrition in your own life.

Keep in mind that these case scenarios are not meant to indicate that students using this textbook are qualified to offer nutritional advice to others. In the real world, only properly trained and licensed health professionals are qualified to provide nutritional counseling.

You will learn more about each of these people in the chapters, but take a moment to read their brief introductions here.

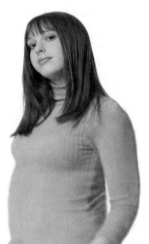

"Hi, I'm Hannah. I'm 18 years old and in my first year at Valley Community College. I haven't made up my mind yet about my major. All I know for sure is that I don't want to work in a hospital like my mom! I got good grades in high school, but I'm a little freaked out by college so far. There's so much homework, plus one of my courses has a lab, plus I have to work part-time because my mom doesn't have the money to put me through school. . . Sometimes I feel like I just can't handle it all. And when I get stressed out, I eat. I've already gained 10 pounds and I haven't even finished my first semester!"

"Hi, I'm Theo. Let's see, I'm 21, and my parents moved to the Midwest from Nigeria 11 years ago. The first time I ever played basketball, in middle school, I was hooked. I won lots of awards in high school and then got a full scholarship to the state university, where I'm a junior studying political science. I decided to take a nutrition course because, last year, I had a hard time making it through the playing season, plus keeping up with my classes and homework. I want to have more energy, so I thought maybe I'm not eating right. Anyway, I want to figure out this food thing before basketball season starts again."

"I'm Liz, I'm 20, and I'm a dance major at the School for Performing Arts. Last year, two other dancers from my class and I won a state championship and got to dance in the New Year's Eve celebration at the governor's mansion. This spring, I'm going to audition for the City Ballet, so I have to be in top condition. I wish I had time to take a nutrition course, but I'm too busy with dance classes and rehearsals and teaching a dance class for kids. But it's okay, because I get lots of tips from other dancers and from the Internet. Like last week, I found a Web site especially for dancers that explained how to get rid of bloating before an audition. I'm going to try it for my audition with the City Ballet!"

"I'm Judy, Hannah's mother, and I'm a nurse's aide at Valley Hospital. Back when Hannah was a baby, I dreamed of going to college so I could be a registered nurse. But then my ex and I split up, and Hannah and I, we've been in survival mode ever since. I'm proud to have raised my daughter without any handouts, and I do good work, but the pay never goes far enough and it's exhausting. I guess that's partly because I'm out of shape, and my blood sugar's high, too. Most nights, I'm so tired at the end of my shift that I just pick up some fast food for supper. I know I should be making home-cooked meals, but like I said, I'm in survival mode."

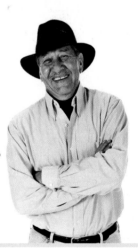

"Hello. My name is Gustavo. Almost 60 years ago, when I was 13, I came to the United States from Mexico with my father and mother and three sisters to pick crops in California, and now I manage a vineyard. They ask me when I'm going to retire, but I can still work as hard as a man half my age. Health problems? None. Well, maybe my doctor tells me my blood pressure is high, but that's normal for my age! I guess what keeps me going is thinking about how my father died 6 months after he retired. He had colon cancer, but he never knew it until it was too late. Anyway, I watch the nightly news and read the papers, so I keep up on what's good for me, "Eat less salt" and all that stuff. I'm doing great!"

New to the Second Edition

For this edition, our goals were to make the book even more practical and make it easier for students to apply the information to their own lives. We also wanted to include more on how to evaluate nutrition information, and to provide the most up-to-date and accurate nutrition information currently available. We have included new journaling features and Nutri-Case characters, and modified many of our box features to be even more practical, often appearing as worksheets or checklists that students can work through. The design and art program have been updated with dynamic colors to add to visual clarity and interest. In order to provide a brief, focused, and easy-to-use text, we've moved the chapter summaries, See for Yourself, and Review Questions 11–15 onto our Companion Website. The See for Yourself feature also appears in the Instructor Manual.

The summary of features on pages vi–vii provides information about the features in the Second Edition. For specific changes to each chapter, please see the following.

Chapter 1

- Revised and updated Test Yourself questions.
- Updated Figure 1.2 with addition of 2006 obesity map.
- Deleted content on Healthy People 2010 and content on the Canadian and UK guidelines for healthy eating.
- Deleted First Edition Table 1.6 (sample diets across four levels of energy intake) and revised the text to reinforce this concept.
- Deleted the MyPyramid Tracker figure (First Edition Figure 1.11).
- Increased coverage of ethnic/religious/cultural influences on why people eat as they do.
- Added a new What About You?: Do You Eat in Response to External or Internal Cues?
- Added a new Figure 1.9 that illustrates using a hand to estimate portion sizes.
- Expanded information on how to evaluate nutrition sources and information and added new Highlight box on Research Study Results: Who Can You Believe?
- Added a new Hannah Nutri-Case about Hannah as a young adult attending college.

Chapter 2

- Revised Test Yourself Question 1.
- Moved hypothalamus information into the main physiology section.
- Added a margin definition of satiation.
- Added information on celiac disease and on gluten allergy.
- Replaced the introductory story.
- Included a new Judy Nutri-Case about hunger and satiation.
- Added a new Nutrition Label Activity: Recognizing Common Allergens in Foods.
- Added a new What About You?: How Well Do You Treat Your GI Tract?
- Updated the Review Questions.

Chapter 3

- Expanded discussion of fiber and included definitions of soluble and insoluble fiber.
- Converted First Edition Table 3.4 (fiber content of common foods) to Figure 3.11 to more clearly illustrate food sources of carbohydrates.

- Converted First Edition Table 3.5 (comparison of two high-carbohydrate diets) to Figure 3.12 to provide a more reader-friendly comparison of two types of high-carbohydrate diets.
- Deleted First Edition Figure 3.11 (nutrients in whole-grain, enriched, and unenriched breads).
- Simplified the mathematical calculations contained in the Nutrition Label Activity.
- Reformatted the Nutrition Label Activity to make it more interactive, encouraging students to "fill in the blanks" and providing the correct answers to allow self-testing of acquired knowledge.
- New Theo Nutri-Case about wanting to eat carbohydrates after a basketball game.
- New Hannah Nutri-Case about eating a low-carb diet.

Chapter 4

- Clarified discussion of distinction between high cholesterol and high blood triglycerides.
- Clarified section on adipose tissue and fat storage.
- Added content on omega-3s and eicosanoids and their roles in the body.
- Clarified the section on fat metabolism.
- Moved the introduction to the essential fatty acids from the Why Do We Need to Eat Fats? section to the What Are Fats? section.
- Updated information and references on fats and cancer.
- Edited the Highlight and What About You? boxes on blood lipids to help students relate to them more.

Chapter 5

- Revised and updated the Test Yourself questions.
- Clarified the coverage of the function of proteins in fluid and electrolyte balance.
- Added information on transport proteins.
- Updated the Highlight boxes on high-protein diets, soy, and mad cow disease.
- Replaced First Edition Table 5.2 (complementary food combinations) with new Figure 5.4.
- Deleted the What About You? box on how to calculate one's protein intake and replaced it with journaling activities at beginning and end of the chapter.

Chapter 6

- Expanded information on vitamin A and the prescription drug Accutane.
- Updated recent recommendations related to cancer, diet, and physical activity.
- Expanded information on food sources of vitamins in Tables 6.1 and 6.2 and Figure 6.1.
- Added Figure 6.13 on phytochemicals.
- Deleted First Edition Table 6.4 (B vitamin food sources) and added food source figures for B vitamins (Figures 6.12–6.14, 6.16–6.18).
- Revised Figure 6.11 to show only one breakfast cereal.
- Added more information on phytochemicals and functional foods.
- Replaced First Edition Table 6.5 with updated Figure 6.13 covering Health Claims and Food Sources of Phytochemicals.
- Deleted First Edition Table 6.6 (groups likely to benefit from vitamin supplementation) and condensed this information into bulleted text.

- Updated and expanded information related to recent controversy on increasing vitamin D recommendations.
- New Hannah Nutri-Case about drinking vitamin C powder.

Chapter 7

- Added a short paragraph on trace minerals of uncertain status.
- Revised the content on myoglobin for clarity.
- Revised the statements about osteoclasts for accuracy.
- Added content about sodium and calcium being involved in muscle contraction and relaxation.
- Added menopause to the discussion of age as a risk factor for osteoporosis.
- Checked tables and narrative to ensure that food sources that are mentioned have good bioavailability.
- Updated the Nutrition Myth or Fact?: Do Zinc Lozenges Help Fight the Common Cold?
- Revised the osteoporosis-risk quiz to be more appropriate for younger readers.
- Added a new Judy Nutri-Case about trying to reduce her sodium intake.

Chapter 8

- Added discussion of the terms intracellular fluid and extracellular fluid.
- Updated recommendations regarding fluid intake.
- Strongly emphasized the importance of water in the All Beverages Are Not Created Equal section.
- Replaced First Edition Table 8.1 (water content of foods) with Figure 8.3.
- Added brief discussions on energy drinks, fortified waters, and the environmental concerns of using bottled water.
- Updated the discussion on the various complications related to maternal consumption of alcohol during pregnancy.
- Added a new Theo Nutri-Case on alcohol consumption.

Chapter 9

- Added more emphasis on tools for portion control, discussed within the section on behavioral strategies.
- Added information on cultural and economic factors influencing weight loss.
- Added more information on strategies for losing weight (including behavioral modification, portion control, setting realistic goals, and various weight loss plans).
- Added a brief section called Set Realistic Goals and another called Eat Smaller Portions of Lower-Fat Foods.
- Added information on weight management after weight loss and the National Weight Control Registry.
- Added Figure 9.11 (photos of good vs. bad fast-food meals).
- Included information on more weight management drugs, such as Orlistat and Alli, and the dangers of dieter's tea and other over-the-counter drugs.
- Reorganized the dieting section.
- Added a new Nutrition Myth or Fact?: Does it Cost More to Eat Right?

Chapter 10

- Updated information on ergogenic aids and emphasized how supplements are not regulated in the same way as drugs/medications.
- Replaced First Edition Table 10.2 with new Figure 10.3 on using the FIT principle to achieve cardiorespiratory and musculoskeletal fitness and flexibility.

- Replaced First Edition Table 10.7 (signs and symptoms of dehydration) with new Figure 10.9.
- Integrated the section A Sound Fitness Program Is Fun into the section on variety and consistency of physical activity.
- Reduced the size and edited content of First Edition Table 10.5 (nutrient composition of various foods and sports bars) to become new Table 10.4.
- Added new Figure 10.6 on the relative contributions of ATP-CP, carbohydrate, and fat to activities of various durations and intensities.
- Added discussion of changing trends in lifestyle contributing to low levels of physical activity in the section Most Americans Are Inactive.

Chapter 11

- Condensed the sections Why Is Nutrition Important Before Conception? and Why Is Nutrition Important During Pregnancy?
- Deleted First Edition Figures 11.1 and 11.3 on embryonic and placental development.
- Condensed the sections called What Are a Toddler's Nutrient Needs? and What Are a Child's Nutrient Needs? to rely more on Table 11.4 for this information.
- Deleted the discussion called Obesity: A Concern Now in the toddler section.
- Deleted the discussion called Body-Image Concerns in the toddler section.
- Added a new Nutrition Myth or Fact?: Is Breakfast the Most Important Meal of the Day?
- Deleted the section on nutrition for middle adults.
- Expanded slightly Table 11.5 on nutrient considerations and condensed the narrative on micronutrient recommendations, referring readers to the table for specific data.
- Expanded the discussion called Interactions Between Medications and Nutrition and added discussion of supplement use among older adults. Added Table 11.6 on drug–nutrient interactions.
- Changed the opening story to focus on obesity and diabetes in a family.

Chapter 12

- Reorganized the section called How Can You Prevent Food-Borne Illness?
- Moved Table 12.3 on preservatives to the section on food additives and updated it to be a bit more comprehensive.
- Added new Figure 12.12 on bioaccumulation.
- Updated the Test Yourself questions and answers.
- Updated the opening story with current information about food-borne illness outbreaks.
- Condensed the Highlight on genetically modified foods.
- Moved the content from the First Edition Highlight on sustainable food production into the text narrative.
- Revised the What About You? box on actions contributing to global food security to be more succinct.

ANCILLARIES HELP STUDENTS AND INSTRUCTORS

Instructors and students have access to a wide variety of ancillary material to facilitate teaching, help learning and retention, and contribute to the classroom experience.

Instructor Ancillaries

Instructor Manual
978-0-321-58135-8/0-321-58135-0
The Instructor Manual contains chapter summaries, lecture outlines, the See for Yourself activities, and other activity ideas, including a diet analysis software activity, for each chapter.

Printed Test Bank
978-0-321-57564-7/0-321-57564-4
The Test Bank contains multiple-choice, true/false, short answer, matching, and essay questions for each chapter of the text. Questions now appear for box content and some questions now incorporate art from the text.

Computerized Test Bank
Created in TestGen, the Computerized Test Bank contains all the questions from the printed Test Bank in a user-friendly, cross-platform CD-ROM. The Computerized Test Bank allows instructors to create and customize quizzes and tests using prewritten questions or inserting questions of their own. The Computerized Test Bank is available as part of the Media Manager.

Media Manager
978-0-321-59645-1/0-321-59645-5
The Media Manager DVD allows instructors to seamlessly integrate the text into their lecture presentations. The Media Manager contains PowerPoint® lecture slides with embedded animations and ABC videos that correspond to each chapter of the book, Jeopardy-style quiz show games for each chapter, PRS-enabled clicker discussion questions, step-edit art for selected figures, full-screen ABC videos, over 130 Transparency Acetate pdf files, the full Computerized Test Bank, Word files of the Instructor ancillaries, and PowerPoint and jpeg files of all the art, tables, and selected photos from the text.

New! Great Ideas: Active Ways to Teach Nutrition
978-0-321-59646-8/0-321-59646-3
This brand-new booklet compiles the best teaching ideas from nutrition instructors across the country. Great Ideas shows you innovative ways to teach a variety of nutrition topics with an emphasis on active learning, and in addition gives general classroom activities that can be used to teach any topic.

MyNutritionLab Instructor Access Kit
978-0-321-58146-4/0-321-58146-6

MyNutritionLab with MyDietAnalysis 3.0 Instructor Access Kit
978-0-321-58095-5/0-321-58095-8
www.mynutritionlab.com
MyNutritionLab is the online course management system that makes it easy to organize your class and push your students' learning to the next level. Organized in an easy student study plan for each chapter, includes links to specific sections of the e-Book, activities, animations created specifically for nutrition, ABC videos, assignable and gradable diet analysis activities, *Get Ready for Nutrition!* math and chemistry study help, Research Navigator, and more. MyNutritionLab with MyDietAnalysis contains single-sign-on to MyDietAnalysis.

Course Management Technologies
Web CT: www.pearsonhighered.com/webct
Blackboard: www.pearsonhighered.com/blackboard
In addition to MyNutritionLab, Web CT and Blackboard are also available. Contact your Pearson sales representative for details.

Nutrition Video Series
Nutrition videos by *Films for the Humanities* include videos on topics such as supplements, diet and cancer, the Food Guide Pyramid, and life in the fast-food lane. Contact your Pearson sales representative for details.

Student Ancillaries

Student Study Guide
Now available on the Companion Website for FREE with each new copy of the text, the Study Guide will help students get the best grade possible with its terminology questions, text outlines, study questions, completion exercises, and critical thinking sections for each chapter.

Companion Website
www.pearsonhighered.com/nutritionplace
The Companion Website offers students the free Study Guide, chapter summaries, chapter and cumulative quizzes with immediate feedback, web links, flashcards, a glossary, RSS feeds of current

news from www.nutrition.gov, Find the Quack features and follow-up questions, critical thinking questions, and answers to Nutri-Case questions.

MyNutritionLab Student Access Kit
978-0-321-58145-7/0-321-58145-8

MyNutritionLab with MyDietAnalysis 3.0 Student Access Kit
978-0-321-58094-8/0-321-58094-X

Provide full student access to MyNutritionLab and MyNutritionLab with MyDietAnalysis.

MyDietAnalysis 3.0
www.mydietanalysis.com

Powered by ESHA Research, Inc., MyDietAnalysis features a database of nearly 20,000 foods and allows students to track diet and activity and create multiple reports and profiles. This easy-to-use program contains serving-size photos, a physical activity self-quiz for accurate assessment of daily activity, and the ability to generate, comment on, and submit reports electronically.

MyDietAnalysis 2.0 CD-ROM
978-0-321-53468-2/0-321-53468-9

Powered by ESHA Research, Inc., MyDietAnalysis features a database of nearly 20,000 foods and allows students to track diet and activity and create multiple reports and profiles.

Eat Right! Healthy Eating in College and Beyond
0-8053-8288-7/978-0-8053-8288-4

This handy, full-color, 80-page booklet provides students with practical guidelines, tips, shopper's

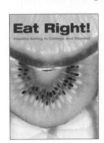

guides, and recipes so they can start putting healthy eating guidelines into action. Topics include healthy eating in the cafeteria, dorm room, and fast-food restaurants; eating on a budget; weight management tips; vegetarian alternatives; and guidelines on alcohol and health.

ACKNOWLEDGMENTS

It is eye opening to author a textbook and to realize that the work of so many people contributes to the final product.

We would like to thank the fabulous staff at Benjamin Cummings for their incredible support and dedication to this book. Our Acquisitions Editors, Deirdre Espinoza and Sandra Lindelof, encouraged us to be authors, and have provided unwavering support and guidance throughout the entire process of writing and publishing this book. Frank Ruggirello, Publisher, has committed extensive resources to ensuring the quality of this text, and his support and enthusiasm has helped us maintain the momentum we needed to complete this project. We could never have written this text without the exceptional writing and editing skills of Laura Bonazzoli, our Developmental Editor. In addition to her content guidance, she wrote the chapter-opening stories, the Nutri-Cases, the Find the Quack scenarios on the Web site, and the margin journaling features. Laura's energy, enthusiasm, and creativity significantly enhanced the quality of this textbook. Marie Beaugureau, our Project Editor, kept us sane with her sense of humor and excellent organizational skills. Jacob Evans and Shannon Cutt, Assistant Editors, provided us with editorial and administrative support that we would have been lost without.

Multiple talented players helped build this book in the production and design process as well. Beth Masse, Production Supervisor, and Norine Strang and the whole group at S4Carlisle Publishing Services, kept manuscripts moving through the entire process, and they never lost track of the minute details. Donna Kalal, Senior Art Editor, supervised the art and photo programs, and Kristin Piljay researched photos. Yvo Riezebos created a beautiful text and cover design.

We can't go without thanking the marketing and sales teams, especially Neena Bali, Senior Marketing Manager, who has been working incredibly hard to get this book out to those who will benefit most from it.

We would also like to extend our gratitude to our contributor, Carole Conn of the University of New Mexico. Carol wrote Chapter 12 for the First Edition and her efforts and personal research experience with global nutrition issues are greatly appreciated.

Our goal of meeting instructor and student needs could not have been realized without the team of educators and editorial staff who worked on the substantial supplements package for *Nutrition for Life*. Kim Aaronson wrote the inventive and useful Student Study Guide; Ruth Reilly and Jesse Morrell, both of the University of New Hampshire, created a comprehensive Test Bank; Linda Fleming, of Middlesex Community College, authored the wonderful Instructor's Manual; all of which were managed by Supplements Editor, Jennifer Cassidento. Amy Marion of New Mexico State University worked on the PowerPoint lecture slides, managed by Assistant Media Producer Lee Ann Doctor. Lee Ann also headed up the coordination and development of the Companion Website to the text, working with content contributors Louise Whitney of Lansing Community College and Karen Meyers of the University of Central Oklahoma.

We would also like to thank the many colleagues, friends, and family members who helped us along the way. Janice would specifically like to thank her family and friends who have been so incredibly wonderful throughout her career. She would also like to thank her colleagues and students who continue to challenge her and contribute significantly to her deep enjoyment of teaching and conducting nutrition-related research. Melinda would specifically like to thank her husband, Steve Carroll, for the patience and understanding he has shown through this process—once again. He has learned that there is always another chapter due! Melinda would also like to thank her family, friends, and professional colleagues for their support and listening ear through this whole process. They have all helped make life a little easier during this incredibly busy time.

Reviewers

Cassandra August
Baldwin-Wallace College

Valerie J. Benedix
Clovis Community College

Anne K. Black
Austin Peay State University

K. Shane Broughton
University of Wyoming

Fay C. Carpenter
Housatonic Community College

Gale Cohen
Mercer County Community College

Paula Cochrane
New Mexico Community College

Johanna Donnenfield
Scottsdale Community College

Sally Ebmeier
Wayne State College

Renee Finnecy
Mercyhurst College

Gary Fosmire
Pennsylvania State University

Anne Holmes
Luzerne County Community College

Caryl Johnson
Eastern New Mexico University

Jayanthi Kandiah
Ball State University

U. Beate Krinke
University of Minnesota

Barbara J. McCahan
Plymouth State University

Karen E. McConnell
Pacific Lutheran University

Karen Meyers
University of Central Oklahoma

Anna M. Page
Johnson County Community College

Roseann L. Poole
Tallahassee Community College

Susan Rippy
Eastern Illinois University

Janet Schwartz
Framingham State College

Jane Burrell Uzcategui
California State University, Los Angeles

Andrea Villarreal
Phoenix College

Green T. Waggener
Valdosta State University

Diane Wagoner
Indiana University of Pennsylvania

Melissa Wdowik
University of North Carolina, Charlotte

Louise Whitney
Lansing Community College

Cynthia A. Wilson
Seattle Central Community College

Maureen Zimmerman
Mesa Community College

BRIEF CONTENTS

CONTENTS

APPENDICES

TEST YOURSELF

Are these statements true or false? Circle your guess.

1 Cookies, ice cream, and other "treats" can be part of a healthful diet.   **TRUE or FALSE**

2 By definition, nutrients provide the body with energy.   **TRUE or FALSE**

3 Calories are a particular type of carbohydrate.   **TRUE or FALSE**

4 A healthful diet should include vitamin supplements.   **TRUE or FALSE**

5 The top nutritional guidelines in the United States encourage abstinence from alcohol.   **TRUE or FALSE**

Test Yourself answers can be found at the end of the chapter.

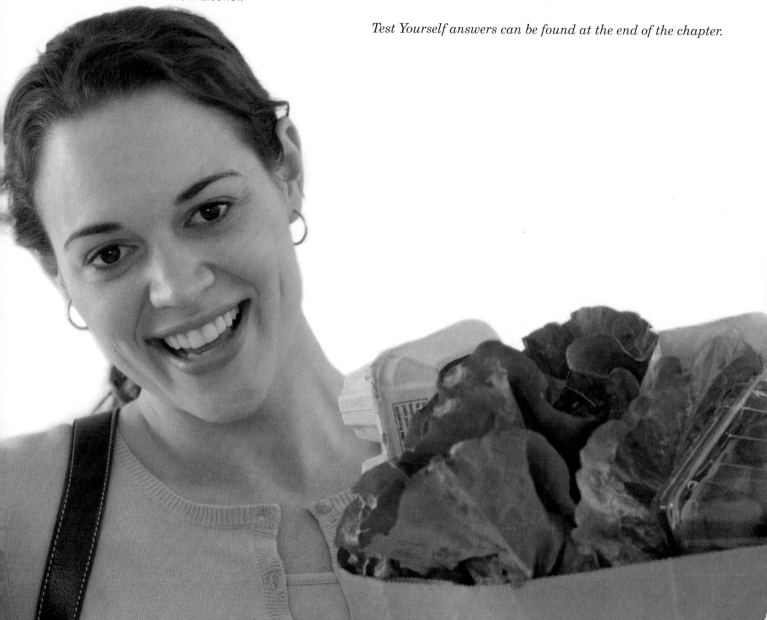

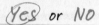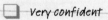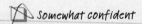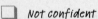
MIGUEL HADN'T EXPECTED that college life would make him feel so tired. After classes, he just wanted to go back to his dorm room and sleep. Plus, he had been having difficulty concentrating and was worried that his first-semester grades would be far below those he'd achieved in high school. Scott, his roommate, had little sympathy. "It's all that junk food you eat!" he insisted. "Let's go down to the organic market for some real food." Miguel dragged himself to the market with Scott but rested at the juice counter while his roommate went shopping. A woman wearing a white lab coat approached him and introduced herself as the market's staff nutritionist. "You're looking a little pale," she said. "Anything wrong?" Miguel explained that he had been feeling tired lately. "I don't doubt it," the woman answered. "I can see from your skin tone that you're anemic. You need to start taking an iron supplement." She took a bottle of pills from a shelf and handed it to him. "This one is the easiest for you to absorb, and it's on special this week. Take it twice a day, and you should start feeling better in a day or two."

Miguel purchased the supplement and began taking it that night with the meal his roommate prepared. He took it twice the next day as well, but didn't feel any better. After 2 more days on the supplement, he visited the university health clinic, where a nurse drew some blood for testing. When the results of the blood tests came in, the physician told him that his thyroid gland wasn't functioning properly. She prescribed a medication and congratulated Miguel for catching the problem early. "If you had waited," she said, "it would only have gotten worse, and you could have become seriously ill." Miguel asked if he should continue taking his iron supplement. The physician looked puzzled. "Where did you get the idea that you needed an iron supplement?"

Like Miguel, you've probably been offered nutrition-related advice from well-meaning friends and self-professed "experts." Perhaps you found the advice helpful, or maybe, as in Miguel's case, it turned out to be all wrong. Where can you go for reliable advice about nutrition? What exactly *is* nutrition anyway? Why do we choose to eat as we do, and how does our diet influence our health? In this chapter, we'll explore these questions and help you begin to design a diet that works for you.

What Is Nutrition, and Why Is It Important?

If you think that the word *nutrition* means pretty much the same thing as **food,** you're right—partially. But the word has a broader meaning that will gradually become clear as you make your way in this course. Specifically, **nutrition** is the science that studies food and how food nourishes our bodies and influences our health. It encompasses how we consume, digest, metabolize, and store nutrients and how these nutrients affect our bodies. Nutrition science also studies the factors that influence our eating patterns, makes recommendations about the amount we should eat of each type of food, and addresses issues related to food safety and the global food supply. You can think of nutrition, then, as the discipline that encompasses everything about food.

Thousands of years ago, people in some cultures believed that the proper diet could cure criminal behavior, cast out devils, and bring us into alignment with the divine. Although modern science has failed to find evidence to support these claims, we do know that proper nutrition can help us improve our health, prevent certain

food The plants and animals we consume.

nutrition The scientific study of food and how food nourishes the body and influences health.

diseases, achieve and maintain a healthy weight, and maintain our energy and vitality. As you'll learn in Chapter 2, you are what you eat: The substances you take into your body are broken down and reassembled into your brain cells, bones, muscles—all of your tissues and organs. Think about it: If you eat three meals a day, then by this time next year, you'll have had more than a thousand chances to influence your body's makeup! Let's take a closer look at how nutrition supports health and wellness.

Nutrition Is One of Several Factors Contributing to Wellness

Wellness can be defined in many ways. Traditionally considered simply the absence of disease, wellness is now described as a multidimensional state of being that includes physical, emotional, and spiritual health (FIGURE 1.1). Wellness is not an end point in our lives but is an active process we work on every day.

In this book, we focus on a critical aspect of wellness: physical health, which is influenced by both our nutrition and our level of physical activity. The two are so closely related that you can think of them as two sides of the same coin: Our overall state of nutrition is influenced by how much energy we expend doing daily activities, and our level of physical activity has a major impact on how we use the nutrients in our food. Several studies have even suggested that healthful nutrition and regular physical activity can increase feelings of well-being and reduce feelings of anxiety and depression. In other words, wholesome food and physical activity just plain feel good!

A Healthful Diet Can Prevent Some Diseases and Reduce Your Risk for Others

Early nutrition science focused on identifying the effect of nutrient deficiencies on human health. Diseases such as scurvy, pellagra, goiter, and rickets occur when an individual consumes a diet deficient in an essential nutrient. For instance, scurvy plagued sailors on long sea voyages who had no access to fresh fruits and vegetables

The study of nutrition encompasses everything about food.

wellness A multidimensional, lifelong process that includes physical, emotional, and spiritual health.

FIGURE 1.1 Many factors contribute to an individual's wellness. Primary among these are a nutritious diet and regular physical activity.

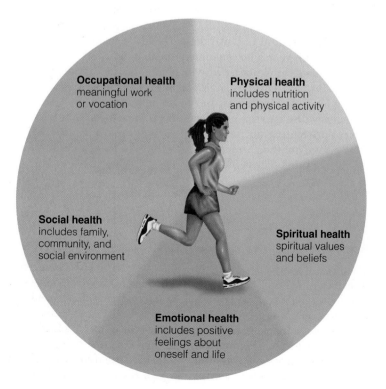

Occupational health
meaningful work
or vocation

Physical health
includes nutrition
and physical activity

Social health
includes family,
community, and
social environment

Spiritual health
spiritual values
and beliefs

Emotional health
includes positive
feelings about
oneself and life

FIGURE 1.2 These diagrams illustrate the increase in obesity rates across the United States from 1985 to 2006 as documented in the Behavioral Risk Factor Surveillance Survey. Obesity is defined as a body mass index greater than or equal to 30, or approximately 30 lbs overweight for a 5′4″ woman.
(Data from BRFSS Behavioral Risk Factor Surveillance System, www.cdc.gov/brfss/; Mokdad, A. H., et al. 1999. *JAMA* 282:16; Mokdad, A. H., et al. 2001. *JAMA* 286:10; Mokdad, A. H., et al. 2003. *JAMA* 289:1; CDC. 2006. *MMWR* 55:985–988. Graphics from Centers for Disease Control and Prevention, U.S. Obesity Trends 1985 to 2006. www.cdc.gov)

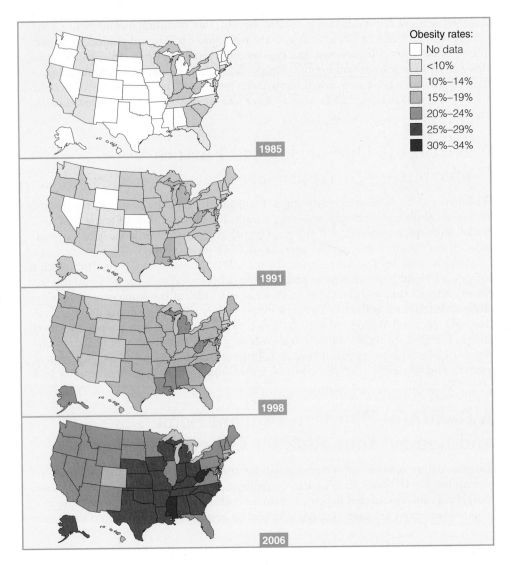

and thus consumed no vitamin C. Until the early 20th century, pellagra killed thousands of Americans each year who consumed a niacin-deficient diet. The severity of nutrient-deficiency diseases explains why following nutrient guidelines such as the Dietary Reference Intakes (DRIs) is so important for our health. An ample food supply and fortifying foods with nutrients have also helped to ensure that the majority of nutrient-deficiency diseases are not of concern in developed countries.

In addition to preventing nutrient-deficiency diseases, a healthful diet can reduce your risk for many of the chronic diseases that are among the top ten causes of death in the United States. These include:

- heart disease
- cancer
- stroke
- type 2 diabetes

Obesity, which in many people results from an imbalance between nutrition and physical activity, is a risk factor in several of these chronic diseases. In the United States and many developed nations, the prevalence of obesity has dramatically increased over the past 20 years (FIGURE 1.2). Obesity is discussed in detail in Chapter 9. Throughout this text, we highlight the role of nutrition and physical activity in the prevention and development of chronic disease.

Nutritional factors also appear to mildly influence the development of many diseases. For instance, poor nutrition is known to play some role in diseases such as os-

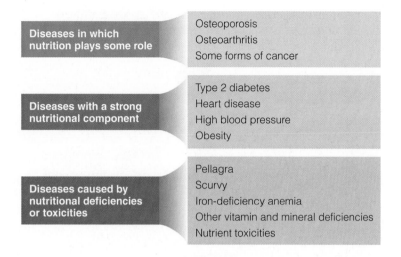

teoporosis and some forms of cancer. More research is needed, however, to clarify the strength of these associations. The varying role of nutrition, from mild influence, to strong association, to directly causing a disease, is illustrated in FIGURE 1.3.

> RECAP *Nutrition is the science that studies food and how food affects our bodies and our health. Both nutrition and physical activity are important components of wellness. Goals of a healthful diet include preventing nutrient-deficiency diseases, lowering the risk for chronic diseases, and lowering the risk of diseases in which nutrition plays some role.*

What Are Nutrients?

A glass of milk or a spoonful of peanut butter may seem as if it is all one substance, but in reality most foods are made up of many different chemicals. Some of these chemicals are not useful to the body, whereas others are critical to human growth and function. These latter chemicals are referred to as **nutrients.** The six groups of nutrients found in the foods we eat are (FIGURE 1.4):

- carbohydrates
- fats and oils (two types of lipids)
- proteins
- vitamins
- minerals
- water

Carbohydrates, Fats, and Proteins Are Macronutrients That Provide Energy

Carbohydrates, fats, and proteins are the only nutrients in foods that provide energy. By this we mean that these nutrients break down and reassemble into a fuel that our bodies use to support physical activity and basic functioning. Although taking a multivitamin and a glass of water might be beneficial in other ways, it will not provide you with the energy you need to do your 20 minutes on the stair-climber! The energy nutrients are also referred to as **macronutrients.** *Macro* means "large," and our bodies need relatively large amounts of these nutrients to support normal function and health.

Alcohol is a chemical found in food, and it provides energy. Nevertheless, it is not technically considered a nutrient because it does not support the regulation of body

nutrients Chemicals found in foods that are critical to human growth and function.

macronutrients Nutrients that our bodies need in relatively large amounts to support normal function and health. Carbohydrates, fats, and proteins are macronutrients.

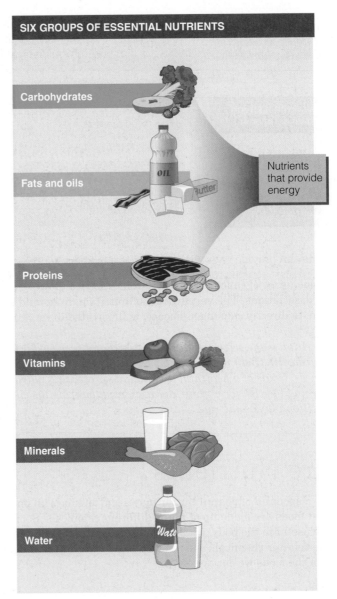

FIGURE 1.4 The six groups of essential nutrients found in the foods we consume.

functions or the building or repairing of tissues. In fact, the alcohol in beverages is technically classified as a narcotic drug. To learn more about alcohol consumption, see Chapter 8.

Nutrition scientists describe the amount of energy in food as units of *kilocalories* (kcal). A kilocalorie is the amount of heat required to raise the temperature of 1 kilogram of water by 1 degree Celsius. *Kilo-* is a prefix used in the metric system to indicate 1,000, so a kilocalorie is technically 1,000 calories. However, for the sake of simplicity, food labels use the term *calories* to indicate kilocalories. Thus, if the wrapping on an ice cream bar states that it contains 150 calories, it actually contains 150 *kilo*calories. In this textbook, we use the term *kilocalories* as a unit of energy; we use the term *calories* when discussing food labels.

Carbohydrates Are a Primary Fuel Source

Carbohydrates are the primary source of fuel for our active bodies, particularly for the brain. They provide 4 kcal per gram. Many carbohydrates are *fiber-rich;* that is, they contain nondigestible parts of plants that offer a variety of health benefits. Many are also rich in *phytochemicals*—plant chemicals that are thought to reduce our risk for cancer and heart disease.

carbohydrates The primary fuel source for our bodies, particularly for the brain and for physical exercise.

Carbohydrates encompass a wide variety of foods. Grains and vegetables contain carbohydrates, as do fruits, legumes (including lentils, dry beans, and peas), seeds and nuts, and milk and other dairy products. Carbohydrates and their role in health are the subject of Chapter 3.

Fats Provide More Energy Than Carbohydrates

Fats are also an important source of energy for our bodies, especially during rest and low-intensity activity. Because they pack together tightly, fats yield more energy per gram than carbohydrates, 9 kcal versus 4 kcal. Dietary fats come in a variety of forms. Solid fats include such foods as butter, lard, and margarine. Liquid fats are referred to as *oils* and include vegetable oils such as canola and olive oils. Cholesterol is a fat that is synthesized in our bodies and is also present in animal foods such as meats and egg yolk. Chapter 4 provides a thorough discussion of fats.

Proteins Support Tissue Growth, Repair, and Maintenance

Although **proteins** can provide energy, they are not a primary source of energy for our bodies. Proteins play a major role in building new cells and tissues, maintaining the structure and strength of bone, repairing damaged structures, and assisting in many body functions. Meats and dairy products are primary sources of proteins for many Americans, but we can also obtain adequate amounts from nuts and seeds, legumes, vegetables, and whole grains. Proteins are described in detail in Chapter 5.

Vitamins and Minerals Are Micronutrients

Vitamins and minerals are referred to as **micronutrients** because we need relatively small amounts of them (*micro-* means "small") to support normal health and body functions.

Vitamins Assist in Regulating Bodily Functions

Vitamins are compounds that contain the substance carbon and assist us in regulating the processes of our bodies. For example, vitamins play a critical role in building and maintaining healthy bone, blood, and muscle tissue, supporting the immune system so we can fight illness and disease, and maintaining healthy vision. Contrary to popular belief, vitamins do not provide energy (kilocalories); however, vitamins do play an important role in assisting our bodies with releasing and using the energy found in carbohydrates, fats, and proteins.

A vitamin's ability to dissolve in water versus fat affects how it is absorbed, transported, stored, and excreted from our bodies. Thus, nutrition experts classify vitamins into two groups (Table 1.1):

- water soluble
- fat soluble

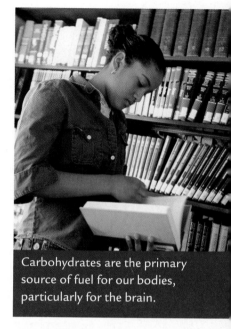

Carbohydrates are the primary source of fuel for our bodies, particularly for the brain.

fats An important energy source for our bodies at rest and during low-intensity exercise.

proteins A macronutrient that the body uses to build tissue and regulate body functions. Proteins can provide energy but are not a primary source.

micronutrients Nutrients needed in relatively small amounts to support normal health and body functions. Vitamins and minerals are micronutrients.

vitamins Micronutrients that contain carbon and assist us in regulating the processes of our bodies. They are classified as water soluble or fat soluble.

TABLE 1.1   Overview of Vitamins

Type	Names	Characteristics
Fat soluble	A, D, E, and K	Soluble in fat Stored in the human body Toxicity can occur from consuming excess amounts, which accumulate in the body
Water soluble	C, B vitamins (thiamin, riboflavin, niacin, vitamin B_6, vitamin B_{12}, pantothenic acid, biotin, and folate)	Soluble in water Not stored to any extent in the human body Excess excreted in urine Toxicity generally only occurs as a result of vitamin supplementation

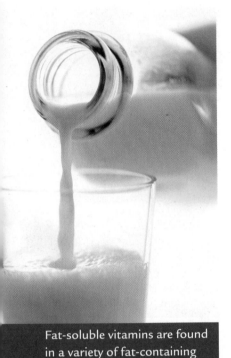

Fat-soluble vitamins are found in a variety of fat-containing foods, including dairy products.

Because our bodies cannot synthesize most vitamins, we must consume them in our diets. Both water-soluble and fat-soluble vitamins are essential for our health and are found in a variety of foods, from animal products, nuts, and seeds to fruits and vegetables. Many vitamins break down upon prolonged exposure to heat and/or light, which explains why vitamin supplements are not sold in clear bottles. Chapter 6 discusses vitamins.

Minerals Are Not Broken Down during Digestion

The sodium in table salt, the calcium in milk, and the iron in red meat are all examples of minerals essential to human health and functioning. **Minerals** are substances that:

- do not contain carbon,
- are not broken down during digestion, and
- are not destroyed by heat or light.

Thus, all minerals maintain their structure no matter what environment they are in. This means that the calcium in our bones is the same as the calcium in the milk we drink, and the sodium in our cells is the same as the sodium in table salt. Among their many important functions, minerals assist in fluid regulation and energy production, are essential to the health of our bones and blood, and help rid our bodies of harmful chemicals. They are classified into two groups according to the amounts we need in our diet and how much of the mineral is found in our bodies (Table 1.2):

- major minerals
- trace minerals

Major minerals earned their name from the fact that we need to consume at least 100 milligrams (mg) per day in our diets and because the total amount found in our bodies is at least 5 grams (or 5,000 mg). **Trace minerals** are those we need to consume in amounts less than 100 mg per day, and the total amount in our bodies is less than 5 grams (or 5,000 mg). Food sources of major and trace minerals are varied and include meats, dairy products, fruits and vegetables, and nuts.

Water Supports All Body Functions

Water is an inorganic nutrient that is vital for our survival. We consume water in its pure form, in juices, soups, and other liquids, and in solid foods such as fruits and vegetables. Adequate water intake ensures the proper balance of fluid both inside and outside of our cells and also assists in the regulation of nerve impulses, muscle contractions, nutrient transport, and excretion of waste products. Because of the key role that water plays in our health, Chapter 8 focuses on water and its function in our bodies.

minerals Micronutrients that do not contain carbon, are not broken down during digestion and absorption, and are not destroyed by heat or light. Minerals assist in the regulation of many body processes and are classified as major minerals or trace minerals.

major minerals Minerals we need to consume in amounts of at least 100 mg per day and of which the total amount in our bodies is at least 5 g.

trace minerals Minerals we need to consume in amounts less than 100 mg per day and of which the total amount in our bodies is less than 5 g.

TABLE 1.2   Overview of Minerals

Type	Names	Characteristics
Major minerals	Calcium, phosphorus, sodium, potassium, chloride, magnesium, sulfur	Needed in amounts greater than 100 mg/day in our diets Amount present in the human body is greater than 5 grams (or 5,000 mg)
Trace minerals	Iron, zinc, copper, manganese, fluoride, chromium, molybdenum, selenium, iodine	Needed in amounts less than 100 mg/day in our diets Amount present in the human body is less than 5 grams (or 5,000 mg)

RECAP *The six essential nutrient groups found in foods are carbohydrates, fats, proteins, vitamins, minerals, and water. Carbohydrates, fats, and proteins are macronutrients, and they provide our bodies with the energy necessary to thrive. Vitamins and minerals are micronutrients that do not provide energy but are essential to human functioning. Adequate water intake ensures the proper balance of fluid both inside and outside of our cells.*

Why Do We Want to Eat What We Want to Eat?

You've just finished eating at your favorite Thai place. As you walk back to the block where you parked your car, you pass a bakery whose window displays several cakes and pies, each of which looks more enticing than the last, and from whose door wafts a complex aroma of coffee, cinnamon, and chocolate. You stop. Are you hungry? You must be, because you go inside and buy a slice of chocolate torte and an espresso. Later that night, when the caffeine from the chocolate and coffee keeps you awake, you wonder why you succumbed.

Food Stimulates Our Senses

One answer is that food stimulates our senses. Foods that are artfully prepared, arranged, or ornamented appeal to our sense of sight. Advertisers know this and spend millions of dollars annually in the United States to promote and package foods in an appealing way.

Our sense of smell is a powerful stimulant to eating. The aromas of foods that comforted us as children, such as freshly baked bread, fried rice, or apple pie, can be especially irresistible. Interestingly, our sense of smell is so acute that a newborn baby can distinguish the scent of its own mother's breast milk from that of other mothers.[1]

Of all our senses, taste is the most important in determining what foods we choose to eat. Much of our ability to taste foods actually comes from our sense of smell. This is why foods are not as appealing when we are sick with a cold. Certain tastes, such as for sweet foods, are almost universally appealing, whereas others, such as the astringent taste of foods like spinach and kale, are quite individual. Because many natural poisons and spoiled foods are bitter, our distaste for bitterness is thought to be protective.[2]

Texture—or "mouth feel"—is also important in food choices, as it stimulates nerve endings sensitive to touch in our mouth and on our tongue: Do you prefer carrot juice, cooked carrots, or raw carrot sticks? Even your sense of hearing can be stimulated by foods, from the fizz of soda to the crunch of peanuts to the "snap, crackle, and pop" of Rice Krispies® cereal.

External Cues Trigger Appetite

Hunger is a physical sensation that drives us to find food and eat. If you've just finished a meal, hunger won't lure you into a bakery . . . but appetite might. **Appetite** is a psychological desire to consume specific foods. It is aroused by external cues—such as the sight of chocolate cake or the smell of coffee—related to pleasant sensations, and is often experienced as strong cravings for particular foods in the absence of hunger. Although we give different definitions for appetite and hunger, many times they do overlap, and symptoms of appetite and hunger are different for many people. Hunger is discussed in more detail in Chapter 2.

External cues also include social events like birthday parties or holidays such as Thanksgiving, which can stimulate us to eat more than usual or to indulge in foods that are normally "forbidden." For some people, being in a certain location can trigger appetite, such as at a baseball game or in a movie theater. Others may be triggered by the time of day or by an activity such as watching television or studying.

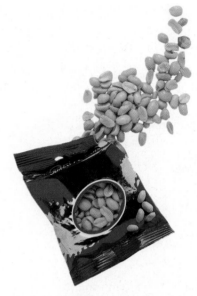

Peanuts are a good source of the major minerals magnesium and phosphorus.

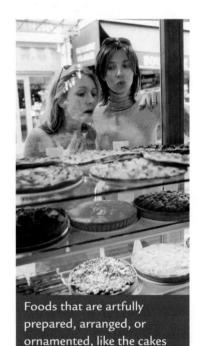

Foods that are artfully prepared, arranged, or ornamented, like the cakes and pies in this bakery display case, appeal to our sense of sight.

hunger A physical sensation that drives us to eat.

appetite A psychological desire to consume specific foods.

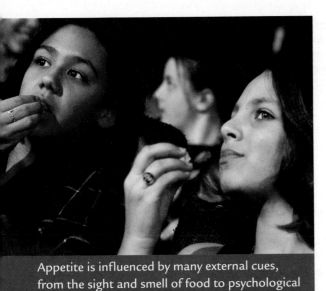

Appetite is influenced by many external cues, from the sight and smell of food to psychological and social associations, such as watching a movie with friends.

Many people feel an increase or decrease in their appetite when they are under stress. And some people's appetite fluctuates according to their companions: Would you eat more if you were having dinner with a date or with a group of friends?

If you are trying to lose weight or to maintain your present weight, it is important to stay aware, as you go through a day, of whether you are truly hungry or whether you simply have an appetite. If you decide it is your appetite, try to get away from the trigger. For instance, in the bakery scenario, you could simply walk away. By the time you reached your car, you'd probably forget the sights and smells of the bakery and would be aware of how full you felt from your Thai meal. Remember that because appetite is a psychological mechanism, you can train yourself to stop or ignore its cues when you want to avoid its consequences.

Culture, Religion, and Learning Also Influence Our Food Choices

Pigs' feet, anyone? What about blood sausage, stewed octopus, or tripe? These are delicacies in various European cultures, whereas the meat of horses, dogs, monkeys, and snakes are enjoyed in different regions of Asia. Would you eat grasshoppers, ants, termites, or tarantulas? If you'd grown up in certain parts of Africa or Central America, you probably would. That's because our preference for particular foods is largely a *learned* response: The cultures in which we are raised teach us what plant and animal products are appropriate to eat. Culture includes our ethnicity, family traditions, and personal values. Thus if your parents fed you cubes of plain tofu throughout your toddlerhood, then you are probably still eating tofu now.

A person's religion can also influence his or her food choices. Many Buddhists, Hindus, and Seventh Day Adventists are vegetarians, and Mormons may limit their meat intake and avoid caffeinated beverages and alcohol. Traditional Roman Catholics do not eat meat on Fridays or during the 40 days prior to Easter, a period called *Lent*. Muslims eat only foods that are considered lawful, referred to as *Halal*. Forbidden foods and beverages, called *Haram*, include alcohol, pork and its byproducts, lard, meat and poultry that are not slaughtered according to Islamic dietary law, and foods containing blood. Jewish dietary laws state that only kosher foods can be consumed. The term *kosher* indicates not only specific types of foods but also the methods used to slaughter and prepare them, and how and when they can be eaten. Foods such as shellfish, pork, and birds of prey are forbidden, and meat and poultry cannot be eaten with dairy products.

When thinking about cultural and religious influences on eating behaviors, bear in mind that these descriptions apply only to groups as a whole—the extent to which an individual of a particular culture or religion follows its food practices can vary considerably. You probably include foods from a variety of cultures in your own diet. Thus, you can't assume you know what people eat just because you know their ethnicity or religious beliefs.

Early introduction to foods is not essential; we can learn to enjoy new foods at any point in our lives. Immigrants from developing nations settling in the United States or Canada often adopt a typical Western diet, especially when their traditional foods, such as certain staple grains, legumes, fruits, and vegetables, are not readily available. This happens temporarily when we travel: the last time you were away from home, you probably enjoyed sampling a variety of dishes that were not normally part of your diet.

Flaxseed on yogurt? Kiwi? Collard greens? Food preferences also change when people learn what foods are most healthful in terms of nutrient density and prevention of chronic diseases. As you read this textbook, chances are you'll quite naturally start including certain foods in your diet as you learn more about their health benefits.

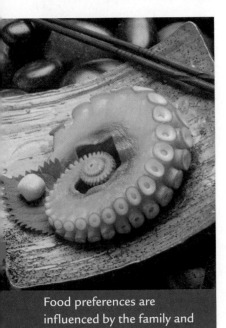

Food preferences are influenced by the family and culture you are raised in.

We can also "learn" to dislike foods we once enjoyed. For example, if we experience an episode of food poisoning after eating undercooked scrambled eggs, we may develop a strong distaste for all types of cooked eggs. Many adults who become vegetarians do so after learning about the treatment of animals in slaughterhouses; they may have eaten meat daily when they were young but could not imagine ever eating it again.

Now that you understand how environment, mood, social factors, culture, religion, and learning all influence our food choices, you might be curious to investigate your own reasons for eating what and when you do. If so, check out the accompanying feature, What About You?: Do You Eat in Response to External or Internal Cues?

> **RECAP** *Our senses of sight, smell, and taste are stimulated by foods. The texture of foods can also stimulate us to eat or may cause some foods to be unappealing. Appetite is a psychological desire to consume certain foods and is generally related to pleasant sensations associated with food. Environment, mood, social factors, culture, and religious beliefs affect food choices and eating patterns. Exposure to new foods, learning about nutrition, and other experiences can change our food choices. For people trying to lose weight, it is important to ignore the cues of appetite to avoid overeating.*

NUTRI-CASE HANNAH

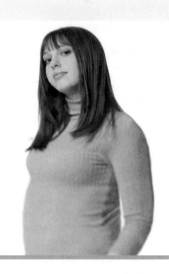

" My friend Kristi has been teasing me about my 'freshman bulge,' but it's not a joke to me! I've gained 10 pounds since I started college a few months ago, and she hasn't gained an ounce! I know what the difference is: when Kristi gets stressed she loses her appetite. For me, it's exactly the opposite—all I want to do is eat. Kristi says, 'Learn some better stress-reduction techniques, like yoga!' Oh right! I'm supposed to twist myself into a pretzel when I can't even touch my toes?"

Look back at the previous discussion of why we want to eat. Would you guess that Hannah eats more frequently in response to physical or psychological cues? Identify at least one strategy she could try that might help her respond more healthfully to stress. (Hint: See the accompanying What About You? feature on page 12.)

What Is a Healthful Diet?

A **healthful diet** provides the proper combination of energy and nutrients. It has four characteristics: it is adequate, moderate, balanced, and varied. No matter if you are young or old, overweight or underweight, healthy or coping with illness, if you keep in mind these characteristics of a healthful diet, you will be able to consciously select foods that provide you with the optimal combination of nutrients and energy each day.

A Healthful Diet Is Adequate

An **adequate diet** provides enough of energy, nutrients, and fiber to maintain a person's health. A diet may be inadequate in many areas or only one. For example, many people in the United States do not eat enough vegetables and therefore are not consuming enough of many of the important nutrients found in vegetables, such as

healthful diet A diet that provides the proper combination of energy and nutrients and is adequate, moderate, balanced, and varied.

adequate diet A diet that provides enough energy, nutrients, and fiber to maintain a person's health.

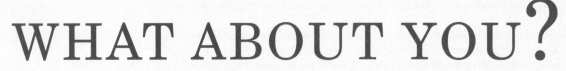

WHAT ABOUT YOU?

Do You Eat in Response to External or Internal Cues?

Whether you're trying to lose weight, gain weight, or maintain your current healthful weight, you'll probably find it intriguing to keep a log of the reasons behind your decisions about what, when, where, and why you eat. Are you eating in response to internal sensations telling you that your body needs food or in response to your emotions, situation, or a prescribed diet? Keeping a "cues" log for 1 full week would give you the most accurate picture of your eating habits, but even logging 2 or 3 days of meals and snacks should increase your cue awareness. That increased awareness is an important step toward making nutrition work for you.

Each day, every time you eat a meal, snack, or beverage other than water, make a quick note of:

- **when you eat.** Many people eat at certain hours (for example, noon, 6 PM, etc.) whether they are hungry or not.
- **what you eat, and how much.** A handful of nuts and a 6-oz glass of orange juice? Or a candy bar and a 12-oz cola?
- **where you eat.** At home watching television, in the student center, riding the subway?
- **with whom you eat.** Are you alone or with others? If with others, are they eating as well? Have they offered you food?
- **your emotions.** Some people overeat when they are happy, others when they are anxious, bored, impatient, or frustrated. Sometimes people eat to distract themselves from feelings they don't want to identify and deal with. For some, food becomes a substitute for emotional fulfillment.
- **your sensations: what you see, hear, or smell.** Are you eating because you just saw a TV commercial for pizza, or smelled chocolate-chip cookies, or . . . ?
- **any diet restrictions.** Are you choosing a particular food because it is allowed on your current diet plan? Or are you hungry for a meal but substituting a diet soda in order to stay within a certain daily allowance of energy?
- **your physiologic hunger.** Rate your hunger on a scale from 1 to 5 as follows:
  - 1 = you feel full or even stuffed;
  - 2 = you feel satiated but not uncomfortably full;
  - 3 = neutral, you feel no discernible fullness nor hunger;
  - 4 = you feel hungry and want to eat;
  - 5 = you feel strong physiologic sensations of hunger and need to eat.

Use a table such as the one here to help you log your food cues. The first row has been filled in for you as an example.

After keeping a log like this for several days, if you become aware of patterns you want to change, such as eating when you are worried or whenever you walk by the snack bar, take positive steps to change those patterns. For instance, instead of stifling your worries with food, sit down with a pen and paper and write down exactly what you are worried about, including steps you are going to take to address your concerns. If you discover that you eat every time you walk past the snack bar, then next time you walk that way, before going in, check in with your gut: are you truly hungry? If so, then purchase a healthful snack: maybe a yogurt, a piece of fruit, or a bag of peanuts. If you're not really hungry, take a moment to acknowledge the strength of this visual cue—and then walk on by.

Date: _____

Time	Food(s)	Location	People	Emotions	Sensations	Diet?	Hunger Rating
10:00, break between classes	Coffee and donut	Coffee cart in student center	With Marcus and Kate	They stopped to get a snack and I wanted to fit in	Coffee smelled great	No	3

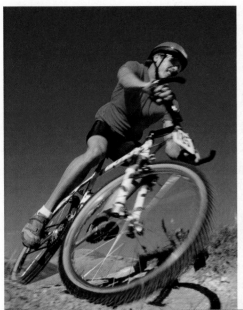
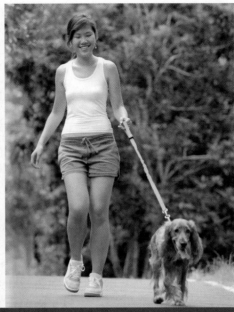

A diet that is adequate for one person may not be adequate for another. A woman who is lightly active may require fewer kilocalories of energy per day than a highly active male.

fiber-rich carbohydrate, vitamin C, beta-carotene, and potassium. Other people may eat only plant-based foods. Unless they supplement or use fortified foods, their diets will be inadequate in a single nutrient, vitamin B$_{12}$.

A Healthful Diet Is Moderate

Moderation refers to eating the right amounts of foods to maintain a healthy weight and to optimize the functioning of our bodies. People who eat too much or too little of certain foods may not be able to reach their health goals. For example, some people drink 60 fluid ounces (or three 20-oz bottles) of soft drinks every day. Drinking this much contributes an extra 765 kcal of energy to a person's diet. To avoid weight gain from these kilocalories, most people would need to reduce their food intake, probably by cutting out healthful food choices. Consuming soft drinks in moderation keeps more energy available for nourishing foods.

A Healthful Diet Is Balanced

A **balanced diet** is one that contains the combinations of foods that provide the proper balance of nutrients. As you will learn in this course, our bodies need many types of foods in varying amounts to maintain health. For example, fruits and vegetables are excellent sources of fiber, vitamin C, beta-carotene, potassium, and magnesium. Meats are not good sources of these nutrients, but they are excellent sources of protein, iron, zinc, and copper. By eating a proper balance of healthful foods, we can be confident that we are consuming enough of the nutrients we need.

A Healthful Diet Is Varied

Variety refers to eating a lot of different foods each day. In many communities in the United States, there are thousands of healthful foods to choose from. By trying new foods on a regular basis, we optimize our chances of consuming the multitude of nutrients our bodies need. In addition, eating a varied diet prevents boredom and avoids our getting into a "food rut."

moderation Eating the right amounts of foods to maintain a healthy weight and to optimize our bodies' functioning.

balanced diet A diet that contains the combinations of foods that provide the proper proportion of nutrients.

variety Eating a lot of different foods each day.

> RECAP *A healthful diet provides adequate nutrients and energy in moderate amounts. A healthful diet also includes an appropriate balance and a wide variety of foods.*

How Can You Design a Diet That Works for You?

Now that you know what the six classes of nutrients are, you are probably wondering how much of each you need each day. To answer this question for yourself, you need to know the current recommended nutrient intakes.

Use the Dietary Reference Intakes to Figure Out Your Nutrient Needs

The lists of dietary standards in both the United States and Canada are called the **Dietary Reference Intakes (DRIs).** These standards identify the amount of a nutrient you need to prevent deficiency disease, but they also consider how much of this nutrient may reduce your risk for chronic disease. The DRIs also establish an upper level of safety for some nutrients.

The DRIs consist of six values (FIGURE 1.5):

- The **Estimated Average Requirement (EAR)** represents the average daily nutrient intake level estimated to meet the requirement of half of the healthy individuals in a particular life stage or gender group.[3] As an example, the EAR for iron for women between the ages of 19 and 30 years represents the average daily intake of iron that meets the requirement of half of the women in this age group.

- The **Recommended Dietary Allowance (RDA)** represents the average daily nutrient intake level that meets the nutrient requirements of 97% to 98% of healthy individuals in a particular life stage and gender group.[3] For example, the RDA for iron is 18 mg per day for women between the ages of 19 and 30 years. This amount of iron will meet the nutrient requirements of almost all women in this age category. Scientists use the EAR to establish the RDA. In fact, if an EAR cannot be determined for a nutrient, then this nutrient cannot have an RDA. When this occurs, an Adequate Intake value is determined for a nutrient.

Dietary Reference Intakes (DRIs) A set of nutritional reference values for the United States and Canada that apply to healthy people.

Estimated Average Requirement (EAR) The average daily nutrient intake level estimated to meet the requirement of half of the healthy individuals in a particular life stage and gender group.

Recommended Dietary Allowance (RDA) The average daily nutrient intake level that meets the nutrient requirements of 97% to 98% of healthy individuals in a particular life stage and gender group.

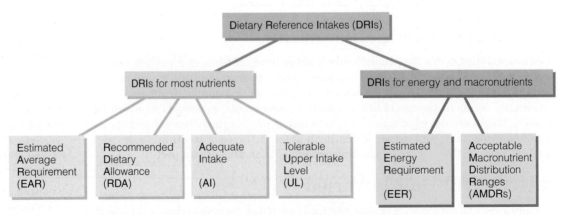

FIGURE 1.5 The Dietary Reference Intakes (DRIs) for all nutrients. Note that the Estimated Energy Requirement (EER) only applies to energy (kilocalories), and the Acceptable Macronutrient Distribution Ranges (AMDRs) only applies to the macronutrients and alcohol.

- The **Adequate Intake (AI)** value is a recommended average daily nutrient intake level based on estimates of nutrient intake by a group of healthy people.[3] These estimates are assumed to be adequate and are used when the evidence necessary to determine an RDA is not available. Numerous nutrients have an AI value, including calcium, vitamin D, vitamin K, and fluoride.

- The **Tolerable Upper Intake Level (UL)** is the highest average daily intake likely to pose no risk of adverse health effects. As intake of a nutrient increases in amounts above the UL, the potential for toxic effects and health risks increases. Note that there is not enough research to define the UL for all nutrients.

- The **Estimated Energy Requirement (EER)** is the average energy (kcal) intake that is predicted to maintain energy balance in a healthy adult. This recommendation considers a person's level of physical activity: the EER for an active person is higher than the EER for an inactive person even if all other factors (age, gender, etc.) are the same.

- The **Acceptable Macronutrient Distribution Range (AMDR)** is a range of intakes for carbohydrate, fat, and protein that is associated with reduced risk of chronic disease and provides adequate levels of essential nutrients. The AMDR is expressed as a percentage of total energy or as a percentage of total calories (Table 1.3).

Many of the DRI values are listed in a table on the inside cover of this book; they are also reviewed with each nutrient as it is introduced throughout this text. To determine your nutrient needs, find your life-stage group and gender in the left-hand column, then simply look across to see each nutrient's value that applies. Using the DRI values in conjunction with diet planning tools such as the Dietary Guidelines for Americans, discussed next, will help ensure a healthful and adequate diet.

Follow the Dietary Guidelines for Americans

The **Dietary Guidelines for Americans** are a set of principles developed by the U.S. Department of Health and Human Services and the U.S. Department of Agriculture to assist Americans in designing a healthful diet and lifestyle (Table 1.4).[4] These guidelines emphasize both food choices and physical activity habits to help reduce our risk for chronic diseases.

The United States is not the only country to develop dietary guidelines. For instance, Canada recently revised its dietary guidelines and the United Kingdom has its own Guidelines for a Healthy Diet.

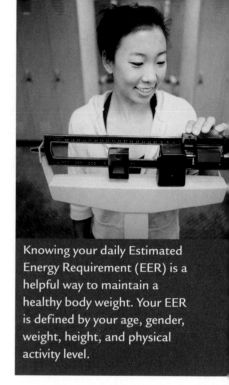

Knowing your daily Estimated Energy Requirement (EER) is a helpful way to maintain a healthy body weight. Your EER is defined by your age, gender, weight, height, and physical activity level.

Adequate Intake (AI) A recommended average daily nutrient intake level based on observed or experimentally determined estimates of nutrient intake by a group of healthy people.

Tolerable Upper Intake Level (UL) The highest average daily nutrient intake level likely to pose no risk of adverse health effects to almost all individuals in a particular life stage and gender group.

Estimated Energy Requirement (EER) The average dietary energy intake that is predicted to maintain energy balance in a healthy adult.

Acceptable Macronutrient Distribution Range (AMDR) A range of intakes for a particular energy source that is associated with reduced risk of chronic disease while providing adequate intake of essential nutrients.

Dietary Guidelines for Americans A set of principles developed by the U.S. Department of Agriculture and the U.S. Department of Health and Human Services to assist Americans in designing a healthful diet and lifestyle.

TABLE 1.3 Acceptable Macronutrient Distribution Ranges (AMDR) for Healthful Diets

Nutrient	AMDR*
Carbohydrate	45–65%
Fat	20–35%
Protein	10–35%

Source: From *Dietary Reference Intakes for Energy, Carbohydrates, Fiber, Fat, Fatty Acids, Cholesterol, Protein, and Amino Acids (Macronutrients).* Reprinted with permission from the National Academies Press. © 2005, National Academy of Sciences.

*AMDR values expressed as percent of total energy or as percent of total kilocalories.

TABLE 1.4 The Dietary Guidelines for Americans, 2005

Topic	Example of Key Recommendations
Adequate Nutrients Within Energy Needs	Consume a variety of nutrient-dense foods and beverages within and among the basic food groups while choosing foods that limit the intake of saturated and *trans* fats, cholesterol, added sugars, salt, and alcohol.
Weight Management	To maintain body weight in a healthy range, balance energy from foods and beverages with energy expended.
Physical Activity	Engage in regular physical activity and reduce sedentary activities to promote health, psychological well-being, and a healthy body weight.
Food Groups to Encourage	Consume a sufficient amount of fruits and vegetables while staying within energy needs. Two cups of fruit and 2½ cups of vegetables per day are recommended for a reference 2,000-kcal intake, with higher or lower amounts depending on the energy level.
Fats	Consume less than 10% of energy from saturated fatty acids and less than 300 mg/day of cholesterol, and keep *trans* fatty acid consumption as low as possible.
Carbohydrates	Choose fiber-rich fruits, vegetables, and whole grains often.
Sodium and Potassium	Consume less than 2,300 mg (approximately 1 tsp. of salt) of sodium per day.
Alcoholic Beverages	Those who choose to drink alcoholic beverages should do so sensibly and in moderation—defined as the consumption of up to one drink per day for women and up to two drinks per day for men.
Food Safety	To avoid microbial food-borne illness, clean hands, food contact surfaces, and fruits and vegetables. Meat and poultry should *not* be washed or rinsed.

Following is a brief description of each of the Dietary Guidelines for Americans. Refer to the accompanying Game Plan for specific examples of how you might alter your current diet and physical activity habits to meet some of these guidelines.

Aim for a Healthy Weight

Being overweight or obese increases our risk for many chronic diseases, including heart disease, type 2 diabetes, stroke, and some forms of cancer. Evaluating your weight includes calculating your body mass index, which is a ratio of your weight to your height. We discuss how to do this in Chapter 9.

Be Physically Active Each Day

Engage in at least 30 minutes of moderate physical activity most days of the week. Moderate physical activity includes walking, riding a bike, mowing the lawn with a push mower, or performing heavy yard work or housework. Other activities that are beneficial include those that build strength, such as lifting weights, and those that increase flexibility, such as yoga. The 30-minute guideline is a minimum; if you are already doing more activity than this, then continue on your healthful path. Also, for people who may need to lose weight, engaging in at least 60 minutes of moderate physical activity most days of the week is recommended. For more information on physical activity, see Chapter 10.

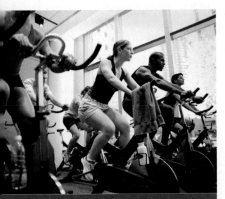

Being physically active for at least 30 minutes each day can reduce your risk for chronic diseases.

GAME PLAN

Ways to Incorporate the Dietary Guidelines for Americans into Your Daily Life

People experience a wide range of reactions when reading the Dietary Guidelines for Americans. Some feel satisfied that they are already following them, but many people see one or more areas where their behaviors could improve. If that sounds like you, and you'd like to make some changes, we recommend

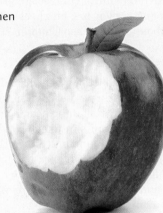

you start small. Substitute just one of these actions for your regular behavior each week, and by the time you finish this course, you'll have made the Dietary Guidelines for Americans part of your healthy life!

IF YOU NORMALLY DO THIS:	TRY DOING THIS INSTEAD:
Watch television when you get home at night	Do 30 minutes of stretching or lifting of hand weights in front of the television
Drive to the store down the block	Walk to and from the store
Go out to lunch with friends	Take a 15- to 30-minute walk with your friends at lunchtime 3 days each week
Eat white bread with your sandwich	Switch to a bread made from whole grains
Eat white rice or fried rice with your meal	Eat brown rice or wild rice
Choose cookies or a candy bar for a snack	Choose a fresh peach, apple, pear, orange, or banana for a snack
Order French fries with your hamburger	Order a green salad with low-fat salad dressing on the side
Spread butter or margarine on your white toast each morning	Spread fresh fruit compote or peanut butter on whole-grain toast
Order a bacon double cheeseburger at your favorite restaurant	Order a grilled chicken sandwich with lettuce and tomato
Drink nondiet soft drinks to quench your thirst	Drink water with a slice of lemon, diet soft drinks, or iced tea
Eat potato chips with your favorite sandwich	Eat baby carrots or slices of sweet red pepper dipped in low-fat ranch dressing

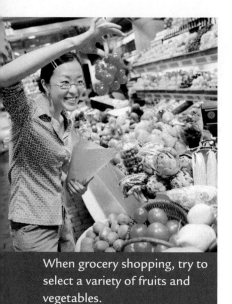

When grocery shopping, try to select a variety of fruits and vegetables.

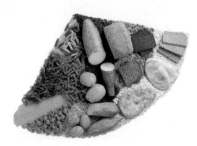

Eating a diet rich in whole-grain foods such as whole-wheat bread and brown rice can enhance your overall health.

Choose a Variety of Healthful Foods

The Dietary Guidelines for Americans recommend eating a variety of fruits and vegetables each day. Two cups of fruit and 2½ cups of vegetables per day are recommended for people consuming 2,000 kcal daily.

Whole grains are healthful food choices because they contain more vitamins, minerals, and fiber than refined grains. Examples of whole-grain foods include brown rice, oatmeal, whole-wheat bread, and popcorn. The guidelines recommend eating at least 3 servings of whole grains each day. Examples of servings are 1 slice of bread, 1 cup of whole-grain cereal, or ½ cup of cooked rice.

The guidelines also recommend consuming adequate amounts of calcium-rich foods. Calcium is a mineral that is important for strong bones. Three cups of low-fat or fat-free milk, or calcium-fortified soy milk, orange juice, or other fortified beverages each day fulfill this recommendation, as does an equivalent amount of low-fat yogurt and/or low-fat cheese (1½ oz of cheese = 1 cup of milk). For more information about calcium, see Chapter 7.

Limit Fats, Salt, and Sugar

Fat is an important part of a healthful diet, as it provides energy and important nutrients. However, eating a diet high in total fat can lead to overweight and obesity, as well as increase your risk for cancer. A healthful diet limits total fat to no more than 35% of total energy, limits intake of solid fats such as butter, lard, and margarine, and includes adequate amounts of healthful fats such as canola oil and olive oil. Fats are the subject of Chapter 4.

Foods high in sugar promote tooth decay and can contribute significantly to overweight and obesity when eaten in excess. These foods should be eaten in small amounts and only on occasion.

Salt contains sodium, a mineral linked to high blood pressure in some people. In addition, eating high amounts of sodium can cause us to lose calcium from our bones, which may increase our risk for bone loss and bone fractures. Much of the salt in our diets comes from processed and prepared foods. Ways to decrease your salt intake include eating foods without salt added either during processing or at the table, limiting your intake of processed meats and snack foods such as chips, and choosing beans, soups, and other foods with labels that say "low-sodium." For more information on sodium, see Chapter 7.

Keep Food Safe to Eat

A healthful diet is one that is safe from food-borne illnesses such as those caused by bacteria, viruses, and other toxins. One of the most important ways to prevent food-borne illness is to wash your hands and kitchen surfaces thoroughly with warm water and detergent before preparing food and after handling raw meats, shellfish, and eggs. Food safety is discussed in detail in Chapter 12.

If You Drink Alcoholic Beverages, Do So in Moderation

Moderate consumption of alcohol has been associated with cardiovascular benefits. In contrast, drinking alcoholic beverages in excess can lead to many health and social problems and increases the risk for accidental injury and death. The Dietary Guidelines for Americans therefore suggest that if you drink alcoholic beverages, do so in moderation. *Moderation* is defined as no more than one drink per day for women and no more than two drinks per day for men. To learn more about alcohol, refer to Chapter 8.

RECAP *The Dietary Reference Intakes (DRIs) are dietary standards for nutrients established for healthy people in a particular life-stage or gender group. The Dietary Guidelines for Americans include achieving a healthy weight, being physically active each day, selecting a variety of healthful foods, limiting fats, salt, and sugar, keeping foods safe to eat, and if you drink alcohol, doing so in moderation.*

Use MyPyramid to Help You Plan Meals and Snacks

The U.S. Department of Agriculture (USDA) food guidance system, called **MyPyramid,** is another tool that can guide you in designing a healthful diet (FIGURE 1.6). MyPyramid is an interactive, personalized guide that people can access on the Internet to assess their current diet and physical activity levels and to obtain a list of recommended changes to make in their food intake and physical activity patterns.

MyPyramid Includes Six Components for Physical Health

The six components of MyPyramid are:

STEP 1. Activity The activity component of MyPyramid, represented by the steps and the person climbing them, reminds us to be physically active every day.

STEP 2. Moderation The moderation component of MyPyramid is represented by the narrowing of each food group from the bottom to the top of the pyramid. The wider base of each food group reminds us to choose more of the most healthful foods in each group. The narrower apex reminds us to choose fewer of the less healthful foods in each group.

STEP 3. Personalization The person on the steps of MyPyramid, and the slogan and Web site (Steps to a Healthier You, www.MyPyramid.gov), encourage each of us to design a diet and determine a level of activity that is healthful for us.

STEP 4. Proportionality Notice that the food group bands differ in width. The differing widths indicate how much food a person should consume from each group, in proportion to the other groups. To find out how many servings *you* should consume from each food group, log onto www.MyPyramid.gov.

STEP 5. Variety The color-coded bands represent the different categories of foods and oils that should be eaten each day.

STEP 6. Gradual Improvement The slogan "Steps to a Healthier You" suggests that people can benefit from taking small steps each day to improve their diet and lifestyle.

When you log onto www.MyPyramid.gov, you'll be assigned a calorie level based on your gender, age, and activity level. Then, from a group of 12 possible pyramids, the program will generate the one that most closely matches your profile.

MyPyramid Emphasizes Healthful Food Choices

The food groups in MyPyramid include grains, vegetables, fruits, oils, milk, and meat and beans. The grains section of MyPyramid emphasizes "making half your grains whole," meaning you should make sure at least half of the grains you eat each day come from whole-grain sources. These foods are good sources of fiber-rich carbohydrates and many micronutrients.

The vegetables section emphasizes "vary your veggies," meaning you should eat a variety of vegetables each day, including dark green and orange vegetables and dry beans and peas. The emphasis of the fruits section is to "focus on fruits," that is, to eat a variety of fruits (including fresh, frozen, canned, or dried) and to go easy on fruit juices. Eating a variety of *both* fruits and vegetables is important in ensuring our consumption of many vital nutrients, including phytochemicals. A detailed explanation of phytochemicals is provided in Chapter 6.

The oils section of MyPyramid emphasizes "know your fats." This message encourages us to find out which fats are most healthful and to select those more often. You'll learn about the health effects of the different types of fats in Chapter 4.

MyPyramid A revised pyramid-based food guidance system developed by the USDA and based on the 2005 Dietary Guidelines for Americans and the Dietary Reference Intakes from the National Academy of Sciences.

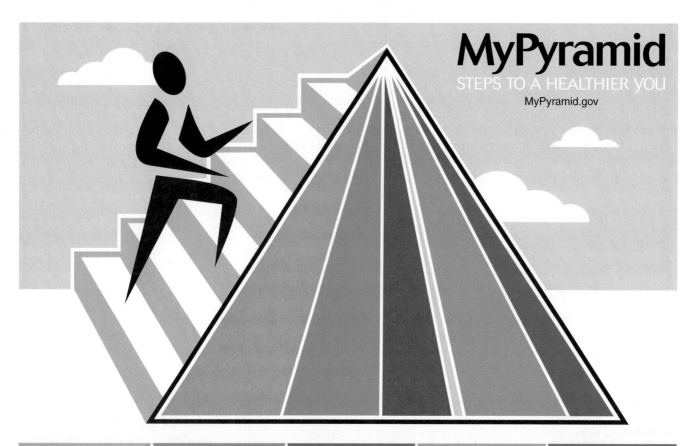

MyPyramid
STEPS TO A HEALTHIER YOU
MyPyramid.gov

GRAINS	VEGETABLES	FRUITS	MILK	MEAT & BEANS
Make half your grains whole	**Vary your veggies**	**Focus on fruits**	**Get your calcium-rich foods**	**Go lean with protein**
Eat at least 3 oz of whole-grain cereals, breads, crackers, rice, or pasta every day	Eat more dark-green veggies like broccoli, spinach, and other dark leafy greens	Eat a variety of fruit	Go low-fat or fat-free when you choose milk, yogurt, and other milk products	Choose low-fat or lean meats and poultry
1 oz is about 1 slice of bread, about 1 cup of breakfast cereal, or $1/2$ cup of cooked rice, cereal, or pasta	Eat more orange vegetables like carrots and sweet-potatoes	Choose fresh, frozen, canned, or dried fruit	If you don't or can't consume milk, choose lactose-free products or other calcium sources such as fortified foods and beverages	Bake it, broil it, or grill it
	Eat more dry beans and peas like pinto beans, kidney beans, and lentils	Go easy on fruit juices		Vary your protein routine—choose more fish, beans, peas, nuts, and seeds

For a 2,000-calorie diet, you need the amounts below from each food group. To find the amounts that are right for you, go to MyPyramid.gov.

Eat 6 oz every day	Eat 2$1/2$ cups every day	Eat 2 cups every day	Get 3 cups every day; for kids aged 2 to 8, it's 2	Eat 5$1/2$ oz every day

Find your balance between food and physical activity
- Be sure to stay within your daily calorie needs.
- Be physically active for at least 30 minutes most days of the week.
- About 60 minutes a day of physical activity may be needed to prevent weight gain.
- For sustaining weight loss, at least 60 to 90 minutes a day of physical activity may be required.
- Children and teenagers should be physically active for 60 minutes every day, or most days.

Know the limits on fats, sugars, and salt (sodium)
- Make most of your fat sources from fish, nuts, and vegetable oils.
- Limit solid fats like butter, margarine, shortening, and lard, as well as foods that contain these.
- Check the Nutrition Facts label to keep saturated fats, trans fats, and sodium low.
- Choose food and beverages low in added sugars. Added sugars contribute calories with few, if any, nutrients.

MyPyramid.gov
STEPS TO A HEALTHIER YOU

U.S. Department of Agriculture
Center for Nutrition Policy and Promotion
April 2005
CNPP-15

USDA is an equal opportunity provider and employer.

FIGURE 1.6 The USDA MyPyramid Food Guidance System. MyPyramid is a personalized guide that people can use to assess their current diet and physical activity levels and to make changes in their food intake and physical activity patterns. To learn more about this pyramid, go to www.MyPyramid.gov.

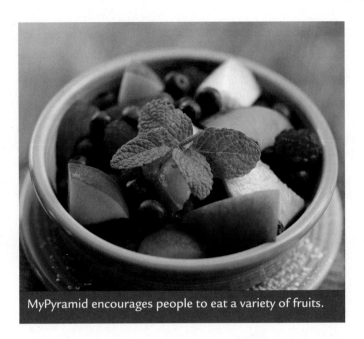

MyPyramid encourages people to eat a variety of fruits.

The milk section, which includes milk, yogurt, and cheese, reminds us to "get your calcium-rich foods." Low-fat or fat-free dairy products and calcium-fortified juices and soy beverages are recommended.

The meat and beans section, which includes meat, poultry, fish, dry beans, eggs, and nuts, emphasizes "go lean on protein." Low-fat or lean meats and poultry are encouraged, as are cooking methods such as baking, broiling, or grilling instead of frying. People are also encouraged to include more fish, beans, nuts, and seeds. Notice that legumes, which include dried beans, peas, and lentils, are included here as well as in the vegetables section. This is because legumes are good sources of fiber and contain many of the vitamins found in vegetables, and they are also good sources of protein and some of the minerals found in meat and poultry.

One new concept introduced in MyPyramid is that of **discretionary calories.** Discretionary calories represent the extra amount of energy you can consume after you have met all of your essential needs. The amount of discretionary calories you can eat depends on your age, gender, and physical activity level, but is typically about 100 to 300 kcal/day. Examples of foods that some people may choose to use up their discretionary calories include butter, margarine, mayonnaise, and cream. High-sugar foods such as desserts and soft drinks are also discretionary items, as are alcoholic beverages. You can also use your discretionary calories to eat more healthful foods.

MyPyramid also helps you decide *how much* of each food you should eat. The number of servings for each section of the pyramid is determined based on your recommended calorie level. FIGURE 1.7 shows the number of daily servings of food from each food group for a 2,000-kcal intake. This example may not be right for you, as people who need more or less energy need to eat more or fewer servings from each section of MyPyramid. Go to www.MyPyramid.gov to determine how many calories and servings of food you should eat each day.

What Does Serving Size Mean in MyPyramid?

What is considered a serving size for the foods listed in MyPyramid? To answer this, you need to know the term **ounce-equivalent** (or oz-equivalent), which defines a serving size that is 1 ounce, or equivalent to an ounce, for the grains and meats and beans sections. Servings in the vegetables, fruits, and milk groups are defined in cups. Refer to Figure 1.7 again—it shows the number of oz-equivalents or cups that

discretionary calories A term used in the MyPyramid food guidance system that represents the extra amount of energy you can consume after you have met all of your essential needs by consuming the most nutrient-dense foods that are low fat or fat free and that have no added sugars.

ounce-equivalent (or oz-equivalent) A term used to define a serving size that is 1 ounce, or equivalent to an ounce, for the grains section and the meats and beans section of MyPyramid.

Food group	Number of cups or oz-equivalents for a 2,000-kcal food intake pattern	Examples of amounts equal to 1 cup or 1 oz-equivalent			
Milk group	3 cups	1 cup (8 fl. oz) milk	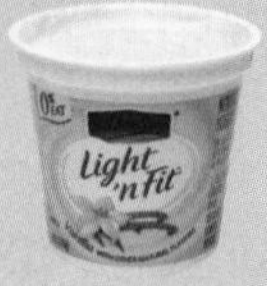 1 cup (8 fl. oz) yogurt	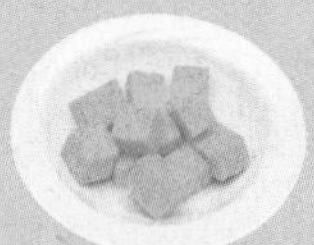 1.5 oz hard cheese	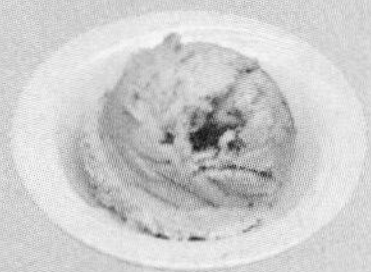 1 cup of ice cream
Meat and beans group	5.5 oz-equivalents	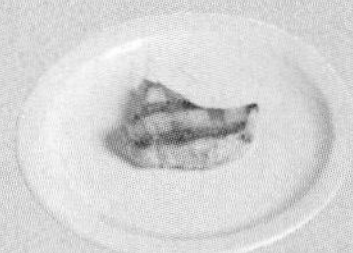 1-oz pork loin chop	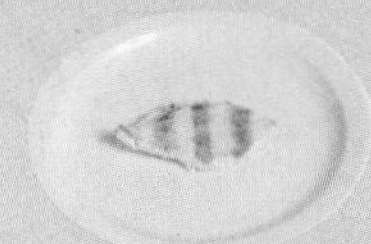 1-oz chicken breast without skin	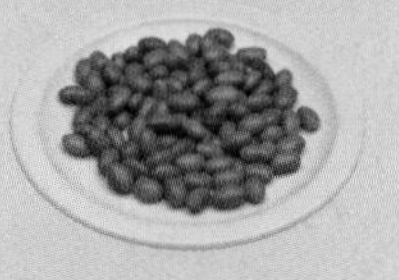 1/4 cup pinto beans	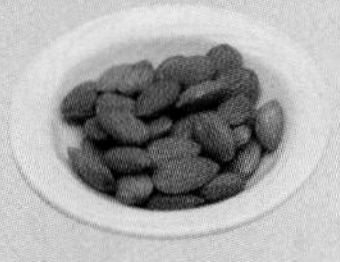 1/2 oz almonds
Vegetables group	2.5 cups	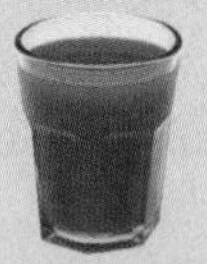 1 cup (8 fl. oz) tomato juice	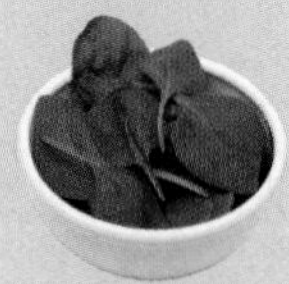 2 cups raw spinach	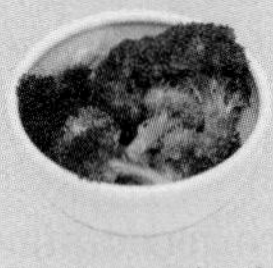 1 cup cooked broccoli	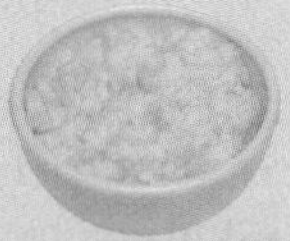 1 cup mashed potatoes
Fruits group	2 cups	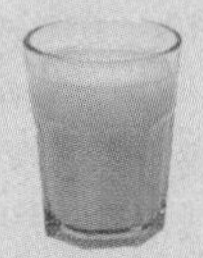 1 cup (8 fl. oz) orange juice	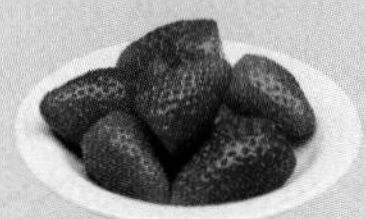 1 cup strawberries	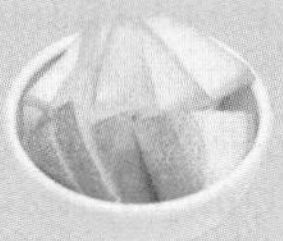 1 cup of pears	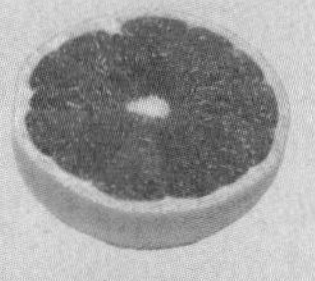 1/2 pink grapefruit
Grains group	6 oz-equivalents	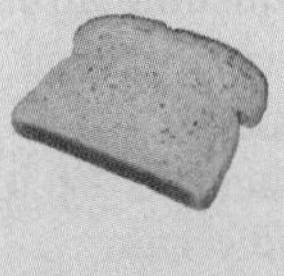 1 (1 oz) slice of whole-wheat bread	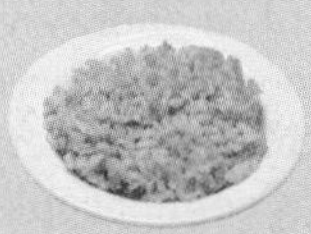 1/2 cup (1 oz) cooked brown rice	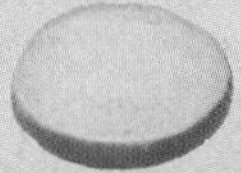 1/2 regular hamburger bun	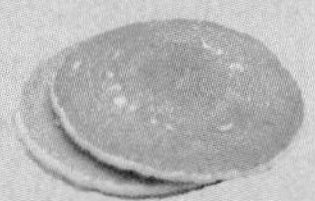 2 pancakes (4 in. diameter)

FIGURE 1.7 Examples of serving sizes for foods in each food group of MyPyramid for a 2,000-kcal food intake pattern.

should be consumed each day for a 2,000-kcal food intake pattern and examples for each food group. FIGURE 1.8 gives you a comparison to your hand that may make it easier to estimate serving size. For example:

- An oz-equivalent from the grain group is defined as 1 slice of bread, 1 cup of ready-to-eat cereal, or ½ cup of cooked rice, pasta, or cooked cereal.

- A cup of most raw or cooked vegetables is in fact 1 cup, but for raw leafy vegetables such as spinach or lettuce, it's defined as 2 cups.

- A serving of meat is just 1 oz-equivalent! When you eat a "quarter pound" burger, you're getting 4 servings! One egg, 1 tablespoon peanut butter, and ¼ cup cooked beans or lentils are also considered 1 oz-equivalent from the meat and beans group.

Although it may seem unnatural and inconvenient to measure your food servings, understanding the size of a serving is crucial to planning a nutritious diet.

It is important to understand that a serving size as defined in MyPyramid may not be equal to a serving size defined on a food label. For instance, the serving size for crackers in MyPyramid is 3 to 4 small crackers, whereas a serving size for crackers on a food label can range from 5 to 18 crackers, depending on the size and weight of the cracker. In addition, the serving sizes in MyPyramid are typically much smaller than the foods we buy for consumption. Although in recent years food manufacturers have labeled serving sizes more realistically, in some cases they still do not match the sizes suggested in MyPyramid. As a result, you must become an educated consumer and learn to read labels skeptically. Try the Nutrition Label Activity to determine whether the serving sizes listed on assorted food labels match the serving sizes that you normally consume.

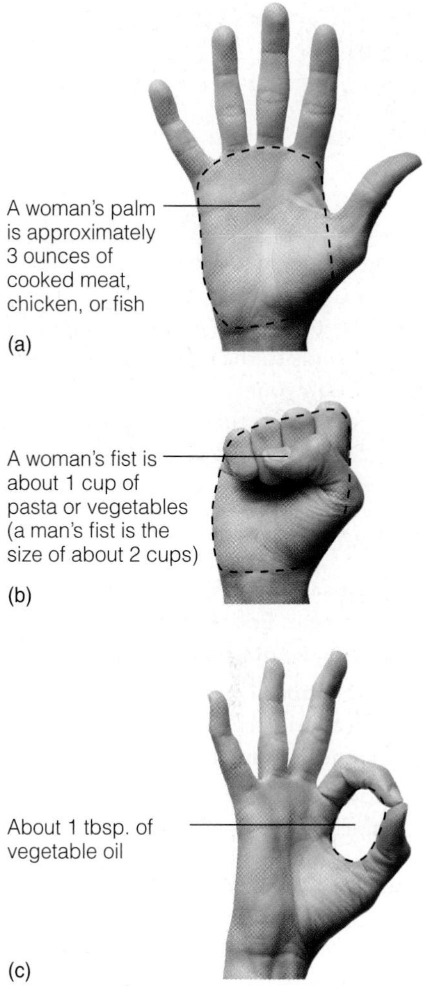

Choose Foods High in Nutrient Density

As a general guideline, you should choose foods high in **nutrient density.** This means eating foods that give you the highest amount of nutrients for the least amount of energy (or calories). An example is discussed in FIGURE 1.9. A helpful analogy for selecting nutrient-dense foods is shopping: most of us look for the best quality we can find at the lowest price. Because you can only "afford" a certain number of calories each day to maintain a healthy weight, it makes sense to maximize the nutrients you can get for each calorie you consume.

Variations of Food Guides Accommodate Individual Food Preferences

As MyPyramid was just released to the general public in 2005, variations are still being developed. However, you can easily select foods that meet your specific ethnic, religious, or other lifestyle preferences and still follow the MyPyramid system. For instance, there are variations of food pyramids available for athletes, vegetarians (see Chapter 5), children, and older adults. There are also many ethnic and cultural variations, such as the Latin American and Asian versions shown in FIGURE 1.10 on page 25. These variations empower us to design a healthful diet that accommodates our individual food preferences.

Compare Your Diet to MyPyramid

Now that you've read about MyPyramid, you might be wondering how your current diet stacks up. For that matter, what is your current diet? Have you ever really thought about it? Try logging on to the MyPyramid Web site (www.MyPyramid.gov) and go to the MyPyramid Tracker. It contains an online food intake assessment tool that scores the overall quality of your diet based on the 2005 Dietary Guidelines for Americans. You can analyze your diet for a single day or up to 1 year. You can also obtain a calculation of your nutrient intake from foods, a comparison of your diet with MyPyramid recommendations, and nutrient information from any dietary supplements you might consume.

Nutrition Scientists Have Identified Limitations of MyPyramid

Although MyPyramid is a useful tool for designing a healthful diet, it does have its limitations. As discussed in the previous section, the serving sizes as defined in MyPyramid are relatively small and do not always coincide with the standard amounts of food we buy, prepare, and serve.

A woman's palm is approximately 3 ounces of cooked meat, chicken, or fish

(a)

A woman's fist is about 1 cup of pasta or vegetables (a man's fist is the size of about 2 cups)

(b)

About 1 tbsp. of vegetable oil

(c)

FIGURE 1.8 Use your hands to help you estimate serving sizes of common foods.

nutrient density The relative amount of nutrients per amount of energy (number of calories).

NUTRITION LABEL ACTIVITY

How Realistic Are the Serving Sizes Listed on Food Labels?

Many people read food labels to determine the energy (i.e., calorie) value of foods but don't pay attention to the actual serving size that corresponds to the listed caloric value. To test how closely your "naturally selected" serving size meets the actual serving size of certain foods, try these two label activities:

ACTIVITY 1:

- Choose a breakfast cereal that you commonly eat. Pour the amount of cereal that you would normally eat into a bowl.

- Before pouring any milk on your cereal, use a measuring cup to measure the actual amount of cereal you poured.

- Now read the label of the cereal and determine the serving size (for example, ¾ cup or 1 cup) and the caloric value listed on the label. How does your "naturally selected" serving size and the label-defined serving size compare?

ACTIVITY 2:

- At the grocery store, locate various boxes of snack crackers such as regular and reduced-fat Triscuits, Ritz crackers, and so on. Look at the number of crackers and total calories per serving listed on the labels of these crackers.

- How do the number of crackers and total calories per serving differ for the serving size listed on each box?

- How do the serving sizes listed in the nutrition facts label compare to how many crackers you would usually eat?

These are just two examples of ways to understand how nutrition labels can assist you in making balanced and healthful food choices. Empowered with knowledge of what constitutes a serving size, you may find it easier to consume the appropriate amount of food for your nutrient needs.

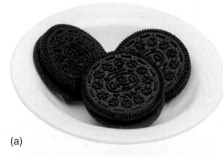
(a)

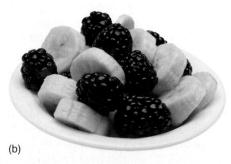
(b)

FIGURE 1.9 Examples of foods that are low or high in nutrient density. (a) Three chocolate sandwich cookies. (b) The combination of one medium banana and ½ cup fresh blackberries. Each bowl of food provides approximately 140 kcal. The cookies provide almost 6 g of fat (52 kcal), 1 g of fiber, and very few vitamins and minerals. The fruit combination provides almost 7 g of fiber and less than a gram of fat (about 7 kcal). The fruit also provides a significant amount of other nutrients such as potassium, vitamin A, and vitamin C. For our limited daily energy budget, the fruit is more nutrient dense and a more healthful choice.
(Data calculated using U.S. Department of Agriculture, Agricultural Research Service. 2007. USDA National Nutrient Database for Standard Reference, Release 20. Nutrient Data Laboratory Home Page, www.ars.usda.gov/ba/bhnrc/ndl.)

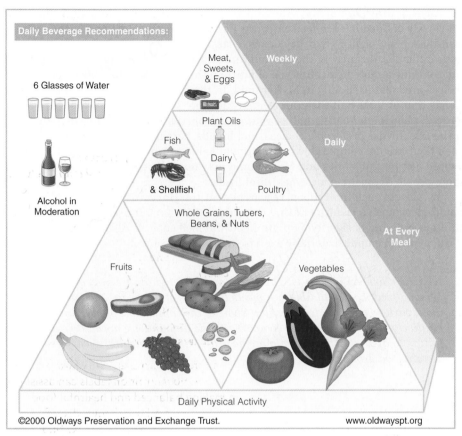

(a) Latin American diet pyramid

FIGURE 1.10 There are dozens of ethnic and cultural variations of food pyramids. Two examples illustrated here are (a) the Latin American diet pyramid and (b) the Asian diet pyramid.
(©2000 Oldways Preservation and Exchange Trust. www.oldwayspt.org.)

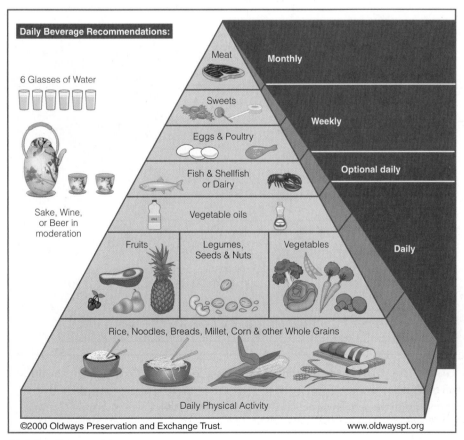

(b) Asian diet pyramid

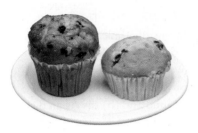

Although the serving size of a "medium" muffin in MyPyramid is 1 oz-equivalent, many muffins sold today range in size from 2 to 8 oz.

Another drawback of MyPyramid is that low-fat and low-calorie food choices are not clearly defined in each food category. For instance, the meat and beans group identifies meat, poultry, fish, dry beans, eggs, and nuts as food choices, but these foods differ significantly in the amount and type of fat they contain. Fish is low in fat and contains a more healthful type of fat than that found in red meats, yet these two choices are treated equally in MyPyramid. In the grains group, MyPyramid recommends that at least half the grains eaten each day should be from whole-grain sources, allowing for eating half of your grain sources from refined foods. Whole grains are always preferable choices, and breads, cereal, and pastas made with refined flour are not comparable in nutritional value to whole-grain foods. Thus, the revised dietary guidelines and MyPyramid may not have gone far enough in encouraging people to consume more healthful foods.

To address such limitations, researchers at the Harvard School of Public Health developed a Healthy Eating Pyramid (FIGURE 1.11). It uses a somewhat different pyramid design to highlight healthful food choices. Also notice that the base of the pyramid emphasizes daily exercise and weight control.

RECAP *You can use the USDA MyPyramid food guidance system to plan a personalized, healthful diet that meets the goals of adequacy, moderation, balance, variety, and nutrient density. Some of the limitations of MyPyramid include relatively small serving sizes compared to the amounts we normally eat and the failure to distinguish between more healthful and less healthful choices within certain food groups.*

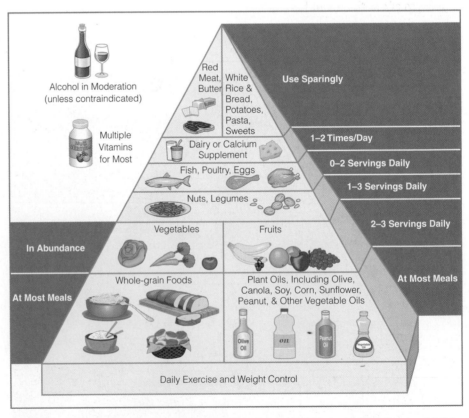

FIGURE 1.11 The Healthy Eating Pyramid is a food guide that highlights healthful food choices.

(Reprinted with the permission of Simon & Schuster Adult Publishing Group from *Eat, Drink, and Be Healthy: The Harvard Medical School Guide to Healthy Eating* by Walter C. Willett, M.D. © 2001 by President and Fellows of Harvard College.)

Read Food Labels

If you want to take control of your food choices, then it's essential to read food labels. That's because food labels give you the facts behind the hype. The U.S. Food and Drug Administration requires all food manufacturers to include complete nutrition information on labels of all packaged foods. Besides fresh produce and meats, which are unpackaged or minimally packaged, the only products exempt from the labeling requirement are foods such as coffee and most spices that contain insignificant amounts of all nutrients.

Five Components Must Be Included on Food Labels

Five primary components of information must be included on food labels (FIGURE 1.12):

1. *A statement of identity:* The common name of the product or an appropriate identification must be prominently displayed on the label.
2. *The net contents of the package:* This information accurately describes the quantity of the food product in the entire package. This information may be listed as weight (e.g., grams), volume (e.g., fluid ounces), or numerical count (e.g., 4 bars).
3. *Ingredient list:* The ingredients must be listed by their common name, in descending order by weight. This means that the first product listed in the ingredient list is the predominant ingredient in that food.
4. *The name and address of the food manufacturer, packer, or distributor:* This information can be used to contact the company.
5. *Nutrition Facts Panel:* This panel is the primary tool to assist you in choosing more healthful foods. The following section provides an explanation of the components of the Nutrition Facts Panel.

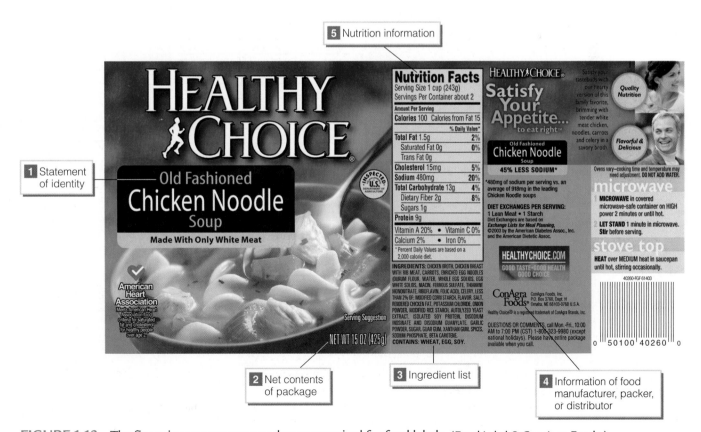

FIGURE 1.12 The five primary components that are required for food labels. (Food Label © Con Agra Foods.)

How to Read and Use the Nutrition Facts Panel

FIGURE 1.13 shows an example of a **Nutrition Facts Panel.** This part of the label includes a variety of information that is useful when designing a healthful diet. Let's start at the top of the panel and work our way down.

1. *Serving size and servings per container:* The FDA has defined serving sizes based on the amounts people typically eat for each food. However, keep in mind that the serving size listed on the package may not be the same as the amount you eat. You must factor in how much of the food you eat when determining the amount of nutrients that this food contributes to your actual diet.

2. *Total calories and calories from fat per serving:* By looking at this section of the label, you can determine if this food is relatively high in fat. For example, one serving of the food on this label contains 320 total calories, with 90 of those calories coming from fat. This means that this food contains approximately 28% of its total calories as fat, making it relatively low in fat.

3. *List of nutrients:* Those nutrients listed toward the top, including total fat, saturated fat, cholesterol, and sodium, are generally nutrients that we strive to limit in a healthful diet. Some of the nutrients listed toward the bottom are those we try to consume more of, including fiber, vitamins A and C, calcium, and iron.

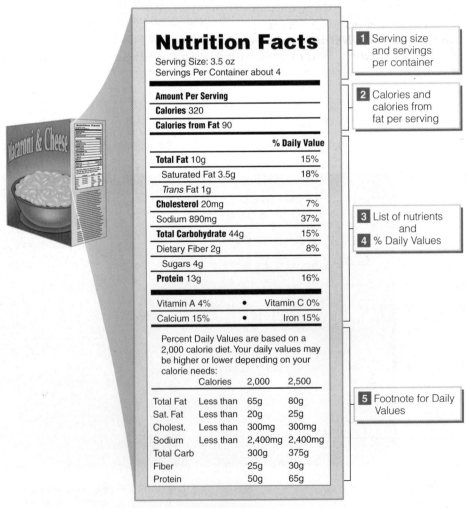

Nutrition Facts Panel The label on a food package that contains the nutrition information required by the FDA.

FIGURE 1.13 The Nutrition Facts Panel contains a variety of information to help you select more healthful food choices.

4. ***The percent daily values (%DV):*** This information tells you how much a serving of food contributes to your overall intake of nutrients listed on the label. Because we are all individuals with unique nutritional needs, it is impossible to include nutrition information that applies to each person consuming this food. Thus, the FDA used standards based on a 2,000-calorie diet when defining the %DV. You can use these percentages to determine whether a food is high or low in a given nutrient, even if you do not consume a 2,000-calorie diet each day. For example, if you are trying to consume more calcium, you might compare the labels of two different brands of fortified orange juice: you read that one contains 10% DV for calcium in an 8-oz serving, whereas the other contains 25% DV for calcium in an 8-oz serving. Thus, you can make your choice between these products without having to know anything about how many calories you need.

5. ***Footnote:*** The footnote includes an explanatory note and a table with Daily Values for a 2,000- and 2,500-calorie diet. This table, which may not be present on the package if the size of the food label is too small, is always the same because the information refers to nutrients, not to a specific food. For instance, it states that someone eating 2,000 calories should strive to eat less than 65 g of fat per day, whereas a person eating 2,500 calories should eat less than 80 g of fat per day.

RECAP *Reading food labels is a necessary skill when planning a healthful diet. Food labels provide the identity of the food, the net contents of the package, the contact information for the food manufacturer or distributor, the ingredients in the food, and a Nutrition Facts Panel. The Nutrition Facts Panel provides specific information about calories, macronutrients, and select vitamins and minerals.*

percent daily values (%DV) Information on a Nutrition Facts Panel that tells you how much a serving of food contributes to your overall intake of nutrients listed on the label. The information is based on an energy intake of 2,000 kcal per day.

NUTRI-CASE GUSTAVO

"Until last night, I hadn't stepped inside of a grocery store for 10 years, maybe more. But then my wife fell and broke her hip and had to go to the hospital. On my way home from visiting her, I remembered that we didn't have much food in the house, so I thought I'd do a little shopping. Was I ever in for a shock. I don't know how my wife does it, choosing between all the different brands, reading those long labels. She never went to school past sixth grade, and she doesn't speak English very well either! I bought a frozen chicken pie for my dinner, but it didn't taste right. So I got the package out of the trash and read all the labels, and that's when I realized there wasn't any chicken in it at all! It was made out of tofu! This afternoon, my daughter is picking me up, and we're going to do our grocery shopping together."

Given what you've learned about FDA food labels, what parts of a food package would you advise Gustavo to be sure to read before he makes a choice? What other advice might you give him to make his grocery shopping easier? Imagine that, like Gustavo's wife, you have only limited skills in mathematics and reading. In that case, what other strategies might you use when shopping for nutritious foods?

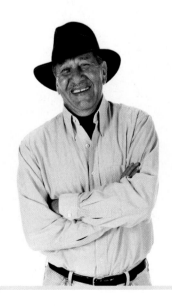

Whom Can You Trust to Help You Choose Foods Wisely?

After reading this chapter, you can see that nutrition plays a critical role in preserving health and preventing and treating disease. As recognition of this vital role has increased over the past few decades, the public has become more and more interested in understanding how nutrition affects health. One result of this booming interest has been the publication of an almost overwhelming quantity of nutritional information and claims on television infomercials, on Web sites, in newspapers, magazines, and journals, on product packages, and via many other forums. Most of us do not have the knowledge or training to interpret and evaluate the reliability of this information and thus are vulnerable to misinformation.

Throughout this text we provide you with information to assist you in becoming a more educated consumer regarding nutrition. You will learn about labeling guidelines, the proper use of supplements, and whether various nutrition topics are myths or facts. In addition, the Companion Website to this book (www.pearsonhighered. com/nutritionplace) contains a feature called *Find the Quack* for each chapter of the book. As you may know, **quackery** is the misrepresentation of a product, program, or service for financial gain. For example, a high-priced supplement may be marketed as uniquely therapeutic when in fact it is only as effective as much less expensive remedies commonly available. Many manufacturers of such products describe them as "patented," but this means only that the product has been registered with the U.S. Patent Office, for a fee. It provides no guarantee of the product's effectiveness or its safety. After considering the information presented in each *Find the Quack* feature, you'll have a chance to decide for yourself: Is this a legitimate product or service, or is it quackery? Armed with the information in this book, plus plenty of opportunities to test your knowledge, you will become more confident when trying to evaluate nutrition claims. Let's start by identifying trustworthy sources of nutrition information.

quackery The promotion of an unproven remedy, such as a supplement or other product or service, usually by someone unlicensed and untrained.

Trustworthy Experts Are Educated and Credentialed

The following is a list of the most common groups of health professionals who provide reliable and accurate nutrition information:

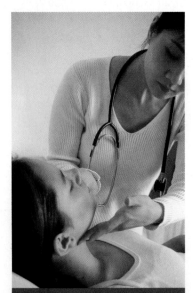

Medical doctors may have limited experience and training in the area of nutrition, but they can refer you to a registered dietitian (RD) or licensed dietitian to assist you in meeting your dietary needs.

- Registered dietitian (or RD): A registered dietitian (RD) is an individual who possesses at least a baccalaureate (bachelor's) degree and has completed a defined content of course work and experience in nutrition and dietetics. This individual also meets the eligibility requirements of the Commission on Dietetic Registration.[5] For a list of individuals who are registered dietitians in your community, you can look in the yellow pages of your phone book or contact the American Dietetic Association at www.eatright.org.

- Licensed dietitian: A licensed dietitian is a dietitian meeting the credentialing requirement of a given state in the United States to engage in the practice of dietetics.[5] Each state in the United States has its own laws regulating dietitians.

- Nutritionist: This term generally has no definition or laws regulating it. In some cases, it refers to a professional with academic credentials in nutrition who may also be an RD.[5] In some states, these professionals are called licensed nutritionists (LN). In other cases, the term *nutritionist* may refer to anyone who thinks he or she is knowledgeable about nutrition. In the chapter-opening scenario, how might Miguel have determined whether or not the "nutritionist" was qualified to give him advice?

- Professional with an advanced degree (a master's degree [MA or MS] or doctoral degree [PhD]) in nutrition: Many individuals hold an advanced degree in nutrition and have years of experience in a nutrition-related career. For instance, they may teach at community colleges or universities or work in fitness or healthcare settings. Unless these individuals are licensed or registered dietitians, they are not certified to provide clinical dietary counseling or treatment for individuals with disease. However, they are reliable sources of information about nutrition and health.

- Physician: The term *physician* encompasses a variety of healthcare professionals. A medical doctor (MD) is educated, trained, and licensed to practice medicine in the United States. However, MDs typically have very limited experience and training in the area of nutrition, as medical students in the United States are not required to take any nutrition courses. If you require a dietary plan to treat an illness or disease, most MDs will refer you to an RD or LN. In contrast, an osteopathic physician, referred to as a doctor of osteopathy (DO), may have studied nutrition extensively, as may a naturopathic physician, a homeopathic physician, or a chiropractor. Thus, it is prudent to determine a physician's level of expertise rather than assuming that he or she has extensive knowledge of nutrition.

Government Sources of Information Are Usually Trustworthy

Many government health agencies address the problem of nutrition-related disease in the United States. These organizations are funded with taxpayer dollars, and many provide financial support for research in the areas of nutrition and health. A few of the most recognized and respected of these government agencies are discussed here.

The Centers for Disease Control and Prevention Protects the Health and Safety of Americans

The *Centers for Disease Control and Prevention (CDC)* is considered to be the leading federal agency in the United States that protects the health and safety of people. The CDC is located in Atlanta, Georgia, and works in the areas of health promotion, disease prevention and control, and environmental health. To learn more about the CDC, go to www.cdc.gov.

The National Institutes of Health Is the World's Leading Medical Research Agency

The *National Institutes of Health (NIH)* is the world's leading medical research center, and it is the focal point for medical research in the United States. The NIH is one of the agencies of the Public Health Service, which is part of the U.S. Department of Health and Human Services. The NIH has many institutes, such as the National Cancer Institute and the National Center for Complementary and Alternative Medicine, that focus on a broad array of nutrition-related health issues. NIH headquarters are located in Bethesda, Maryland. To find out more about the NIH, go to www.nih.gov.

Professional Organizations Provide Reliable Nutrition Information

There are a number of professional organizations whose members are qualified nutrition professionals, scientists, and educators. These organizations publish cutting-edge

HIGHLIGHT

Research Study Results: Whom Can You Believe?

"Reduce your fat intake! Make sure at least 60% of your diet comes from carbohydrates!"

"Eat more protein and fat! Carbohydrates cause obesity!"

Do you ever feel overwhelmed by the abundant and often conflicting advice in media reports related to nutrition? If so, you're not alone. In addition to the "high-carb, low-carb" controversy, we've had mixed messages about the effectiveness of calcium supplements in preventing bone loss, high fluid intake in preventing constipation, and high fiber intake in preventing colon cancer. And after decades of warnings that coffee and tea could be bad for our health, it now appears that both contain chemicals that can be beneficial! When even nutrition researchers don't seem to agree, whom can we believe?

Nutrition is a relatively young science, and relies in part on the discoveries of other relatively young sciences such as biochemistry and genetics. New experiments are being designed every day to determine how nutrition affects our health, and new discoveries are being made. Viewing con-flicting evidence as essential to the advancement of our understanding may help you to feel more comfortable with the contradictions. In fact, controversy is what stimulates researchers to explore unknown areas and attempt to solve the mysteries of nutrition and health.

In addition, it's important to recognize that media reports rarely include a thorough review of the research findings on a given topic. Typically, they focus only on the most recent study. Thus, one report on the nightly news should never be taken as absolute fact on any topic. To become a more educated consumer and informed critic of nutrition reports in the media, you need to understand the research process and how the results of different types of studies should be interpreted. So let's take a closer look.

Research Involves Applying the Scientific Method

The *scientific method* is a multistep process that involves observation, experimentation, and development of a theory (Figure 1.14). Its standardized procedures minimize

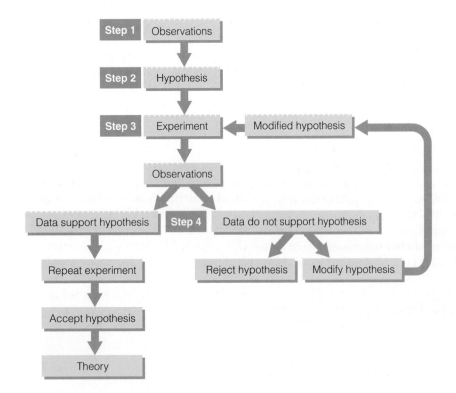

FIGURE 1.14 The scientific method, which forms the framework for scientific research. Step 1: Observations are made regarding some phenomenon, which lead researchers to ask a question. Step 2: A hypothesis is generated to explain the observations. Step 3: An experiment is conducted to test the hypothesis. Observations are made during the experiment, and data are generated and documented. Step 4: The data may either support or refute the hypothesis. If the data support the hypothesis, more experiments are conducted to test and confirm support for the hypothesis. A hypothesis that is supported after repeated testing may be called a theory. If the data do not support the hypothesis, the hypothesis is either rejected or modified and then retested.

Research Study Results: Whom Can You Believe? *(continued)*

the influence of personal prejudices and biases on our understanding of natural phenomena. Thus, this method is used to perform quality research studies in any discipline, including nutrition.

Observation of a Phenomenon Initiates the Research Process

The first step in the scientific method is observing and describing a phenomenon. As an example, let's say you are working in a healthcare office that caters to mostly elderly clients. You have observed that many of the elderly have high blood pressure, but there are some who have normal blood pressure. After talking with a large number of elderly clients, you notice a pattern developing in that the clients who report being more physically active are also those having lower blood pressure readings. This observation leads you to question the relationship that might exist between physical activity and blood pressure. Your next step is to develop a *hypothesis,* or possible explanation for your observation.

A Hypothesis Is a Possible Explanation for an Observation

A hypothesis states an assumption you want to test. It is also sometimes referred to as a research question. In this example, your hypothesis would be something like, "Regular physical activity lowers blood pressure in elderly people." You must generate a hypothesis before you can conduct experiments to determine what factors may explain your observation.

Experiments Are Conducted to Test Research Hypotheses

An *experiment* is a scientific process that tests a research question or hypothesis. In the case of your hypothesis, we could design a variety of research studies to determine the impact of regular physical activity on blood pressure in elderly people. Later in this highlight, we will review the different types of research that can be done to assist us in answering your question.

A well-designed experiment attempts to control for factors that may coincidentally influence the results. In the case of your research study, it is well-known that weight loss can reduce blood pressure in people with high blood pressure. Thus, in performing your experiment on the effects of exercise on blood pressure, you would want to control for weight loss. You could do this by making sure people eat enough food so that they do not lose weight during your study and weighing them regularly to verify weight maintenance.

It is important to emphasize that one research study does not prove or disprove a hypothesis. Ideally, multiple experiments are conducted over many years to thoroughly examine a hypothesis. Science exists to allow us to continue to challenge existing hypotheses and expand what we currently know.

A Theory May Be Developed After Extensive Research

If multiple experiments do not support a hypothesis, then the hypothesis is rejected or modified. On the other hand, if the results of multiple experiments consistently support a hypothesis, then it is possible to develop a theory. A *theory* represents a hypothesis or group of related hypotheses that have been confirmed through repeated scientific experiments. Theories are strongly accepted principles, but they can be challenged and changed as a result of applying the scientific method. Remember that centuries ago, it was theorized that the earth was flat. People were so convinced of this that they refused to sail beyond known boundaries because they believed they would fall off the edge. Only after multiple explorers challenged this theory was it discovered that the earth is round. We continue to apply the scientific method today to test hypotheses and challenge theories.

Various Types of Research Studies Tell Us Different Stories

You have just learned how the scientific method is applied to test a hypothesis. Establishing nutrition guidelines and understanding the role of nutrition in health involves constant experimentation. Depending on how the research study is designed, we can gather information that tells us different stories. Let's now learn more about the different types of research conducted and what they tell us.

Epidemiological Studies Inform Us of Existing Relationships

Epidemiological studies are also referred to as *observational studies.* These types of studies are helpful in assessing nutritional habits, disease trends, or other health phenomena of large populations and determining the factors that may influence these phenomena. However, these studies can only indicate *relationships* between factors; they do not suggest the data are linked by cause and effect. For instance, smoking and low vegetable intake appear to be related in some studies, but this does not mean that smoking cigarettes causes people to eat fewer vegetables, or that eating fewer vegetables causes people to smoke.

(continued)

Research Study Results: Whom Can You Believe? *(continued)*

Animal Studies

In many cases, studies involving animals provide preliminary information that assists scientists in designing human studies. Animal studies also are used to conduct research that cannot be done with humans. For instance, researchers can cause a nutrient deficiency in an animal and study its adverse health effects over the animal's life span, but this type of experiment with humans is not acceptable. Drawbacks of animal studies include ethical concerns and the fact that the results may not apply directly to humans.

Human Studies

The two primary types of studies conducted with humans include case-control studies and clinical trials. *Case-control studies* involve comparing a group of individuals with a particular condition (for instance, 100 elderly people with high blood pressure) to a similar group without this condition (for instance, 100 elderly people with normal blood pressure). This comparison allows the researcher to identify factors other than the defined condition that differ between the two groups. By identifying these factors, researchers can gain a better understanding of things that may cause and help prevent disease. For example, researchers may find that 75% of the people in their normal blood pressure group are physically active but that only 20% of the people in their high blood pressure group are physically active. Again, this would not prove that physical activity prevents high blood pressure. It would merely suggest a relationship between these two factors.

Clinical trials are tightly controlled experiments in which an intervention is given to determine its effect on a given disease or health condition. Interventions may include medications, nutritional supplements, controlled diets, or exercise programs. In clinical trials, people in an experimental group are given the intervention, and people in a control group are not. The responses of the two groups are compared. In the case of the blood-pressure experiment, researchers could assign one group of elderly people with high blood pressure to an exercise program and assign a second group of elderly people with high blood pressure to a program where no exercise is done. Over the next few weeks, months, or even years, researchers could measure the blood pressure of the people in each group. If the blood pressure of those who exercised decreased and the blood pressure of those who did not exercise rose or remained the same, the influence of exercise on lowering blood pressure would be supported.

There are other important things to consider when evaluating the quality of a clinical trial. Ideally, researchers should *randomly* assign research participants to intervention groups (who get the treatment) and control groups (who do not get the treatment). Randomizing participants is like flipping a coin or drawing names from a hat; it reduces the possibility of showing favoritism toward any participants and also ensures the groups are similar on the factors or characteristics you are measuring in the study. These types of studies are called *randomized clinical trials.*

If possible, it is also important to "blind" both researchers and participants to the treatment being given. A *single-blind experiment* is one in which the participants are blinded to the treatment, but the researchers know which group is getting the treatment and which group is not. A *double-blind experiment* is one in which neither researchers nor participants know which group is really getting the treatment. Double blinding helps prevent the researcher from seeing only the results he or she wants to see, even if these results do not actually occur. In the case of testing medications or nutrition supplements, the blinding process can be assisted by giving the control group a placebo. A *placebo* is an imitation treatment that has no effect on participants; for instance, a sugar pill may be given in place of a vitamin supplement. Studies like this are referred to as *double-blind randomized clinical trials.*

Use Your Knowledge of Research to Help You Evaluate Media Reports

How can all of this research information assist you in becoming a better consumer and critic of media reports? By having a better understanding of the research process and types of research conducted, you are more capable of discerning the truth or fallacy within media reports. Keep the following points in mind when examining any media report:

Research Study Results: Whom Can You Believe? *(continued)*

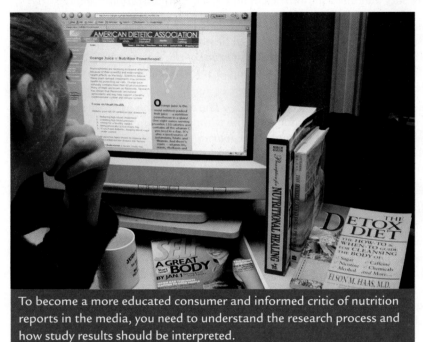

To become a more educated consumer and informed critic of nutrition reports in the media, you need to understand the research process and how study results should be interpreted.

science and are capable of misinterpreting research results.

● Is the report based on reputable research studies? Did the research follow the scientific method, and were the results reported in a reputable scientific journal? Ideally, the journal is peer-reviewed; that is, the articles are critiqued by other specialists working in the same scientific field. A reputable report should include the reference, or source of the information, and should identify researchers by name. This allows the reader to investigate the original study and determine its merit. Examples of reputable journals include the *American Journal of Clinical Nutrition, Journal of Nutrition, Journal of the American Dietetic Association,* the *New England Journal of Medicine,* and the *Journal of the American Medical Association* (*JAMA*).

● Is the report based on testimonials about personal experiences? Are sweeping conclusions made from only one study? Be wary of personal testimonials, as they are fraught with bias. In addition, one study cannot answer all of our questions or prove any hypothesis, and the findings from individual studies should be placed in their proper perspective.

● Who conducted the research, and who paid for it? Was the study funded by a company that stands to profit from certain results? Are the researchers receiving goods, personal travel funds, or other perks from the research sponsor, or do they have investments in companies or products related to their study? If the answer to these questions is yes, there exists a *conflict of interest* between the researchers and the funding agency. If a conflict of interest does exist, it may seriously compromise the researchers' ability to conduct unbiased research and report the results in an accurate and responsible manner.

● Who is reporting the information? Is it an article in a newspaper, magazine, or on the Internet? If the report is made by a person or group who may financially benefit from you buying their products, you should be skeptical of the reported results. Also, many people who write for popular magazines and newspapers are not trained in

● Are the claims in the report too good to be true? Are claims made about curing disease or treating a multitude of conditions? If something sounds too good to be true, it probably is. Claims about curing diseases or treating many conditions with one product should be a signal to question the validity of the report.

Throughout this text, we provide you with information to assist you in evaluating research studies and marketing statements about nutrition-related products and services. You will learn about labeling guidelines, the proper use of supplements, and whether various nutrition claims are myths or facts. Armed with this knowledge, you will become more confident when trying to determine what to buy and whom to trust.

nutrition research studies and educational information in journals that are accessible in most university and medical libraries. Some of these organizations include:

- The American Dietetic Association (ADA): This is the largest organization of food and nutrition professionals in the United States and the world. The ADA publishes a professional journal called the *Journal of the American Dietetic Association;* information about ADA can be found at www.eatright.org. The Canadian equivalent is Dietitians of Canada.

- The American Society for Nutrition (ASN): The ASN is the premier research society dedicated to improving quality of life through the science of nutrition. ASN publishes two professional journals, the *Journal of Nutrition* and the *American Journal of Clinical Nutrition* (AJCN). Information about ASN can be found at www.nutrition.org.

- The American College of Sports Medicine (ACSM): The ACSM is the leading sports medicine and exercise science organization in the world. *Medicine and Science in Sports and Exercise* is the professional journal of the ACSM. You can learn more about the ACSM at www.acsm.org.

If you aren't sure whether or not the source of your information is reliable or can't tell whether the results of a particular study apply to you, how do you find out? What if two studies seem sound, but their findings contradict each other? The accompanying Highlight explains how you can become a more informed and critical consumer of nutrition-related research.

RECAP *The most common groups of health professionals who provide reliable and accurate nutrition information include registered dietitians, licensed dietitians, licensed nutritionists, professionals with an advanced degree in nutrition, and some physicians. The term* nutritionist *is not a guarantee that the individual has any training in nutrition. The Centers for Disease Control and Prevention is the leading federal agency in the United States that protects the health and safety of people. The National Institutes of Health is the leading medical research agency in the world.*

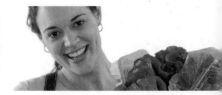

REVIEW QUESTIONS

Circle the correct choice.

1. Which of the following foods contains all six nutrient groups?
   a. strawberry ice cream
   b. an egg-salad sandwich
   c. creamy tomato soup
   d. all of the above

2. An adequate diet
   a. provides enough energy to meet minimum daily requirements.
   b. provides enough of the energy, nutrients, and fiber necessary to maintain the person's health.
   c. provides a sufficient variety of nutrients to maintain a healthy weight and to optimize the body's functioning.
   d. contains combinations of foods that provide healthful proportions of nutrients.

3. The Dietary Guidelines for Americans recommend which of the following?
   a. Choosing and preparing all foods without salt.
   b. Consuming two alcoholic beverages per day.
   c. Being physically active each day.
   d. Consuming a fat-free diet.

4. MyPyramid recommends
   a. drinking a variety of fruit juices each day.
   b. eating more dark green and orange vegetables.
   c. consuming at least one 8-oz glass of whole milk each day.
   d. baking, broiling, or frying meats.

5. The Nutrition Facts Panel on packaged foods provides information about the micronutrients
   a. vitamin A, sodium, potassium, and calcium.
   b. vitamin A, vitamin C, sodium, iron, and calcium.
   c. vitamin C, sodium, and calcium.
   d. No micronutrient information is included on the Nutrition Facts Panel.

6. True or False? Fat-soluble vitamins provide energy.

7. True or False? The Recommended Dietary Allowance represents the average daily intake level that meets the requirements of almost all healthy individuals in a given life stage or gender group.

8. True or False? Alcohol can be part of a healthful diet.

9. True or False? Eating a variety of foods ensures that your diet is healthful.

10. True or False? The serving size listed on a Nutrition Facts Panel is based on the amount people typically eat of that food.

WEB LINKS

www.fda.gov
U.S. Food and Drug Administration (FDA)

Learn more about the government agency that regulates our food and first established regulations for nutrition information on food labels.

www.healthierus.gov/dietaryguidelines
Dietary Guidelines for Americans 2005

Use these guidelines to make changes in your food choices and physical activity habits to help reduce your risk for chronic disease.

www.MyPyramid.gov
USDA MyPyramid Steps to a Healthier You

Use the MyPyramid Tracker on this Web site to assess the overall quality of your diet based on the USDA MyPyramid.

www.oldwayspt.org
Oldways Preservation and Exchange Trust

Find different variations of ethnic and cultural food pyramids.

www.hsph.harvard.edu
The Harvard School of Public Health

Search this site to learn more about the Healthy Eating Pyramid.

www.eatright.org
American Dietetic Association (ADA)

Obtain a list of registered dietitians in your community from the largest organization of food and nutrition professionals in the United States. Information about careers in dietetics is also available at this site. Visit the food and nutrition information section of this Web site for additional resources to help you achieve a healthy lifestyle.

www.cdc.gov
Centers for Disease Control and Prevention (CDC)

Visit this site for additional information about the leading federal agency in the United States that protects the health and safety of people.

www.nih.gov
National Institutes of Health (NIH)

Find out more about the National Institutes of Health, an agency under the U.S. Department of Health and Human Services.

http://hp2010.nhlbihin.net/portion
The National Institutes of Health (NIH) Portion Distortion Quiz

Take this short quiz to see if you know how today's food portions compare to those of 20 years ago.

www.nutrition.org
The American Society for Nutrition (ASN)

Learn about the mission and membership requirements for the American Society for Nutrition, and explore future scientific meetings and articles in the *Journal of Nutrition* and the *American Journal of Clinical Nutrition.*

www.acsm.org
American College of Sports Medicine (ACSM)

Obtain information about the world's leading sports medicine and exercise science organization.

www.naaso.org
The Obesity Society

Learn about this interdisciplinary society and its work to develop, extend, and disseminate knowledge in the field of obesity.

TEST YOURSELF ANSWERS

1. **True.** Although nutrition guidelines recommended that we consume these types of foods only occasionally, they can be included in moderation as part of a healthful diet.

2. **False.** Not all nutrients provide energy; the primary energy sources for our bodies are carbohydrates and fats.

3. **False.** Calories are a measure of the energy in foods. More precisely, a kilocalorie is the amount of heat required to raise the temperature of 1 kilogram of water by 1 degree Celsius.

4. **False.** A diet that is adequate, moderate, balanced, and varied may not require supplementation. However, certain individuals may need to supplement based on specific health concerns.

5. **False.** The top nutritional guidelines published in the United States, the 2005 Dietary Guidelines for Americans, state that moderate alcohol consumption can be part of a healthful diet. Moderate alcohol consumption is defined as one drink per day for women and two drinks per day for men.

REFERENCES

1. Gardner, S. L., and E. Goldson. 2002. The neonate and the environment: Impact on development. In: Merenstein, G. G., and S. L. Gardner, eds., *Handbook of Neonatal Intensive Care,* 5th ed. St. Louis: Mosby, pp. 219–282.
2. Marieb, E. 2004. *Human Anatomy and Physiology,* 6th ed. San Francisco: Benjamin Cummings, pp. 556–557.
3. Institute of Medicine, Food and Nutrition Board. 2003. *Dietary Reference Intakes: Applications in Dietary Planning.* Washington, DC: National Academies Press.
4. USDHHS and USDA. 2005. Dietary Guidelines for Americans 2005: Key recommendations for the general population. Available at www.health.gov/dietaryguidelines/dga.../recommendations.
5. Winterfeldt, E. A., M. L. Bogle, and L. L. Ebro. 2005. *Dietetics. Practice and Future Trends.* 2nd ed. Sudbury, MA: Jones and Bartlett Publishers.

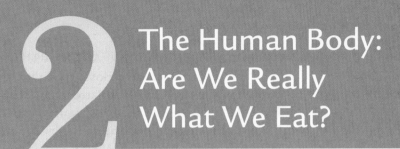

TEST YOURSELF

Are these statements true or false? Circle your guess.

1 Your stomach is the primary organ responsible for telling you when you are hungry.

TRUE or **FALSE**

2 The entire process of digestion and absorption of one meal takes about 24 hours.

TRUE or **FALSE**

3 Some types of bacteria actually help keep our digestive system healthy.

TRUE or **FALSE**

4 Most ulcers result from a type of infection.

TRUE or **FALSE**

5 Irritable bowel syndrome is a rare disease that mostly affects older people.

TRUE or **FALSE**

Test Yourself answers can be found at the end of the chapter.

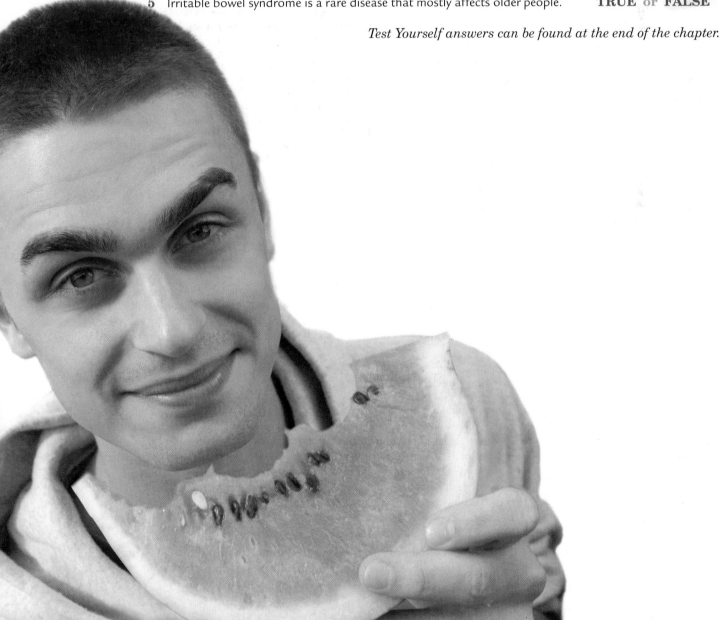

TWO MONTHS AGO, ANDREA'S lifelong dream of becoming a lawyer came one step closer to reality: she moved out of her parents' home in the Midwest to attend law school in Boston. Unfortunately, the adjustment to a new city, new friends, and her intensive coursework was more stressful than she'd imagined, and Andrea has been experiencing insomnia and exhaustion. What's more, her always "sensitive stomach" has been getting worse: after almost every meal, she gets cramps so bad she can't stand up, and twice she has missed classes because of sudden attacks of pain and diarrhea. She suspects that the problem is related to stress, and wonders if she is going to experience it throughout her life. She is even thinking of dropping out of school if that would make her feel well again.

Almost everyone experiences brief periods of abdominal pain, diarrhea, or other symptoms of gastrointestinal distress from time to time. Such episodes are usually caused by food poisoning or an infection such as influenza. But do you know anyone who experiences these symptoms periodically for days, weeks, or even years? If so, has it made you wonder why? What are the steps in normal digestion and absorption of food, and at what points can the process break down?

We begin this chapter by touring the cells, tissues, and organs of the human body. We then explore how the body breaks down and absorbs foods and eliminates waste products. Finally, we discuss some common disorders that affect these processes.

Are We Really What We Eat?

You've no doubt heard the saying that "you are what you eat." But is this scientifically true? To answer that question, and to better understand how we digest and process foods, we'll need to look at how our bodies are organized (FIGURE 2.1).

Atoms Bond to Form Molecules

Like all substances on Earth, our bodies are made up of *atoms*. Atoms are the smallest units of matter, and they cannot be broken down by natural means. Atoms almost constantly bind to each other in nature to form groups called *molecules*. For example, a molecule of water is composed of two atoms of hydrogen and an atom of oxygen, which is abbreviated H_2O.

During digestion, we break our food down into small molecules that can be easily transported in the bloodstream. From there, these food molecules cross into our cells to help build the structures of our bodies and provide the energy we need to live and move.

Molecules Join to Form Cells

Whereas atoms are the smallest units of matter and make up both living and nonliving things, **cells** are the smallest units of life. That is, cells can grow, reproduce themselves, take in nutrients, and excrete wastes. The human body is composed of billions of cells that are continually being replaced. To support the construction of new cells, we need a steady supply of nutrient molecules from the breakdown of foods. Nutrient molecules also provide the fuel that cells need to perform their function in the body.

Cells Are Encased in a Membrane

The contents of a cell are enclosed by a **cell membrane** (FIGURE 2.2). This thin outer coat defines the cell's boundaries. Cell membranes are *semipermeable*: some mole-

cell The smallest unit of matter that exhibits the properties of living things, such as growth, reproduction, and the taking in of nutrients.

cell membrane The boundary of an animal cell that separates its internal cytoplasm, nucleus, and other structures from the external environment.

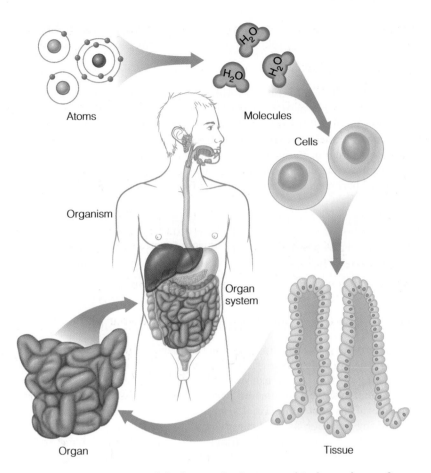

Atoms

Molecules

Cells

Organism

Organ system

Organ

Tissue

FIGURE 2.1   The organization of the human body. Atoms bind together to form molecules. The cells of our bodies are constructed using molecules made from the foods we eat. Cells join to form tissues, one or more types of which form organs. Body systems, such as the gastrointestinal system shown here, are made up of several organs, each of which performs a discrete function. The human organism has 11 such organ systems.

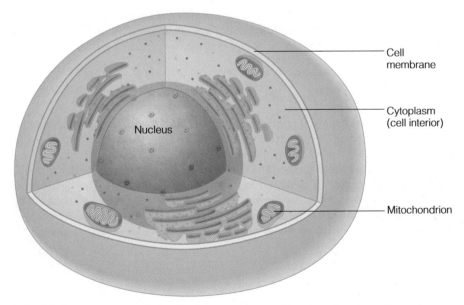

Cell membrane

Cytoplasm (cell interior)

Nucleus

Mitochondrion

FIGURE 2.2   Representative cell of the small intestine, showing the cell membrane, the cytoplasm, the nucleus, and several mitochondria.

cules can easily flow through them, whereas others cannot. This quality enables the cell membrane to act as a gatekeeper, controlling what goes into and out of the cell.

Cells Contain Fluid and Tiny Structures That Support Life

Enclosed by the cell membrane is a fluid called **cytoplasm.** Floating in the cytoplasm are many tiny structures that accomplish some surprisingly sophisticated functions. For instance, the cell *nucleus* is where our genetic information, in the form of DNA (deoxyribonucleic acid), is located. A cell's DNA contains the instructions that the cell uses to make proteins. Cells that have high energy needs, such as muscle cells, also contain lots of *mitochondria.* You can think of mitochondria as a cell's "powerhouse," because they produce energy from food molecules.

Cells Join to Form Tissues and Organs

Cells of a single type, such as muscle cells, join together to form **tissues** (see Figure 2.1). Several types of tissues join together to form **organs,** which are sophisticated structures that perform a unique body function. The stomach is an organ, for example, as is the small intestine.

Organs Make Up Functional Systems

Organs are further grouped into **systems** that perform integrated functions (see Figure 2.1). For example, the gastrointestinal system is responsible for digesting food, absorbing nutrients, and excreting food wastes. The stomach is one organ of the gastrointestinal system. It holds and partially digests food, but it can't perform all the functions of the gastrointestinal system by itself. These functions require several organs working together, as we'll see shortly.

Finally, many organ systems together make up the human **organism**—that is, a complete living being that can function independently of other living beings. All organisms must take in nutrients in order to survive, and complex organisms, like us, experience a sensation called hunger that doesn't let us ignore this need for long! We explore hunger in the next section.

> RECAP *Atoms, the smallest units of matter, group together to form molecules. Digestion breaks down food into molecules small enough to be easily absorbed into the body and transported to our cells. Cells, the smallest units of life, are encased in a cell membrane that acts as a gatekeeper. Cells of the same type join together to make tissues. Different tissue types give rise to different kinds of organs. Body systems, such as the gastrointestinal system, depend on many different organs to carry out their functions. Many systems are present in an organism.*

What Makes Us Hungry?

Think back to the last time you were *really hungry*. Maybe you felt a sort of gnawing emptiness in your gut, or were a little cranky or spaced out. Whatever your sensations, they probably compelled you to stop your other activities and eat! In Chapter 1, we defined *hunger* as a physical sensation that drives us to find food and eat. Because it's so strong, hunger is typically experienced as an unpleasant sensation. The signal arises from within us, not because we saw or smelled something in our environment. Also, hunger isn't associated with a specific food: when we're really hungry, a lot of different foods appeal to us. Now that we know what hunger is, let's look at what causes it.

Signals from the Brain Cause Hunger and Satiation

The primary organ producing the sensation of hunger is the brain. That's right—it's not the stomach, but the brain that tells us when we're hungry. The region of brain tissue that is responsible for prompting us to seek food is called the **hypothalamus.**

cytoplasm The liquid within an animal cell.

tissue A sheet or other grouping of like cells that performs like functions, for example, muscle tissue.

organ A body structure composed of two or more tissues and performing a specific function, for example, the esophagus.

system A group of organs that work together to perform a unique function, for example, the gastrointestinal system.

organism A complete and independent living being.

hypothalamus A region of the forebrain where visceral sensations such as hunger and thirst are regulated.

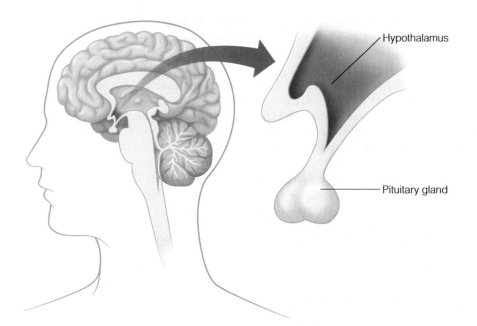

Hypothalamus

Pituitary gland

FIGURE 2.3 The hypothalamus triggers hunger by integrating signals from nerve cells throughout the GI tract, as well as messages carried by hormones.

It's located above the pituitary gland in the forebrain, a part of the brain that regulates involuntary (nonconscious) activity (FIGURE 2.3). We don't consciously decide to feel hungry; rather, hunger arises and grows stronger until our conscious, cognitive brain notices it.

The hypothalamus continually monitors the body for data indicating whether or not we are hungry. When the data suggest we need food, the hypothalamus triggers the sensation of hunger. The two primary sources of this data are nerve cells and certain chemicals called *hormones*:

- Special nerve cells lining the stomach and small intestine sense whether these organs are empty or distended with food. They then communicate this information to the hypothalamus. If you have not eaten for many hours and your stomach and small intestine do not contain food, these lining cells signal the hypothalamus that it is "time to eat."

- **Hormones** are chemical messengers that are secreted into the bloodstream by one of the many *glands* of the body. Glands are organs that release hormones in response to internal body conditions, such as falling or rising levels of fuels within the blood. Glucose, which comes from the breakdown of carbohydrates, is the body's most readily available fuel. So it's not surprising that the body continually monitors the level of glucose in the blood. When we have not eaten for a while, blood glucose levels fall, triggering a change in the level of certain hormones. The hypothalamus responds to this hormonal change by prompting us to feel hungry.

After we eat, the hypothalamus picks up the sensations of a distended stomach and small intestine and detects a change in hormone levels that indicates a rise in blood glucose. When it integrates these signals, we experience **satiation**—in other words, we feel full.

The Amount and Type of Food We Eat Can Also Affect Hunger and Satiation

A food or nutrient is said to contribute to satiation if that food makes us feel full and causes us to stop eating. Foods containing protein have the highest satiety value.[1] This means that a ham sandwich will cause us to feel satiated for a longer period of time than will a tossed salad and toast, even if both meals have exactly the same number of calories. Also, the energy density of a food contributes significantly to

hormone Chemical messenger that is secreted into the bloodstream by one of the many glands of the body.

satiation State of satisfaction, especially with food intake; fullness.

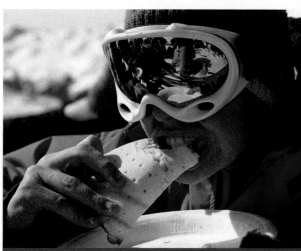

Our bodies feel hunger when we haven't eaten for many hours or our blood glucose is low.

satiation: because fats are more energy dense (kcal/g) than carbohydrate and protein, meals that contain a lot of fat are typically quite filling.

Another factor affecting hunger is how bulky the meal is; that is, how much fiber and water is within the food. Bulky meals tend to stretch the stomach and small intestine quickly. As we just discussed, this distention sends signals back to the hypothalamus telling us that we are full—so we stop eating. Beverages tend to be less satisfying than semisolid foods, and semisolid foods have a lower satiety value than solid foods. For example, if you were to eat a bunch of grapes, you would feel fuller than you would if you were to drink a glass of grape juice.[2]

RECAP *In contrast to appetite, hunger is a physiologic sensation triggered by the hypothalamus in response to data about stomach and intestinal distention, and levels of certain hormones that change in response to falling or rising blood glucose. High-protein foods cause us to feel satiated for a longer period of time, and bulky foods fill us up quickly, causing the distention that signals the hypothalamus that we are full.*

NUTRI-CASE JUDY

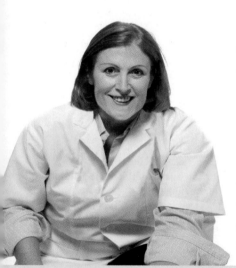

"My doctor tells me I've got to lose some weight—at least 20 pounds, he says, to get my blood sugar down. But every time I try, I just end up feeling so hungry. Like yesterday at work, I ate a tuna sandwich and a teensy bag of French fries from the cafeteria at lunch, and when I got home I just had a can of chicken soup for dinner. But then I was watching TV and there was this ad for a Mexican restaurant, and that made me realize how hungry I was for *real* food! So I fixed myself a bowl of chili and cheese, and that filled me up. And I don't feel guilty about it either! I mean, if you're hungry, then that means you need to eat!"

What aspects of this scenario suggest that Judy's decision to fix herself a bowl of chili was prompted more by appetite than physical hunger? On the other hand, why do you think she didn't feel satiated after dinner, but the chili and cheese "filled her up"? What could Judy add to her chicken soup tonight that might turn it into a meal that is both healthful and satisfying?

digestion The process by which foods are broken down into their component molecules, both mechanically and chemically.

absorption The physiologic process by which molecules of food are taken from the GI tract into the body.

elimination The process by which the undigested portions of food and waste products are removed from the body.

What Happens to the Food We Eat?

We're now ready to discover what happens when we answer the call of hunger and eat. Of course we all know that the food we consume is digested, then the useful nutrients are absorbed, and, finally, the waste products are eliminated. Here are some useful definitions for these three steps:

- **Digestion** is the process by which foods are broken down into their component molecules, either mechanically or chemically.
- **Absorption** is the process of taking the products of digestion through the wall of the intestine.
- **Elimination** is the process by which the undigested portions of food and waste products are removed from the body.

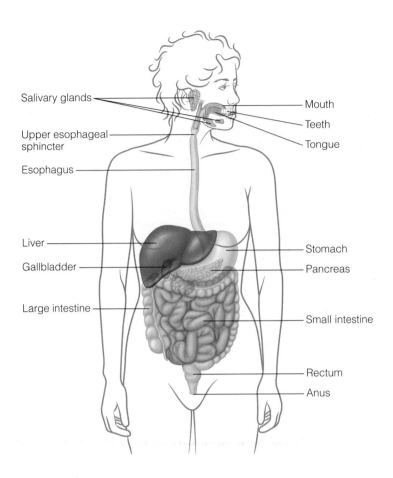

FIGURE 2.4 An overview of the gastrointestinal (GI) tract. The GI tract begins in the mouth and ends at the anus and is composed of numerous organs.

gastrointestinal (GI) tract A long, muscular tube consisting of several organs: the mouth, esophagus, stomach, small intestine, and large intestine.

sphincter A tight ring of muscle separating organs of the GI tract that opens in response to nerve signals indicating that food is ready to pass into the next section.

The processes of digestion, absorption, and elimination occur within the **gastrointestinal (GI) tract,** a long tube beginning at the mouth and ending at the anus: if held out straight, an adult GI tract would be close to 30 feet in length (FIGURE 2.4). It is composed of several distinct organs, including the mouth, the esophagus, the stomach, the small intestine, and the large intestine. These organs work together to process foods but are kept somewhat separated by muscular **sphincters,** which are tight rings of muscle that open when a nerve signal indicates that food is ready to pass into the next section.

Now let's take a look at the role of each of these organs. Imagine that you eat a turkey sandwich for lunch today. It contains two slices of bread spread with mayonnaise, some turkey, two lettuce leaves, and a slice of tomato. Let's travel along with the sandwich and see what changes it undergoes within your GI tract.

Digestive Juices Begin to Flow Even before We Eat

Believe it or not, your body starts preparing to digest food even before you take your first bite. In response to the sight, smell, or thought of food, the nervous system stimulates the release of digestive juices that help prepare the GI tract for the breakdown of food. Sometimes we even experience some involuntary movement of the GI tract commonly called "hunger pangs."

Chewing Moistens and Breaks Down Food

Now it's time to take that first bite and chew. Chewing is very important because it moistens the food and mechanically breaks it down into pieces small enough to swallow (FIGURE 2.5). The tough lettuce fibers and tomato seeds are also broken open. Thus, chewing initiates the mechanical digestion of food.

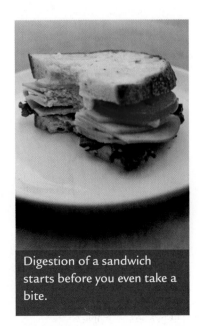

Digestion of a sandwich starts before you even take a bite.

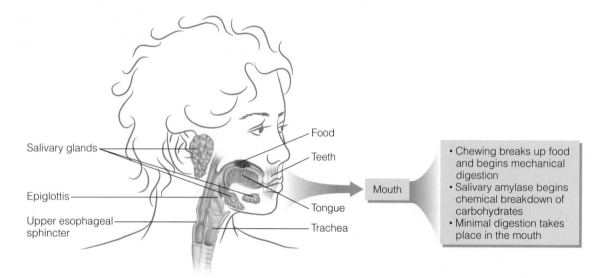

FIGURE 2.5 Where your food is now: the mouth. Chewing moistens food and mechanically breaks it down into pieces small enough to swallow, while salivary amylase begins chemical digestion of carbohydrates.

As our teeth cut and grind the different foods in the sandwich, more surface area is exposed to the digestive juices in our mouth. Foremost among these is **saliva,** which we secrete from our **salivary glands.** Saliva not only moistens food but also begins the process of chemical digestion. Saliva contains *amylase,* a chemical that begins to break apart carbohydrate molecules. Saliva also contains other components such as antibiotics that protect the body from germs entering the mouth and keep the oral cavity free from infection.

Salivary amylase is the first of many *enzymes* that assist the body in digesting and absorbing food. Because we will encounter many enzymes on our journey through the GI tract, let's discuss them briefly here. **Enzymes** are chemicals, usually proteins, that induce chemical changes in other substances to speed up body processes. Imagine them as facilitators: a chemical reaction that might take hours to occur independently can happen in seconds with the help of one or more enzymes. Digestion—as well as many other biochemical processes that go on in the body—could not happen without them. By the way, enzyme names typically end in *-ase* (as in amylase), so they are easy to recognize as we discuss the digestive process.

In reality, very little digestion occurs in the mouth. We don't hold food in our mouths for long, and very few of the enzymes needed to break down food are present in saliva. Salivary amylase starts the digestion of carbohydrates, but this ends when food reaches the stomach. That's because the acidic environment of the stomach destroys this enzyme.

The Esophagus Transports Food into the Stomach

Now that our sandwich is soft and moist, it's time to swallow (**FIGURE 2.6**). Most of us take swallowing for granted, but it's a very complex process. As the bite of sandwich moves to the very back of the mouth, the brain is sent a signal to raise the soft palate. This temporarily closes the openings to the nasal passages, preventing aspiration of food or liquid into the sinuses. The brain also receives a signal to close off the *epiglottis,* a tiny flap of tissue that is like a trapdoor covering the entrance to the trachea (or "windpipe"). The epiglottis is normally open, allowing us to breathe freely. When it closes during swallowing, food and liquid cannot enter the trachea. Sometimes this protective mechanism goes awry, for instance when we try to eat and talk at the same time, and food or liquid "goes down the wrong way." When this hap-

saliva A mixture of water, mucus, enzymes, and other chemicals that moistens the mouth and food, binds food particles together, and begins the digestion of carbohydrates.

salivary glands Group of glands found under and behind the tongue and beneath the jaw that release saliva continually as well as in response to the thought, sight, smell, or presence of food.

enzymes Chemicals, usually proteins, that act on other chemicals to speed up body processes.

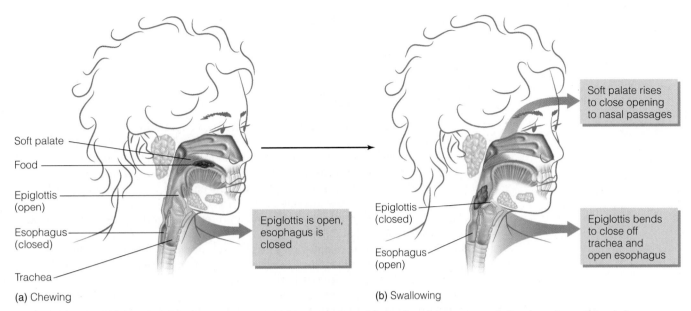

Soft palate

Food

Epiglottis
(open)

Esophagus
(closed)

Trachea

(a) Chewing

Epiglottis is open,
esophagus is
closed

Soft palate rises
to close opening
to nasal passages

Epiglottis
(closed)

Esophagus
(open)

Epiglottis bends
to close off
trachea and
open esophagus

(b) Swallowing

FIGURE 2.6 Chewing and swallowing are complex processes. (a) During the process of chewing, the epiglottis is open and the esophagus is closed so that we can continue to breathe as we chew. (b) During swallowing, the epiglottis closes so that food does not enter the trachea and obstruct our breathing. The soft palate rises to seal off our nasal passages to prevent aspiration of food or liquid into the sinuses.

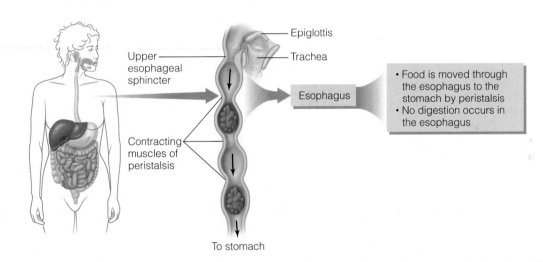

Epiglottis

Trachea

Upper
esophageal
sphincter

Esophagus

• Food is moved through
the esophagus to the
stomach by peristalsis
• No digestion occurs in
the esophagus

Contracting
muscles of
peristalsis

To stomach

FIGURE 2.7 Where your food is now: the esophagus. Peristalsis, the rhythmic contraction and relaxation of both circular and longitudinal muscles in the esophagus, propels food toward the stomach. Peristalsis occurs throughout the GI tract.

pens, we experience the sensation of choking, and we cough until the offending food or liquid is expelled.

As the trachea closes, the *upper esophageal sphincter* opens. This allows food to pass from the back of the throat into the **esophagus,** the muscular tube that propels food toward the stomach (**FIGURE 2.7**). It does this by contracting two sets of muscles: inner sheets of circular muscle squeeze the food, while outer sheets of longitudinal muscle push food along. Together, these rhythmic waves of squeezing and pushing are called **peristalsis.** We will see shortly that peristalsis occurs throughout the GI tract.

Gravity also helps food move down the esophagus. Together, peristalsis and gravity can transport a bite of food from the mouth to the opening of the stomach in 5 to 8 seconds. At the end of the esophagus is another sphincter muscle, the *gastroesophageal sphincter* (*gastro-* indicates the stomach), that is normally tightly

esophagus Muscular tube of the GI tract connecting the back of the mouth to the stomach.

peristalsis Waves of squeezing and pushing contractions that move food in one direction through the length of the GI tract.

closed. When food reaches the end of the esophagus, this sphincter relaxes to allow it to pass into the stomach. In some people, this sphincter is continually somewhat relaxed. Later in the chapter, we'll discuss this disorder and why it causes the unpleasant sensation of heartburn.

The Stomach Mixes, Digests, and Stores Food

The J-shaped **stomach** is a sack-like organ that can expand in some people to hold several cups of food (FIGURE 2.8). Before any food reaches the stomach, the brain sends signals telling it to be ready for the food to arrive. The stomach gets ready for your sandwich by secreting **gastric juice,** which contains several important compounds, including *hydrochloric acid (HCl)* and the enzyme *pepsin,* which start to break down proteins, and the enzyme *gastric lipase,* which begins to break down fats. The stomach also secretes *mucus,* which protects its lining from being digested by the hydrochloric acid and pepsin.

In addition to chemical digestion, the stomach performs mechanical digestion, mixing and churning the food until it becomes a liquid called **chyme.** Enzymes can access this liquid chyme more easily than solid food.

Although most absorption occurs in the small intestine, the stomach lining does begin absorbing a few substances. These include water, some minerals and some fats, and certain drugs, including aspirin and alcohol.

Another of your stomach's jobs is to store your sandwich (or what's left of it!) until the next part of the digestive tract, the small intestine, is ready for it. Remember that the stomach can hold several cups of food. This amount would overwhelm the small intestine if it were released all at once. Instead, food stays in your stomach about 2 hours before it is released a little at a time, as chyme, into the small intestine. Regulating this release is the *pyloric sphincter.*

stomach J-shaped organ where food is partially digested, churned, and stored until released into the small intestine.

gastric juice Acidic liquid secreted within the stomach that contains hydrochloric acid, pepsin, and other chemicals.

chyme Semifluid mass consisting of partially digested food, water, and gastric juices.

small intestine The largest portion of the GI tract where most digestion and absorption take place.

> RECAP *Chewing initiates mechanical and chemical digestion. During swallowing, our nasal passages close and the epiglottis covers the trachea. The esophagus is a muscular tube that transports food from the mouth to the stomach via rhythmic waves called* peristalsis. *The stomach secretes gastric juice, which begins the breakdown of proteins and fats, as well as mucus to protect its lining. It mixes food into chyme, which is released into the small intestine through the pyloric sphincter.*

Most Digestion and Absorption Occurs in the Small Intestine

The **small intestine** is the longest portion of the GI tract, accounting for about two-thirds of its length. However, at only an inch in diameter, it is comparatively narrow.

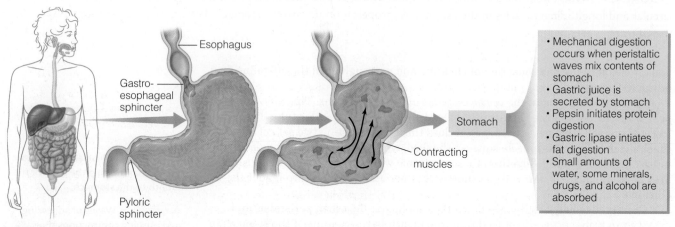

- Mechanical digestion occurs when peristaltic waves mix contents of stomach
- Gastric juice is secreted by stomach
- Pepsin initiates protein digestion
- Gastric lipase intiates fat digestion
- Small amounts of water, some minerals, drugs, and alcohol are absorbed

Esophagus

Gastro-esophageal sphincter

Pyloric sphincter

Contracting muscles

Stomach

FIGURE 2.8 Where your food is now: the stomach. In the stomach, the protein and fat in your sandwich begin to be digested. Your meal is churned into chyme and stored until released into the small intestine.

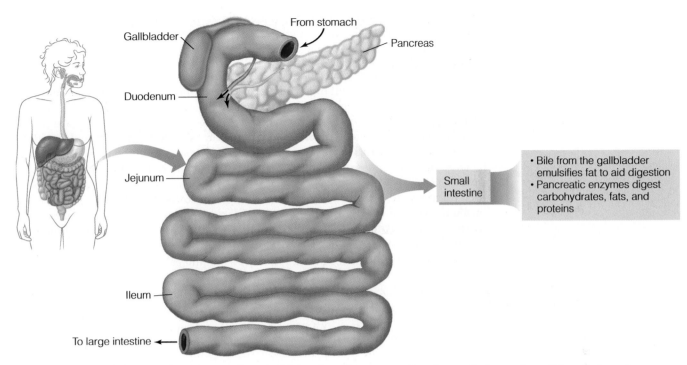

Gallbladder
From stomach
Pancreas
Duodenum
Jejunum
Ileum
To large intestine

Small intestine

- Bile from the gallbladder emulsifies fat to aid digestion
- Pancreatic enzymes digest carbohydrates, fats, and proteins

FIGURE 2.9 **Where your food is now: the small intestine. Here, most digestion and absorption of the nutrients in your sandwich take place.**

The small intestine is composed of three sections (FIGURE 2.9):

- The first section is the *duodenum.* It is connected via the pyloric sphincter to the stomach.
- The *jejunum* is the middle portion of the small intestine.
- The *ileum* is the last portion. It is connected to the large intestine at another sphincter, called the *ileocecal valve* (*ileo-* refers to the ileum and *-cecal* refers to the cecum, the first portion of the large intestine).

Most digestion and absorption takes place in the small intestine. Here, food is broken down into its smallest components, molecules that the body can then absorb into its internal environment. In this next section, we review a variety of *accessory organs* (organs that assist digestion but are not part of the gastrointestinal tract), enzymes, and unique anatomical features of the small intestine that allow for maximal absorption of most nutrients.

The Gallbladder and Pancreas Aid in Digestion

As the fat from the turkey and mayonnaise enters the small intestine, an accessory organ, the **gallbladder,** contracts. The gallbladder is located beneath the liver (see Figure 2.4) and stores a greenish fluid produced by the liver called **bile.** Contraction of the gallbladder sends bile into the duodenum. Bile then *emulsifies* the fat—that is, it breaks it up into smaller particles that are more accessible to digestive enzymes. If you've ever noticed how a drop of liquid detergent breaks up a film of fat floating at the top of a basin of greasy dishes, you understand the function of bile.

The **pancreas,** an accessory organ located behind the stomach, manufactures, holds, and secretes digestive enzymes (see Figure 2.4). These pancreatic enzymes continue the digestion of carbohydrates, fats, and proteins. The pancreas is also responsible for manufacturing hormones that are important in the conversion of food into energy.

Now the protein, carbohydrate, and fat in your sandwich have been processed into a liquid that contains molecules of nutrients small enough for absorption. This molecular "soup" continues to move along the small intestine via peristalsis, encountering the absorptive cells of the intestinal lining all along the way.

gallbladder A sack of tissue beneath the liver that stores bile and secretes it into the small intestine.

bile Fluid produced by the liver and stored in the gallbladder that emulsifies fats in the small intestine.

pancreas Gland located behind the stomach that secretes digestive enzymes.

A Specialized Lining Enables the Small Intestine to Absorb Food

The lining of the small intestine is especially well suited for absorption. If you looked at it under a microscope, you would notice that it is heavily folded (FIGURE 2.10). Within these folds are small finger-like projections called *villi,* whose constant movement helps them to encounter and trap nutrient molecules. Covering the villi are even tinier hair-like structures called *microvilli.* The microvilli form a surface somewhat like the bristles on a hairbrush and are often referred to as the **brush border.** Together, these absorptive features increase the surface area of the small intestine by more than 500 times, allowing it to absorb many more nutrients than it could if it were smooth.

Nutrients enter the body by passing through the cells of the brush border. Once inside the villi, the nutrients encounter *capillaries* (tiny blood vessels) and a *lacteal,* which is a small lymph vessel (see Figure 2.10). These vessels soak up the final products of digestion and begin their transport.

Intestinal Cells Readily Absorb Vitamins, Minerals, and Water

The turkey sandwich you ate contained several vitamins and minerals in addition to the protein, carbohydrate, and fat. These vitamins and minerals are not really

brush border Term that describes the microvilli of the small intestine's lining, which tremendously increase its absorptive capacity.

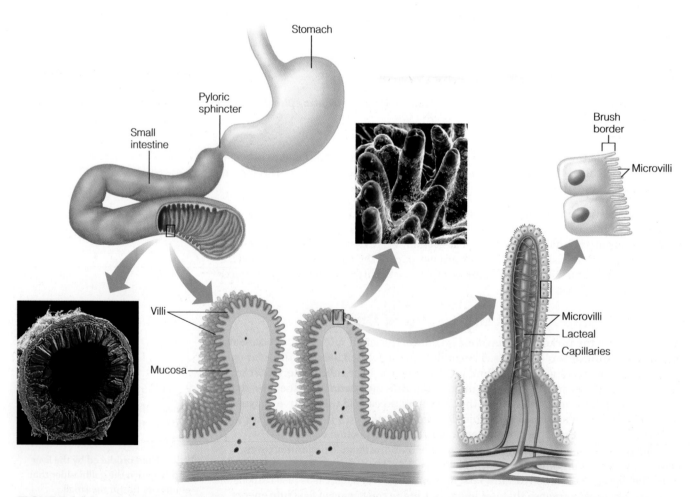

FIGURE 2.10 Absorption of nutrients occurs via the specialized lining of the small intestine. The lining of the small intestine is heavily folded and has thousands of finger-like projections called *villi.* The cells covering the villi end in hair-like projections called *microvilli* that together form the brush border. These features significantly increase the absorptive capacity of the small intestine.

"digested" the same way that macronutrients are. They do not have to be broken down because they are small enough to be readily absorbed by the small intestine.

Finally, a large component of food is water, and of course you also drink lots of water throughout the day. Water is absorbed along the entire length of the GI tract because it is a small molecule that can easily pass through the cell membrane. However, as we will see shortly, a significant percentage of water is absorbed in the large intestine.

Blood and Lymph Transport Nutrients

Our bodies have two main fluids that transport nutrients (including water) and waste products throughout the body. These fluids are blood and lymph. Blood travels through the cardiovascular system, and lymph travels through the lymphatic system (FIGURE 2.11).

As blood travels through the GI tract, it picks up the nutrients that were absorbed through the villi of the small intestine and then carries them to the liver for processing. The waste products picked up by the blood as it circulates around the body are filtered and excreted by the kidneys.

The lymphatic vessels pick up most fats and fat-soluble vitamins and transport them in lymph. This lymph eventually returns to an area near the heart where the lymphatic and blood vessels join together.

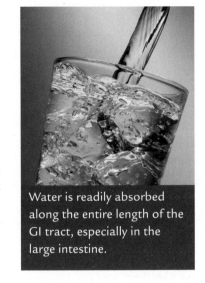

Water is readily absorbed along the entire length of the GI tract, especially in the large intestine.

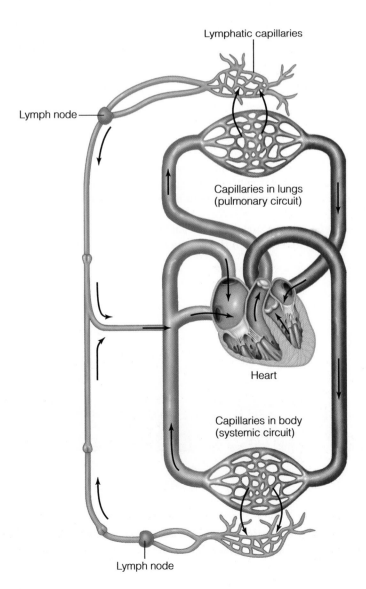

Lymphatic capillaries

Lymph node

Capillaries in lungs (pulmonary circuit)

Heart

Capillaries in body (systemic circuit)

Lymph node

FIGURE 2.11 Blood travels through the cardiovascular system to transport nutrients and fluids and pick up waste products. Lymph travels through the lymphatic system and transports most fats and fat-soluble vitamins.

The Liver Regulates Blood Nutrients

Most nutrients absorbed from the small intestine enter the *portal vein,* which carries them to the **liver.** Another accessory digestive organ, the liver is a triangular wedge that rests almost entirely within the protection of the lower rib cage, on the right side of the body (see Figure 2.4). The liver is the largest digestive organ; it is also one of the most important organs in the body, performing more than 500 discrete functions. One of these functions is to receive the products of digestion and then release into the bloodstream those nutrients needed throughout the body. The liver also plays a major role in processing, storing, and regulating the blood levels of the energy nutrients.

Have you ever wondered why people who abuse alcohol are at risk for damaging their liver? That's because another of its functions is to filter the blood, removing potential toxins like alcohol and other drugs. As we discuss in Chapter 8, the liver can filter the blood of alcohol at the rate of approximately one drink per hour. When someone exceeds this rate, the liver becomes overwhelmed by the excessive alcohol, which damages its cells. With chronic alcohol abuse, scar tissue forms. The scar tissue blocks the free flow of blood through the liver, so that any further toxins accumulate in the blood. This can lead to confusion, coma, and even death.

Another important job of the liver is to synthesize many of the chemicals used by the body in carrying out digestion. For example, the liver synthesizes bile, which, as we just discussed, is then stored in the gallbladder until needed to emulsify fats.

The Large Intestine Stores Food Waste until It Is Excreted

liver The largest organ of the GI tract and one of the most important organs of the body. Its functions include production of bile and processing of nutrient-rich blood from the small intestine.

large intestine Final organ of the GI tract consisting of the cecum, colon, rectum, and anal canal, and in which most water is absorbed and feces are formed.

The **large intestine** is a thick tube-like structure that frames the small intestine on three-and-a-half sides (FIGURE 2.12). It begins with a sack of tissue called the *cecum,* which explains the name of the sphincter—the *ileocecal valve*—that connects it to the ileum of the small intestine. From the cecum, it continues up the right side of the abdomen as the *ascending colon.* The *transverse colon* runs across the top of the small intestine, and then the *descending colon* comes down on the left side of the abdomen. The *sigmoid colon* is the last segment and extends from the bottom left corner to the *rectum.* The rectum ends in the *anal canal,* which is just over an inch long.

What has happened to our turkey sandwich? When any undigested and unabsorbed food components and water in the chyme finally reach the large intestine,

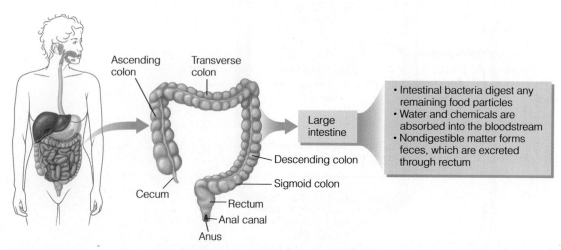

FIGURE 2.12 Where your food is now: the large intestine. Most water absorption occurs here, as does the formation of food wastes into semisolid feces. Peristalsis propels the feces out of the body.

they mix with intestinal bacteria. These bacteria are normal and helpful residents, as they finish digesting any remaining particles left from your sandwich. In fact, the bacteria living in the large intestine are so helpful that, as discussed in the accompanying Highlight on page 54, many people consume them deliberately!

No other digestion occurs in the large intestine. Instead, its main functions are to store the chyme for 12 to 24 hours and during that time to absorb chemicals and water from it, leaving a semisolid mass called *feces*. Weak waves of peristalsis move the feces through the colon, except for one or more stronger waves each day that force the feces more powerfully toward the rectum for elimination.

RECAP *Most digestion and absorption occurs in the small intestine with the help of bile, which emulsifies fats, and pancreatic enzymes that break down carbohydrates, fats, and proteins. The lining of the small intestine contains villi and microvilli that trap and absorb nutrients. The liver processes all nutrients absorbed from the small intestine. Bacteria in the large intestine assist with digestion of any remaining digestible food products. The large intestine stores chyme, from which it absorbs water and any other remaining nutrients, leaving a semisolid mass, called feces, that is then eliminated from the body.*

The Nervous System Coordinates and Regulates Digestion

The nervous system in your body is like the central command desk. Nerves relay messages between the various organs and glands, allowing the transfer of data about when to start and stop various functions, how to operate, and what the body needs. The nerves serving the GI tract are known as **enteric nerves.**

Enteric nerves can often respond independently to signals produced within the GI tract without first relaying them to the brain for interpretation or assistance. On the other hand, many jobs require the involvement of the brain. For instance, when enteric nerves pick up signals indicating that the tissues lining the GI tract are stretched, they signal the brain that your digestive tract is full, and then your brain sends out messages that prompt you to stop eating.

All along the gastrointestinal tract are a series of glands that secrete digestive juices, mucus, and water. These secretions are also controlled by nerves. For example, as chyme moves from the stomach into the small intestine, nerve signals are sent to stimulate the pancreas and gallbladder to secrete digestive enzymes and bile.

Now that you know what happens to the food you eat, you might have a new appreciation for the amazing complexity of your GI tract. Did you know that your everyday behaviors can assist its functioning—or make its job a lot harder? How well do you treat your GI tract? See the What About You? box on page 55 to find out.

RECAP *The coordination and regulation of digestion is directed by the nervous system. The enteric nerves of the GI tract work with the brain to achieve digestion, absorption, and elimination of food.*

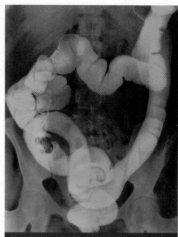

The large intestine is a thick tube-like structure that stores the undigested mass leaving the small intestine and absorbs any remaining nutrients and water.

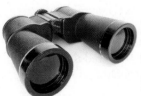

HEALTHWATCH
What Disorders Are Related to Digestion, Absorption, and Elimination?

Considering the complexity of digestion, absorption, and elimination, it's no wonder that sometimes things go wrong. Let's look at some GI tract disorders and what you might be able to do if any of these problems affect you.

enteric nerves The nerves of the GI tract.

HIGHLIGHT

Probiotics: What Are They, Can They Improve Gastrointestinal Health, and Should You Eat Them?

The last time you ate a cup of creamy, fruity yogurt, did you think about the fact that you were also eating *bacteria*? Don't worry—these microorganisms won't harm you; they'll help your body to function. They are one of a group of substances called *probiotics:* live microorganisms found in, or added to, fermented foods that optimize the bacterial environment of the large intestine.

Interest in probiotics was sparked in the early 1900s with the work of Elie Metchnikoff, a Nobel Prize–winning scientist. Dr. Metchnikoff linked the long, healthy lives of Bulgarian peasants with their consumption of fermented milk products such as yogurt. Subsequent research identified the bacteria in fermented milk products as the factor that promoted health. These bacteria were given the name *probiotics,* meaning "pro-life."

In the United States foods that contain probiotics include fortified milk, yogurt, and a creamy beverage called *kefir* that is made from fermented milk. Probiotics are also sold in supplement form. The bacterial species most frequently used in these foods and supplements are *Lactobacillus* and *Bifidobacterium.*

When a person consumes a product containing probiotics, the bacteria adhere to the intestinal wall for a few days, exerting their beneficial actions. Because their activity is short-lived, they probably need to be consumed on a daily basis to be most effective. The exact means by which probiotics benefit human health is currently being researched. One theory is that they increase the number and activity of immune cells that help us fight infections. However, although they appear to improve immune function, there is still limited research on how this occurs.[3,4]

Some health problems that may be successfully treated with probiotics include [5-7]:

- Diarrhea caused by certain infectious microorganisms or associated with use of antibiotic medications
- Infections in children in daycare
- Traveler's diarrhea
- Irritable bowel syndrome (IBS) and inflammatory bowel diseases
- Infection from *Helicobacter pylori,* which is the bacteria associated with conditions such as peptic ulcers, gastritis, and gastric cancer

- Lactose intolerance (inability to digest milk sugar)
- Allergy risk reduction in infants
- Eczema in children
- Urinary and genital tract infections in women

Although the research supporting the potential of probiotics to successfully treat these conditions is promising, more research is needed before we can identify with certainty the circumstances under which probiotics enhance human health.

It is important to remember that in order to be effective, a minimum number of bacteria must be present in foods. Although the exact number of bacteria is not known, it is estimated that a daily dose of at least 1 to 10 billion bacteria is needed to be effective.[8] To put this in perspective, commercial yogurts meeting the National Yogurt Association Standards contain 100 million live and active cultures per gram. So a 1-cup serving (8 oz, or 227 g) of yogurt contains more than 22 billion bacteria, or more than the estimated effective dose.

Bacteria only live for a short time. This means that foods and supplements containing probiotics have a limited shelf life and must be properly stored and consumed within a relatively brief period of time to confer maximal benefit. In general, refrigerated foods containing probiotics have a shelf-life of 3 to 6 weeks, whereas the shelf life for supplements containing probiotics is about 12 months. However, because the probiotic content in refrigerated foods is much more stable than that in supplements, the more perishable forms may be a better health bet.

Based on what you have just learned about probiotics, do you think products containing them should be consumed on a daily basis? Are you interested in adding probiotics to your diet? How do you think food labels can be improved to assist consumers in identifying key aspects of probiotic-containing foods? As the number of probiotic-containing foods increases in the U.S. market, these are just some of the questions that need to be answered to assist consumers in making healthful food choices.

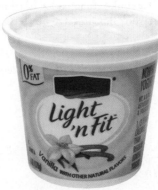

Probiotics can be found in yogurt and other fermented milk products.

WHAT ABOUT YOU?

How Well Do You Treat Your GI Tract?

You might not realize it, but little things you do each day can help keep your GI tract working properly, or can contribute to GI problems. How well do you treat your GI tract? For each of the following questions, circle Yes or No, then see the explanation to find out:

- Do you frequently overeat (have to loosen your clothes, feel discomfort, etc.)?
  YES or NO

- Do you typically eat quickly (for example, eat a full meal in a few minutes)?
  YES or NO

- Do you drink more than three caffeine-containing beverages a day (coffee, tea, colas)?
  YES or NO

- Do you smoke cigarettes?
  YES or NO

- Do you routinely get fewer than seven hours of sleep a night?
  YES or NO

- Do you eat fewer than five servings of fruits and vegetables a day?
  YES or NO

- Do you drink fewer than nine cups (for women) or 13 cups (for men) of water and other fluids a day?
  YES or NO

- Do you engage in fewer than 30 minutes of physical activity a day?
  YES or NO

- Do you use antacids, bowel stimulants, or other GI medications more than once a week?
  YES or NO

- Do you engage in binge-drinking (consuming five or more alcoholic drinks on one occasion)?
  YES or NO

If you answered "No" to all of the above questions, congratulations! You're contributing to the health and functioning of your GI tract. "Yes" answers mean your GI tract is working harder than it should, and the more "Yes" answers you gave, the greater your risk for GI problems.

The behaviors identified in the first five questions—eating too large a meal at one sitting, eating too quickly, drinking too much caffeine, smoking, and failing to get enough sleep—all can contribute to indigestion. The next three questions relate to bowel function: Eating plenty of fruits and vegetables (which provide dietary fiber) and drinking plenty of fluids are behaviors that help move food through the GI tract. In addition, many researchers believe that inadequate physical activity can inhibit proper bowel function, as can overuse of calcium-containing antacids and overreliance on bowel stimulants. The last question asks about binge-drinking, which results in inflammation of the delicate tissue lining the GI tract. In fact, alcohol abuse is a risk factor for several cancers of the GI tract, and both alcohol abuse and smoking damage the liver.

Our recommendations? Make a note of any questions to which you answered "Yes," then change your behavior. The better you treat your GI tract, the better it'll treat you.

Heartburn Is Caused by Reflux of Stomach Acid

heartburn The painful sensation that occurs over the sternum when hydrochloric acid backs up into the lower esophagus.

gastroesophageal reflux disease (GERD) A painful type of heartburn that occurs more than twice per week.

When you eat food, your stomach secretes hydrochloric acid (HCl) to start the digestion process. In some people, the gastroesophageal sphincter becomes irritated or overly relaxed. In either case, the result is that HCl seeps back up into the esophagus (FIGURE 2.13). Although the stomach is protected from HCl by a thick coat of mucus, the esophagus does not have this coating. Thus, the HCl burns it. When this happens, a person experiences a painful sensation in the center of the chest. This condition is commonly called **heartburn.** People often take over-the-counter "antacids" to neutralize the hydrochloric acid, thereby relieving the heartburn. A nondrug approach is to repeatedly swallow: this action causes any acid within the esophagus to be swept down into the stomach, eventually relieving the symptoms.

Gastroesophageal reflux disease (GERD) is a more painful type of heartburn that occurs more than twice per week. GERD affects about 19 million Americans and, like heartburn, occurs when HCl flows back into the esophagus. Although people who experience occasional heartburn usually have no structural abnormalities, many people with GERD have an overly relaxed esophageal sphincter or damage to the esophagus itself. Symptoms of GERD include persistent heartburn and acid regurgitation. Some people have GERD without heartburn and instead experience chest pain, trouble swallowing, burning in the mouth, the feeling that food is stuck in the throat, and/or hoarseness in the morning.[9]

The exact causes of GERD are unknown. However, a number of factors may contribute, including cigarette smoking, alcohol use, overweight, pregnancy, lying down after a meal, and certain foods. In addition, a *hiatal hernia,* in which the upper part of the stomach lies above the diaphragm muscle, can contribute. Controlling these fac-

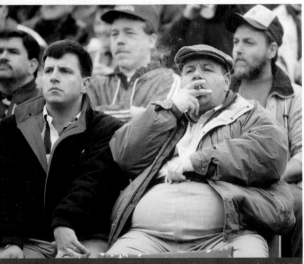

Although the exact causes of gastroesophageal reflux disease (GERD) are unknown, smoking and being overweight may be contributing factors.

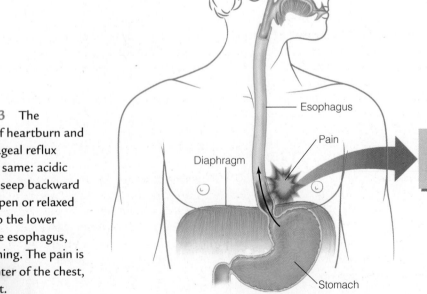

FIGURE 2.13 The mechanism of heartburn and gastroesophageal reflux disease is the same: acidic gastric juices seep backward through an open or relaxed sphincter into the lower portion of the esophagus, burning its lining. The pain is felt in the center of the chest, over the heart.

Esophagus

Pain

Diaphragm

Gastroesophageal sphincter remains partially opened, allowing gastric juice to seep backward and burn the esophageal lining

Stomach

tors, for instance by avoiding lying down for 3 hours after a meal, can prevent or reduce symptoms. Taking an antacid before meals can also help, and many other medications are now available to treat GERD.

An Ulcer Is an Area of Erosion in the GI Tract

A **peptic ulcer** is an area of the GI tract that has been eroded away by a combination of hydrochloric acid and the enzyme pepsin (FIGURE 2.14). In almost all cases, it is located in the stomach area (*gastric ulcer*) or the part of the duodenum closest to the stomach (*duodenal ulcer*). It causes a burning pain in the abdominal area, typically 1 to 3 hours after eating a meal. In serious cases, eroded blood vessels bleed into the GI tract, causing vomiting of blood and/or blood in the stools, as well as anemia. If the ulcer entirely perforates the tract wall, stomach contents can leak into the abdominal cavity, causing a life-threatening infection called *peritonitis*.

You might have heard the advice that people with an ulcer should try to reduce their stress and avoid caffeine and spicy foods. But do stress and certain foods really cause or contribute to ulcers? See the Nutrition Myth or Fact? box below for a discussion of this question.

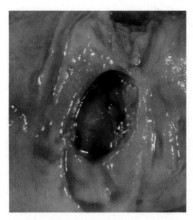

FIGURE 2.14   A peptic ulcer.

peptic ulcer   Area of the GI tract that has been eroded away by the acidic gastric juice of the stomach. The two main causes of peptic ulcers are an *H. pylori* infection or use of nonsteroidal anti-inflammatory drugs.

RECAP *Heartburn is caused by seepage of gastric juices into the esophagus. Gastroesophageal reflux disease (GERD) is a more painful type of heartburn that occurs more than twice per week. A peptic ulcer is an area of erosion of the stomach lining caused by gastric juices.*

NUTRITION MYTH OR FACT?

Are Ulcers Caused by Stress, Alcohol, or Spicy Foods?

For decades, physicians believed that experiencing high levels of stress, drinking alcohol, and eating spicy foods were the primary factors responsible for ulcers. But in 1982, Australian gastroenterologists Robin Warren and Barry Marshall detected the same species of bacteria in the majority of their ulcer patients' stomachs.[10] Treatment with an antibiotic effective against the bacterium, *Helicobacter pylori* (*H. pylori*), cured the ulcers. It is now known that *H. pylori* plays a key role in development of most peptic ulcers.[11] The hydrochloric acid in gastric juice kills most bacteria, but *H. pylori* is unusual in that it thrives in acidic environments.[12] Approximately 40% of people have this bacterium in their stomach, but most people do not develop ulcers. The reason for this is not known.

Prevention of infection with *H. pylori,* as with any infectious microorganism, includes regular hand washing and safe food-handling practices (for more on food safety, see Chapter 12). Because of the role of *H. pylori* in ulcer development, treatment usually involves antibiotics and acid-suppressing medications. Special diets and stress-reduction techniques are no longer typically recommended because they do not reduce acid secretion. However, people with ulcers should avoid specific foods they identify as causing them discomfort.

Although most peptic ulcers are caused by *H. pylori* infection, some are caused by prolonged use of nonsteroidal anti-inflammatory drugs (NSAIDs); these drugs include pain relievers such as aspirin, ibuprofen, and naproxen sodium. They appear to cause ulcers by suppressing the secretion of mucus and bicarbonate, which normally protect the stomach from its acidic gastric juice. Ulcers caused by NSAIDs use generally heal once a person stops taking the medication.[13]

NUTRITION LABEL ACTIVITY

Recognizing Common Allergens in Foods

The U.S. Food and Drug Administration (FDA) requires food labels to clearly identify any ingredients containing protein derived from the eight major allergenic foods.[14] Manufacturers must identify "in plain English" the presence of ingredients that contain protein derived from:

- milk
- eggs
- fish
- crustacean shellfish (crab, lobster, shrimp, and so on)
- tree nuts (almonds, pecans, walnuts, and so on)
- peanuts
- wheat
- soybeans

Although more than 160 foods have been identified as causing food allergies in sensitive individuals, the FDA requires labeling for only these eight foods because together they account for over 90% of all documented food allergies in the United States and represent the foods most likely to result in severe or life-threatening reactions.[15]

These eight allergenic foods must be indicated in the list of ingredients; alternatively, adjacent to the ingredients list, the label must say "Contains" followed by the name of the food. For example, the label of a product containing the milk-derived protein casein would have to use the term "milk" in addition to the term "casein" so that those with milk allergies would clearly understand the presence of an allergen they need to avoid.[15] Any food product found to contain an undeclared allergen is subject to recall by the FDA.

Look at the ingredients list from an energy bar, shown below, and try the following questions:

- **Which of the FDA's eight allergenic foods does this bar definitely contain?** _____
- **If you were allergic to peanuts, would eating this bar pose any risk to you?**
  YES or NO
- **If you were allergic to almonds, would eating this bar pose any risk to you?**
  YES or NO
  (Answers can be found at the end of this chapter.)

Ingredients: Soy protein isolate, rice flour, oats, milled flaxseed, brown rice syrup, evaporated cane juice, sunflower oil, soy lecithin, cocoa, nonfat milk solids, salt.

Contains soy and dairy. May contain traces of peanuts and other nuts.

Some People Experience Disorders Related to Specific Foods

You check out the ingredients list on your energy bar, and you notice that it says, "Produced in a facility that processes peanuts." The package on your microwave dinner cautions: "Contains wheat, milk, and soy." Why all the warnings about these foods? The reason is that, to some people, consuming these foods can be dangerous, even life-threatening. To learn more about product labeling for potential food offenders, see the Nutrition Label Activity.

Disorders related to specific foods can be clustered into three main groupings: food intolerances, food allergies, and a genetic disorder called celiac disease. We discuss these separately.

Food Intolerance

food intolerance A cluster of GI symptoms that occur following consumption of a particular food but are not caused by an immune system response.

A **food intolerance** is a cluster of GI symptoms (often gas, pain, and diarrhea) that occur following consumption of a particular food. The immune system plays no role in intolerance, and although episodes are unpleasant, they are usually transient, resolving after the offending food has been eliminated from the body. An example is lactose intolerance. It occurs in people whose bodies do not produce sufficient quantities of the enzyme lactase, which is needed for the breakdown of the milk sugar lactose. (Lactose intolerance is discussed in more detail in Chapter 3.) People can also have an intolerance to wheat, soy, and other foods, but as with lactose intolerance, the symptoms pass once the offending food is out of the person's system.

Food Allergy

A **food allergy** is a hypersensitivity reaction of the immune system to a particular component (usually a protein) in a food. This reaction causes the immune cells to release chemicals that cause either limited or body-wide inflammation. About 5% of infants and young children and 2% of adults experience food allergies.[14] Although this makes them much less common than food intolerances, food allergies can be far more serious. Approximately 30,000 consumers require emergency room treatment and 150 Americans die each year because of allergic reactions to foods.[14]

You may have heard stories of people being allergic to foods as common as peanuts. This is the case for Liz. She was out to dinner with her parents, celebrating her birthday, when the dessert cart came around. The caramel custard looked heavenly and was probably a safe choice, but she asked the waiter just to be sure that it contained no peanuts. He checked with the chef, then returned and assured her that, yes, the custard was peanut-free—but within minutes of consuming it, Liz's skin became flushed, and she struggled to breathe. As her parents were dialing 911, she lost consciousness. Fortunately, the paramedics arrived within minutes and were able to resuscitate her. It was subsequently determined that, unknown to the chef, the spoon that his prep cook had used to scoop the baked custard into serving bowls had been resting on a cutting board where he had chopped peanuts for a different dessert. Just this small exposure to peanuts was enough to cause a severe allergic reaction in Liz.

How can a food that most people consume regularly, such as peanuts, shellfish, eggs, or milk, cause another person's immune system to react so violently? In Liz's case, a trace amount of peanut stimulated immune cells throughout her body to release their inflammatory chemicals. In some people, the inflammation is localized, so the damage is limited. For instance, some people's mouth and throat itch when they eat cantaloupe, whereas others develop a rash whenever they eat eggs. What made Liz's experience so terrifyingly different was that the inflammation was widespread, affecting essentially all of her body systems and sending her into a state called *anaphylactic shock*. Left untreated, anaphylactic shock is nearly always fatal, so many people with known food allergies carry with them a kit containing an injection of a powerful stimulant called epinephrine. This drug can reduce symptoms long enough to buy the victim time to get emergency medical care.

Celiac Disease

Celiac disease, also known as *celiac sprue*, is a digestive disease that severely damages the lining of the small intestine and interferes with absorption of nutrients.[16] As in food allergy, the body's immune system causes the disorder. However, because there is a strong genetic predisposition to celiac disease, with the risk now linked to specific gene markers, it is also classified as a genetic disorder.[16]

In celiac disease, the offending food component is a protein called *gluten* that is found in wheat, rye, and barley. Note, however, that celiac disease is not the same as a gluten allergy: many people believe they are allergic to gluten because they experience symptoms (a runny nose, a skin rash, etc.) when they eat wheat products, but they do not have the intestinal damage characteristic of celiac disease. That is, when people with celiac disease eat gluten, their immune system triggers an inflammatory response that erodes the villi of the small intestine. If the person is unaware of the disorder and continues to eat gluten, repeated immune reactions cause the villi to become greatly decreased. As a result, the person becomes unable to absorb certain nutrients properly—a condition known as *malabsorption*. Over time malabsorption can lead to malnutrition (poor nutrient status).[17]

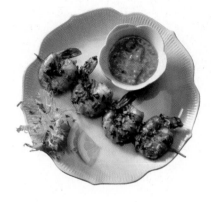

For some people, eating a meal of grilled shrimp with peanut sauce would cause a severe allergic reaction.

food allergy An inflammatory reaction caused by an immune system hypersensitivity to a protein component of a food.

celiac disease A genetic disorder characterized by an inability to absorb a protein called gluten. This causes an inflammatory immune response that damages the lining of the small intestine.

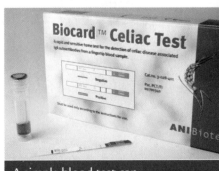

A simple blood test can identify celiac disease.

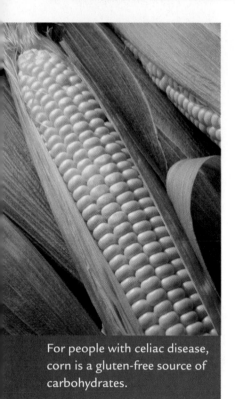

For people with celiac disease, corn is a gluten-free source of carbohydrates.

Symptoms of celiac disease can mimic those of other intestinal disturbances, and so the condition is often misdiagnosed. Some of the symptoms include fatty stools (due to poor fat absorption); frequent stools, either watery or hard; cramping; anemia; pallor; and weight loss. Other puzzling symptoms do not appear to involve the GI tract. These include an intensely itchy rash called *dermatitis herpetiformis*, osteoporosis (poor bone density), infertility, seizures, anxiety, depression, and migraine headaches, among others.[17]

Diagnostic tests for celiac disease include a variety of blood tests that screen for the presence of immune proteins called antibodies, or for the genetic markers of the disease. However, the "gold standard" for diagnosis is a biopsy of the small intestine showing atrophy of the intestinal villi. Because long-term complications of undiagnosed celiac disease include an increased risk for cancer of the small intestine, early diagnosis can be life-saving. Unfortunately, celiac disease is currently thought to be widely underdiagnosed in the United States.[17]

Currently there is no cure for celiac disease. Treatment is with a special gluten-free diet that excludes all forms of wheat, rye, and barley. The diet is challenging, but many gluten-free foods are now available, including breads, pasta, and other products made from corn, rice, soy, and even garbanzo bean flours.

> **RECAP** *Food intolerance is a condition in which a person experiences gastrointestinal discomfort following consumption of certain foods, but the symptoms are not prompted by the immune system. In contrast, both food allergies and celiac disease are caused by an immune response. Food allergies cause inflammation that results in localized problems such as skin rash or systemic problems such as life-threatening anaphylactic shock. Celiac disease is a genetic disorder that causes damage to the intestinal villi following consumption of gluten, a protein found in wheat, rye, and barley.*

NUTRI-CASE LIZ

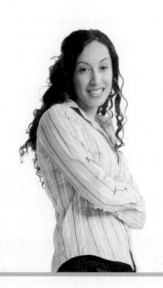

"I used to think of my peanut allergy as no big deal, but ever since my experience at that restaurant last year, I've been pretty obsessive about it. For months afterward, I refused to eat anything that I hadn't prepared myself. I do eat out now, but I always insist that the chef prepare my food personally, with clean utensils. Shopping is a lot harder too, because I have to check every label. The worst, though, is eating at my friends' houses. I have to ask them whether they keep peanuts or peanut butter in their homes. Some of them are really sympathetic, but others look at me as if I'm a hypochondriac! I wish I could think of something to say to them to make them understand that this isn't something I have any control over."

What could Liz say in response to friends who don't understand the cause and seriousness of her food allergy? Do you think it would help Liz to share her fears with her doctor and discuss possible strategies? If so, why? In addition to shopping, dining out, and eating at friends' houses, what other situations might require Liz to be cautious about her food choices?

Diarrhea Results When Food Is Expelled Too Quickly

Diarrhea is the passage of loose, watery stools, often three or more times a day. Other symptoms may include cramping, abdominal pain, bloating, nausea, fever, and bloody stools. Diarrhea is usually caused by an infection of the gastrointestinal tract, a chronic disease, stress, food intolerances, reactions to medications, or as a result of a bowel disorder.[18]

Acute diarrhea lasts less than 3 weeks and is usually caused by an infection from bacteria, a virus, or a parasite. Chronic diarrhea is usually caused by allergies to cow's milk, celiac disease, irritable bowel syndrome, or some other disorder. Whatever the cause, diarrhea can be harmful because the person can lose large quantities of water and minerals like sodium and become severely dehydrated. Diarrhea is particularly dangerous in infants and young children. In fact, each year millions of children worldwide die from dehydration caused by diarrhea. Oral rehydration with specially formulated fluids can reverse dehydration and allow for the introduction of yogurt, rice, banana, and other mild foods.

A condition referred to as *traveler's diarrhea* has become a common health concern because of the expansion in global travel. The accompanying Game Plan provides tips for avoiding traveler's diarrhea.

Constipation Results When Food Wastes Are Expelled Too Slowly

Constipation is typically defined as a condition in which no stools are passed for 2 or more days; however, it is important to recognize that many people normally experience bowel movements only every second or third day. Thus, the definition of constipation varies from one person to another. In addition to being infrequent, the stools are difficult to pass and usually hard and small.

Many people experience temporary constipation at some point in their lives in response to a variety of causes. Often, people have trouble with it when they travel, when their schedule is disrupted, if they change their diet, or if they are on certain medications. Neural factors are thought to be responsible in some people, as explained in the following discussion of irritable bowel syndrome. Treatment with a short course of laxatives or bowel stimulants is often effective. Many healthcare professionals recommend increasing the consumption of fruits, vegetables, and fluids as well as the amount of physical activity; however, the effect of increased fiber, fluid, and physical activity on constipation is the subject of some controversy.[19]

Irritable Bowel Syndrome Causes Intense Pain after Eating

Irritable bowel syndrome (IBS) is a bowel disorder that interferes with normal functions of the colon. Symptoms include abdominal cramps, bloating, and either constipation or diarrhea. Approximately 20% of Americans are diagnosed with IBS, which affects twice as many women as men.[20,21] IBS typically first appears around 20 years of age.

Although no definitive cause of IBS is known, recent studies indicate that the syndrome may arise from an abnormality in the way the brain interprets information from the colon or from abnormal functioning of a chemical called *serotonin*. In the brain, serotonin is thought to influence mood, but in the colon, where 95% of the body's serotonin is found, it promotes peristalsis.[22] Whatever the cause, peristalsis appears to be disrupted. In some people with IBS, food moves too quickly through the colon, and fluid cannot be absorbed fast enough, which causes diarrhea. In others, the movement of the colon is too slow, and too much fluid is absorbed, leading to constipation.

diarrhea Condition characterized by the frequent passage of loose, watery stools.

constipation Condition characterized by the absence of bowel movements for a period of time that is significantly longer than normal for the individual. When a bowel movement does occur, stools are usually small, hard, and difficult to pass.

irritable bowel syndrome (IBS) A bowel disorder that interferes with normal functions of the colon. IBS causes abdominal cramps, bloating, and constipation or diarrhea.

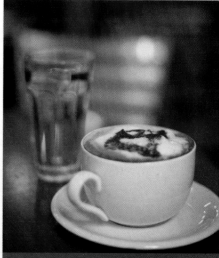

Consuming caffeinated drinks is one of several factors that may be linked with irritable bowel syndrome (IBS), a disorder that interferes with normal functions of the colon.

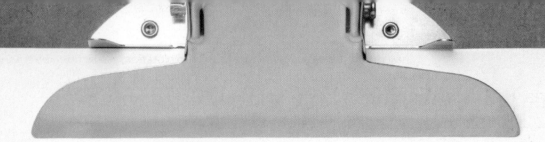

GAME PLAN

Tips for Avoiding Traveler's Diarrhea

Diarrhea is the rapid movement of fecal matter through the large intestine, often accompanied by large volumes of water. *Traveler's diarrhea* (also called *dysentery*), which is experienced by people traveling to regions where clean drinking water is not readily available, is usually caused by viral or bacterial infections. Diarrhea represents the body's way of ridding itself of the invasive agent. The large intestine and even some of the small intestine become irritated by the microbes and the body's defense against them. This irritation leads to increased secretion of fluid and increased peristalsis of the large intestine, causing watery stools and a higher-than-normal frequency of bowel movements.

People generally get traveler's diarrhea from consuming water or food that is contaminated with fecal matter. High-risk destinations include developing countries in Africa, Asia, Latin America, and the Middle East. However, hikers and others traveling in any remote regions are at increased risk if they drink untreated water from lakes, rivers, and streams.

Traveler's diarrhea usually starts about 5 to 15 days after you arrive at your destination. Symptoms include fatigue, lack of appetite, abdominal cramps, and watery diarrhea. In some cases, you may also experience nausea, vomiting, and low-grade fever. Usually, the diarrhea passes within 4 to 6 days, and people recover completely. What can you do to prevent traveler's diarrhea? The following tips should help[22]:

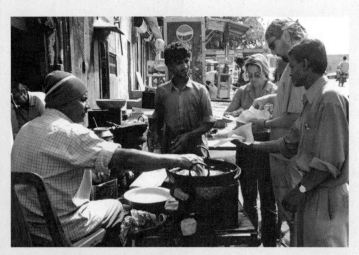

When traveling in developing countries, it is wise to avoid food from street vendors.

❑ Drink only brand-name bottled beverages, including water, wine, beer, and sodas. Use bottled water even for brushing your teeth. In general, it is smart to assume that all local water, even if bottled, is unsafe. Also avoid foods and beverages exposed to or cleaned with local water.

❑ Wipe the bottle or can clean before drinking the beverage.

❑ Do not drink beverages with ice. Freezing does not kill all bacteria.

❑ To render local water safe, boil it for several minutes. Beverages such as tea and coffee made with boiled water are safe.

❑ "Boil it, peel it, cook it, or forget it."[22] All food should be well cooked. Do not eat raw meat, fish, shellfish, or vegetables, including salad greens. Do not eat raw fruits unless they've been washed in boiled or bottled water, and then peeled. Do not eat fruits without peels, such as strawberries or raspberries.

❑ Avoid eating food purchased from street vendors, as well as any cooked food that is no longer hot in temperature.

❑ Prior to traveling to a high-risk country, discuss your trip with your physician for current recommendations for prevention and treatment.

If you do suffer from traveler's diarrhea, it is important to replace the fluid and nutrients lost as a result of the illness. There are specially formulated oral rehydration solutions available to help replenish vital nutrients that are lost; these solutions are usually available in most countries at local pharmacies or stores. Antibiotics may also be needed to kill the bacteria. Once treatment is initiated, the diarrhea should cease within 2 to 3 days. If the diarrhea persists for more than 10 days after the initiation of treatment, or if there is blood in your stools, you should see a physician immediately to determine the cause and get appropriate treatment to avoid serious medical consequences.

Emotional and physiologic stress is currently thought to contribute to symptoms of IBS. Foods linked to physiologic stress include caffeinated beverages, alcohol, dairy products, wheat, large meals, and certain medications. Treatment options include medications that treat diarrhea or constipation, stress management, regular physical activity, and dietary management. Probiotics, which were discussed in the Highlight on page 54, have also been shown to reduce symptoms of IBS.[3]

At this point, you might be wondering whether Andrea, in our chapter opener, has IBS. Without a full medical examination, it's impossible to say. That's because IBS and celiac disease can present with very similar symptoms. In fact, some researchers are now advising that all patients with symptoms suggestive of IBS be screened for celiac disease.[23]

RECAP *Diarrhea is frequent passage of loose or watery stools, whereas constipation is failure to have a bowel movement for 2 or more days or within a time period that is normal for the individual. Irritable bowel syndrome (IBS) causes abdominal cramps, bloating, and constipation or diarrhea. The causes of IBS are unknown; however, emotional and physiologic stress are implicated.*

Where I'm at now...

At the beginning of this chapter, we asked if you experience problems with your digestive system, and if so, if you've seen a doctor about it. Now that you've read about the potentially serious consequences of failing to diagnose and treat GERD, ulcers, food allergies, and celiac disease, we're hoping that you don't let embarrassment or other excuses keep you from getting to the root of the problem. Choose the statement below that best describes where you're at now:

☐ I don't have any digestive problems, but if I ever develop any, I'll see a doctor.

☐ I do have a digestive problem, and I've consulted a doctor about it.

☐ I do have a digestive problem, and I'm making an appointment to see a doctor about it today!

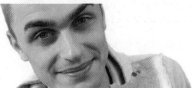

REVIEW QUESTIONS

Circle the correct choice.

1. Enzymes are
   a. chemical messenger molecules released from glands.
   b. chemicals that help speed up body processes.
   c. acids found in the cell nucleus that instruct cells in the building of proteins.
   d. acids that begin the breakdown of proteins in the mouth.

2. Bile is a greenish fluid that
   a. is stored by the pancreas.
   b. is produced by the gallbladder.
   c. breaks down proteins.
   d. emulsifies fats.

3. The region of brain tissue that is responsible for prompting us to seek food is the
   a. pituitary gland.
   b. pancreas.
   c. hypothalamus.
   d. thalamus.

4. Heartburn is caused by
   a. seepage of gastric acid into the esophagus.
   b. seepage of gastric acid into the cardiac muscle.
   c. seepage of bile into the chest cavity.
   d. seepage of salivary amylase into the stomach.

5. Most digestion of carbohydrates, fats, and proteins takes place in the
   a. mouth.
   b. stomach.
   c. small intestine.
   d. large intestine.

6. True or False? Atoms are the smallest units of life.

7. True or False? Nutrients absorbed through the cells of the brush border are transported to the liver.

8. True or False? The nerves of the GI tract are collectively known as the enteric nervous system.

9. True or False? Vitamins and minerals are digested in the small intestine.

10. True or False? Undiagnosed irritable bowel syndrome increases the risk for cancer of the small intestine.

WEB LINKS

www.digestive.niddk.nih.gov
National Digestive Diseases Information Clearinghouse (NDDIC)

Explore this site to learn more about diarrhea, irritable bowel syndrome (IBS), heartburn, and gastroesophageal reflux disease (GERD).

www.nlm.nih.gov/medlineplus
MEDLINE Plus Health Information

Search for "food allergies" to obtain additional resources as well as the latest news about food allergies.

www.healthfinder.gov
Health Finder

Search this site to learn more about disorders related to digestion, absorption, and elimination.

www.foodallergy.org
The Food Allergy and Anaphylaxis Network (FAAN)

Visit this site to learn more about common food allergens.

www.americanceliac.org/cd.htm
American Celiac Disease Alliance

Learn more about the diagnosis and treatment of celiac disease, ongoing research, and living with celiac disease.

www.csaceliacs.org
Celiac Sprue Association—National Celiac Disease Support Group

This national educational organization provides information and referral services for people with celiac disease.

www.ibsassociation.org
Irritable Bowel Syndrome Association

Visit this site for information on diagnosis, treatment, and clinical studies on irritable bowel syndrome, as well as for other Internet links.

TEST YOURSELF ANSWERS

1. **False.** Your brain, not your stomach, is the primary organ responsible for telling you when you are hungry.

2. **True.** Although there are individual variations in how we respond to food, the entire process of digestion and absorption of one meal usually takes about 24 hours.

3. **True.** Certain bacteria are normal and helpful residents of the large intestine, where they assist in digestion. They also appear to protect the tissue lining the intes-

tinal walls and may improve immune function. Food products and supplements containing these bacteria are called *probiotics*.

4. **True.** Most ulcers result from an infection of the bacterium *Helicobacter pylori*. Contrary to popular belief, ulcers are not caused by stress, alcohol, or spicy foods.

5. **False.** Irritable bowel syndrome is a relatively common disease that affects 20% of the U.S. population. It typically appears by early adulthood.

NUTRITION LABEL ACTIVITY ANSWERS

1. Which of the FDA's eight allergenic foods does this bar definitely contain? **Milk (dairy) and soybeans**

2. If you were allergic to peanuts, would eating this bar pose any risk to you? **Yes, because the bar "May contain traces of peanuts."**

3. If you were allergic to almonds, would eating this bar pose any risk to you? **Yes, because the bar also may contain "traces of other nuts." Since these nuts are not specified, it would not be entirely safe for someone allergic to almonds to eat the bar.**

REFERENCES

1. Bell E. A., and B. J. Rolls. 2001. Regulation of energy intake: Factors contributing to obesity. In: Bowman B. A., and R. M. Russell, eds., *Present Knowledge in Nutrition*. 8th ed. Washington, DC: ILSI Press.
2. Zorrilla, G. 1998. Hunger and satiety: Deceptively simple words for the complex mechanisms that tell us when to eat and when to stop. *J. Am. Diet. Assoc.* 98:1111.
3. Kerr, M. 2003. Probiotics significantly reduce symptoms of IBS, ulcerative colitis. *Medscape Medical News 2003*. Available at www.medscape.com/viewarticle/455964_print.
4. Kopp-Hoolihan, L. 2001. Prophylactic and therapeutic uses of probiotics: A review. *J. Am. Diet. Assoc.* 101:229–238, 241.
5. Saier, M. H., Jr., and N. M. Mansour. 2005. Probiotics and prebiotics in human health. *J. Mol. Microbiol. Biotechnol.* 10(1):22–25.
6. Doron, S., and S. L. Gorbach. 2006. Probiotics: their role in the treatment and prevention of diseases. *Expert Rev. Anti-Infect. Ther.* 4(2):261–275.
7. Ezendam, J., and H. van Loveren. 2006. Probiotics: Immunomodulation and evaluation of safety and efficacy. *Nutr. Rev.* 64(1):1–14.
8. Sanders, M. E., D. C. Walker, K. M. Walker, K. Aoyama, and T. R. Klaenhammer. 1996. Performance of commercial cultures in fluid milk applications. *J Dairy Sci.* 79:943–955.
9. National Digestive Diseases Information Clearinghouse (NDDIC). 2003. Heartburn, hiatal hernia, and gastroesophageal reflux disease (GERD). NIH Publication No. 03–0882. Available at http://digestive.niddk.nih.gov/ddiseases/pubs/gerd/index.htm.
10. Bauman, R. 2004. *Microbiology*. San Francisco: Benjamin Cummings, p. 617.
11. Chan, F. K. L., and W. K. Leung. 2002. Peptic-ulcer disease. *Lancet* 360:933–941.
12. Germann, W. J., and C. L. Stanfield. 2002. *Principles of Human Physiology*. San Francisco: Benjamin Cummings, p. 622.
13. National Digestive Diseases Information Clearinghouse (NDDIC). 2004. NSAIDs and peptic ulcers. NIH Publication No. 04–4644. Available at http://digestive.niddk.nih.gov/ddiseases/pubs/nsaids/index.htm.
14. U.S. Food and Drug Administration (FDA). December 20, 2005. FDA to Require Food Manufacturers to List Food Allergens. FDA News. Available at www.fda.gov/bbs/topics/NEWS/2005/NEW01281.html.
15. U.S. Food and Drug Administration (FDA). July 18, 2006. Information for Consumers: Food Allergen Labeling and Consumer Protection Act of 2004 Questions and Answers. Available at www.cfsan.fda.gov/~dms/alrgqa.html.
16. National Digestive Diseases Information Clearinghouse (NDDIC). October 2005. Celiac Disease. NIH Publication No. 06-4269. Available at http://digestive.niddk.nih.gov.
17. National Institutes of Health. June 2004. NIH Consensus Development Conference on Celiac Disease. Available at http://consensus.nih.gov/2004/2004CeliacDisease118html.htm.
18. National Digestive Diseases Information Clearinghouse (NDDIC). 2003. Diarrhea. NIH Publication No. 04–2749. Available at http://digestive.niddk.nih.gov/ddiseases/pubs/diarrhea/index.htm.
19. Bakalar, N. 2005. Is fiber the answer? Researchers doubt it. *New York Times*, January 18, p. D7.
20. National Digestive Diseases Information Clearinghouse (NDDIC). 2003. Irritable bowel syndrome. NIH Publication No. 03–693. Available at http://digestive.niddk.nih.gov/ddiseases/pubs/ibs/index.htm.
21. Duenwald, M. 2004. New remedies for a frustrating illness. But do they work? *New York Times*, January 18, p. D5.
22. Stanley, S. L. 1999. Advice to travelers. In: Yamada, T., ed., *Textbook of Gastroenterology*. Vol. 1. 3rd ed. Philadelphia: Lippincott Williams & Wilkins.
23. National Institutes of Health. March 12, 2002. Celiac Disease Meeting Summary. DDICC Meeting Minutes. Available at http://digestive.niddk.nih.gov/federal/ddicc/minutes_3-12-02.pdf.

3

Carbohydrates: Plant-Derived Energy Nutrients

TEST YOURSELF

Are these statements true or false?
Circle your guess.

1 The terms carbohydrate and sugar mean the same thing.   **TRUE** or **FALSE**

2 Diets high in sugar cause hyperactivity in children and diabetes.   **TRUE** or **FALSE**

3 Carbohydrates are the primary fuel source for our brain and body tissues.   **TRUE** or **FALSE**

4 Carbohydrates are fattening.   **TRUE** or **FALSE**

5 Alternative sweeteners, such as aspartame, are safe to consume.   **TRUE** or **FALSE**

Test Yourself answers can be found at the end of the chapter.

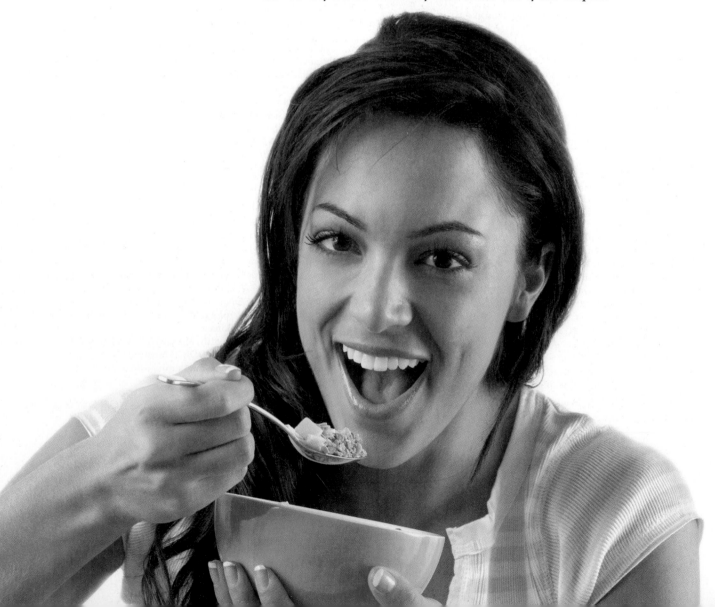

J ASMINE SKIPPED SCHOOL again today. When her Mom asked her why, she said she had a headache. That is only partly true: her real "headache" is the thought of explaining to her friends why, all of a sudden, she can't have the sodas and snacks they've always consumed at school. She and her friends admit they're overweight, but they've always had fun together, so their weight hasn't bothered them. Jasmine doesn't want her friends to find out that things are different now—that she has to change her diet, exercise regularly, and lose weight. She doesn't want to admit that she's just been diagnosed with the same disease her grandmother has: type 2 diabetes.

Does the consumption of soft drinks and other sugary foods lead to diabetes, or, for that matter, to obesity or any other disorder? Several popular diets, including The Zone Diet, Sugar Busters, and Dr. Atkins' New Diet Revolution, claim that refined carbohydrates can be harmful to your health.[1-3] Is this true? If you noticed that a friend regularly consumed four or five soft drinks a day, plus candy and other sweet snacks, would you say anything? Are carbohydrates a health menace, and is one type of carbohydrate as bad as another?

In this chapter, we explore the differences between simple and complex carbohydrates and learn why some carbohydrates really are better than others. You'll learn how the body breaks down carbohydrates and uses them for fuel and find out how much carbohydrate you should eat each day. We'll end the chapter with a look at diabetes, a serious health problem that occurs when the body loses its ability to process the carbohydrates we eat. One form, type 2 diabetes, used to be considered a disease of older people but is now increasingly diagnosed in overweight and obese teens and young adults in the United States.

What Are Carbohydrates?

As we mentioned in Chapter 1, **carbohydrates** are one of the three macronutrients. They are an important energy source for the entire body and are the preferred energy source for nerve cells, including those of the brain. We will say more about their functions shortly.

The term carbohydrate literally means "hydrated carbon." You know that water (H_2O) is made of hydrogen and oxygen, and that when something is said to be hydrated, it contains water. The chemical abbreviation for carbohydrate is CHO. These three letters stand for the three components of a molecule of carbohydrate: carbon, hydrogen, and oxygen.

Most Carbohydrates Come from Plant Foods

We obtain carbohydrates predominantly from plant foods such as fruits, vegetables, and grains. Plants make the most abundant form of carbohydrate, called glucose, through a process called **photosynthesis.** During photosynthesis, the green pigment of plants, called chlorophyll, absorbs sunlight, which provides the energy needed to fuel the manufacture of glucose. As shown in FIGURE 3.1, water absorbed from the earth by the roots of plants combines with carbon dioxide present in the leaves to produce glucose. Plants continually store glucose and use it to support their own growth. Then, when we eat plant foods, our bodies digest, absorb, and use the stored glucose.

The only nonplant sources of carbohydrates are foods derived from milk. For instance, breast milk, cow's milk, cheese, and ice cream all contain a carbohydrate called lactose.

carbohydrate   One of the three macronutrients, a compound made up of carbon, hydrogen, and oxygen. It is derived from plants and provides energy.

photosynthesis   Process by which plants use sunlight to fuel a chemical reaction that combines carbon and water into glucose, which is then stored in their cells.

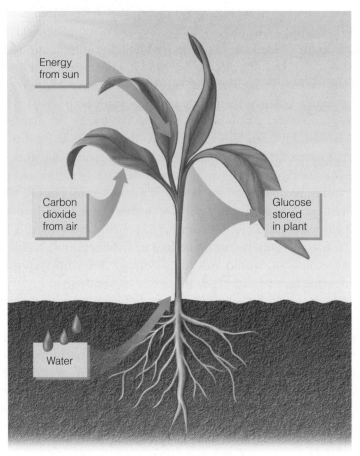

FIGURE 3.1 Plants make carbohydrates through the process of photosynthesis. Water, carbon dioxide, and energy from the sun are combined to produce glucose.

simple carbohydrate Commonly called *sugar;* a monosaccharide or disaccharide such as glucose.

monosaccharide The simplest of carbohydrates: consists of one sugar molecule, the most common form of which is glucose.

disaccharide A carbohydrate compound consisting of two sugar molecules joined together.

glucose The most abundant sugar molecule: a monosaccharide generally found in combination with other sugars. The preferred source of energy for the brain and an important source of energy for all cells.

fructose The sweetest natural sugar; a monosaccharide that occurs in fruits and vegetables. Also called *levulose,* or *fruit sugar.*

galactose A monosaccharide that joins with glucose to create lactose, one of the three most common disaccharides.

Simple Carbohydrates Are Sugars

Carbohydrates can be classified as *simple* or *complex.* As you might expect, simple carbohydrates are made up of only one or two molecules, whereas complex carbohydrates contain long chains of hundreds or even thousands of molecules.

Simple carbohydrates are commonly referred to as *sugars.* Six sugars are common in our diet. Three of these sugars are called **monosaccharides** because they consist of only a single sugar molecule (*mono* means "one," and *saccharide* means "sugar"). The other three sugars are **disaccharides** and consist of two molecules of sugar joined together (*di* means "two").

The Three Monosaccharides Are Glucose, Fructose, and Galactose

Glucose, fructose, and *galactose* are the three monosaccharides in our diet (FIGURE 3.2A). Because plants manufacture **glucose,** it probably won't surprise you to discover that glucose is the most abundant sugar in our diets and in our bodies. Glucose does not generally occur by itself in foods; instead, it is usually attached to other sugars in larger molecules. In our bodies, glucose is the preferred source of energy for the brain, and it is a very important source of energy for all cells.

Fructose, the sweetest natural sugar, is found in fruits and vegetables. Fructose is also called *levulose,* or *fruit sugar.* In many processed foods, it comes in the form of *high-fructose corn syrup.* This syrup is made from corn and is used to sweeten soft drinks, desserts, candies, and jellies.

Galactose does not occur alone in foods. It joins with glucose to create lactose, one of the three most common disaccharides.

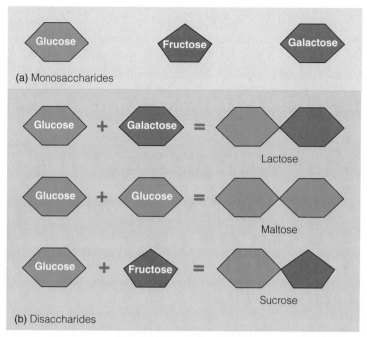

FIGURE 3.2   The simple carbohydrates. (a) The three most common monosaccharides in the diet are glucose, fructose, and galactose. (b) These join together to make the disaccharides lactose, maltose, and sucrose.

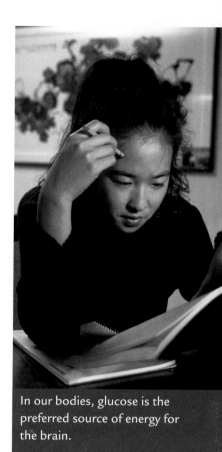

In our bodies, glucose is the preferred source of energy for the brain.

The Three Disaccharides Are Lactose, Maltose, and Sucrose

The three most common disaccharides found in foods are *lactose, maltose,* and *sucrose* (FIGURE 3.2B). **Lactose** (also called *milk sugar*) is made up of glucose and galactose. Interestingly, human breast milk has a higher amount of lactose than cow's milk and therefore tastes sweeter.

Maltose (also called *malt sugar*) consists of two molecules of glucose. It does not generally occur by itself in foods but rather is bound together with other molecules. As our bodies break these larger molecules down, maltose results as a by-product. Maltose is also the sugar that is fermented during the production of beer and liquor products. Contrary to popular belief, very little maltose remains in alcoholic beverages after the fermentation process; thus, alcoholic beverages are not good sources of carbohydrate.

Sucrose is composed of glucose and fructose. Because sucrose contains fructose, it is sweeter than lactose or maltose. Sucrose provides much of the sweet taste found in honey, maple syrup, fruits, and vegetables. Table sugar, brown sugar, powdered sugar, and many other products are made by refining the sucrose found in sugarcane and sugar beets. Are naturally occurring forms of sucrose more healthful than manufactured forms? The Nutrition Myth or Fact? feature on page 70 investigates the common belief that honey is more nutritious than table sugar.

Complex Carbohydrates Are Starches and Fiber

Complex carbohydrates, the second major type of carbohydrate, generally consist of long chains of glucose molecules. The technical name for complex carbohydrates is **polysaccharides** (*poly* means "many"). Complex carbohydrates exist in foods as either starches or fiber. A third complex carbohydrate, glycogen, is not obtained from our diets (FIGURE 3.3). Each of these three types is discussed in more detail shortly.

lactose   Also called *milk sugar;* a disaccharide consisting of one glucose molecule and one galactose molecule. Found in milk, including human breast milk.

maltose   A disaccharide consisting of two molecules of glucose. Does not generally occur independently in foods but results as a by-product of digestion. Also called *malt sugar.*

sucrose   A disaccharide composed of one glucose molecule and one fructose molecule. Sweeter than lactose or maltose.

complex carbohydrate   A nutrient compound consisting of long chains of glucose molecules, such as starch, glycogen, and fiber.

polysaccharide   A complex carbohydrate consisting of long chains of glucose.

NUTRITION MYTH OR FACT?

Is Honey More Nutritious Than Table Sugar?

Liz's friend Tiffany is dedicated to eating healthful foods. She advises Liz to avoid white sugar and to eat foods that contain honey, molasses, or raw sugar. Like many people, Tiffany believes these sweeteners are more natural and nutritious than refined table sugar. How can Liz sort sugar fact from fiction?

Remember that sucrose consists of one glucose molecule and one fructose molecule joined together. From a chemical perspective, honey is almost identical to sucrose, as honey also contains glucose and fructose molecules in almost equal amounts. However, enzymes in the "honey stomachs" of bees separate some of the glucose and fructose molecules, resulting in honey looking and tasting slightly different from sucrose. As you know, bees store honey in combs and fan it with their wings to reduce its moisture content. This also alters the appearance and texture of honey.

Honey does not contain any more nutrients than sucrose, so it is not a more healthful choice than sucrose. In fact, per tablespoon, honey has more calories (or energy) than table sugar. This is because the crystals in table sugar take up more space on a spoon than the liquid form of honey, so a tablespoon contains less sugar. However, some people argue that honey is sweeter, so you use less.

It is important to note that honey commonly contains bacteria that can cause fatal food poisoning in infants. The more mature digestive system of older children and adults is immune to the effects of these bacteria, but babies younger than 12 months should never be given honey.

Are raw sugar and molasses more healthful than table sugar? Actually, the "raw sugar" available in the United States is not really raw. Truly raw sugar is made up of the first crystals obtained when sugar is processed. Sugar in this form contains dirt, parts of insects, and other by-products that make it illegal to sell in the United States. The raw sugar products in American stores have actually gone through more than half of the same steps in the refining process used to make table sugar.

Molasses is the syrup that remains when sucrose is made from sugarcane. Molasses is darker and less sweet than table sugar. It does contain some iron, but this iron does not occur naturally. It is a contaminant from the machines that process the sugarcane!

The truth is, no added sugars contain many nutrients that are important for health. This is why highly sweetened products are referred to as "empty calories."

Starches Are Stored in Plants

Plants store glucose not as single molecules but as complex carbohydrates called **starches.** Excellent food sources of starches include grains (wheat, rice, corn, oats, and barley), legumes (peas, beans, and lentils), and tubers (potatoes and yams). Our cells cannot use starch molecules exactly as they occur in plants. Instead, our bodies must break them down into the monosaccharide glucose from which we can then fuel our energy needs.

Fiber Gives Plants Their Structure

starch   A polysaccharide stored in plants; the storage form of glucose in plants.

fiber   The nondigestible carbohydrate parts of plants that form the support structures of leaves, stems, and seeds.

Fiber is the nondigestible parts of plants that form the support structures of leaves, stems, and seeds. Like starches, fiber consists of long polysaccharide chains. The body easily breaks apart the chains in starches; however, the bonds that connect fiber molecules are not easily broken. This means that most forms of fiber pass through the digestive system without being broken down and absorbed, and so fiber contributes little or no energy to our diet. However, fiber offers many health benefits, as we discuss shortly (pages 74–75).

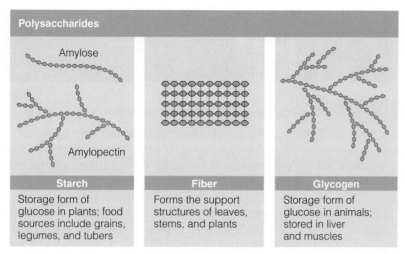

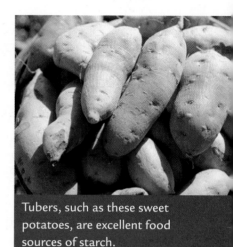

Tubers, such as these sweet potatoes, are excellent food sources of starch.

FIGURE 3.3 The complex carbohydrates, or polysaccharides, include starches and fiber. Glycogen is a storage form of glucose found in animals and is not a dietary source of carbohydrate.

Nutrition experts and food producers use several terms to distinguish among different types of fiber. We discuss these terms here, as they're important for understanding the contribution of fiber to our health.

Dietary vs. Functional Fiber   Fiber that occurs naturally in foods is called **dietary fiber.** In a sense, you can think of dietary fiber as the plant's "skeleton." Good food sources of dietary fiber include fruits, vegetables, seeds, legumes, and whole grains. We frequently hear the recommendation to eat whole grains, but is grain ground into flour and baked into bread still whole? Maybe, maybe not! So what does the term *whole grain* really mean? Find out in the Highlight: What Makes a Whole Grain Whole? feature on page 72.

Another type of fiber, called **functional fiber,** is manufactured and added to foods and fiber supplements. Examples of functional fiber sources you might see on nutrition labels include cellulose, guar gum, pectin, and psyllium. **Total fiber** is the sum of dietary fiber and functional fiber in a particular food. On the Nutrition Facts Panel, the term *Dietary Fiber* actually represents the total amount of fiber in that food, and includes the dietary fiber that occurs naturally and any functional fiber that may have been added to a particular food.

Soluble vs. Insoluble Fiber   Fiber can also be classified according to its chemical and physical properties as soluble or insoluble. **Soluble fibers** dissolve in water. They are also **viscous,** which means they form a gel when wet. Though the digestive tract cannot independently digest soluble fibers, they are easily digested by bacteria present in the colon. Soluble fibers are typically found in citrus fruits, berries, oat products, and beans. Research suggests that regular consumption of soluble fibers reduces the risks for cardiovascular disease and type 2 diabetes by lowering blood cholesterol and blood glucose levels.

Insoluble fibers are those that do not typically dissolve in water. These fibers are usually nonviscous and typically cannot be easily digested by bacteria in the colon. Insoluble fibers are generally found in whole grains such as wheat, rye, and brown rice and are also found in many vegetables. These fibers are not associated with reducing cholesterol levels but are known for promoting regular bowel movements, alleviating constipation, and reducing the risk for a disorder called diverticulosis (discussed later in this chapter).

Fiber-Rich Carbohydrates   Materials written for the general public commonly avoid referring to the carbohydrates found in foods as complex or simple; instead, recommendations such as the *Dietary Guidelines for Americans* (2005) emphasize

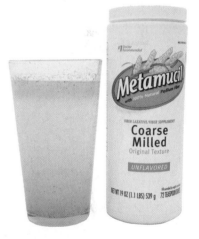

Dissolvable laxatives can be examples of soluble fibers.

dietary fiber   The type of fiber that occurs naturally in foods.

functional fiber   The nondigestible forms of carbohydrate that are extracted from plants or manufactured in the laboratory and have known health benefits.

total fiber   The sum of dietary fiber and functional fiber.

soluble fibers   Fibers that dissolve in water.

viscous   Term referring to a gel-like consistency; viscous fibers form a gel when dissolved in water.

insoluble fibers   Fibers that do not dissolve in water.

HIGHLIGHT

What Makes a Whole Grain Whole?

Grains are grasses that produce edible kernels. A kernel of grain is the seed of the grass: if you were to plant a kernel of barley, a blade of grass would soon shoot up. Kernels of different grains all share a similar design. As shown in the figure, they consist of three parts (Figure 3.4):

- The outermost covering, called the *bran,* is very high in fiber and contains most of the grain's vitamins and minerals.
- The *endosperm* is the grain's midsection and contains most of the grain's carbohydrates and protein.
- The *germ* sits deep in the base of the kernel, surrounded by the endosperm, and is rich in healthful fats and some vitamins.

Whole grains are kernels that retain all three of these parts.

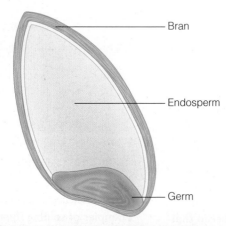

FIGURE 3.4   A whole grain includes the bran, endosperm, and germ.

The kernels of some grains also have a *husk* (or hull): a thin, dry coat that is inedible. Removing the husk is always the first step in milling (grinding) these grains for human consumption.

People worldwide have milled grain for centuries, usually using heavy stones. Minimal milling removes only a small amount of the bran, leaving a crunchy grain suitable for cooked cereals. For example, cracked wheat and hulled barley retain much of the kernel's bran. Whole-grain flours are produced when whole grains are ground and then recombined. Because these hearty flours retain a portion of the bran, endosperm, and germ, foods such as breads made with them are rich in fiber and a wide array of vitamins and minerals.

With the advent of modern technology, processes for milling grains became more sophisticated, with seeds being repeatedly ground and sifted into increasingly finer flours retaining little or no bran and therefore little fiber and few vitamins and minerals. For instance, white wheat flour, which consists almost entirely of endosperm, is high in carbohydrate but retains only about 25% of the wheat's fiber, vitamins, and minerals. In the United States, manufacturers of breads and other baked goods made with white flour are required by law to enrich their products with vitamins and minerals to replace some of those lost in processing. However, enrichment replaces only a handful of nutrients and leaves the bread low in fiber.

When choosing breads, crackers, and other baked goods, look for whole wheat, whole oats, or similar whole grains on the ingredient list. This ensures that the product contains the fiber and micronutrients that nature packed into the plant's seed.

---

fiber-rich carbohydrates   A group of foods containing either simple or complex carbohydrates that are rich in dietary fiber. These foods, which include most fruits, vegetables, and whole grains, are typically fresh or only moderately processed.

glycogen   A polysaccharide stored in animals; the storage form of glucose in animals.

eating **fiber-rich carbohydrates** such as fruits, vegetables, and whole grains.[4] This term is important to nutritional recommendations because fiber-rich carbohydrates are known to contribute to good health, but not all complex carbohydrate foods are fiber-rich. For example, potatoes that have been processed into frozen hash browns retain very little of their original fiber. On the other hand, some foods rich in simple carbohydrates (such as fruits) are also fiber-rich. So when you're reading labels, it pays to check the grams of dietary fiber per serving. And by the way, if the food you're considering is fresh produce and there's no label to read, that almost guarantees it's fiber-rich.

Glycogen Is a Polysaccharide Stored by Animals

Glycogen is the storage form of glucose for animals, including humans. We store glycogen in our muscles and liver, and we can break it down very quickly into glucose when we need it for energy. Very little glycogen exists in food; thus, glycogen is not a dietary source of carbohydrate.

> RECAP *Carbohydrates are energy-providing macronutrients that contain carbon, hydrogen, and oxygen. Plants make one type of carbohydrate, glucose, through the process of photosynthesis. Simple carbohydrates include the monosaccharides glucose, fructose, and galactose, and the disaccharides lactose, maltose, and sucrose. All complex carbohydrates are polysaccharides. They include starch, glycogen, and fiber. Starch is the storage form of glucose in plants, whereas glycogen is the storage form of glucose in animals. Fiber forms the support structures of plants; our bodies cannot readily digest fiber.*

Why Do We Need to Eat Carbohydrates?

We have seen that carbohydrates are an important energy source for our bodies. Let's learn more about this and some other functions of carbohydrates.

Carbohydrates Provide Energy

Carbohydrates, an excellent source of energy for all our cells, provide 4 kilocalories (kcal) of energy per gram. Some of our cells can also use fat and even protein for energy if necessary. However, our red blood cells, as well as our brains and nerve cells, rely on glucose. This is why you get tired, irritable, and shaky when you have not eaten carbohydrates for a prolonged period of time.

Carbohydrates Fuel Activity and Exercise

As shown in **FIGURE 3.5**, our bodies always use some combination of carbohydrates and fat to fuel daily activities. Fat is the predominant energy source used by most of our cells at rest and during low-intensity activities such as sitting, standing, and walking. Even during rest, however, our brain cells and red blood cells still rely on glucose.

When we exercise, whether running, briskly walking, bicycling, or performing any other activity that causes us to breathe harder and sweat, we begin to use more glucose than fat. When you are exercising at maximal effort, carbohydrates are providing almost 100% of the energy your body requires.

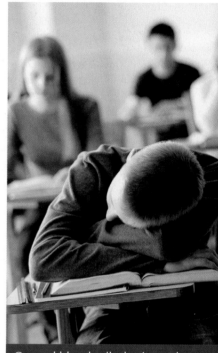

Our red blood cells, brain, and nerve cells primarily rely on glucose. This is why you get tired, irritable, and shaky when you have not eaten for a prolonged period of time.

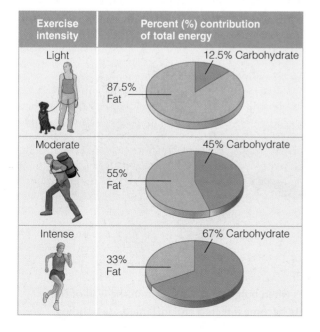

FIGURE 3.5 Amounts of carbohydrate and fat used during light, moderate, and intense exercise.
(Adapted from J. A. Romijn, E. F. Coyle, L. S. Sidossis, A. Gastaldelli, J. F. Horowitz, E. Endert, and R. R. Wolfe. 1993. Regulation of endogenous fat and carbohydrate metabolism in relation to exercise intensity and duration. *Am. J. Physiol.* 265 [*Endocrinol. Metab.* 28]: E380–E391. Used with permission by the American Physiological Society.)

Low Carbohydrate Intake Can Lead to Ketoacidosis

When we do not eat enough carbohydrate, the body begins to break down fat for energy. This process, called **ketosis,** produces an alternative fuel called **ketones.** In people who are fasting or starving, ketosis is an important mechanism for providing energy to the brain. However, if inadequate carbohydrate intake continues for an extended period of time, the body will produce excessive amounts of ketones. Because many ketones are acids, high ketone levels make the blood very acidic, a condition called **ketoacidosis.** Ketoacidosis most commonly occurs when a person has uncontrolled diabetes (diabetes is discussed later in this chapter). The high acidity of the blood interferes with basic body functions and damages many body tissues. Ketoacidosis can even lead to coma and death.

Carbohydrates Spare Protein

If the diet does not provide enough carbohydrate, the body will make glucose from protein. This involves breaking down the proteins in blood and tissues into amino acids, then converting them to glucose. This process is called **gluconeogenesis** (or "generating new glucose").

When the body uses proteins for energy, the proteins cannot be used to make new cells, repair tissues, or perform any of their other functions. During periods of carbohydrate deprivation, the body will take amino acids from the blood first and then from other tissues such as the muscles, heart, liver, and kidneys. Using amino acids in this manner over a prolonged period of time can seriously damage these organs.

Fiber-Rich Carbohydrates Have Health Benefits

A diet rich in fiber may possibly reduce the risk of gastrointestinal diseases such as colon cancer and help prevent hemorrhoids, constipation, and other motility problems by keeping stools moist and soft. Fiber gives gut muscles "something to push on" and makes it easier to eliminate stools. For the same reason, fiber reduces the risk of *diverticulosis,* a condition that is caused in part by trying to eliminate small, hard stools. A great deal of pressure must be generated in the large intestine (colon) to pass hard stools. This increased pressure weakens intestinal walls, causing them to bulge outward and form pockets (FIGURE 3.6). Feces and fibrous materials can get trapped in these pockets, which become infected and inflamed. This is a painful condition that must be treated with antibiotics or surgery.

Other health benefits of eating fiber-rich carbohydrates include:

- Reduced overall risk for obesity. Eating a high-fiber diet causes a person to feel more full, which may help people to eat less and maintain a healthful weight.

- Reduced risk of heart disease. Fiber can delay or block the absorption of dietary cholesterol into the bloodstream.

When we exercise or perform any other activity that causes us to breathe harder and sweat, we begin to use more glucose than fat.

ketosis The process by which the breakdown of fat during fasting states results in the production of ketones.

ketones Substances produced during the breakdown of fat when carbohydrate intake is insufficient to meet energy needs. Provide an alternative energy source for the brain when glucose levels are low.

ketoacidosis A condition in which excessive ketones are present in the blood, causing the blood to become very acidic, which alters basic body functions and damages tissues. Untreated ketoacidosis can be fatal. This condition is found in individuals with untreated diabetes mellitus.

gluconeogenesis The generation of glucose from the breakdown of proteins into amino acids.

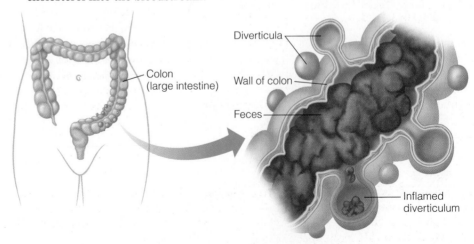

FIGURE 3.6 Diverticulosis occurs when bulging pockets form in the wall of the large intestine (colon). These pockets become infected and inflamed, demanding proper treatment.

- Decreased risk for type 2 diabetes. Fiber absorbs water, expands in the intestine, and slows the movement of food through the upper part of the digestive tract. In slowing digestion, fiber also slows the release of glucose into the blood and may thereby lower the risk of type 2 diabetes (discussed in detail later in this chapter).

> RECAP *Carbohydrates are an excellent energy source at rest and during exercise and provide 4 kcal of energy per gram. Carbohydrates are necessary in the diet to spare body protein and prevent ketoacidosis. Complex carbohydrates contain fiber and phytochemicals that can reduce the risk for obesity, heart disease, diabetes, cancer, and other health problems.*

NUTRI-CASE THEO

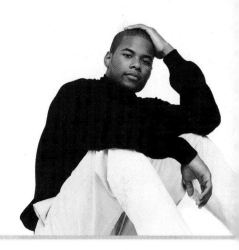

"Right after a game, I just crave carbs. Problem is, by the time the game is over and I've showered and changed, it's late, and the only places that are open are fast-food joints. I don't want to eat pizza or burgers and fries right before I go to bed, so most nights I just go back to my dorm room and make myself a peanut-butter sandwich. I have it with a banana and a carton of milk, and that seems to help me get to sleep, but I have to admit, when I wake up the morning after a game, I'm always ravenous!"

Why do you think Theo craves carbohydrates after a basketball game? Without precisely calculating their nutrient composition, which postgame meal do you guess would be more healthful: pepperoni pizza and a soft drink; a burger, fries, and a vanilla shake; or a peanut butter sandwich on whole-wheat bread, a banana, and a carton of milk? Why? Is Theo's hunger the morning after a game a signal that something about his postgame meal or about his general daily food intake needs to change?

What Happens to the Carbohydrates We Eat?

Because glucose is the form of sugar that our bodies use for energy, the primary goal of carbohydrate digestion is to break down polysaccharides and disaccharides into monosaccharides that can then be converted to glucose. Chapter 2 provided an overview of digestion. Here, we focus in a bit more detail on the digestion and absorption of carbohydrates. FIGURE 3.7 provides a visual tour of carbohydrate digestion.

Digestion Breaks Down Most Carbohydrates into Monosaccharides

Carbohydrate digestion begins in the mouth (Figure 3.7, step 1). The starch in the foods you eat mixes with your saliva during chewing. Saliva contains an enzyme called **salivary amylase,** which breaks starch into smaller particles and eventually into the disaccharide maltose.

As the bolus of food leaves the mouth and enters the stomach, all digestion of carbohydrates ceases. This is because the acid in the stomach inactivates most of the salivary amylase enzyme (Figure 3.7, step 2).

salivary amylase An enzyme in saliva that breaks starch into smaller particles and eventually into the disaccharide maltose.

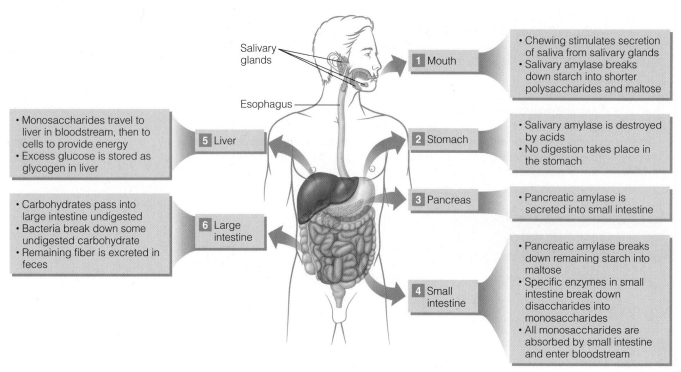

Salivary glands

Esophagus

1 Mouth
- Chewing stimulates secretion of saliva from salivary glands
- Salivary amylase breaks down starch into shorter polysaccharides and maltose

2 Stomach
- Salivary amylase is destroyed by acids
- No digestion takes place in the stomach

3 Pancreas
- Pancreatic amylase is secreted into small intestine

4 Small intestine
- Pancreatic amylase breaks down remaining starch into maltose
- Specific enzymes in small intestine break down disaccharides into monosaccharides
- All monosaccharides are absorbed by small intestine and enter bloodstream

5 Liver
- Monosaccharides travel to liver in bloodstream, then to cells to provide energy
- Excess glucose is stored as glycogen in liver

6 Large intestine
- Carbohydrates pass into large intestine undigested
- Bacteria break down some undigested carbohydrate
- Remaining fiber is excreted in feces

FIGURE 3.7 A review of carbohydrate digestion and absorption.

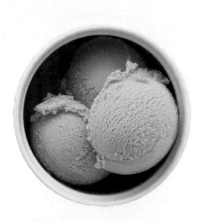

Milk products, such as ice cream, are hard to digest for people who are lactose intolerant.

pancreatic amylase An enzyme secreted by the pancreas into the small intestine that digests any remaining starch into maltose.

lactose intolerance A disorder in which the body does not produce sufficient lactase enzyme and therefore cannot digest foods that contain lactose, such as cow's milk.

The majority of carbohydrate digestion occurs in the small intestine. As the contents of the stomach enter the small intestine, an enzyme called **pancreatic amylase** is secreted by the pancreas into the small intestine (Figure 3.7, step 3). This enzyme digests any remaining starch into maltose. Additional enzymes in the mucosal cells that line the intestinal tract work to break down disaccharides into monosaccharides (Figure 3.7, step 4). All monosaccharides are then absorbed into the mucosal cells lining the small intestine, from which they enter into the bloodstream.

In some people, the small intestine does not produce enough of an enzyme called *lactase,* which is necessary to break down the disaccharide lactose found in milk products. People with this condition, called **lactose intolerance,** therefore cannot digest dairy foods properly. Lactose intolerance should not be confused with a milk allergy: people who are allergic to milk experience an immune reaction to the proteins found in cow's milk. Lactose intolerance is not caused by an immune response but rather by an enzyme deficiency.

Symptoms of lactose intolerance include intestinal gas, bloating, cramping, nausea, diarrhea, and discomfort after consuming dairy foods. Not everyone experiences these symptoms to the same extent. Some people can digest small amounts of dairy products, whereas others cannot tolerate any. Many people can tolerate specially formulated milk products that are low in lactose, whereas others take pills or use drops that contain the lactase enzyme when they eat dairy products. Some lactose-intolerant people can also digest yogurt and aged cheese, as the bacteria or molds used to ferment these products break down the lactose during processing.

The Liver Converts All Monosaccharides into Glucose

After they are absorbed into the bloodstream, monosaccharides travel to the liver, where any nonglucose monosaccharides are converted to glucose (Figure 3.7, step 5). If needed immediately for energy, the liver releases glucose into the bloodstream, which carries it throughout the body to provide energy to cells. If there is no immediate demand by the body for glucose, it is stored as glycogen in the liver and muscles. The liver can store 70 g (or 280 calories) of glycogen, and our muscles can normally

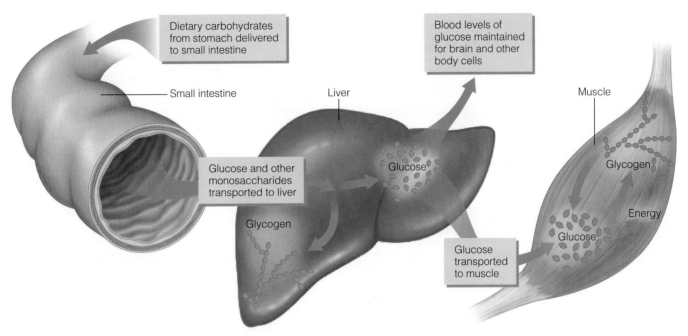

Dietary carbohydrates from stomach delivered to small intestine

Small intestine

Liver

Blood levels of glucose maintained for brain and other body cells

Muscle

Glucose and other monosaccharides transported to liver

Glucose

Glycogen

Glycogen

Glucose transported to muscle

Glucose

Glycogen

Energy

FIGURE 3.8 Glucose is stored as glycogen in both the liver and muscles. The glycogen stored in the liver maintains blood glucose between meals; muscle glycogen provides immediate energy to the muscle during exercise.

store about 120 g (or 480 calories) of glycogen. Between meals, the body draws on liver glycogen reserves to maintain blood glucose levels and support the needs of cells, including those of the brain, spinal cord, and red blood cells (**FIGURE 3.8**).

The glycogen stored in our muscles provides energy to the muscles during intense exercise. Endurance athletes can increase their storage of muscle glycogen from two to four times the normal amount through a process called *glycogen,* or *carbohydrate, loading* (see Chapter 10).

Fiber Is Excreted from the Large Intestine

We do not possess enzymes that can break down fiber. Thus, fiber passes through the small intestine undigested and enters the large intestine, or colon. Once in the large intestine, bacteria break down some previously undigested carbohydrates including soluble fiber, causing the production of gas and a few fatty acids. The cells of the large intestine use these fatty acids for energy. The fiber remaining in the colon adds bulk to stools and is excreted (Figure 3.7, step 6) in feces. In this way, fiber assists in maintaining bowel regularity.

> RECAP *Carbohydrate digestion starts in the mouth and continues in the small intestine. Glucose and other monosaccharides are absorbed into the bloodstream and travel to the liver, where nonglucose sugars are converted to glucose. Glucose is either used by the cells for energy or is converted to glycogen and stored in the liver and muscle for later use. Lactose intolerance results from the inability to digest lactose due to insufficient amounts of lactase.*

Insulin and Glucagon Regulate the Level of Glucose in Blood

Our bodies continually regulate the level of glucose in the blood within a fairly narrow range that meets the body's needs. Two hormones, insulin and glucagon, assist the body with maintenance of blood glucose. Specialized cells in the pancreas synthesize, store, and secrete both hormones.

When we eat a meal, our blood glucose level rises. But glucose in the blood cannot help nerve, muscle, and other cells function unless it can cross into them.

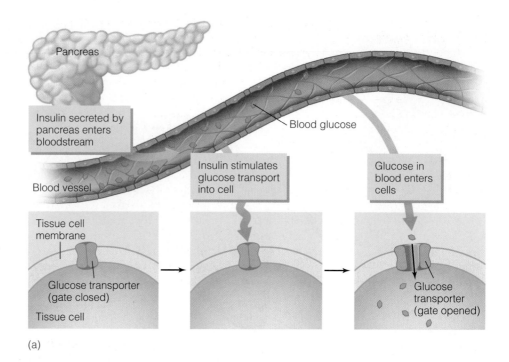

Pancreas

Insulin secreted by pancreas enters bloodstream

Blood glucose

Blood vessel

Insulin stimulates glucose transport into cell

Glucose in blood enters cells

Tissue cell membrane

Glucose transporter (gate closed)

Tissue cell

Glucose transporter (gate opened)

(a)

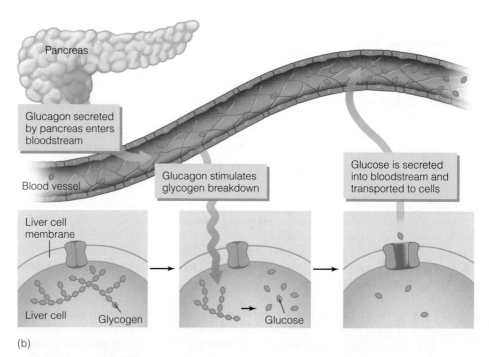

Pancreas

Glucagon secreted by pancreas enters bloodstream

Blood vessel

Glucagon stimulates glycogen breakdown

Glucose is secreted into bloodstream and transported to cells

Liver cell membrane

Liver cell   Glycogen

Glucose

(b)

FIGURE 3.9 Regulation of blood glucose by the hormones insulin and glucagon. (a) When blood glucose levels increase after a meal, the pancreas secretes insulin. Insulin opens gates in the cell membrane to allow the passage of glucose into the cell. (b) When blood glucose levels are low, the pancreas secretes glucagon. Glucagon enters liver cells, where it stimulates the breakdown of stored glycogen into glucose. This glucose is then released into the bloodstream.

insulin Hormone secreted by the beta cells of the pancreas in response to increased blood levels of glucose. Facilitates uptake of glucose by body cells.

Glucose molecules are too large to cross cell membranes independently. To get in, glucose needs assistance from the hormone **insulin,** which is secreted by the beta cells of the pancreas (FIGURE 3.9A). Insulin can be thought of as a key that opens a gate in the cell membrane and carries the glucose into the cell interior, where it can be used for energy. Insulin also stimulates the liver and muscles to take up glucose and store it as glycogen.

When you have not eaten for some period of time, your blood glucose levels decline. This decrease in blood glucose stimulates the alpha cells of the pancreas to secrete another hormone, **glucagon** (FIGURE 3.9B). Glucagon acts in an opposite way to insulin: it causes the liver to convert its stored glycogen into glucose, which is then secreted into the bloodstream and transported to the cells for energy. Glucagon also assists in the breakdown of body proteins to amino acids so the liver can stimulate *gluconeogenesis,* or the production of new glucose from amino acids.

Typically, the effects of insulin and glucagon balance each other to maintain blood glucose within a healthy range. If this balance is altered, it can lead to health conditions such as diabetes (see pages 92–94) or hypoglycemia. In **hypoglycemia,** blood glucose falls to lower-than-normal levels. One cause of hypoglycemia is excessive production of insulin, which lowers blood glucose too far. The symptoms usually appear about 1 to 3 hours after a meal and include nervousness, shakiness, anxiety, sweating, irritability, headache, weakness, and rapid or irregular heartbeat. Although many people believe they experience these symptoms, true hypoglycemia is rare. People with diabetes can develop hypoglycemia if they inject too much insulin or when they exercise and fail to eat enough carbohydrates. It can also be caused by a pancreatic tumor, liver infection, or other underlying disorder.

RECAP *Two hormones, insulin and glucagon, are involved in regulating blood glucose. Insulin lowers blood glucose levels by facilitating the entry of glucose into cells. Glucagon raises blood glucose levels by stimulating gluconeogenesis and the breakdown of glycogen stored in the liver. Hypoglycemia is a lower-than-normal blood glucose level.*

The Glycemic Index Shows How Foods Affect Our Blood Glucose Levels

The **glycemic index** refers to the potential of foods to raise blood glucose levels. Foods with a high glycemic index cause a sudden spike in blood glucose. This in turn triggers a surge in insulin, which may be followed by a dramatic drop in blood glucose. Foods with a low glycemic index cause low to moderate fluctuations in blood glucose. When foods are assigned a glycemic index value, they are often compared with the glycemic effect of pure glucose.

The glycemic index of a food is not always easy to predict. FIGURE 3.10 ranks certain foods according to their glycemic index. Do any of these rankings surprise you? Most people assume that foods containing simple sugars have a higher glycemic index than starches, but this is not always the case. For instance, compare the glycemic index for apples and instant potatoes. Although instant potatoes are a starchy food, they have a glycemic index value of 83, whereas the value for an apple is only 36! Nutritious, low-glycemic-index foods include beans and lentils, fresh vegetables, and whole-wheat bread.

The **glycemic load** of a food is the amount of carbohydrate it contains multiplied by its glycemic index. The glycemic load is thought by some nutrition experts to be a better indicator of the effect of a food on a person's glucose response, as it factors in both the glycemic index and the total grams of carbohydrate of the food that is consumed. For instance, raw carrots have a relatively high glycemic index but very little total carbohydrate and thus a low glycemic load. Thus, a serving of raw carrots is unlikely to cause a significant rise in glucose and insulin.

Why do we care about the glycemic load? Meals with a lower glycemic load are a better choice for someone with diabetes, for instance, because they will not trigger dramatic fluctuations in blood glucose. Even among healthy people, consuming a low-glycemic-load diet may reduce the risk of heart disease and colon cancer, because low-glycemic-load foods generally contain more fiber and help decrease fat levels in the blood.

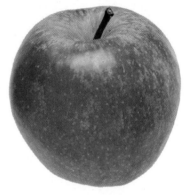

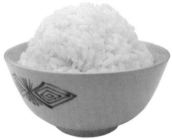

An apple (36) has a much lower glycemic index than a serving of white rice (56).

glucagon   Hormone secreted by the alpha cells of the pancreas in response to decreased blood levels of glucose. Causes breakdown of liver stores of glycogen into glucose.

hypoglycemia   A condition marked by blood glucose levels that are below normal fasting levels.

glycemic index   Rating of the potential of foods to raise blood glucose and insulin levels.

glycemic load   The amount of carbohydrate contained in a particular food, multiplied by its glycemic index.

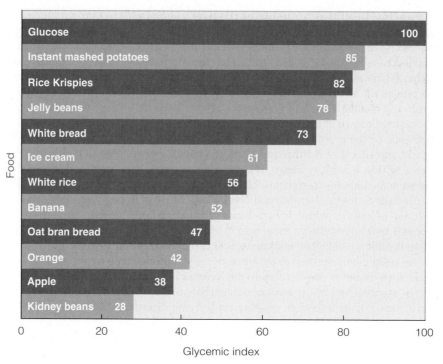

FIGURE 3.10 Glycemic index values for various foods as compared to pure glucose.
(Values derived from K. Foster-Powell, S. H. A. Holt, and J. C. Brand-Miller. 2002. International table of glycemic index and glycemic load values. *Am. J. Clin. Nutr.* 76: 5–56.)

> **RECAP** *The glycemic index is a value that indicates the potential of foods to raise blood glucose and insulin levels. The glycemic load of a food is the amount of carbohydrate it contains multiplied by its glycemic index.*

How Much Carbohydrate Should We Eat?

Carbohydrates are an important part of a balanced, healthy diet. The Recommended Dietary Allowance (RDA) for carbohydrate is based on the amount of glucose the brain uses.[5] The current RDA for carbohydrate for adults 19 years of age and older is 130 g of carbohydrate per day. It is important to emphasize that this RDA does not cover the amount of carbohydrate needed to support daily activities; it only covers the amount of carbohydrate needed to supply adequate glucose to the brain.

As we mentioned in Chapter 2, carbohydrates and the other macronutrients have been assigned an Acceptable Macronutrient Distribution Range (AMDR). This is the range of intake associated with a decreased risk of chronic diseases. The AMDR for carbohydrates is 45% to 65% of total energy intake. Table 3.1 compares the carbohydrate recommendations from the Institute of Medicine with the *Dietary Guidelines for Americans* related to carbohydrate-containing foods.[4,5] As you can see, the Institute of Medicine provides specific numeric recommendations, whereas the *Dietary Guidelines for Americans* are general suggestions about foods high in complex carbohydrates. Most health agencies agree that most of the carbohydrates you eat each day should be complex, fiber-rich, and unprocessed carbohydrates. Eating the recommended amount of whole grains and fruits and vegetables each day will ensure that you get enough fiber and other complex carbohydrates in your diet.

TABLE 3.1 Dietary Recommendations for Carbohydrates

Institute of Medicine Recommendations*	Dietary Guidelines for Americans†
Recommended Dietary Allowance (RDA) for adults 19 years of age and older is 130 g of carbohydrate per day.	Choose fiber-rich fruits, vegetables, and whole grains often.
The Acceptable Macronutrient Distribution Range (AMDR) for carbohydrate is 45% to 65% of total daily energy intake.	Choose and prepare foods and beverages with little added sugars or caloric sweeteners, such as amounts suggested by the USDA Food Guide and the DASH eating plan.
Added sugar intake should be 25% or less of total energy intake each day.	Reduce the incidence of dental caries by practicing good oral hygiene and consuming sugar- and starch-containing foods and beverages less frequently.

*Data from Dietary Reference Intakes for Energy, Carbohydrates, Fiber, Fat, Fatty Acids, Cholesterol, Protein, and Amino Acids (Macronutrients). © 2005, National Academy of Sciences, courtesy of the National Academies Press, Washington, DC.

†U.S. Department of Health and Human Services (USDHHS) and U.S. Department of Agriculture (USDA). 2005. *Dietary Guidelines for Americans, 2005*. 6th ed. Washington, DC: U.S. Government Printing Office, www.healthierus.gov/dietaryguidelines.

RECAP *The RDA for carbohydrate is 130 g per day; this amount is only sufficient to supply adequate glucose to the brain. The AMDR for carbohydrate is 45% to 65% of total energy intake.*

Most Americans Eat Too Much Refined Carbohydrate

The average carbohydrate intake in the United States is approximately 50%. For some people, almost half of this amount consists of simple sugars. Where does all this sugar come from? Some sugar comes from healthful food sources, such as fruits and milk. Some comes from foods made with refined grains, such as soft white breads, saltine crackers, and pastries. Much of the rest comes from *added sugars*. **Added sugars** are defined as sugars and syrups that are added to foods during processing or preparation.[5] For example, many processed foods include high-fructose corn syrup, an added sugar.

The most common source of added sugars in the U.S. diet is sweetened soft drinks; we drink an average of 40 gallons per person each year. Consider that one 12-oz sugared cola contains 38.5 g of sugar, or almost 10 teaspoons. If you drink the average amount, you are consuming more than 16,420 g of sugar (about 267 cups) each year! Other common sources of added sugars include cookies, cakes, pies, fruit drinks, fruit punches, and candy, but even many nondessert items, such as some peanut butters, yogurts, and even salad dressings, contain added sugars.

If you want a quick way to figure out the amount of sugar in a processed food, check the Nutrition Facts Panel for the line that identifies "Sugars." You'll notice that the amount of sugar in a serving is identified in grams. Divide the grams by 4 to get teaspoons. For instance, one national brand of yogurt contains 21 g of sugar in a half-cup serving. That's more than 5 teaspoons of sugar! Doing this mental math before you buy may help you choose between different versions of the same food.

Added sugars are not chemically different from naturally occurring sugars. However, foods and beverages with added sugars have lower levels of vitamins, minerals, and fiber than fruits and other foods that naturally contain simple sugars. That's why most healthcare organizations recommend that we limit our consumption of added sugars.

To prevent weight gain and tooth decay, many people choose sugar-free versions of soft drinks, jams, flavored yogurts, desserts, chewing gum, and other foods. These products are typically made with alternative sweeteners. The accompanying Highlight on pages 82–83 identifies the most common alternative sweeteners in use today and examines the controversy about their safety.

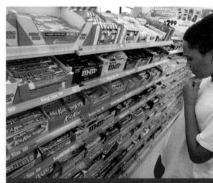

Foods with added sugars, like candy, have lower levels of vitamins, minerals, and fiber than foods that naturally contain simple sugars.

added sugars Sugars and syrups that are added to food during processing or preparation.

HIGHLIGHT

What's the Story on Alternative Sweeteners?

Most of us love sweets but want to avoid the extra calories and tooth decay that go along with them. That's why foods with alternative sweeteners have become staples in the diets of many Americans. But what are alternative sweeteners, and are they safe to consume?

Remember that all carbohydrates contain 4 kcal of energy per gram. Because sweeteners such as sucrose, fructose, honey, and brown sugar contribute calories (or energy), they are called **nutritive sweeteners.** Other nutritive sweeteners include the *sugar alcohols* such as mannitol, sorbitol, isomalt, and xylitol. These are popular in sugar-free gums and mints, because they do not support the bacteria that cause tooth decay. However, at 2 to 4 kcal of energy per gram, they are not calorie-free.

Alternative Sweeteners Are Non-Nutritive

A number of other products have been developed to sweeten foods without promoting tooth decay and weight gain. As these products provide little or no energy, they are called **non-nutritive,** or *alternative,* **sweeteners.**

Limited Use of Alternative Sweeteners Is Not Harmful

Research has shown alternative sweeteners to be safe for adults, children, and individuals with diabetes. Women who are pregnant should discuss the use of alternative sweeteners with their healthcare provider. In general, it appears safe for pregnant women to consume alternative sweeteners in amounts within the Food and Drug Administration (FDA) guidelines.[6] These amounts, known as the **acceptable daily intake** (ADI), are estimates of the amount of a sweetener that someone can consume each day over a lifetime without adverse effects. The estimates are based on studies conducted on laboratory animals, and they include a 100-fold safety factor: actual intake by humans is typically well below the ADI.

Many Alternative Sweeteners Are in Our Foods

Alternative sweeteners available on the market today include saccharin, acesulfame-K, aspartame, sucralose, and neotame.

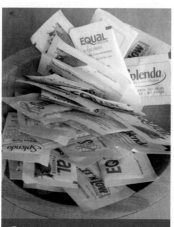

Contrary to recent reports claiming severe health consequences related to consumption of alternative sweeteners, major health agencies have determined that these products are safe for us to consume.

Discovered in the late 1800s, *saccharin* is about 300 times sweeter than sucrose. Evidence to suggest that saccharin may cause bladder tumors in rats surfaced in the 1970s, but more than 20 years of scientific research has shown that saccharin is not related to bladder cancer in humans. Based on this evidence, in May 2000 the National Toxicology Program of the U.S. government removed saccharin from its list of products that may cause cancer. Saccharin is used in foods and beverages and as a tabletop sweetener. It is sold as Sweet n' Low in the United States.

Acesulfame-K (or acesulfame potassium) is marketed under the names Sunette and Sweet One. It is a calorie-free sweetener that is 175 times sweeter than sugar. It is used to sweeten gums, candies, beverages, instant tea, coffee, gelatins, and puddings. The taste of acesulfame-K does not change when it is heated, so it can be used in cooking.

Aspartame, also called Equal and NutraSweet, is one of the most popular alternative sweeteners currently in use. Although aspartame contains 4 kcal of energy per gram, it is 200 times sweeter than sucrose, so only small amounts are necessary. Thus, it ends up contributing almost no energy. A significant amount of research has been done to test the safety of aspartame: Table 3.2 shows how many servings of aspartame-sweetened foods have to be consumed to exceed the ADI. Notice, however, that children who consume many diet sodas and other aspartame-sweetened products could potentially exceed this amount. People with the disease *phenylketonuria (PKU)* should not consume aspartame at all. PKU is a genetic disorder that prevents the breakdown of the amino acid phenylalanine, a component of aspartame. In people with PKU, phenylalanine builds up in the tissues of the body and causes irreversible brain damage. Thus, people with PKU must follow a phenylalanine-limited diet.

The FDA has recently approved the use of *sucralose* as an alternative sweetener. Marketed under the brand name Splenda, it is 600 times sweeter than sucrose and is stable when heated, so it can be used in cooking. It has been approved for use in many foods, including chewing gum, salad dressings, beverages, gelatin and pudding

What's the Story on Alternative Sweeteners? *(continued)*

products, canned fruits, frozen dairy desserts, and baked goods.

The FDA has also recently approved *neotame* as an alternative sweetener. It is 7,000 to 13,000 times sweeter than sugar and can be used in many foods such as beverages, dairy products, frozen desserts, baked goods, and chewing gums.

TABLE 3.2 The Amount of Food that a 50-lb Child and a 150-lb Adult Would Have to Consume Each Day to Exceed the ADI for Aspartame

Food	50-Pound Child	150-Pound Adult
12 fl. oz carbonated soft drink	7	20
8 fl. oz powdered soft drink	11	34
4 fl. oz gelatin dessert	14	42
Packets of tabletop sweetener	32	97

Source: Adapted from International Food Information Council. 2003. *Food Safety and Nutrition Information. Sweeteners. Everything You Need to Know About Aspartame.* Reprinted with permission.

Using Artificial Sweeteners Does Not Necessarily Prevent Weight Gain

We keep emphasizing throughout this book that to prevent weight gain, you need to balance the total number of calories you consume against the number you expend. If you're expending an average of 2,000 calories a day and you consume about 2,000 calories a day, then you'll neither gain nor lose weight. But if, in addition to your normal diet, you regularly indulge in "treats," you're bound to gain weight, whether those "treats" are sugar-free or not. Consider the calorie count of these artificially sweetened foods:

One piece of sugar-free hard candy	22 calories
One cup of nonfat chocolate frozen yogurt with artificial sweetener	199 calories
One sugar-free chocolate-chip cookie (24 g)	100 calories
One serving of no-sugar-added hot cocoa	55 calories

Do the number of calories in these foods surprise you? Remember, sugar-free doesn't mean calorie-free. Make it a habit to check the Nutrition Facts Panel to find out how much energy is really in your food!

The Atkins Diet, the Sugar Busters diet, and many other diet plans blame sugar for many of our health problems, from tooth decay to hyperactivity to obesity. Does sugar deserve its bad reputation? Let's examine the facts behind the accusations.

Sugar Causes Tooth Decay

Simple carbohydrates, both naturally occurring and in processed foods, play a role in dental problems because the bacteria that cause tooth decay thrive on them. These bacteria produce acids that eat away at tooth enamel and can eventually cause cavities and gum disease (FIGURE 3.11). Eating sticky foods that adhere to teeth, such as caramels, crackers, sugary cereals, and licorice, and sipping sweetened beverages over a period of time increase the risk of tooth decay. This means that people shouldn't slowly sip soda or juice and that babies should not be put to sleep with a bottle unless it contains water. As we have seen, even breast milk contains sugar, which can slowly drip onto the baby's gums. As a result, infants should not routinely be allowed to fall asleep at the breast.

To reduce your risk for tooth decay, brush your teeth after each meal and especially after drinking sugary drinks and eating candy. Drinking fluoridated water and using a fluoride toothpaste also will help protect your teeth.

There Is No Proven Link between Sugar and Hyperactivity in Children

Although many people believe that eating sugar causes hyperactivity and other behavioral problems in children, there is little scientific evidence to support this claim. Some children actually become less active shortly after a high-sugar meal! However, it is important to emphasize that most studies of sugar and children's behavior have only looked at the effects of sugar a few hours after ingestion. We know very little about the long-term effects of sugar intake on the behavior of children. Behavioral

nutritive sweeteners Sweeteners such as sucrose, fructose, honey, and brown sugar that contribute calories (or energy).

non-nutritive sweeteners Also called *alternative sweeteners;* manufactured sweeteners that provide little or no energy.

acceptable daily intake (ADI) An estimate made by the Food and Drug Administration of the amount of a non-nutritive sweetener that someone can consume each day over a lifetime without adverse effects.

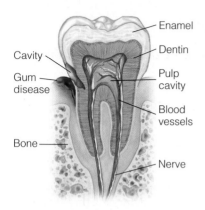

FIGURE 3.11 Eating simple carbohydrates can cause an increase in cavities and gum disease. This is because bacteria in the mouth consume simple carbohydrates present on the teeth and gums and produce acids, which eat away at these tissues.

and learning problems are complex issues, most likely caused by a multitude of factors. Because of this complexity, the Institute of Medicine has stated that overall, there currently does not appear to be enough evidence to suggest that eating too much sugar causes hyperactivity or other behavioral problems in children.[5] Thus, a Tolerable Upper Intake Level for sugar has not been set.

High Sugar Intake Can Lead to Unhealthful Levels of Blood Lipids

Many low-carbohydrate diet plans claim that North Americans' overconsumption of simple sugars is partly responsible for our high rates of heart disease. But is this claim valid? There is research evidence suggesting that consuming a diet high in simple sugars can lead to unhealthful changes in blood lipids. You will learn more about blood lipids (including cholesterol and lipoproteins) in Chapter 4. Briefly, higher intakes of simple sugars are associated with *increases* in blood lipids that contribute to heart disease and *decreases* in blood lipids that are considered protective against heart disease.[5,7] Although there is not enough scientific evidence at the present time to state with confidence that eating a diet high in simple sugars causes heart disease, it is prudent for those at risk for heart disease to eat a diet low in simple sugars.

High Sugar Intake Does Not Cause Diabetes but May Contribute to Obesity

There is no scientific evidence that eating a diet high in sugar causes diabetes. In fact, studies examining the relationship between sugar intake and type 2 diabetes report either no association between sugar intake and diabetes or a decreased risk of diabetes with increased sugar intake.[8] However, people who have diabetes need to moderate their intake of sugar and closely monitor their blood glucose levels.

To date, there is no evidence to prove that sugar intake causes obesity; however, some studies suggest that there may be a link, especially in children. For example, a recent study found that overweight children consumed more sugared soft drinks than did children of normal weight.[9] Another study found that for every extra sugared soft drink consumed by a child per day, the risk of obesity increases by 60%.[10] We do know that if you consume more energy than you expend, you will gain weight. It makes intuitive sense that people who consume extra energy from high-sugar foods are at risk for obesity, just as people who consume extra energy from fat gain weight. In addition to the increased potential for obesity, another major concern about high-sugar diets is that they are inadequate in nutrients critical to maintain our health. Although we cannot state with certainty that consuming a high-sugar diet causes obesity, it is important to optimize your intake of nutrient-dense foods and limit added sugars.

> RECAP *Added sugars include sucrose, high-fructose corn syrup, and other sugars and syrups added to foods during processing or preparation. Sugar causes tooth decay but does not appear to cause hyperactivity in children. Higher intakes of simple sugars are associated with increases in blood lipids that are associated with heart disease. Diets high in sugar cause unhealthful changes in blood sugar but do not cause diabetes. The relationship between added sugars and obesity is controversial.*

Most Americans Eat Too Little Fiber-Rich Carbohydrate

Do you get enough fiber-rich carbohydrates each day? If you are like most people in the United States, you eat only about 2 servings of fruits or vegetables each day; this is far below the amount recommended in MyPyramid. Do you eat whole grains and legumes every day? Many people eat plenty of breads, pastas, and cereals, but most do not consistently choose whole-grain products. As we explained earlier, whole-grain foods have a lower glycemic index than simple carbohydrates; thus, they prompt a more gradual release of insulin and result in less severe fluctuations in both insulin and glucose. Whole-grain foods also provide more nutrients and fiber than foods made with enriched flour.

Table 3.3 defines terms commonly used on nutrition labels for breads and cereals. Read the label for the bread you eat—does it list *whole-wheat flour* or just *wheat flour?* Although most labels for breads and cereals list wheat flour as the first ingredient, this term actually refers to enriched white flour, which is made when wheat flour is processed. Don't be fooled—becoming an educated consumer will help you select whole grains instead of processed foods.

We Need at Least 25 Grams of Fiber Daily

How much fiber do we need? The Adequate Intake for fiber is 25 g per day for women and 38 g per day for men, or 14 g of fiber for every 1,000 kcal per day that a person eats.[5] Most people in the United States eat only 12 to 18 g of fiber each day, getting only half of the fiber they need. Although fiber supplements are available, it is best to get fiber from food because foods contain additional nutrients such as vitamins and minerals.

Eating the amounts of whole grains, vegetables, fruits, nuts, and legumes recommended in MyPyramid will ensure that you eat adequate fiber. FIGURE 3.12 lists some common foods and their fiber content. Think about how you can design your own diet to include high-fiber foods.

It is also important to drink more water as you increase your fiber intake, as fiber binds with water to soften stools. Inadequate water intake with a high-fiber diet can actually result in hard, dry stools that are difficult to pass through the colon.

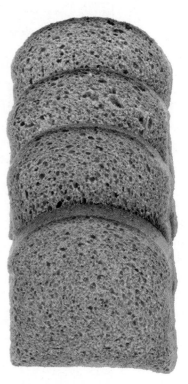

Whole-grain foods provide more nutrients and fiber than foods made with enriched flour.

TABLE 3.3 Terms Used to Describe Grains and Cereals on Nutrition Labels

Term	Definition
Brown bread	Bread that may or may not be made using whole-grain flour. Many brown breads are made with white flour with brown (caramel) coloring added.
Enriched (or fortified) flour or grain	Enriching or fortifying grains involves adding nutrients back to refined foods. In order to use this term in the United States, a minimum amount of iron, folate, niacin, thiamin, and riboflavin must be added. Other nutrients can also be added.
Refined flour or grain	Refining involves removing the coarse parts of food products; refined wheat flour is flour in which all but the internal part of the kernel has been removed. Refined sugar is made by removing the outer portions of sugar beets or sugarcane.
Stone ground	Refers to a milling process in which limestone is used to grind any grain. Stone ground does not mean that bread is made with whole grain, as refined flour can be stone ground.
Unbleached flour	Flour that has been refined but not bleached; it is very similar to refined white flour in texture and nutritional value.
Wheat flour	Any flour made from wheat; includes white flour, unbleached flour, and whole-wheat flour.
White flour	Flour that has been bleached and refined. All-purpose flour, cake flour, and enriched baking flour are all types of white flour.
Whole-grain flour	A grain that is not refined; whole grains are milled in their complete form, with only the husk removed.
Whole-wheat flour	An unrefined, whole-grain flour made from whole wheat kernels.

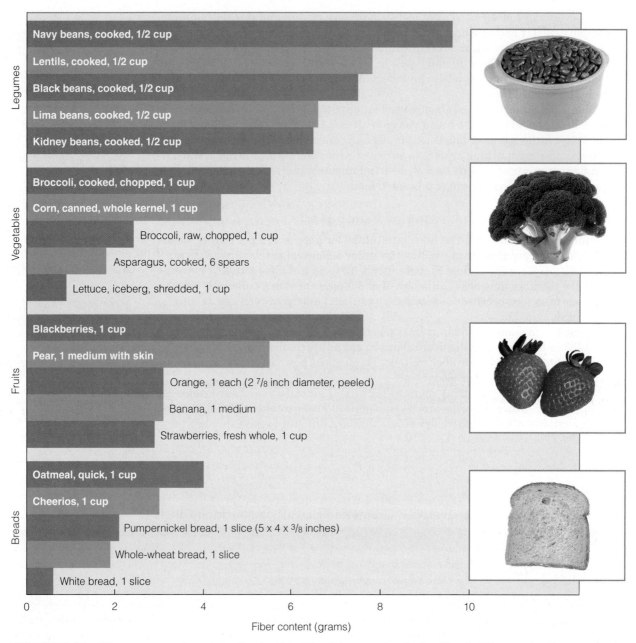

FIGURE 3.12 Fiber content of common foods. *Note:* The Adequate Intake for fiber is 25 g per day for women and 38 g per day for men.
Source: U.S. Department of Agriculture, Agricultural Research Service. 2007. USDA National Nutrient Database for Standard Reference, Release 20. Nutrient Data Laboratory Home Page, www.ars.usda.gov/ba/bhnrc/ndl.

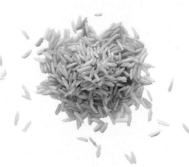

Brown rice is a good food source of dietary fiber.

Can you eat too much fiber? Excessive fiber consumption can lead to problems such as:

- intestinal gas, bloating, and constipation.
- dehydration. Because fiber binds with water, it causes the body to eliminate more water, so a very-high-fiber diet could result in dehydration.
- reduced absorption of certain nutrients. Because fiber binds many vitamins and minerals, a high-fiber diet can reduce our absorption of important nutrients such as iron, zinc, and calcium.
- malnutrition in groups such as children, some elderly, the chronically ill, and other at-risk populations. In these groups excess fiber intake can lead to malnu-

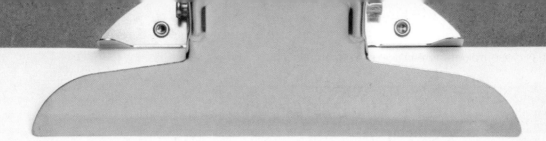

GAME PLAN

Tips for Increasing Your Fiber Intake One Step at a Time

Gradually increasing your fiber intake gives your gastrointestinal organs time to adjust to the increased bulk in your diet. This is especially important if you've been eating a very-low-fiber diet (fewer than 10 g of fiber per day) for many years. Here's how to increase your fiber intake one step at a time:

Step 1.

Incorporate just one of the strategies listed below each day for 1 week.

Step 2.

Make sure you drink plenty of fluids. The best way to make sure you're well hydrated is to track your output: if your urine is clear to pale yellow, you're getting enough fluid.

Step 3.

Keep a record of your total daily fiber intake and of how you're feeling.

Step 4.

If you adjust well to the increased fiber, then go ahead and incorporate two strategies a day the following week.

Step 5.

Continue until you reach your optimal daily fiber intake.

Here are some strategies to choose from:

❑ Switch from a low-fiber breakfast cereal to one that has at least 4 g of fiber per serving.

❑ Switch to whole-grain bread for morning toast or lunchtime sandwiches. Two slices of whole-grain bread provide 4–6 g of fiber. (Check the Nutrition Facts Panel for the whole-grain bread you're using.)

❑ For a midmorning snack, mix 1–2 tablespoons of bran or whole ground flaxseed meal (4 g of fiber) into a cup of lowfat yogurt. These products are available at most health-food stores and many large supermarkets.

❑ Instead of chips with your sandwich, have a side of carrot sticks or celery sticks (approximately 2 g of fiber per serving).

❑ For an afternoon snack, choose an apple or pear, with the skin on (approximately 5 g of fiber).

❑ Eat one serving of beans or other legumes at dinner (approximately 6 g of fiber).

❑ Don't forget the vegetables! A cup of boiled chopped okra or beet greens provides about 4 g of fiber, and acorn squash a whopping 9 g! Raw veggies are fiber-rich, too, so a large salad is a good source of fiber.

❑ For dessert, switch from cookies, cake, or ice cream to a serving of fresh, frozen, or dried fruit. A half cup of fresh or frozen blackberries or raspberries provides 4–5 g of fiber, and a single ounce of dried mixed fruit (prunes, apricots, etc.) provides 2 g.

❑ For an evening snack, try a mixture of popcorn, peanuts, and raisins: one cup of popcorn (1 g of fiber) with ¼ cup of peanuts (3 g) and ¼ cup of raisins (2 g) provides a total of 6 g of fiber.

If you incorporate one of these strategies and experience diarrhea, constipation, or excess intestinal gas that causes discomfort, then your body may not be adjusting well to the increased fiber. Back off a little, perhaps by cutting the serving size or incorporating a strategy only every other day. Try this for 2 weeks, then try to increase gradually again.

NUTRI-CASE HANNAH

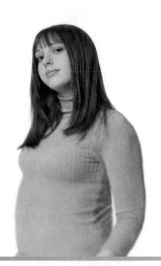

" Last night, my mom called and said she'd be late getting home from work, so I made dinner. I was tired after my classes and I had a lot of homework to get to, so I kept it simple. I made us each a cheeseburger—no bun!—served with frozen French fries and some carrot sticks with guacamole on the side. We both had a cola, too. Later that night, though, when I was studying, I got a snack attack and raided a package of sugar-free cookies. I ate maybe three or four, but I didn't think it was a big deal because they're sugar-free. Then when I checked the package label this morning, I found out that each cookie has 90 calories! It bummed me out—until those cookies, I'd been doing pretty well on my new low-carb diet!"

Hannah takes public transportation to the community college she attends, and does not engage in regular physical activity. Without analyzing the precise grams of carbohydrate or number of calories in Hannah's meal, would you agree that before the cookies she'd been "doing pretty well" on her low-carb diet? In other words, would you describe her meal as low carb? Would you characterize her meal as low in energy? About how many grams of dietary fiber do you think were in the meal?

trition because they feel full before they have eaten enough to provide adequate energy and nutrients.

Do you want to increase the amount of fiber you consume each day? If so, it's important to go slowly, giving your system time to adjust to the increased bulk in your new diet. Otherwise, you might experience some of the symptoms of excessive fiber consumption described earlier. To avoid stressing your body, check out the Game Plan on page 87 for tips on increasing your fiber intake one step at a time.

Shopper's Guide: Hunting for Complex Carbohydrates

FIGURE 3.13 compares the food and fiber content of two diets: one high in fiber-rich carbohydrates and the other high in refined carbohydrates. Here are some hints for selecting healthful carbohydrate sources:

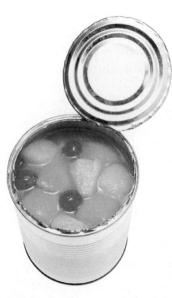

Check to make sure that canned fruits are packed in their own juices and not syrup.

- Select breads and cereals that are made with whole grains such as wheat, oats, barley, and rye (make sure the label says "whole" before the word *grain*). Choose foods that have at least 2 or 3 g of fiber per serving.
- Buy fresh fruits and vegetables whenever possible. When appropriate, eat foods such as potatoes, apples, and pears with the skin left on.
- Frozen vegetables and fruits can be a healthful alternative when fresh produce is not available. Check frozen selections to make sure there is no extra sugar or salt added.
- Be careful when buying canned fruits and vegetables, as many are high in sodium and added sugar. Foods that are packed in their own juice are more healthful than those packed in syrup.
- Eat legumes frequently; every day if possible. Canned or fresh beans, peas, and lentils are excellent sources of complex carbohydrates, fiber, vitamins, and minerals. Add them to soups, casseroles, and other recipes—it is an easy way to eat more of them. If you are trying to consume less sodium, rinse canned beans to remove extra salt or choose low-sodium alternatives.

High Fiber-Rich Carbohydrate Diet	High Refined Carbohydrate Diet

Breakfast:
1 1/2 cups Cheerios
1 cup skim milk
2 slices whole-wheat toast
  with 1 tbsp. light margarine
1 medium banana
8 fl. oz fresh orange juice

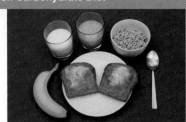

Breakfast:
1 1/2 cups Fruit Loops cereal
1 cup skim milk
2 slices white bread toasted,
  with 1 tbsp. light margarine
8 fl. oz fresh orange juice

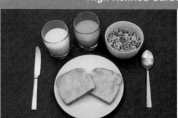

Lunch:
8 fl. oz low-fat blueberry
  yogurt
Tuna sandwich (2 slices
  whole-wheat bread; 1/4 cup
  tuna packed in water,
  drained; 1 tsp. Dijon mustard;
  2 tsp. low-calorie
  mayonnaise)
2 carrots, raw, with peel
1 cup raw cauliflower
1 tbsp. peppercorn ranch
  salad dressing
  (for dipping vegetables)

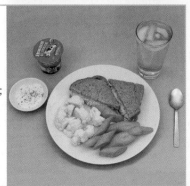

Lunch:
McDonald's Quarter
  Pounder—1 sandwich
1 large order French fries
16 fl. oz cola beverage
30 jelly beans

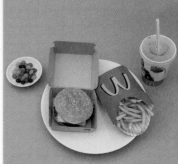

Snack:
3 cups nonfat popcorn

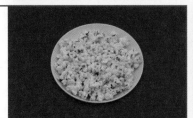

Snack:
1 cinnamon raisin bagel (3 1/2 -
  inch diameter)
2 tbsp. cream cheese
8 fl. oz low-fat strawberry
  yogurt

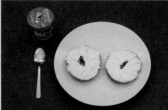

Dinner:
1/2 chicken breast roasted
1 cup brown rice, cooked
1 cup cooked broccoli
Spinach salad
(1 cup chopped spinach,
  1 whole egg white, 2 slices
  turkey bacon, 3 cherry
  tomatoes, and 2 tbsp. creamy
  bacon salad dressing)
2 baked apples (no added
  sugar)

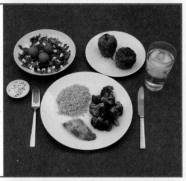

Dinner:
1 whole chicken breast,
  roasted
2 cups mixed green salad
2 tbsp. ranch salad dressing
1 serving macaroni and
  cheese
12 fl. oz cola beverage
Cheesecake (1/9 of cake)

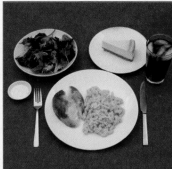

(No Snack)

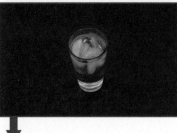

Late-Night Snack:
2 cups gelatin dessert
  (cherry flavored)
3 raspberry oatmeal no-fat
  cookies

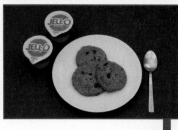

Nutrient Analysis:
2150 kcal
60% of energy from carbohydrates
22% of energy from fat
18% of energy from protein
38 grams of dietary fiber

Nutrient Analysis:
4012 kcal
60% of energy from carbohydrates
25% of energy from fat
15% of energy from protein
18.5 grams of dietary fiber

FIGURE 3.13 Comparison of two high-carbohydrate diets. *Note:* Diets were analyzed using Food Processor Version 7.21 (ESHA Research, Salem, OR).

NUTRITION LABEL ACTIVITY

Recognizing Carbohydrates on the Label

Figure 3.14 shows labels for two breakfast cereals. The cereal on the left (a) is processed and sweetened, whereas the one on the right (b) is a whole-grain product with no added sugar. Which is the better breakfast choice? Fill in the label data below to find out!

- **Check the center of each label to locate the amount of total carbohydrate.**

  For the sweetened cereal, the total carbohydrate is _26_ g.

  For the whole-grain cereal, the total carbohydrate is _27_ g for a smaller serving size.

- **Look at the information listed as subgroups under Total Carbohydrate. The label for the sweetened cereal lists all types of carbohydrates in the cereal: dietary fiber, sugars, and other carbohydrate (which refers to starches). Notice that this cereal contains 13 g of sugar—half of its total carbohydrates.**

  How many grams of dietary fiber does the sweetened cereal contain? _1_

- **The label for the whole-grain cereal lists only 1 g of sugar, which is less than 4% of its total carbohydrates.**

  How many grams of dietary fiber does the whole-grain cereal contain? _4_

  Notice that on this label there is no amount listed for starches (or "Other Carbohydrate"). In this case, the amount of starch is the difference between the 27 g of total carbohydrate and the sum of dietary fiber plus sugars.

  How much starch is in the whole-grain cereal? _22_

  (Hint: Plug in the numbers: 27 g of total carbohydrate – _4_ g of dietary fiber plus sugars = _22_ g of starch.)

- **Now look at the percent values listed to the right of the Total Carbohydrate section. For both cereals (without milk), their percent contribution to daily carbohydrate is 9%. This does not mean that 9% of the calories in these cereals come from carbohydrates. Instead, this percentage refers to the Daily Values listed at the bottom of each label. For a person who eats 2,000 calories, the recommended amount of carbohydrate each day is 300 g. One serving of each cereal contains 26–27 g, which is about 9% of 300 g.**

(Answers can be found at the end of this chapter.)

Which cereal should you choose? Check the ingredients list for the sweetened cereal. Remember that the ingredients are listed in the order from highest to lowest amount. The second and third ingredients listed are sugar and brown sugar, and the corn and oat flours are not whole-grain flours. Now look at the ingredients for the other cereal—it contains whole-grain oats. Although the sweetened product is enriched with more B vitamins, iron, and zinc, the whole-grain cereal packs 4 g of fiber per serving and contains no added sugars. Overall, it is a more healthful choice.

Nutrition Facts

Serving Size: 3/4 cup (30g)
Servings Per Package: About 14

Amount Per Serving	Cereal	Cereal With 1/2 Cup Skim Milk
Calories	120	160
Calories from Fat	15	15

	% Daily Value**	
Total Fat 1.5g*	2%	2%
Saturated Fat 0g	0%	0%
Trans Fat 0g		
Polyunsaturated Fat 0g		
Monounsaturated Fat 0.5g		
Cholesterol 0mg	0%	1%
Sodium 220mg	9%	12%
Potassium 40mg	1%	7%
Total Carbohydrate 26g	9%	11%
Dietary Fiber 1g	3%	3%
Sugars 13g		
Other Carbohydrate 12g		
Protein 1g		
Vitamin A	0%	4%
Vitamin C	0%	2%
Calcium	0%	15%
Iron	25%	25%
Thiamin	25%	25%
Riboflavin	25%	35%
Niacin	25%	25%
Vitamin B6	25%	25%
Folate	25%	25%
Zinc	25%	25%

* Amount in cereal. One-half cup skim milk contributes an additional 65mg sodium, 6g total carbohydrate (6g sugars), and 4g protein.

** Percent Daily Values are based on a 2,000 calorie diet. Your daily values may be higher or lower depending on your calorie needs:

	Calories	2,000	2,500
Total Fat	Less than	65g	80g
Sat. Fat	Less than	20g	25g
Cholesterol	Less than	300mg	300mg
Sodium	Less than	2,400mg	2,400mg
Potassium		3,500mg	3,500mg
Total Carbohydrate		300g	375g
Dietary fiber		25g	30g

Calories per gram:		2,500
Fat 9 • Carbohydrate 4 • Protein 4		

INGREDIENTS: Corn Flour, Sugar, Brown Sugar, Partially Hydrogenated Vegetable Oil (Soybean and Cottonseed), Oat Flour, Salt, Sodium Citrate (a flavoring agent), Flavor added [Natural & Artificial Flavor, Strawberry Juice Concentrate, Malic Acid (a flavoring agent)], Niacinamide (Niacin), Zinc Oxide, Reduced Iron, Red 40, Yellow 5, Red 3, Yellow 6, Pyridoxine Hydrochloride (Vitamin B6), Riboflavin (Vitamin B2), Thiamin Mononitrate (Vitamin B1), Folic Acid (Folate) and Blue 1.

(a)

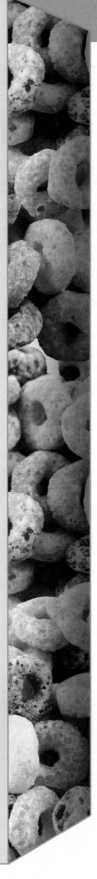

Nutrition Facts

Serving Size: 1/2 cup dry (40g)
Servings Per Container: 13

Amount Per Serving	
Calories	150
Calories from Fat	25

	% Daily Value*
Total Fat 3g	5%
Saturated Fat 0.5g	2%
Trans Fat 0g	
Polyunsaturated Fat 1g	
Monounsaturated Fat 1g	
Cholesterol 0mg	0%
Sodium 0mg	0%
Total Carbohydrate 27g	9%
Dietary Fiber 4g	15%
Soluble Fiber 2g	
Insoluble Fiber 2g	
Sugars 1g	
Protein 5g	
Vitamin A	0%
Vitamin C	0%
Calcium	0%
Iron	10%

* Percent Daily Values are based on a 2,000 calorie diet. Your daily values may be higher or lower depending on your calorie needs:

	Calories	2,000	2,500
Total Fat	Less than	65g	80g
Sat. Fat	Less than	20g	25g
Cholesterol	Less than	300mg	300mg
Sodium	Less than	2,400mg	2,400mg
Total Carbohydrate		300g	375g
Dietary fiber		25g	30g

INGREDIENTS: 100% Natural Whole Grain Rolled Oats.

(b)

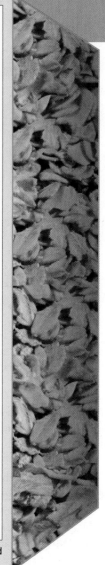

FIGURE 3.14 Labels for two breakfast cereals: (a) sweetened cereal, (b) whole-grain cereal.

Try the Nutrition Label Activity on the next page to learn how to recognize various carbohydrates on food labels. Armed with this knowledge, you are now ready to make more healthful food choices.

> RECAP *The Adequate Intake for fiber is 25 g per day for women and 38 g per day for men. Most Americans eat only half of the fiber they need each day. Foods high in fiber include whole grains and cereals, fruits, and vegetables. The more processed the food, the less fiber it is likely to contain.*

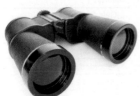

HEALTHWATCH

What Is Diabetes, and Why Has It Become a Public Health Concern?

Diabetes is a chronic disease in which the body can no longer regulate glucose within normal limits, and blood glucose levels become dangerously high or fall dangerously low. These fluctuations in glucose injure tissues throughout the body. If not controlled, diabetes can lead to blindness, seizures, kidney failure, nerve disease, amputations, stroke, and heart disease. In severe cases, it can be fatal.

Approximately 16 million people in the United States—6% of the total population—are diagnosed with diabetes. It is speculated that another 5 million people have the disease but don't know it. FIGURE 3.15 shows the percentage of adults with diabetes from various ethnic groups in the United States.[11] As you can see, diabetes is more common in African Americans, Mexican Americans, American Indians, and Alaska Natives. It is also more common in older adults than in younger adults or children.

There are two main forms of diabetes: type 1 and type 2. Some women develop a third form, *gestational diabetes,* during pregnancy; we will discuss this in more detail in Chapter 11.

diabetes   A chronic disease in which the body can no longer regulate glucose.

FIGURE 3.15   The percentage of adults from various ethnic and racial groups with type 2 diabetes.
(Data from the National Diabetes Information Clearinghouse [NDIC]. 2005. National Diabetes Statistics. National Institutes of Health [NIH] Publication No. 06-3892. http://diabetes.niddk.nih.gov/dm/pubs/statistics/index.htm. Accessed November 2007.)

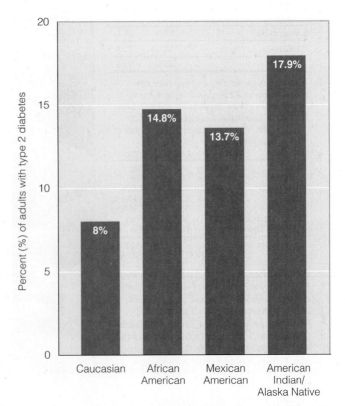

In Type 1 Diabetes, the Body Does Not Produce Enough Insulin

Approximately 10% of people with diabetes have **type 1 diabetes,** in which the body cannot produce enough insulin. When people with type 1 diabetes eat a meal and their blood glucose rises, the pancreas is unable to secrete insulin in response. Glucose levels soar, and the body tries to expel the excess glucose by excreting it in the urine. In fact, the medical term for the disease is *diabetes mellitus* (from the Greek *diabainein,* "to pass through," and Latin *mellitus,* "sweetened with honey"), and frequent urination is one of its warning signs (see Table 3.4 for other symptoms). If blood glucose levels are not controlled, a person with type 1 diabetes will become confused and lethargic and have trouble breathing. This is because the person's brain is not getting enough glucose to function properly. Uncontrolled diabetes can lead to ketoacidosis, which was discussed earlier; left untreated, the ultimate result is coma and death.

The cause of type 1 diabetes is unknown, but it may be an *autoimmune disease.* This means that the body's immune system attacks and destroys its own tissues: in this case, the beta cells of the pancreas.

Most cases of type 1 diabetes are diagnosed in adolescents around 10 to 14 years of age, although the disease can appear in younger children and adults. It occurs more often in families, so siblings and children of those with type 1 diabetes are at greater risk.

The only treatment for type 1 diabetes is daily insulin injections. Insulin is a hormone composed of protein, so it would be digested in the intestine if taken as a pill. Individuals with type 1 diabetes must monitor their blood glucose levels closely, using a *glucometer,* and administer injections of insulin several times a day to maintain their blood glucose levels in a healthful range (**FIGURE 3.16**).

In Type 2 Diabetes, Cells Become Less Responsive to Insulin

In **type 2 diabetes,** body cells become *resistant,* or less responsive, to insulin. This type of diabetes develops progressively, meaning that the biological changes resulting in the disease occur over a long period of time.

In most cases, obesity is the trigger for a cascade of changes that eventually result in the disorder. Specifically, the cells of many obese people exhibit a condition called *insulin insensitivity* (or *insulin resistance*). The pancreas attempts to compensate for this insensitivity by secreting more insulin. Over time, a person who is insulin insensitive will have to circulate very high levels of insulin to use glucose for energy. Eventually, the pancreas becomes incapable of secreting such excessive amounts, and the beta cells stop producing the hormone altogether.

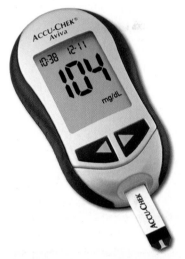

FIGURE 3.16 Monitoring blood glucose requires pricking a finger each day and measuring the blood using a glucometer.

TABLE 3.4   Symptoms of Type 1 and Type 2 Diabetes

Type 1 Diabetes	Type 2 Diabetes*
Frequent urination	Any of the type 1 symptoms
Unusual thirst	Blurred vision
Extreme hunger	Cuts/bruises that are slow to heal
Unusual weight loss	Tingling/numbness in the hands or feet
Extreme fatigue	Recurring skin, gum, or bladder infections
Irritability	

Source: Symptoms of Type 1 and Type 2 Diabetes. © 2005 American Diabetes Association. Reprinted with permission.

*Some people with type 2 diabetes experience no symptoms.

type 1 diabetes Disorder in which the body cannot produce enough insulin.

type 2 diabetes Progressive disorder in which body cells become less responsive to insulin or the body does not produce enough insulin.

WHAT ABOUT YOU?

Calculate Your Risk for Type 2 Diabetes

To calculate your risk for developing type 2 diabetes, circle your answers to the following questions:

- I am overweight.
  YES or NO

- I am sedentary (I exercise fewer than three times a week).
  YES or NO

- I have a close family member with type 2 diabetes.
  YES or NO

- I am a member of one of the following groups:
  YES or NO
  - African American
  - Hispanic American (Latino)
  - Native American
  - Pacific Islander

- I have had gestational diabetes, or I gave birth to at least one baby weighing more than 9 lb.
  YES or NO

- My blood pressure is 140/90 or higher, or I have been told that I have high blood pressure.
  YES or NO

- My cholesterol levels are not normal. (See the discussion of cholesterol in Chapter 4.)
  YES or NO

The more "yes" responses you give, the higher your risk of developing type 2 diabetes. You cannot change your ethnicity or your family members' health, but you can take steps to maintain a healthful weight and increase your physical activity. For tips, see Chapters 9 and 10.

Data from the National Diabetes Information Clearinghouse (NDIC). Available at http://diabetes.niddk.nih.gov.

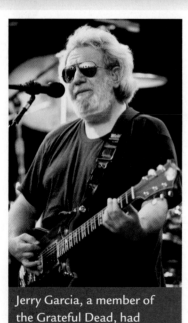

Jerry Garcia, a member of the Grateful Dead, had type 2 diabetes.

Many factors can cause type 2 diabetes. Genetics plays a role, so relatives of people with type 2 diabetes are at increased risk. Obesity and physical inactivity also increase the risk. Indeed, diabetes is thought to have become an epidemic in the United States because of a combination of our poor eating habits, sedentary lifestyles, increased obesity, and an aging population.

Most cases of type 2 diabetes develop after age 45, and almost 20% of Americans 65 years of age and older have diabetes. Once commonly known as *adult-onset diabetes,* type 2 diabetes in children was virtually unheard of until recently. Unfortunately, the disease is increasing dramatically among children and adolescents, posing serious health consequences for them and their future children.[12] Because type 2 diabetes in children and adolescents is a relatively new phenomenon, accurate statistics regarding the number of cases have not been generated; however, the American Diabetes Association states that type 2 diabetes is being diagnosed more frequently in children and adolescents, particularly among those of American Indian, African American, and Hispanic heritage.[13]

Lifestyle Choices Can Help Control or Prevent Type 2 Diabetes

Type 2 diabetes can be treated in a variety of ways. Weight loss, healthful eating patterns, and regular exercise can control symptoms in some people. More severe cases may require oral medications. These drugs work in either of two ways: they improve the sensitivity of body cells to insulin or reduce the amount of glucose the liver produces. If a person with type 2 diabetes can no longer secrete enough insulin, the patient must take daily injections of insulin just like a person with type 1 diabetes.

People with diabetes should follow most of the same dietary guidelines recommended for those without diabetes. One difference is that people with diabetes may need to eat less carbohydrate and slightly more fat or protein to help regulate their blood glucose levels. Typically, a registered dietitian develops an individualized diet plan based on each patient's responses to foods.

In addition, people with diabetes should avoid alcoholic beverages, which can cause hypoglycemia. The symptoms of alcohol intoxication and hypoglycemia are very similar. The person with diabetes, his or her companions, and healthcare professionals may confuse these conditions; this can result in a potentially life-threatening situation.

Although there is no cure for type 2 diabetes, many cases could be prevented or their onset delayed. We cannot control our family history, but we can use the following strategies to decrease our risk:

- Eat a balanced diet with plenty of whole grains, fruits, legumes, and vegetables.
- Exercise regularly: moderate daily exercise may prevent the onset of type 2 diabetes more effectively than dietary changes alone.[14]
- Maintain an appropriate body weight: studies show that losing only 10 to 30 lb can reduce or eliminate the symptoms of type 2 diabetes.[15]

What's your risk of developing diabetes? Check out What About You?: Calculate Your Risk for Type 2 Diabetes to find out.

> RECAP *Diabetes is a disease that results in dangerously high levels of blood glucose. In type 1 diabetes, the pancreas cannot secrete sufficient insulin, so insulin injections are required. Type 2 diabetes develops over time and may be triggered by obesity: body cells are no longer sensitive to the effects of insulin or the pancreas no longer secretes sufficient insulin for bodily needs. Supplemental insulin may or may not be needed to treat type 2 diabetes. Diabetes causes tissue damage and increases the risk of heart disease, blindness, kidney disease, and amputations. Many cases of type 2 diabetes could be prevented or delayed with a balanced diet, regular exercise, and achieving and maintaining a healthful body weight.*

Where I'm at now...

Now that you've read this chapter, would you say you've been getting enough fiber most days?

Yes or No

Do you plan to increase your intake of fiber-rich carbohydrates?

Yes or No

Do you plan to decrease your intake of simple carbohydrates?

Yes or No

What other changes—if any—do you plan to make in your food choices?

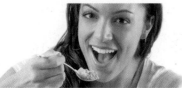

REVIEW QUESTIONS

Circle the correct choice.

1. The glycemic index rates
   a. the acceptable amount of alternative sweeteners to consume in one day.
   b. the potential of foods to raise blood glucose and insulin levels.
   c. the risk of a given food for causing diabetes.
   d. the ratio of soluble to insoluble fiber in a complex carbohydrate.

2. Carbohydrates contain
   a. carbon, nitrogen, and water.
   b. carbonic acid and a sugar alcohol.
   c. hydrated sugar.
   d. carbon, hydrogen, and oxygen.

3. The most common source of added sugar in the American diet is
   a. table sugar.
   b. white flour.
   c. alcohol.
   d. sweetened soft drinks.

4. Glucose, fructose, and galactose are
   a. monosaccharides.
   b. disaccharides.
   c. polysaccharides.
   d. complex carbohydrates.

5. Obesity is thought to be a common trigger of
   a. hypoglycemia.
   b. type 1 diabetes.
   c. type 2 diabetes.
   d. lactose intolerance.

6. True or False? Children and teens with diabetes almost invariably have type 1 diabetes.

7. True or False? High-fructose corn syrup is both a simple carbohydrate and a refined carbohydrate.

8. True or False? A person with lactose intolerance is allergic to milk.

9. True or False? Plants store glucose as glycogen.

10. True or False? Salivary amylase breaks down starches into galactose.

WEB LINKS

www.eatright.org
American Dietetic Association

Visit this Web site to learn more about diabetes, low- and high-carbohydrate diets, and general healthful eating habits.

www.ific.org
International Food Information Council Foundation (IFIC)

Search this site to find out more about sugars and low-calorie sweeteners.

www.ada.org
American Dental Association

Go to this site to learn more about tooth decay as well as other oral health topics.

www.nidcr.nih.gov
National Institute of Dental and Craniofacial Research (NIDCR)

Find out more about recent oral and dental health discoveries and obtain statistics and data on the status of dental health in the United States.

www.diabetes.org
American Diabetes Association

Find out more about the nutritional needs of people living with diabetes.

www2.niddk.nih.gov
National Institute of Diabetes and Digestive and Kidney Diseases (NIDDK)

Learn more about diabetes, including treatment, complications, U.S. statistics, clinical trials, and recent research.

TEST YOURSELF ANSWERS

1. **False.** The term *carbohydrate* refers to both simple and complex carbohydrates. The term *sugar* refers to the simple carbohydrates: monosaccharides and disaccharides.

2. **False.** There is no evidence that diets high in sugar cause hyperactivity in children or diabetes.

3. **True.** Our brains rely almost exclusively on glucose for energy, and our body tissues use glucose for energy both at rest and during exercise.

4. **False.** At 4 kcal/g, carbohydrates have less than half the energy of a gram of fat. Eating a high-carbohydrate diet will not cause people to gain body fat unless their total diet contains more energy (or calories) than they

expend. In fact, eating a diet high in complex, fiber-rich carbohydrates is associated with a lower risk for obesity.

5. **True.** Contrary to recent reports claiming severe health consequences related to consumption of alternative sweeteners, major health agencies have determined that these products are safe for most of us to consume in limited quantities.

NUTRITION LABEL ACTIVITY ANSWERS

1. For the sweetened cereal, the total carbohydrate is **26 g.**

2. For the whole-grain cereal, the total carbohydrate is **27 g** for a smaller serving size.

3. How many grams of dietary fiber does the sweetened cereal contain? **1g**

4. How many grams of dietary fiber does the whole-grain cereal contain? **4g**

5. How much starch is in the whole-grain cereal? **22 g**

REFERENCES

1. Sears, B. 1995. *The Zone. A Dietary Road Map.* New York: HarperCollins Publishers.
2. Steward, H. L., M. C. Bethea, S. S. Andrews, and L. A. Balart. 1995. *Sugar Busters! Cut Sugar to Trim Fat.* New York: Ballantine Books.
3. Atkins, R. C. 1992. *Dr. Atkins' New Diet Revolution.* New York: M. Evans & Company, Inc.
4. U.S. Department of Agriculture (USDA). U.S. Department of Health and Human Services. 2005. *Dietary Guidelines for Americans,* 5th ed. Home and Garden Bulletin No. 232. Washington, DC: U.S. Government Printing Office.
5. Institute of Medicine, Food and Nutrition Board. 2002. *Dietary Reference Intakes for Energy, Carbohydrates, Fiber, Fat, Protein and Amino Acids (Macronutrients).* Washington, DC: The National Academy of Sciences.
6. International Food Information Council Foundation. 2004. Gestational Diabetes and Low-Calorie Sweeteners: Answers to Common Questions. Available at www.ific.org/publications/brochures/upload/gestationaldiabetes.pdf. (Accessed November 2007.)
7. Howard, B. V., and J. Wylie-Rosett. 2002. Sugar and cardiovascular disease. A statement for healthcare professionals from the Committee on Nutrition of the Council on Nutrition, Physical Activity, and Metabolism of the American Heart Association. *Circulation* 106:523–527.
8. Meyer, K. A., L. H. Kushi, D. R. Jacobs, J. Slavin, T. A. Sellers, and A. R. Folsom. 2000. Carbohydrates, dietary fiber, and incident of type 2 diabetes in older women. *Am. J. Clin. Nutr.* 71:921–930.
9. Troiano, R. P., R. R. Briefel, M. D. Carroll, and K. Bialostosky. 2000. Energy and fat intakes of children and adolescents in the United States: Data from the National Health and Nutrition Examination Surveys. *Am. J. Clin. Nutr.* 72:1343S–1353S.
10. Ludwig, D. S., K. E. Peterson, and S. L. Gortmaker. 2001. Relation between consumption of sugar-sweetened drinks and childhood obesity: A prospective, observational analysis. *Lancet* 357:505–508.
11. National Diabetes Information Clearinghouse (NDIC). 2005. National Diabetes Statistics. National Institutes of Health Publication No. 06–3892. Available at http://diabetes.niddk.nih.gov/dm/pubs/statistics/index.htm. (Accessed November 2007.)
12. Rosenbloom, A. L., D. V. House, and W. E. Winter. 1998. Non-insulin dependent diabetes mellitus (NIDDM) in minority youth: Research priorities and needs. *Clin Pediatr.* 37:143–152.
13. American Diabetes Association. 2005. Diabetes statistics for youth. Available at www.diabetes.org/diabetes-statistics/prevalence.jsp.
14. Pan, X.-P., G.-W. Li, Y.-H. Hu, J. X. Wang, W. Y. Yang, Z. X. An, Z. X. Hu, J. Lin, J. Z. Xiao, H. B. Cao, P. A. Liu, X. G. Jiang, Y. Y. Jiang, J. P. Wang, H. Zheng, H. Zhang, P. H. Bennett, and B. V. Howard. 1997. Effects of diet and exercise in preventing NIDDM in people with impaired glucose tolerance. *Diabetes Care* 20:537–544.
15. American College of Sports Medicine (ACSM). 2000. Position stand: Exercise and type 2 diabetes. *Med. Sci. Sports Exerc.* 32:1345–1360.

4 Fats: Essential Energy-Supplying Nutrients

TEST YOURSELF

Are these statements true or false? Circle your guess.

1 Cholesterol is unhealthful, and we should consume as little dietary cholesterol as possible.   **TRUE or FALSE**

2 Fat is an important fuel source during rest and exercise.   **TRUE or FALSE**

3 Fried foods can be high in unhealthful fats even if fried with vegetable shortening.   **TRUE or FALSE**

4 Certain fats protect against heart disease.   **TRUE or FALSE**

5 High-fat diets are the primary cause of cancer.   **TRUE or FALSE**

Test Yourself answers can be found at the end of the chapter.

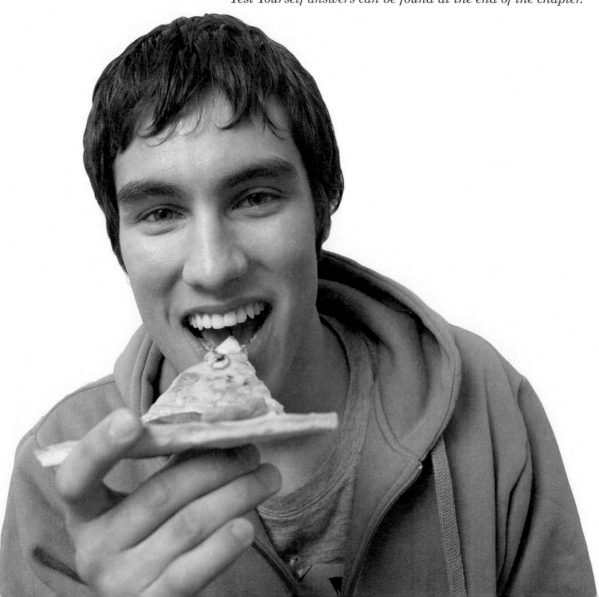

SHIVANI AND HER parents moved to the United States from India when Shivani was 6 years old. Although slender in comparison to her American peers, Shivani was healthy and energetic, excelling in school and riding her new bike in her suburban neighborhood. By the time Shivani entered high school, her weight had caught up to that of her American classmates. Now a sophomore in college, she is struggling with obesity.

Shivani explains, "In India, the diet is mostly rice, lentils, and vegetables. Many people are vegetarians, or they'll eat only fish and poultry. Breakfast is typically fruit and yogurt, not eggs and sausage. And for many families, desserts are only for special occasions. When we moved to America, I wanted to eat like all the other kids: hamburgers, French fries, ice cream, cookies . . . I gained a lot of weight on that diet, and now my doctor says my blood pressure is high and I need to have a cholesterol test to see if I'm at risk for heart disease. It freaks me out thinking some day I might have a heart attack! I wish I could start eating like my relatives back in India again, but they don't serve rice and lentils at the dorm cafeteria."

What causes heart disease, and how can you calculate your risk? Is a high-fat diet always to blame? Can a low-fat diet prevent it? When was the last time you heard anything good about dietary fat? If Shivani were your best friend and you noticed her regularly eating high-fat foods, would you say anything about it? If so, what would you say?

Although some people think of dietary fat as something to be avoided, a certain amount of fat is absolutely essential for good health. In this chapter, we'll discuss the function of fat in the human body and help you distinguish between beneficial and harmful types of dietary fat. You'll also assess how much fat you need in your diet and learn about the relationship between different types of dietary fat and the development of heart disease and other disorders.

What Are Fats?

Fats are just one form of a much larger and more diverse group of substances called **lipids** that are distinguished by the fact that they are insoluble in water. Think of a salad dressing made with vinegar and olive oil—a lipid. Shaking the bottle *disperses* the oil but doesn't *dissolve* it: that's why it separates back out again so quickly. Lipids are found in all sorts of living things, including plants, animals, and human beings. In fact, their presence on your skin explains why you can't clean your face with water alone: you need some type of soap to break down the insoluble lipids before you can wash them away. In this chapter, we focus on the small group of lipids that are found in foods.

Fats and oils are two different types of lipids found in foods. Fats such as butter are solid at room temperature, whereas oils such as olive oil are liquid at room temperature. Because most people are more comfortable with the term *fats* instead of *lipids,* we will use that term generically throughout this book, including when we are referring to oils.

Three types of fats are commonly found in foods:

- Triglycerides
- Phospholipids
- Sterols

Most of the fat we eat (95%) is in the form of triglycerides, which is the same way most of the fat in our body is stored. In addition, the types of triglycerides we choose to eat can have a significant impact—positive or negative—on our health. So let's begin this discussion with a closer look at triglycerides. We'll discuss phospholipids and sterols on pages 105–107.

Where I'm starting from ...

How many times a week would you say you consume fried foods (fried eggs, burgers, French fries, etc.)?

What's wrong with fried foods, anyway? Jot down your best guess here:

Have you ever heard of essential fatty acids?

Yes or NO

If so, do you think you get enough of these nutrients each day?

Yes or NO

If YES, what makes you say so?

lipids A diverse group of organic substances that are insoluble in water; lipids include triglycerides, phospholipids, and sterols.

Triglycerides Can Contain Saturated or Unsaturated Fatty Acid Chains

As reflected in the prefix *tri,* a **triglyceride** is a molecule consisting of *three* fatty acids attached to a *three*-carbon glycerol backbone. **Fatty acids** are long chains of carbon atoms bound to each other as well as to hydrogen. They are acids because they contain an acid group at one end of their chain. **Glycerol,** the backbone of a triglyceride molecule, is an alcohol composed of three carbon atoms. One fatty acid chain attaches to each of these three carbons to make the triglyceride (FIGURE 4.1).

You've probably heard the recommendation that you should reduce your intake of saturated and *trans* fatty acids and increase your intake of unsaturated and essential fatty acids. All of these are components of triglycerides, so why are some better than others? The difference lies mainly in how their carbon atoms are bound to hydrogen. As we explain next, this simple factor varies their shape and their effect in our bodies quite dramatically.

Saturated Fats Contain the Maximum Amount of Hydrogen

An atom of carbon has four "attachment sites." It will be unstable until it has bonded to four other atoms—that is, until all four of its attachment sites are filled. In fatty acids, two of these four sites are typically bound to adjacent carbon atoms. These bonds form the carbon chain.

In saturated fatty acids, the two remaining attachment sites are always filled by hydrogen atoms:

$$
\begin{array}{c}
\text{H} \\
| \\
\text{H} - \text{C} - \text{H} \\
| \\
\text{H}
\end{array}
$$

Thus, the saturated fatty acid chain is simply a long chain of carbon atoms bonded to other carbon atoms (two attachment sites) and to hydrogen atoms (two more attachments sites). You can see this in the long chain shown in FIGURE 4.2A. When you look at this chain, notice how regular it is.

In contrast, look at the chain in FIGURE 4.2C. At one point it has a *double bond* between adjacent carbon atoms. (Chemists indicate double bonds between atoms with

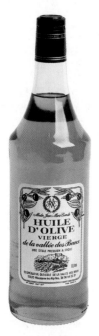

Some fats, such as olive oil, are liquid at room temperature.

triglyceride A molecule consisting of three fatty acids attached to a three-carbon glycerol backbone.

fatty acids Long chains of carbon atoms bound to each other as well as to hydrogen atoms.

glycerol An alcohol composed of three carbon atoms; it is the backbone of a triglyceride molecule.

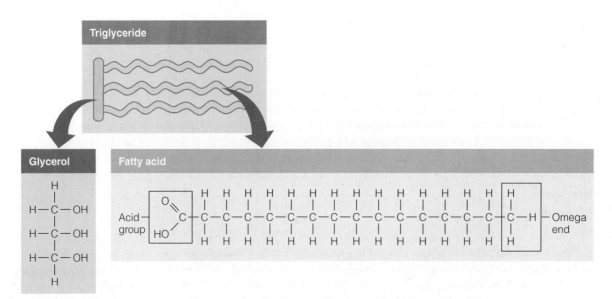

FIGURE 4.1 A triglyceride consists of three fatty acid chains attached to a three-carbon glycerol backbone.

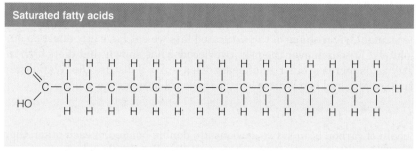

(a)

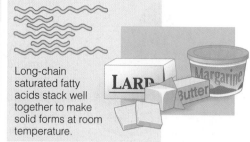

Long-chain saturated fatty acids stack well together to make solid forms at room temperature.

(b)

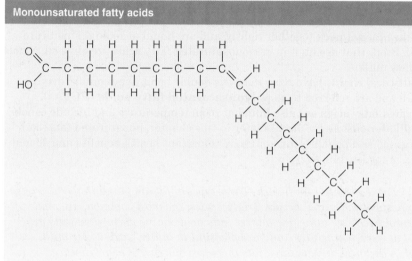

(c)

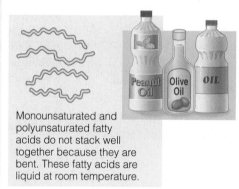

Monounsaturated and polyunsaturated fatty acids do not stack well together because they are bent. These fatty acids are liquid at room temperature.

(d)

FIGURE 4.2 Level of saturation affects the shape of fatty acids. (a) In saturated fats, each carbon atom in the fatty acid chain is singly bonded to two other carbon atoms and two hydrogen atoms. (b) Saturated fats have straight fatty acid chains packed tightly together and are solid at room temperature. (c) In monounsaturated fats, somewhere along the fatty acid chain, two carbon atoms are doubly bonded to each other. This double carbon bond excludes hydrogen at this area of the molecule and produces one kink in the chain. Polyunsaturated fats have two or more such kinks in their fatty acid chain. (d) The kinks in the fatty acid chains of monounsaturated and polyunsaturated fats prevent them from packing tightly together; they are liquid at room temperature.

two parallel lines, like an equal sign [C = C]). This double bond fills two attachment sites, one of which would otherwise be filled by hydrogen. Notice that each of the carbons at this site has just one hydrogen attached, not two. Thus, the total amount of hydrogen is lower in a fatty acid chain with one or more double carbon bonds.

A fatty acid with no double carbon bonds, like the one in Figure 4.2a, is referred to as a **saturated fatty acid (SFA).** This is because the chain is *saturated* with hydrogen: it has the maximum amount of hydrogen bound to it. Some foods that are high in saturated fatty acids are butter, lard, cream, whole milk, many cheeses, beef, coconut oil, and palm kernel oil.

Double carbon bonds give fatty acids chains a "kink" wherever they occur. Molecules of saturated fat have no such bonds, so they always form straight, rigid chains. This quality allows them to pack together densely in fats like butter and lard. To understand why, it might help to imagine a box of toothpicks. Have you ever noticed how many toothpicks are packed into a small box? A hundred? More? But if you were to break a bunch of toothpicks into V shapes anywhere along their length, how many could you then fit into the same box? It would be very few because the bent toothpicks would jumble together, taking up much more space. Like straight toothpicks,

saturated fatty acids (SFA) Fatty acids that have no carbons joined together with a double bond; these types of fatty acids are generally solid at room temperature.

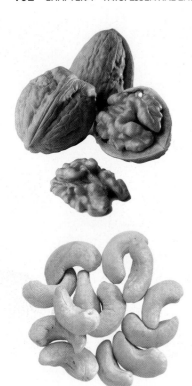

Walnuts and cashews are high in monounsaturated fatty acids.

saturated fatty acid chains can pack together tightly (FIGURE 4.2B). That is why saturated fats, such as the fat in meats and butter, are solid at room temperature.

Does the straight, rigid shape of the saturated fats we eat have any effect on our health? Absolutely! Research over the past two decades has shown that diets high in saturated fatty acids increase our risk of heart disease. We'll discuss the relationship between saturated fats and heart disease in more detail later in this chapter.

Unsaturated Fats Contain Less Hydrogen

If, within a chain of carbon atoms, two carbons are double-bonded to each other, then hydrogen is excluded at this point in the chain (see Figure 4.2c). This lack of hydrogen at *one* part of the molecule results in a fatty acid chain that is referred to as *monounsaturated* (recall from Chapter 3 that the prefix *mono-* means "one"). **Monounsaturated fatty acids (MUFAs)** are usually liquid at room temperature, because their one double carbon bond produces one kink in their chain. Like broken toothpicks, they cannot pack together tightly, and are liquid at room temperature (FIGURE 4.2D). Foods that are high in monounsaturated fatty acids are olive oil, canola oil, and cashew nuts.

If the fatty acid chains have *more than one* double bond, they contain even less hydrogen and are referred to as **polyunsaturated fatty acids (PUFAs).** Polyunsaturated fatty acids are also liquid at room temperature and include canola, corn, and safflower oils. As we discuss later in this chapter, unsaturated fats (both monounsaturated and polyunsaturated) have important health benefits and should be consumed in moderation every day.

> RECAP *Fat is essential for health. Three types of fat are found in foods: triglycerides, phospholipids, and sterols. Triglycerides, the most common, are made up of a glycerol backbone attached to three fatty acid chains. Saturated fatty acids are solid at room temperature and are plentiful in butter, lard, whole milk, and beef. A diet high in saturated fats increases our risk of heart disease. Monounsaturated and polyunsaturated fatty acids are liquid at room temperature and are plentiful in vegetable oils, nuts, and many fish. These fats have important health benefits and should be consumed daily.*

Different Forms of Triglycerides Can Damage or Preserve Our Health

As we will discuss throughout the rest of this chapter, the types of fats we choose to eat can have a greater effect on our health than the amount of fat in our diet.

Both Saturated and *Trans* Fats Are Harmful to Our Health

For several years, food companies from McDonald's to Dunkin' Donuts have been under attack for using *trans* fats in their foods. In 2005, even officials of the Girl Scouts of the United States were forced to respond to concerns of parents and nutrition experts about the high level of *trans* fats found in many of their cookies.[1] But what's behind all the fuss? What are *trans* fats, and why are they harmful?

The type of unsaturated fatty acid that occurs most commonly in nature is kinked, as we just described. In contrast, *trans* fats are rigid, just like saturated fats. (The term *trans* fat describes the diagonally opposite positioning of the hydrogen atoms in the fatty acid chain.) These fats occur rarely in nature; extremely small amounts are found only in dairy foods, beef, and lamb. In contrast, they are abundant in margarines, commercial frying fats, shortenings, and any processed foods or fast foods made with these products. Health concerns about *trans* fats began to arise with research linking high-*trans*-fat diets with heart disease and early death.

The trouble began in the late 19th century when food manufacturers identified the need for a fat that could be produced cheaply and abundantly from vegetable oils, that could be sold in a solid form, and that resisted rancidity. (As you may know,

monounsaturated fatty acids (MUFA) Fatty acids that have two carbons in the chain bound to each other with one double bond; these types of fatty acids are generally liquid at room temperature.

polyunsaturated fatty acids (PUFA) Fatty acids that have more than one double bond in the chain; these types of fatty acids are generally liquid at room temperature.

most fats and oils cannot be stored for long without going rancid.) They developed a process called **hydrogenation,** in which pressurized hydrogen is inserted into the double carbon bonds in the unsaturated fatty acid chains of vegetable oils. Hydrogenation straightens out the chains, making the liquid fat more solid at room temperature—and also more saturated. The extra hydrogen also helps the fat resist rancidity.

One of the most common uses of hydrogenation is to produce margarines. Not surprisingly, stick margarines tend to be higher in *trans* fats (about 4 g per tablespoon) than the less-solid tub margarines (about 1 g per tablespoon). Other products commonly containing *trans* fats are French fries, doughnuts, cakes, crackers, pie crusts, and, yes, cookies.

Research has shown that *trans* fats are more detrimental to our health than saturated fats, because they change the way our cell membranes function and reduce the removal of cholesterol from the blood. For these reasons, the 2005 *Dietary Guidelines for Americans* as well as the Institute of Medicine recommend keeping consumption of *trans* fats to an absolute minimum.[2,3] In addition, because of the concerns related to *trans* fatty acid consumption and heart disease, the U.S. Food and Drug Administration (FDA) now requires food manufacturers to list the amount of *trans* fatty acids per serving on the Nutrition Facts Panel. In response to market pressures, many food manufacturers have begun offering products free of *trans* fatty acids, and they clearly state this claim on the label. Additionally, legislators and food policy organizations around the United States are lobbying for the labeling of *trans* fats on restaurant menus, or for the total elimination of artificial *trans* fats from restaurant foods. But in order to improve public health, we need to make sure that food manufacturers and restaurants don't simply substitute saturated fats. We need to switch to unsaturated fats to decrease our risk for heart disease.

Despite the process of hydrogenation, *trans* fats are still less saturated than saturated fats. So margarine is still a more healthful choice than butter, right? The Nutrition Myth or Fact? box on page 105 explores this question.

Essential Fatty Acids Protect Our Health

Although many people think that all dietary fats should be avoided, we must consume certain fats if we are to survive. These **essential fatty acids (EFAs)** are incorporated into the many phospholipids in our body (described shortly) and are needed to make a number of important biological compounds called *eicosanoids*. In the body, eicosanoids help regulate some key functions, including gastrointestinal tract motility, blood clotting, the expanding and contracting of our blood vessels to regulate blood pressure, the permeability of our blood vessels to fluid and large molecules, and the regulation of inflammation—just to name a few. Since they play an important role in regulating biological processes, we need a balance of the various eicosanoids and thus a balance of EFAs. For example, we need just the right amount of blood clotting at the right time—too much and we get excessive blood clotting and too little and we get excessive bleeding.

EFAs are called "essential" because they must be consumed in the diet and cannot be made in our bodies. The two EFAs required in our diet are linoleic acid and alpha-linolenic acid (**FIGURE 4.3**).

Linoleic Acid **Linoleic acid** is found in vegetable and nut oils such as sunflower, safflower, corn, soy, and peanut oil. If you eat lots of vegetables or use vegetable oil–based margarines or vegetable oils, you are probably getting adequate amounts of this essential fatty acid in your diet. In the body, linoleic acid is transformed into arachidonic acid, which is in turn used to make compounds that regulate body functions such as blood clotting and blood pressure.

Linoleic acid is often referred to as *omega-6 fatty acid.* In order to understand the reason for this name, you need to know that chemists call the final carbon in a fatty acid chain the *omega carbon* (omega [ω] is the last letter in the Greek alphabet). In the fatty acid illustrated in Figure 4.1, the omega end is shown. Omega-6 refers to the sixth carbon in a fatty acid chain when counting back from the omega carbon. In omega-6 fatty acids, the end-most double carbon bond occurs at this

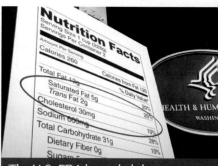

The U.S. FDA has ruled that *trans* fatty acids, or *trans* fat, must be listed as a separate line item on Nutrition Facts Panels for conventional foods and some dietary supplements. Research studies show that diets high in *trans* fatty acids can increase the risk of cardiovascular disease.

hydrogenation The process of adding hydrogen to unsaturated fatty acids, making them more saturated and therefore more solid at room temperature.

essential fatty acids (EFA) Fatty acids that must be consumed in the diet because they cannot be made by our bodies. The two essential fatty acids are linoleic acid and alpha-linolenic acid.

linoleic acid An essential fatty acid found in vegetable and nut oils; also known as omega-6 fatty acid.

FIGURE 4.3 The two essential fatty acids: linoleic acid (omega-6 fatty acid) and alpha-linolenic acid (omega-3 fatty acid).

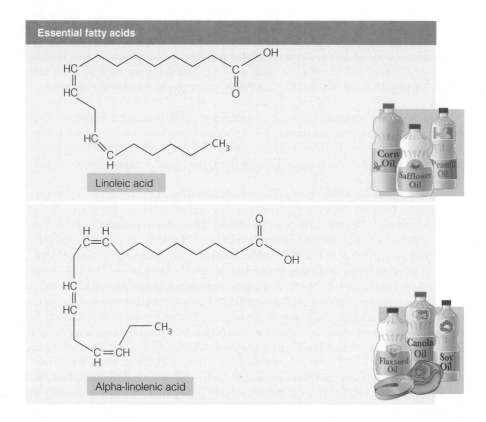

Essential fatty acids

Linoleic acid

Alpha-linolenic acid

carbon. The body cannot make fatty acids with double carbon bonds this close to the omega end of the chain, and so linoleic acid is an essential fatty acid.

Alpha-Linolenic Acid   The second essential fatty acid is **alpha-linolenic acid,** an *omega-3 fatty acid*, which was recognized as being essential about 20 years ago. Its outermost double carbon bond is even further along the chain, at the omega-3 carbon. In addition, its many double carbon bonds make this fatty acid highly kinked and therefore highly fluid. Alpha-linolenic acid is found primarily in leafy green vegetables, flax seeds and flax seed oil, soy oil and foods, canola oil, and fish products and fish oils (see Figure 4.3).

You may have read news reports of the health benefits of the omega-3 fatty acids found in many fish. Two of these fatty acids, **eicosapentaenoic acid (EPA)** and **docosahexaenoic acid (DHA),** are found in especially high levels in cold-water fish such as wild salmon, sardines, and tuna, where their high degree of unsaturation helps keep the fish cell membranes flexible even in extremely cold temperatures. Research indicates that EPA and DHA are protective against heart disease.[4,5] These fatty acids play a role in improving vascular function, and they reduce inflammatory responses, blood clotting, blood pressure, cardiac arrhythmias, and plasma triglycerides, all of which are associated with a reduction in heart disease.[6]

Getting enough of these essential fatty acids is important for health. Because the omega-6 and omega-3 fatty acids are metabolized by the same enzymes, their ratio has also been an issue of concern. But a large body of research suggests that it is more important to get adequate amounts of these fatty acids in your diet than to attempt to consume some precise balance between the two types.[4] By consuming adequate amounts of these EFAs, you can reduce the negative health impact of saturated and *trans* fatty acids. Dietary recommendations for the EFAs are discussed later in this chapter (see page 113).

Many Foods Contain a Variety of Fatty Acids

As shown in **FIGURE 4.4**, foods typically contain a variety of fatty acids. For example, animal fats provide approximately 40% to 60% of their energy from saturated fats

alpha-linolenic acid   An essential fatty acid found in leafy green vegetables, flax seed oil, soy oil, fish oil, and fish products; an omega-3 fatty acid.

eicosapentaenoic acid (EPA)   A type of omega-3 fatty acid that can be made in the body from alpha-linolenic acid and found in our diet primarily in marine plants and animals.

docosahexaenoic acid (DHA)   Another type of omega-3 fatty acid that can be made in the body from alpha-linolenic acid and found in our diet primarily in marine plants and animals; together with EPA, it appears to reduce our risk of a heart attack.

NUTRITION MYTH OR FACT?

Is Margarine More Healthful Than Butter?

Your toast just popped up! Which will it be: butter or margarine? Butter is 65% saturated fat, and as you'll learn throughout this chapter, a diet high in saturated fats is associated with an increased risk of heart disease. In contrast, corn oil margarine is just 2% saturated fat. But what about those 4 g of *trans* fat? Which is the lesser of two evils, the saturated fats in the butter, or the *trans* fat in the margarine?

You're not the only one asking this question. Over the past several years, researchers have determined that *trans* fats raise blood levels of so-called "bad" cholesterol and lower levels of "good" cholesterol. They say that the *trans* fats in margarine are more harmful to health than the saturated fats in butter. So does that mean that butter is the better choice? A decade ago, that may have been the case, but over the past 10 years, several food manufacturers have introduced *trans*-fat-free margarines.

Some of these margarines include plant sterols, which can reduce the level of "bad" cholesterol in the blood by up to 15%. These types of margarines are sold under the brand names of TakeControl® and Benacol®.

The American Heart Association advises that consumers choose soft margarines (liquid or tub varieties) as a substitute for butter and look for "0 g *trans* fat" on the Nutrition Facts panel.[4] Others point out that *trans*-fat-free margarines are still "nonfoods" and recommend that those who prefer whole foods choose unprocessed nut butters (peanut butter, walnut butter, etc.). These natural alternatives are rich in essential fatty acids and other heart-healthy unsaturated fats.

but also provide some unsaturated fats. Most plant fats provide 80% to 90% of their energy from monounsaturated and polyunsaturated fats. For this reason, diets higher in plant foods will usually be lower in saturated fats than diets high in animal products.

> RECAP *The consumption of high levels of saturated fatty acids and* trans *fatty acids is associated with an increased risk of heart disease. In contrast, essential fatty acids are critical to our health. The body cannot synthesize EFAs, so we must consume them. Most foods provide a variety of types of fatty acids.*

Phospholipids Combine Lipids with Phosphate

Along with the triglycerides just discussed, two other types of fats, phospholipids and sterols, are present in the foods we eat. **Phospholipids** consist of a glycerol backbone bound to two fatty acids. In place of the third fatty acid found in triglycerides, phospholipids have a compound that contains *phosphate,* a chemical that is soluble in water (**FIGURE 4.5**). This substitution of a phosphate compound makes phospholipids soluble in water, a property that enables them to assist in transporting fats in our bloodstream (blood is about 50% water). We discuss the transport of fats in more detail later in this chapter (page 110). Also, as shown in Figure 4.5, phospholipids are an important component of the outer membrane of every cell in the body and thus help to regulate the transport of substances into and out of our cells.

Phospholipids are present in peanuts, egg yolk, and some processed foods with dispersed fats, such as salad dressings. However, because our bodies manufacture them, they are not essential for us to include in our diets.

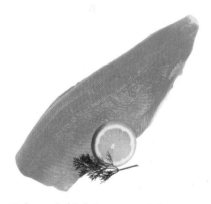

Salmon is high in omega-3 fatty acid content.

phospholipids A type of lipid in which a fatty acid is combined with another compound that contains phosphate; unlike other lipids, phospholipids are soluble in water.

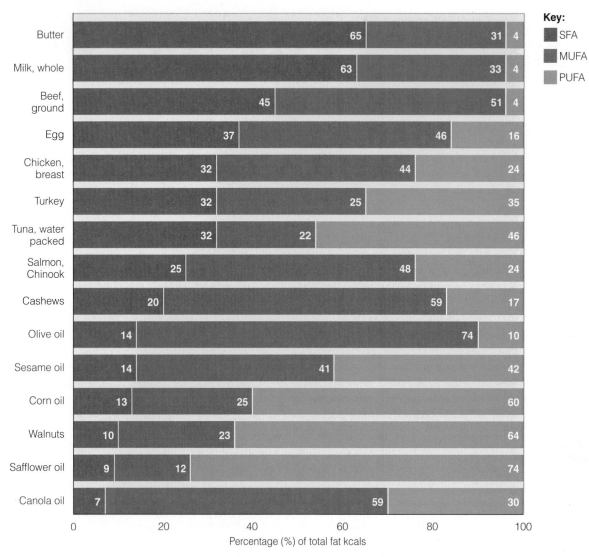

Key:
- SFA
- MUFA
- PUFA

Butter — 65, 31, 4
Milk, whole — 63, 33, 4
Beef, ground — 45, 51, 4
Egg — 37, 46, 16
Chicken, breast — 32, 44, 24
Turkey — 32, 25, 35
Tuna, water packed — 32, 22, 46
Salmon, Chinook — 25, 48, 24
Cashews — 20, 59, 17
Olive oil — 14, 74, 10
Sesame oil — 14, 41, 42
Corn oil — 13, 25, 60
Walnuts — 10, 23, 64
Safflower oil — 9, 12, 74
Canola oil — 7, 59, 30

Percentage (%) of total fat kcals

FIGURE 4.4 Major sources of dietary fat.

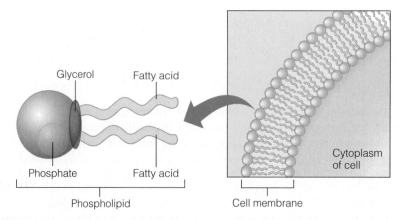

Glycerol
Fatty acid
Phosphate
Fatty acid
Phospholipid
Cytoplasm of cell
Cell membrane

FIGURE 4.5 Structure of a phospholipid. Phospholipids consist of a glycerol backbone attached to two fatty acids and a compound that contains phosphate. They are an important component of our cell membranes and are also found in certain foods, such as peanuts, egg yolks, and some processed foods that contain dispersed fats.

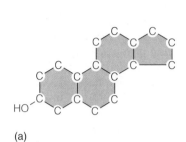

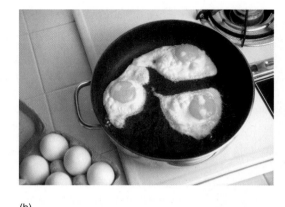

(a)

(b)

FIGURE 4.6 Sterol structure. (a) Cholesterol and other sterols are lipids that contain multiple ring structures. (b) Cholesterol is the most commonly occurring sterol in the diet. It is found in meats, fish, egg yolks, and dairy products.

Sterols Have a Ring Structure

Sterols are also a type of lipid found in foods and in the body, but their multiple-ring structure is quite different from that of triglycerides or phospholipids (**FIGURE 4.6A**). Sterols are found in both plant and animal foods and are produced in the body.

Cholesterol is the most commonly occurring sterol in the diet (**FIGURE 4.6B**). Cholesterol is found only in the fatty part of animal products such as butter, egg yolks, whole milk, meats, and poultry. Egg whites, skim milk, and lean meats have little or no cholesterol. Dietary cholesterol has earned a bad reputation because it is found primarily in foods high in saturated fatty acids, which can increase our blood cholesterol levels. As you will read later in this chapter, elevated blood cholesterol levels suggest an increased risk of cardiovascular disease.

We don't need to consume cholesterol in our diet because our body continually synthesizes it, mostly in the liver and intestines. This continuous production is vital to our health because cholesterol is part of every cell membrane, where it works in conjunction with fatty acids to help maintain cell membrane integrity. It is particularly plentiful in the neural cells that make up the brain, spinal cord, and nerves. The body also uses cholesterol to synthesize several important sterol compounds, including sex hormones (estrogen, androgen, and progesterone), adrenal hormones, bile, and vitamin D. Thus, despite cholesterol's bad reputation, it is absolutely essential to human health.

> RECAP *Phospholipids combine two fatty acids and a glycerol backbone with a phosphate-containing compound that makes them soluble in water. They help transport fats in our bloodstream and are found in the cell membrane. Sterols have a multiple-ring structure; cholesterol is the most commonly occurring sterol in our diets.*

Why Do We Need to Eat Fats?

Dietary fat provides energy and helps our bodies perform some essential internal functions.

Fats Provide Energy

Dietary fat is a primary source of energy. Fat provides 9 kcal/g, while carbohydrate and protein provide only 4 kcal/g. This means that fat is much more energy-dense. For example, 1 tablespoon of butter or oil contains approximately 100 kcal, whereas

sterols A type of lipid found in foods and the body that has a ring structure; cholesterol is the most common sterol that occurs in our diets.

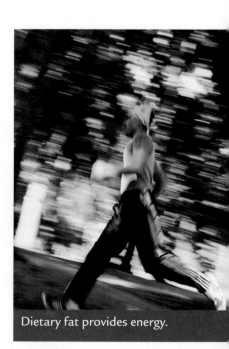

Dietary fat provides energy.

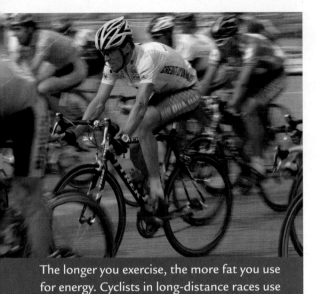

The longer you exercise, the more fat you use for energy. Cyclists in long-distance races use fat stores for energy.

it takes 2.5 cups of steamed broccoli or 1 slice of whole wheat bread to provide 100 kcal.

When we are at rest, approximately 30% to 70% of the energy used by our muscles and organs comes from fat.[6] The exact amount of fat you burn when you are at rest depends on how much fat you are eating in your diet, how physically active you are, and whether you are gaining or losing weight.

Fat is also a major energy source during physical activity. In fact, one of the best means of losing body fat is regular aerobic exercise. During exercise, the body begins to break down fat stores to fuel the working muscles. The amount and source of the fat used depend on your level of fitness; the type, intensity, and duration of the exercise; and what and how much you've eaten before you exercise. Because the body has only a limited supply of stored carbohydrate as glycogen in muscle tissue, the longer you exercise, the more fat you use for energy.

Fats Store Energy for Later Use

Our bodies store extra energy as fat in our *adipose tissue,* which then can be used for energy at rest, during exercise, or during periods of low energy intake. Having a readily available energy source in the form of fat means the body has an energy source even when we choose not to eat (or are unable to eat), when we are exercising, and while we are sleeping. Our bodies have little stored carbohydrate—only enough to last about 1 to 2 days—and there is no place that our body can store extra protein. We cannot consider our muscles and organs as a place where "extra" protein is stored! For these reasons, the fat stored in our adipose and muscle tissues is necessary to keep the body going. Although we do not want too much stored adipose tissue, some is essential to good health.

Fats Enable the Transport of Fat-Soluble Vitamins

Dietary fat enables the transport of the fat-soluble vitamins. These are vitamins A, D, E, and K. Vitamin A is important for vision, vitamin D helps maintain bone health, vitamin E prevents and repairs damage to cells, and vitamin K is important for blood clotting and bone health. Without an appropriate intake of dietary fat, our bodies can become deficient in these important vitamins.

Fats Help Maintain Cell Function and Provide Protection to the Body

Fats are a critical part of every cell membrane. There, they help determine what substances are transported in and out of the cell and regulate what substances can bind to the cell; thus, fats strongly influence the function of the cell. In addition, fats help maintain cell fluidity and other physical properties of the cell membrane. Fats enable our red blood cells, for example, to be flexible enough to bend and move through the smallest capillaries in our body, delivering oxygen to all our cells.

Stored body fat pads the body and protects our organs, such as the kidneys and liver, when we fall or are bruised. The fat under our skin acts as insulation to help us retain body heat. Although we often think of body fat as "bad," it does play an important role in keeping our bodies healthy and functioning properly.

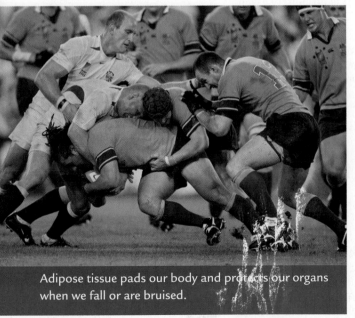

Adipose tissue pads our body and protects our organs when we fall or are bruised.

Fats Contribute to the Flavor and Texture of Foods

Dietary fat adds texture and flavor to foods. Fat makes salad dressings smooth and ice cream "creamy," and it gives cakes and cookies their moist, tender texture. Frying foods in fat, as with doughnuts or French fries, gives them a crisp, flavorful coating. On the other hand, foods containing fats, such as cookies, crackers, chips, and breads, become rancid quickly if they are not stored properly. Manufacturers add preservatives to increase the shelf life of foods with fats.

Fats Help Us to Feel Satiated

Fats in foods help us feel satisfied after a meal. Two factors probably contribute to this effect: first, as we noted earlier, fat has a much higher energy density than carbohydrate or protein. An amount of butter weighing the same number of grams as a medium apple would contain 840 calories! Second, fat takes longer to digest than protein or carbohydrate because more steps are involved in the digestion process. This may help you feel satisfied for a longer period of time because energy is slowly being released into your body.

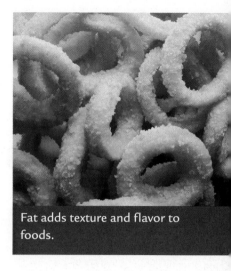

Fat adds texture and flavor to foods.

> RECAP *Dietary fats provide twice the energy of protein and carbohydrate, at 9 kcal/g, and the majority of energy required at rest. Fats are also a major fuel source during exercise. Dietary fats help transport the fat-soluble vitamins into the body and help regulate cell function and maintain membrane integrity. Stored body fat in the adipose tissue helps protect vital organs and pad the body. Fats contribute to the flavor and texture of foods and the satiety we feel after a meal.*

What Happens to the Fats We Eat?

Because fats are not soluble in water, they cannot enter our bloodstream easily from the digestive tract. Thus, fats must be digested, absorbed, and transported within the body differently from carbohydrates and proteins, which are water soluble. The digestion and absorption of fat were discussed in detail in Chapter 2, but we briefly review the process here (FIGURE 4.7).

The Mouth and Stomach Have Limited Roles in Fat Digestion

Dietary fats usually come mixed with other foods in our diet, which we chew and then swallow. Water, mucus, and a salivary enzyme called lingual lipase mix with the fats in the mouth, but this enzyme has a limited role in the breakdown of fats until they reach the stomach (Figure 4.7, step 1). Once in the stomach, lingual lipase and gastric lipase, which is secreted by the stomach, can digest about 10% of fats present. But the primary role of the stomach in fat digestion is to mix and break up the fat into droplets (Figure 4.7, step 2). Because they are not soluble in water, these fat droplets typically float on top of the watery digestive juices in the stomach until they are passed into the small intestine.

The Gallbladder, Liver, and Pancreas Assist in Fat Breakdown

Because fat is not soluble in water, its digestion requires the help of mixing compounds from the gallbladder and digestive enzymes from the pancreas. Recall that the gallbladder is a sac attached to the underside of the liver, and the pancreas is an oblong-shaped organ sitting below the stomach. Both have a duct connecting them to the small intestine.

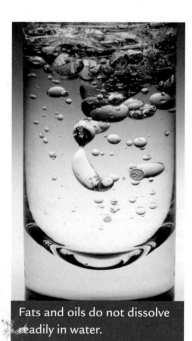

Fats and oils do not dissolve readily in water.

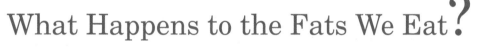

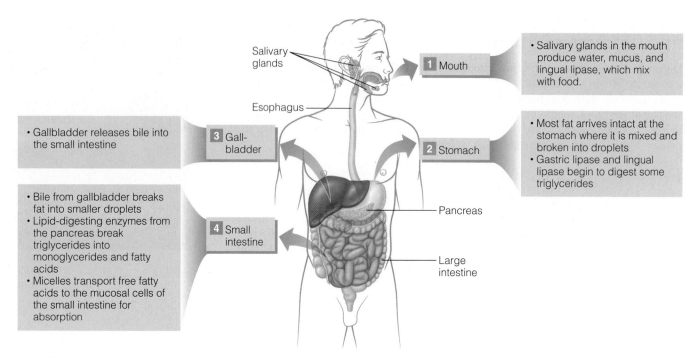

FIGURE 4.7 The process of fat digestion.

As fat enters the small intestine from the stomach, the gallbladder contracts and releases a substance called bile (Figure 4.7, step 3). Bile is produced in the liver from cholesterol and is stored in the gallbladder until needed. Bile contains bile salts that are detergents and, much like soap, break up the fat into smaller and smaller droplets. At the same time, lipid-digesting enzymes produced in the pancreas travel through the pancreatic duct into the small intestine. Once bile has broken the fat into small droplets, these pancreatic enzymes take over, breaking up the triglycerides by removing some of the fatty acids away from the glycerol backbone. Each triglyceride molecule is eventually broken down into two free fatty acids and one *monoglyceride,* which is the glycerol backbone with one fatty acid still attached.

Most Fat Is Absorbed in the Small Intestine

The free fatty acids and monoglycerides next need to be transported to the cells that make up the wall of the small intestine (Figure 4.7, step 4), so that they can be absorbed into the body. This trip requires the help of *micelles,* globules of bile and phospholipids that trap the free fatty acids and monoglycerides and transport them to the intestinal cell wall. Once there, shorter fatty acids can pass directly across the intestinal cell membrane. Longer fatty acids first bind to a special carrier protein and then are absorbed into the cells.

After absorption into the intestinal cells, the shortest fatty acids cross unassisted into the bloodstream and are then transported to the liver. In contrast, the longer fatty acids and monoglycerides are reformulated back into triglycerides. As you know, triglyceride molecules don't mix with water, so they can't cross independently into the bloodstream. Once again, their movement requires special packaging, this time in the form of lipoproteins. A **lipoprotein** is a spherical compound in which triglycerides cluster deep in the center and phospholipids and proteins, which are water soluble, form the surface of the sphere (**FIGURE 4.8**). The specific lipoprotein that transports fat from a meal is called a **chylomicron.** Packaged as chylomicrons, dietary fat finally arrives in your blood.

lipoprotein A spherical compound in which fat clusters in the center and phospholipids and proteins form the outside of the sphere.

chylomicron A lipoprotein produced in the mucosal cell of the intestine; transports dietary fat out of the intestinal tract.

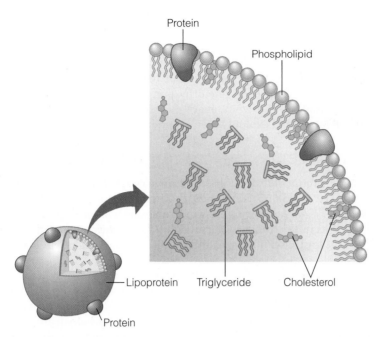

FIGURE 4.8   Structure of a lipoprotein. Notice that the fat clusters in the center of the molecule and the phospholipids and proteins, which are water soluble, form the outside of the sphere. This enables lipoproteins to transport fats in the bloodstream.

Fat Is Stored in Adipose Tissues for Later Use

The chylomicrons, which are filled with dietary fat, are transported to the liver, which can release them into the circulating blood where the fatty acids in the chylomicrons can be taken up by cells. There are three primary fates of this dietary fat:

- If your body needs the fat for energy, it will be quickly transported into your cells and used as fuel.
- The liver can use the fat to make lipid-containing compounds such as certain hormones and bile.
- Alternatively, the fat can be taken up by the muscle or adipose tissue, where it is repackaged as triglyceride and stored for later use.

If you are physically active, your body will preferentially store this extra fat in the muscle tissue first, so the next time you go out for a run, the fat is readily available for energy. That is why people who engage in regular physical activity are more likely to have extra fat stored in the muscle tissue and to have less adipose tissue—something many of us would prefer. Of course, fat stored in the adipose tissue can also be used for energy during exercise, but it must be broken down first and then transported to the muscle cells.

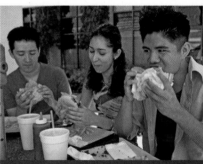

The fat we eat can be transported to our cells, used by the liver, or stored in adipose tissue.

RECAP *Fat digestion begins when fats are broken into droplets by enzymes in the stomach and bile in the small intestine. Enzymes from the pancreas subsequently digest the triglycerides into two free fatty acids and one monoglyceride. These end products of digestion are then transported to the intestinal cells for absorption with the help of micelles. Once inside the intestinal cells, triglycerides are re-formed and packaged into lipoproteins called chylomicrons. The chylomicrons transport the triglycerides to the liver, which can release the chylomicrons back into the blood whenever the body needs the fat within the chylomicrons for energy. Fat stored in the muscle tissue is used as a source of energy during physical activity. Excess fat is stored in the adipose tissue and can be used whenever the body needs energy.*

How Much Fat Should We Eat?

Without a doubt, Americans think dietary fat is bad! Yet, because fat plays such an important role in keeping our bodies healthy, our diet should include a moderate amount of energy from fat. But what, exactly, is a moderate amount? And what foods contain healthful fats? We'll explore these questions here.

Dietary Reference Intake for Total Fat

The Acceptable Macronutrient Distribution Range (AMDR) for fat is 20% to 35% of total energy intake.[3] At 2,000 kcal per day, this amounts to 400 to 700 kcal or approximately 45 to 77 g of fat. For reference, a tablespoon of butter is 11 g of fat and about 100 kcal. Within this range of fat intake, it is also recommended that we minimize our intake of saturated and *trans* fatty acids; these changes will lower our risk of heart disease.

Because carbohydrate is essential in replenishing glycogen, athletes and other physically active people are advised to consume less fat and more carbohydrate than sedentary people. Specifically, it is recommended that athletes consume 20% to 25% of their total energy from fat, 55% to 60% of energy from carbohydrate, and 12% to 15% of energy from protein.[7] This level of fat intake represents approximately 45 to 55 g per day of fat for an athlete consuming 2,000 kcal per day, and 78 to 97 g per day of fat for an athlete consuming 3,500 kcal per day.

Although many people trying to lose weight greatly restrict their consumption of fat, this practice may do more harm than good, especially if they are also eating fewer than 1,500 kcal per day. Research suggests that very-low-fat diets (those with less than 15% of energy from fat) do not provide additional health or performance benefits over moderate-fat diets and are usually very difficult to follow.[8] In fact, most people find they feel better, are more successful in weight maintenance, and are less preoccupied with food if they keep their fat intakes at 20% to 25% of energy intake.

Additionally, people attempting to reduce their dietary fat frequently eliminate food groups, such as meat, dairy, eggs, and nuts. In doing so, they also eliminate potential sources of protein and many essential vitamins and minerals important for good health and maintaining an active lifestyle. Diets low in fat may also be deficient in essential fatty acids.

NUTRI-CASE LIZ

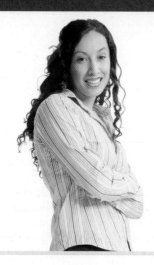

"Lately I'm hungry all the time. I read on a Web site last night that if I limit my total fat intake to no more than 10% of my total calories, I can eat all the carbohydrate and protein that I want, and I won't gain weight. So I went right out to the yogurt shop down the street and ordered a large sundae with non-fat vanilla yogurt and fat-free chocolate syrup. I have to admit, though, that an hour or so after I ate it, I was hungry again. Maybe it's stress . . ."

What do you think of Liz's approach to her persistent hunger? What have you learned in this chapter about the role of fats that might be important information for Liz to know?

Dietary Reference Intakes for Essential Fatty Acids

For the first time, Dietary Reference Intakes (DRIs) for the two essential fatty acids were set in 2002.[3] The adequate intakes are:

- linoleic acid: 14 to 17 g per day for adult men and 11 to 12 g per day for women 19 years and older. Using the typical energy intakes for adult men and women, this translates into an AMDR of 5% to 10% of total energy.
- alpha-linolenic acid: 1.6 g per day for adult men and 1.1 g per day for adult women. This translates into an AMDR of 0.6% to 1.2% of total energy.

For example, an individual consuming 2,000 kcal per day should consume about 11 to 22 g per day of linoleic acid and about 1.3 to 2.6 g per day of alpha-linolenic acid.

Most Americans Eat Too Much Saturated and *Trans* Fat

Of the dietary fat we eat, saturated and *trans* fats are most highly correlated with an increased risk of heart disease because they increase blood cholesterol levels by altering the way cholesterol is removed from the blood. Thus, the recommended intake of saturated fat is less than 7% of our total energy; unfortunately, our average intake of saturated fats is between 11% and 12% of energy.[9]

The *Dietary Guidelines for Americans* and the Institute of Medicine recommend that we keep our intake of *trans* fatty acids to an absolute minimum.[2] Determining the actual amount of *trans* fatty acids consumed in America has been hindered by the lack of an accurate and comprehensive database of foods containing *trans* fatty acids. At the present time, a best guess comes from a recent national survey, which estimated our average intake at 2.6% of our total fat intake.[10]

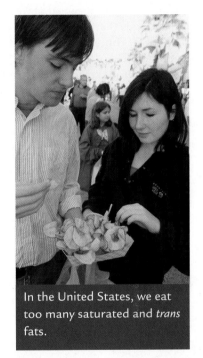

In the United States, we eat too many saturated and *trans* fats.

RECAP *The Acceptable Macronutrient Distribution Range (AMDR) for total fat is 20% to 35% of total energy. The adequate intake (AI) for linoleic acid is 14 to 17 g per day for adult men and 11 to 12 g per day for adult women. The AI for alpha-linolenic acid is 1.6 g per day for adult men and 1.1 g per day for adult women. Because saturated and* trans *fatty acids can increase the risk of heart disease, health professionals recommend that we reduce our intake of saturated fat to less than 7% of our total energy intake and reduce our intake of trans fatty acids to the absolute minimum.*

Shopper's Guide: Choosing Foods with Healthful Fats

The last time you popped a frozen dinner into the microwave, did you stop and read the Nutrition Facts Panel on the box? If you had, you might have been shocked to learn how much saturated fat was in the meal. As we discuss here, many processed foods are hidden sources of fat, especially saturated and *trans* fats. In contrast, many whole foods, such as oils, fish, and nuts, are rich sources of the healthful unsaturated fats our bodies need.

Visible versus Invisible Fats

At breakfast this morning, did you add cream to your coffee? Spread butter on your toast? These added fats, such as oils, butter, margarine, cream, shortening, mayonnaise, or salad dressings, are called **visible fats** because we can easily see that we are adding them to our food.

When we add fat to foods ourselves, we know how much we are adding and what kind. When fat is added in the preparation of a frozen dinner or a fast-food burger and fries, we are less aware of how much or what type of fat is actually

visible fats Fat we can see in our foods or see added to foods, such as butter, margarine, cream, shortening, salad dressings, chicken skin, and untrimmed fat on meat.

HIGHLIGHT

Low-Fat, Reduced-Fat, Non-Fat . . . What's the Difference?

Although most of us enjoy high-fat foods, we also know that eating a lot of fat isn't good for our health or our waistlines. Because of this concern, food manufacturers have produced a host of modified fat foods—so you can have your cake and eat it too! In fact, it is now estimated that there are more than 5,000 different fat-modified foods on the market.[11] This means that we have similar foods that come in a wide range of fat contents. For example, you can purchase full-fat, low-fat, or fat-free milk, ice cream, sour cream, cheese, and yogurt.

In Table 4.1, we list a number of full-fat foods with their lower-fat alternatives. If you incorporate these products in your diet on a regular basis, you can significantly reduce the amount of fat you consume, but watch out! You might not be reducing the number of kcals you consume!

For example, drinking nonfat milk (86 kcal and 0.5 g of fat per serving) instead of whole milk (150 kcal and 8.2 g of fat per serving) will dramatically reduce both fat and energy intake. However, eating fat-free Fig Newton cookies (3 cookies have 204 kcal and 0 g of fat) instead of regular Fig Newton cookies (3 cookies have 210 kcal and 4.5 g of fat) will not reduce your energy intake dramatically, even though it will reduce your fat intake by 4.5 g per serving.

The reduced fat is often replaced with added carbohydrate, as is the case with the reduced-fat peanut butter listed in Table 4.1. As another example, a 6-oz cup of plain nonfat yogurt provides about 82 kcals, but a 6-oz cup of fruit-flavored nonfat yogurt provides 140 kcals due to the added carbohydrate! So if you want to significantly reduce both the amount of fat and the number of calories you consume, you must read the labels of modified-fat foods carefully before you buy.

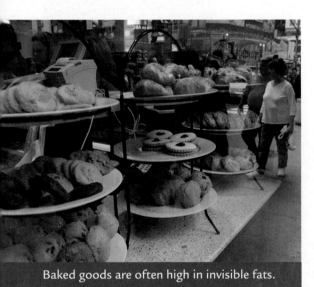

Baked goods are often high in invisible fats.

invisible fats Fats that are hidden in foods, such as the fats found in baked goods, regular-fat dairy products, marbling in meat, and fried foods.

there. In fact, unless we read food labels carefully, we might not be aware that a food contains any fat at all. We call fats in prepared and processed foods **invisible fats** because they are hidden within the food. In fact, their invisibility often tricks us into choosing them over more healthful foods. For example, a slice of yellow cake is much higher in fat (40% of total energy) than a slice of angel food cake (1% of total energy). Yet, many consumers just assume the fat content of these foods is the same, as both are cake. For most of us, the majority of the fat in our diets comes from invisible fat. Foods that can be high in invisible fats are baked goods, regular-fat dairy products, processed meats or meats that are not trimmed, and most convenience and fast foods, such as hamburgers, hot dogs, chips, ice cream, French fries, and other fried foods.

Because high-fat diets have been associated with obesity and heart disease, many Americans have tried to reduce their total fat intake. Food manufacturers have been more than happy to provide consumers with low-fat alternatives to their favorite foods. However, these lower-fat foods may not always have fewer calories. Read the Highlight box above and Table 4.1 to learn how to be a better consumer of reduced-fat foods.

Food Sources of Beneficial Fats

Americans appear to get adequate amounts of omega-6 fatty acids, probably because of the high amount of salad dressings, vegetable and nut oils, margarine, and may-

TABLE 4.1 Comparison of Full-Fat, Reduced-Fat, and Low-Fat Foods

Product and Serving Size	Version	Energy (kcal)	Protein (g)	Carbohydrate (g)	Fat (g)
Milk, 8 oz	Whole, 3.3% fat	150	8.0	11.4	8.2
	2% fat	121	8.1	11.7	4.7
	1% fat	102	8.0	11.7	2.6
	Skim (nonfat)	86	8.4	11.9	0.5
Cheese, cheddar, 1 oz	Regular	111	7.1	0.5	9.1
	Low-fat	81	9.1	0.0	5.1
	Nonfat	41	6.8	4.0	0.0
Mayonnaise, 1 tbsp.	Regular	100	0.0	0.0	11.0
	Light	50	0.0	1.0	5.0
	Fat-free	10	0.0	2.0	0.0
Margarine, corn oil, 1 tbsp.	Regular	100	0.0	0.0	11.0
	Reduced-fat	60	0.0	0.0	7.0
Peanut butter, 1 tbsp.	Regular	95	4.1	3.1	8.2
	Reduced-fat	81	4.4	5.2	5.4
Cream cheese, 1 tbsp.	Soft regular	50	1.0	0.5	5.0
	Soft light	35	1.5	1.0	2.5
	Soft nonfat	15	2.5	1.0	0.0
Wheat Thins, 18 crackers	Regular	158	2.3	21.4	6.8
	Reduced-fat	120	2.0	21.0	4.0
Cookies, Oreo, 3 cookies	Regular	160	2.0	23.0	7.0
	Reduced-fat	130	2.0	25.0	3.5
Cookies, Fig Newton, 3 cookies	Regular	210	3.0	30.0	4.5
	Fat-free	204	2.4	26.8	0.0
Breakfast bars, 1 bar	Regular	140	2.0	27.0	2.8
	Fat-free	110	2.0	26.0	0.0

Source: Data from Food Processor-SQL, Version 9.9, ESHA Research, Salem, OR.

The Food and Drug Administration and the U.S. Department of Agriculture have set specific regulations on allowable product descriptions for reduced-fat products. The following claims are defined for 1 serving: **Fat-free:** less than 0.5 gram of fat; **Low-fat:** 3 grams or less of fat; **Reduced** or **less fat:** at least 25% less fat as compared to a standard serving; **Light:** one-third fewer calories or 50% less fast as compared with a standard serving size.

onnaise we eat; however, our consumption of omega-3 fatty acids is more variable and can be low in the diets of people who do not eat fish or walnuts, drink soy milk, or use soybean, canola, or flaxseed oil. Table 4.2 on page 118 identifies the omega-3 fatty acid content of various foods.

In general, it's best to switch to foods with healthful fats without increasing total fat intake. For example, use olive and canola oil in place of butter and margarine and select fish more often instead of hot dogs, hamburgers, or sausage. Select low- and nonfat milk and yogurt, and reduce your intake of full-fat cheeses and cheese spreads. Read the Nutrition Label Activity: How Much Fat Is in This Food? on the following page to learn how to calculate the fat calories in the foods you buy.

NUTRITION LABEL ACTIVITY

How Much Fat Is in This Food?

How do you know how much fat is in a food you buy? One simple way to determine the amount of fat in foods is to read the Nutrition Facts Panel on the label. By becoming a better label reader, you can make more healthful food selections.

Two cracker labels are shown in Figure 4.9: one cracker is higher in fat than the other. Because the serving size for these crackers is the same, you can tell which has more fat by comparing the total calories from fat in each serving.

Look at the first two lines under **Amount Per Serving** and enter the following data:

- **For the regular Wheat Crackers, the total calories per serving =** __150__.
- **The calories from fat =** __50__.

If you've entered the data correctly, you'll be able to see that one-third of the total number of calories in the regular Wheat Crackers comes from fat.

- **For the Reduced-Fat Wheat Crackers, the total calories from fat =** __35__.

- **The total calories per serving =** __150__.

If you've entered the data correctly, you'll be able to see that about one-fourth of the total number of calories in the Reduced-Fat Wheat Crackers comes from fat.

(Answers can be found at the end of this chapter.)

In short, although the total number of calories per serving is not very different between these two crackers, the level of fat is quite different.

If the total calories per serving from fat are not given on the label, you can compare the two crackers by looking at the total grams of fat per serving. The regular Wheat Crackers have 6 g of fat per serving, whereas the Reduced-Fat Wheat Crackers have only 4 g of fat per serving.

Table 4.1 lists regular, reduced-fat, and fat-free versions of several foods. Notice that the serving sizes for foods within a group are the same (for example, 8 oz of different types of milk, 1 tablespoon of various spreads, etc.). Thus, you can easily compare the total grams of fat for the different foods within each group.

FIGURE 4.9 Labels for two types of wheat crackers. (a) Regular wheat crackers. (b) Reduced-fat wheat crackers.

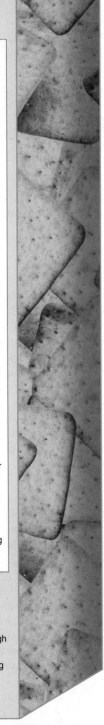

Wheat Crackers

- No Cholesterol

Nutrition Facts

Serving Size: 16 Crackers (31g)
Servings Per Container: About 9

Amount Per Serving

Calories	150
Calories from Fat	50

	% Daily Value*
Total Fat 6g	9%
Saturated Fat 1g	6%
Polyunsaturated Fat 0g	
Monounsaturated Fat 2g	
Trans Fat 0g	
Cholesterol 0mg	0%
Sodium 270mg	11%
Total Carbohydrate 21g	7%
Dietary Fiber 1g	4%
Sugars 3g	
Protein 2g	
Vitamin A	0%
Vitamin C	0%
Calcium	2%
Iron	6%

* Percent Daily Values are based on a 2,000 calorie diet. Your daily values may be higher or lower depending on your calorie needs:

	Calories	2,000	2,500
Total Fat	Less than	65g	80g
Sat. Fat	Less than	20g	25g
Cholesterol	Less than	300mg	300mg
Sodium	Less than	2,400mg	2,400mg
Total Carbohydrate		300g	375g
Dietary Fiber		25g	30g

INGREDIENTS: Enriched Flour (Wheat Flour, Niacin, Reduced Iron, Thiamine Mononitrate (Vitamin B1), Riboflavin (Vitamin B2), Folic Acid), Partially Hydrogenated Soybean Oil, Defatted Wheat Germ, Sugar, Cornstarch, High Fructose Corn Syrup, Salt, Corn Syrup, Malt Syrup, Leavening (Calcium Phosphate, Baking Soda), Vegetable Colors (Annatto Extract, Turmeric Oleoresin), Malted Barley Flour.

(a)

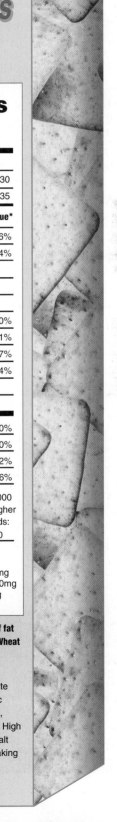

Reduced-Fat Wheat Crackers

- **No Cholesterol**
- **Low Saturated Fat**
  Contains 4g Fat Per Serving

Nutrition Facts

Serving Size: 16 Crackers (29g)
Servings Per Container: About 9

Amount Per Serving

Calories	130
Calories from Fat	35

	% Daily Value*
Total Fat 4g	6%
Saturated Fat 1g	4%
Polyunsaturated Fat 0g	
Monounsaturated Fat 1.5g	
Trans Fat 0g	
Cholesterol 0mg	0%
Sodium 260mg	11%
Total Carbohydrate 21g	7%
Dietary Fiber 1g	4%
Sugars 3g	
Protein 2g	
Vitamin A	0%
Vitamin C	0%
Calcium	2%
Iron	6%

* Percent Daily Values are based on a 2,000 calorie diet. Your daily values may be higher or lower depending on your calorie needs:

	Calories	2,000	2,500
Total Fat	Less than	65g	80g
Sat. Fat	Less than	20g	25g
Cholesterol	Less than	300mg	300mg
Sodium	Less than	2,400mg	2,400mg
Total Carbohydrate		300g	375g
Dietary Fiber		25g	30g

Reduced-Fat Wheat Crackers have 4 grams of fat per serving compared to 6 grams in Original Wheat Crackers.

INGREDIENTS: Enriched Flour (Wheat Flour, Niacin, Reduced Iron, Thiamine Mononitrate (Vitamin B1), Riboflavin (Vitamin B2), Folic Acid), Partially Hydrogenated Soybean Oil, Defatted Wheat Germ, Sugar, Cornstarch, High Fructose Corn Syrup, Corn Syrup, Salt, Malt Syrup, Leavening (Calcium Phosphate, Baking Soda), Vegetable Colors (Annatto Extract, Turmeric Oleoresin), Malted Barley Flour.

(b)

TABLE 4.2 Omega-3 Fatty Acid Content of Selected Foods

Food Item	Omega-3 Fatty Acid (grams per serving)
Flaxseed oil, 1 tbsp.	7.25
Salmon oil (fish oil), 1 tbsp.	4.39
Sardine oil, 1 tbsp.	3.01
Flaxseed, whole, 1 tbsp.	2.50
Herring, Atlantic, broiled, 3 oz	1.83
Herring oil, 1 tbsp.	1.53
Canola oil, 1 tbsp.	1.30
Sardines, Atlantic, w/ bones and oil, 3 oz	1.26
Shrimp, broiled, 3 oz	1.11
Trout, rainbow fillet, baked, 3 oz	1.00
Walnuts, English, 1 tbsp.	0.68
Salmon, smoked Chinook, 3 oz	0.50
Halibut, fillet, baked, 3 oz	0.47
Tuna, white, in oil, 3 oz	0.38
Crab, Dungeness, steamed, 3 oz	0.34
Scallops, broiled, 3 oz	0.26
Tuna, light, in water, 3 oz	0.23

Source: Data from Food Processor SQL, Version 9.9, ESHA Research, Salem, OR.

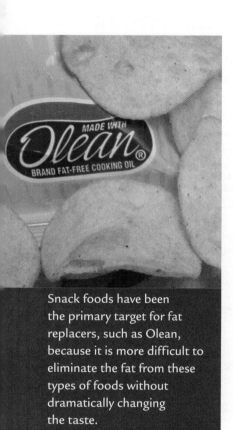

Snack foods have been the primary target for fat replacers, such as Olean, because it is more difficult to eliminate the fat from these types of foods without dramatically changing the taste.

It is important to recognize that there can be some risk associated with eating large amounts of certain types of fish on a regular basis. Some species of fish contain high levels of environmental contaminants such as mercury and polychlorinated biphenyls (PCBs). These contaminants can accumulate in the bodies of individuals who regularly consume contaminated fish. Women who are pregnant or breastfeeding, women who may become pregnant, and small children are at particularly high risk for toxicity from these contaminants.

Sport-caught fish and predator fish such as shark, swordfish, and king mackerel tend to have higher levels of contaminants. Types of fish that are currently considered safe to consume include salmon (except from the Great Lakes region), farmed trout, flounder, sole, mahi mahi, and cooked shellfish. For more information on seafood contamination, see Chapter 12.

Fat Replacers

One way manufacturers lower the fat content of foods like chips, muffins, cakes, and cookies is by replacing the fat with a *fat replacer.* Snack foods have been the primary target for fat replacers, as it is difficult to significantly reduce or eliminate the fat from such products without dramatically changing the taste. Some fat replacers, such as olestra (brand name Olean), may cause gastrointestinal distress in some sensitive individuals or if used in large quantities. Until recently, foods containing olestra had to bear a label warning of potential gastrointestinal side effects. In 2003, the FDA announced that this warning is no longer necessary, as recent research indicates that olestra causes only mild, infrequent discomfort. The safety testing on olestra was extensive, with over 100 animal and 40 human studies reviewed by the FDA, which recently reaffirmed that there were no significant adverse health consequences associated with olestra consumption.

Fat replacers were introduced to the market in the 1990s and may be helpful in reducing overall fat intake, but have not helped to reduce caloric intake or overall obesity rates.[12] These products, however, may be helpful tools for weight loss if combined with a well-balanced energy-restricted diet.

> **RECAP** *Visible fats can be easily recognized, such as fat on meats. Invisible fats are those fats added to food during the manufacturing or cooking process. Common food sources of omega-6 fatty acids include vegetables and vegetable oils, nuts and nut oils, salad dressings, margarine, and mayonnaise. Food sources of omega-3 fatty acids include fish, walnuts, soy milk, and soybean, canola, or flaxseed oil. Fat replacers are those substances used to replace the typical fats found in foods to reduce the amount of fat in the food.*

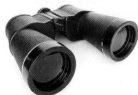

HEALTHWATCH

What Role Do Fats Play in Cardiovascular Disease and Cancer?

We know that a diet high in saturated and *trans* fatty acids can contribute to chronic disease. But just how significant a factor is diet, and what other factors also play a role?

Cardiovascular disease is a general term used to refer to any abnormal condition involving dysfunction of the heart (*cardio* means "heart") and blood vessels (another word for vessels is *vasculature*). A common form of this disease occurs when blood vessels supplying the heart (the *coronary arteries*) become blocked or constricted; such blockage reduces blood flow to the heart or brain and so can result in a heart attack or a stroke. According to the Centers for Disease Control and Prevention, cardiovascular disease is the leading cause of death in the United States across racial and ethnic groups and is a major cause of permanent disability (FIGURE 4.10).[13]

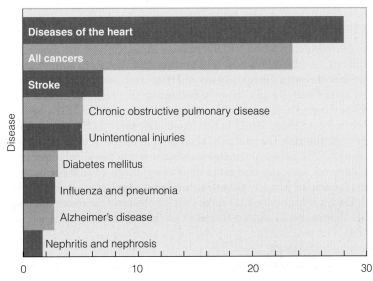

FIGURE 4.10 Cardiovascular disease, which includes heart disease, is the leading cause of death in the United States.
Source: Data from National Center for Health Statistics. 2004. Fast Stats A to Z. Deaths—Leading Causes. Available at www.cdc.gov/nchs/faststats/lcod.htm.

cardiovascular disease
A general term that refers to abnormal conditions involving dysfunction of the heart and blood vessels; cardiovascular disease can result in heart attack or stroke.

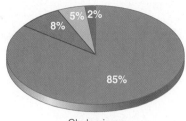

Chylomicron

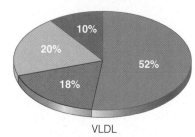

VLDL

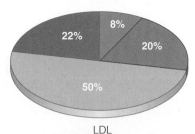

LDL

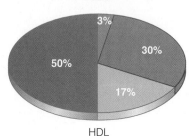

HDL

Key:

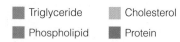

Triglyceride Cholesterol
Phospholipid Protein

FIGURE 4.11 The chemical components of chylomicrons, very-low-density lipoproteins (VLDLs), low-density lipoproteins (LDLs), and high-density lipoproteins (HDLs) blood lipids. Notice that chylomicrons contain the highest proportion of triglycerides, making them the least dense, while HDLs have the highest proportion of protein, making them the most dense.

Dietary Fats Play an Important Role in Cardiovascular Disease

Recall that lipids are transported in the blood by lipoproteins made up of a lipid center and a protein outer coat. Because lipoproteins are soluble in blood, they are commonly called *blood lipids.* In addition to the chylomicrons introduced earlier in this chapter, three lipoproteins are important to consider in any discussion of cardiovascular health and disease:

- very-low-density lipoproteins (VLDLs)
- low-density lipoproteins (LDLs)
- high-density lipoproteins (HDLs)

The density of a lipoprotein refers to its ratio of lipid, which is less dense, to protein, which is very dense. Thus, a very-low-density lipoprotein contains mostly lipid and little protein. The chemical composition of various lipoproteins is compared in FIGURE 4.11. Our blood contains a different mix of these blood lipids according to our diet, our fitness, and whether we have been eating or fasting. Let's look at each of these blood lipids in more detail to determine how they are linked to heart disease risk.

Very-Low-Density Lipoproteins

Very-low-density lipoproteins (VLDLs) are made up mostly of triglyceride. The liver is the primary source of VLDLs, but they are also produced in the intestines. VLDLs are primarily transport vehicles ferrying triglycerides, which are produced in the liver or intestine, to other cells of the body. If their triglyceride load is not needed for fuel, the fatty acids can be released and taken up by the adipose cells for storage.

Diets high in saturated fat, simple sugars, and extra energy tend to increase blood levels of VLDLs, because they increase the production of triglycerides in the liver. Conversely, diets high in omega-3 fatty acids can help reduce VLDL levels because they inhibit the synthesis of triglycerides, which are the primary component of VLDLs. In addition, exercise can reduce VLDLs because the triglycerides transported in the VLDLs can be used for energy instead of remaining to circulate in the blood.

Low-Density Lipoproteins

The lipoproteins resulting when VLDLs release their triglyceride load are much higher in cholesterol, phospholipids, and protein and therefore somewhat more dense. These **low-density lipoproteins (LDLs)** circulate in the blood until they are absorbed by the body's cells, thereby delivering their cholesterol to the cells. Diets high in saturated and *trans* fats *decrease* the removal of LDLs by body cells and therefore increase their levels in the blood. The more LDLs circulating in the blood, the greater the risk that some of their cholesterol will adhere to the walls of the blood vessels. This adhesion causes *scavenger* white blood cells to rush to the site and bind cholesterol. As more and more cholesterol binds to these cells, they burst to form a fatty patch, or *plaque,* that eventually hardens, blocking the artery (FIGURE 4.12). Because high blood levels of LDL-cholesterol increase the risk of heart disease, LDL-cholesterol is often referred to as "bad cholesterol."

High-Density Lipoproteins

High-density lipoproteins (HDLs) are small, dense lipoproteins with a very low cholesterol content and a high protein content. They are produced in the liver, then released to circulate in the blood, picking up cholesterol from dying cells and arterial plaques or transferring it to other lipoproteins. When HDLs deliver their newly acquired cholesterol to the liver, they remove it from the circulatory system. You can see why high blood levels of HDLs are therefore associated with a low risk of coronary artery disease and why HDL-cholesterol is often referred to as "good cholesterol." Incidentally, one of the ways in which omega-3 fatty acids decrease our risk of

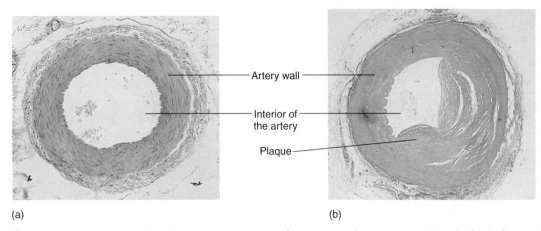

(a)   (b)

FIGURE 4.12   These light micrographs show a cross section of (a) a normal artery containing little cholesterol-rich plaque and allowing adequate blood flow through the heart and (b) an artery that is partially blocked with cholesterol-rich plaque, which can lead to a heart attack.

heart disease is by increasing HDL-cholesterol.[5] There is also some evidence that participating in regular physical exercise can modestly increase HDL-cholesterol levels.

Total Serum Cholesterol

For a small percentage of individuals, the level of dietary cholesterol eaten can influence serum (blood) cholesterol levels. Normally, as the dietary level of cholesterol increases, the body decreases the amount of cholesterol it makes, which keeps the body's level of cholesterol constant. Unfortunately, this feedback mechanism does not work well in everyone. For some individuals, eating dietary cholesterol doesn't decrease the amount of cholesterol produced in the body, and their total body cholesterol levels rise. This in turn increases the levels of cholesterol in the blood. These individuals benefit from reducing their intake of dietary cholesterol, typically by limiting intake of animal products or selecting low-fat animal products. Research also indicates that high intakes of saturated and *trans* fatty acids can increase the total serum cholesterol.

The Role of *Trans* Fatty Acids

Recent research indicates that *trans* fatty acids can raise blood LDL-cholesterol levels as much as saturated fat.[3,14] Thus, to reduce the risk of heart disease, we must reduce our intake of both high-fat animal products and foods that contain vegetable shortening or partially hydrogenated oil, because these are *trans* fats. Don't forget that foods fried in hydrogenated oils, such as French fries and doughnuts, are high in *trans* fatty acids, so these types of foods should also be avoided. Finally, if you use margarine and shortening, look for products that contain no *trans* fatty acids. Choose olive oil, nut butters, and other healthful fats often.

Calculating Your Risk for Cardiovascular Disease

A simple laboratory analysis of your blood can tell you your blood lipid levels, specifically your LDL-cholesterol, HDL-cholesterol, and total serum cholesterol. If you do not know this information about yourself, there are easy ways to find out. Many college and university health centers offer blood lipid screenings at low cost or even free of charge. Or, the next time you visit your physician, ask to have your blood lipids measured. You should also have your blood pressure checked regularly. Blood pressure screening is typically offered at student health centers, at health fairs, and even in many drug stores. It is especially important to take these steps if you have a family history of heart disease.

   If you know your blood pressure and blood lipid levels, then you can estimate your risk of developing cardiovascular disease. Check out What About You? Calculate

very-low-density lipoprotein (VLDL)   Large lipoprotein made up mostly of triglyceride. Functions primarily to transport triglycerides from their source to the body's cells, including to adipose tissues for storage.

low-density lipoprotein (LDL)   Molecule resulting when a VLDL releases its triglyceride load. Higher cholesterol and protein content makes LDLs somewhat more dense than VLDLs.

high-density lipoprotein (HDL)   Small, dense lipoprotein with a very low cholesterol content and a high protein content.

WHAT ABOUT YOU?

Calculate Your Risk for Cardiovascular Disease

If you know your blood lipid numbers, you can use the calculation matrix in Figure 4.13 from the National Institutes of Health to estimate your 10-year risk for cardiovascular disease. Simply answer the questions, enter your points, then total your score. Apply your score to the green grid for females or the blue grid for males. For example, a female with a score of 17 has a 5% chance of developing cardiovascular disease in the next 10 years. If you're reading this and don't know your numbers, now would be a great time to find out what they are.

Your Risk for Cardiovascular Disease, and then compare your total points to the points in the 10-year risk column. You can also do this quick assessment on family members or friends to help them become more aware of their risk factors for cardiovascular disease. There is also an online version of this risk calculator at http://hin.nhlbi.nih.gov/atpiii/calculator.asp?usertype=prof.

You Can Reduce Your Risk for Cardiovascular Disease

The Centers for Disease Control and Prevention (CDC), the Expert Panel on Detection, Evaluation, and Treatment of High Blood Cholesterol in Adults (ATP III), and the American Heart Association have all made recommendations for diet, physical activity, and other lifestyle factors that can improve blood lipid levels and reduce your risk of cardiovascular disease:[8, 15]

- Aim for recommended levels of LDL-cholesterol, HDL-cholesterol, and triglycerides, by:
  - Maintaining total fat intake to within 20% to 35% of energy, and keeping intake of saturated and *trans* fatty acids low (IOM, 2005). Polyunsaturated fats (for example, soy and canola oil) can comprise up to 10% of total energy intake, while monounsaturated fats (for example, olive oil) can comprise up to 20% of total energy intake. For some people, a lower fat intake may help to maintain a healthful body weight.
  - Decreasing dietary saturated fat to less than 7% of total energy intake. Decrease cholesterol intake to less than 300 mg per day, and keep *trans* fatty acid intake at an absolute minimum. Lowering the intakes of these fats will lower your LDL-cholesterol level. Replace saturated fat (e.g., butter, margarine, vegetable shortening, or lard) with more healthful cooking oils, such as olive or canola oil.
  - Increasing dietary intakes of whole grains, fruits, and vegetables so that total dietary fiber is 20 to 30 g per day. Foods high in fiber decrease blood LDL-cholesterol levels.
  - Scheduling regular physical check ups to help you monitor your lipid levels and determine if values are within normal limits

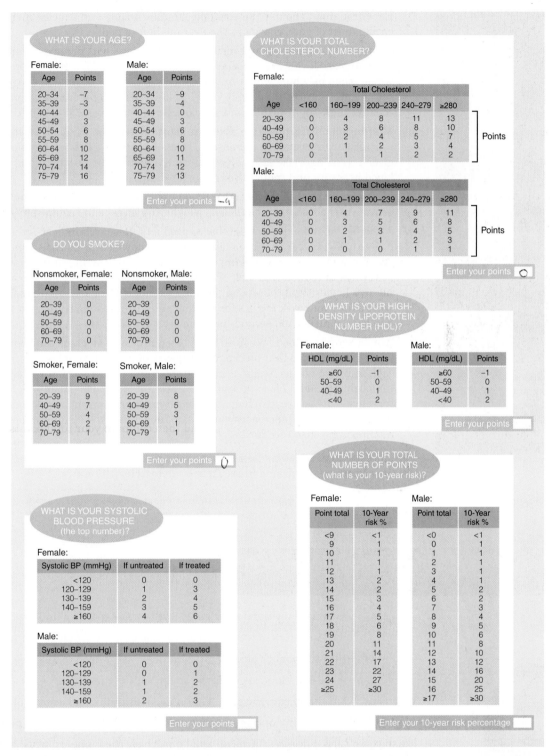

FIGURE 4.13 Calculation matrix to estimate the 10-year risk for cardiovascular disease for men and women.
Source: National Institutes of Health. 2005. High Blood Cholesterol: What You Need to Know. NIH publication No. 05-3290. Available at www.nhlbi.nih.gov/health/public/heart/chol/hbc_what.htm.

- Consume a healthful diet overall. The relationship between diet and cardiovascular disease is multifaceted and complicated by one's genetic risk of getting the disease. Consuming a healthful diet will help you maintain a healthy body weight, and keep your blood lipids, glucose, and blood pressure within healthy limits.

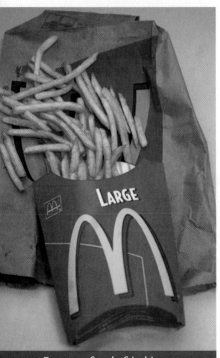

Because foods fried in hydrogenated vegetable oils, such as French fries, are high in *trans* fatty acids, these types of foods should be avoided.

- Eat throughout the day (for example, smaller meals and snacks) instead of eating most of your energy in the evening before bed.

- Maintain blood glucose and insulin concentrations within normal ranges. High blood glucose levels are associated with high blood triglycerides. Consume foods whole (such as whole-wheat breads and cereals, whole fruits and vegetables, and beans and legumes), and limit your intake of high-sugar foods (for example, cookies, high-sugar drinks and snacks, candy, etc.).

- Maintain an active lifestyle. Exercise most days of the week for 30 to 60 minutes if possible. Exercise will increase HDL-cholesterol while lowering blood triglyceride levels. Exercise also helps maintain a healthy body weight and a lower blood pressure and reduces your risk for diabetes.

- Maintain a healthy body weight. Blood lipids and glucose levels typically improve when obese individuals lose weight and engage in regular physical activity.

- Avoid use of and exposure to tobacco products. Research indicates that smokers have a 70% greater chance of developing cardiovascular disease than nonsmokers. Without question, smoking cessation or never starting initially is one of the best ways to reduce your risk of cardiovascular disease. People who stop smoking live longer than those who continue to smoke, and a 15-year cessation period will reduce your risk factors for cardiovascular disease to those of a nonsmoker. You should also avoid second-hand smoke.

- Aim for normal blood pressure. High blood pressure stresses the heart and increases the chance that blockage or rupture of a blood vessel will occur. A diet high in whole grains, fruits, and vegetables and low in sodium will help you maintain a normal blood pressure. Maintaining a healthy body weight and staying physically active also help keep blood pressure normal. Smoking increases blood pressure and increases your risk of heart disease. Regular blood pressure monitoring is also recommended.

For more dietary strategies for reducing your risk of cardiovascular disease, check out the accompanying Game Plan: Tips for Heart-Healthy Eating.

NUTRI-CASE JUDY

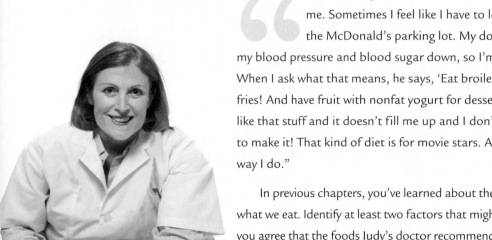

" Ever since my last doctor's visit, I've felt as if there's a 'food cop' spying on me. Sometimes I feel like I have to look over my shoulder when I pull into the McDonald's parking lot. My doctor says I need to lose weight and get my blood pressure and blood sugar down, so I'm supposed to switch to healthy fats. When I ask what that means, he says, 'Eat broiled fish! And salad instead of French fries! And have fruit with nonfat yogurt for dessert!' I didn't bother telling him I don't like that stuff and it doesn't fill me up and I don't have the money to buy it or the time to make it! That kind of diet is for movie stars. All the real people I know eat the same way I do."

In previous chapters, you've learned about the many factors influencing why we eat what we eat. Identify at least two factors that might be affecting Judy's food choices. Do you agree that the foods Judy's doctor recommended are not for "real people" like Judy? Why or why not?

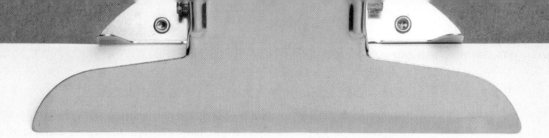

GAME PLAN
Tips for Heart-Healthy Eating

When shopping for and preparing meals at home, as well as when dining out, try these simple strategies to tip the balance of your diet toward heart-healthy fats.

At Home

❑ Boost the nutrient profile of your favorite breakfast cereal by adding 1 tablespoon of ground flaxseed meal.

❑ Select whole-grain breads, and try peanut, almond, or walnut butter as a spread for your toast.

❑ If you normally eat two eggs for breakfast, discard the yolk from one egg for half the cholesterol. Do the same in recipes calling for two eggs.

❑ Select low-fat or nonfat milk, coffee creamers, yogurt, cream cheese, cottage cheese, sour cream, mayonnaise, and salad dressings.

❑ Substitute lower-fat cheeses such as parmesan for higher-fat cheeses such as cheddar.

❑ If you use margarine, select one that is made from a high-omega-3 oil, such as canola oil, and is *trans-* fat free.

❑ Start meals with a salad dressed with olive oil and vinegar or a fat-free soup.

❑ Select lean cuts of meat. Load your plate with vegetables, and make meat a "condiment."

❑ Instead of frying meats, fish, and vegetables, bake or broil them.

❑ Trim all visible fat from meats and poultry before cooking. Eat poultry without the skin.

❑ Instead of buttering your bread, dip it in a mixture of olive oil and a dribble of balsamic vinegar.

❑ Make sure that any crackers or cookies you buy are low in saturated fats and free of *trans* fatty acids.

❑ Choose ice milk, sorbet, or low-fat or nonfat yogurt and fruit for dessert instead of high-fat ice cream.

❑ For snacks, substitute raw vegetables, whole and dried fruits, pretzels, or air-popped popcorn for potato chips or sweets.

❑ Choose water, skim milk, soy milk, or unsweetened beverages over sugar-sweetened beverages.

❑ Read food labels. Select high-fat foods less often or use them in moderation.

❑ Control your portion size, especially when consuming high-fat foods.

Eating Out

❑ When dining out, select a high-omega-3 fatty acid fish, like salmon, or try a vegetarian entrée made with tofu or tempeh. If you do choose meat, ask that it be trimmed of fat and broiled rather than fried.

❑ Consider splitting an entrée with your dinner companion and complement it with a side salad.

❑ On your salad, choose olive oil and vinegar instead of a high-fat dressing. Also use olive oil and vinegar instead of butter for your bread.

❑ Order a baked potato or rice instead of French fries or potatoes *au gratin.*

❑ Skip dessert or choose a fat-free sorbet.

❑ The next time you order a fast-food meal, either skip the French fries or order the kid's meal for portion control.

❑ Order pizza with vegetable toppings instead of pepperoni or sausage.

❑ Order coffee drinks with skim milk instead of cream or whole milk, and accompany them with a biscotti instead of a brownie.

Where I'm at now...

At the beginning of this chapter, you jotted down your guess about what's "wrong" with fried foods. Has your answer changed? If so, how?

Do you now plan to eat fried foods less often?

Yes or **NO** or

Didn't eat much to begin with

Now that you've learned about the benefits of omega-6 and omega-3 essential fatty acids, and their food sources, would you say you get enough of these nutrients each day?

Yes or **NO**

If not, what foods do you plan to add or increase in your diet?

Does a High-Fat Diet Cause Cancer?

Cancer develops as a result of a poorly understood interaction between the environment and genetic factors. In addition, most cancers take years to develop, so examining the impact of diet on cancer development can be a long and difficult process. Diet and lifestyle are two of the most important environmental factors that have been identified in the development of cancer.[16, 17] Three types of cancer that have been studied extensively for their possible relationship to dietary fat intake are breast cancer, colon cancer, and prostate cancer:

- Breast cancer. Currently no clinical trials show a link between the amount of fat consumed and increased risk for breast cancer.[18-20]

- Colon cancer. Recent research shows that a Western diet high in red meat, fat, refined grains, and desserts is associated with a greater recurrence of colon cancer compared to a diet high in fruits, vegetables, poultry, and fish.[21] Because we now know that physical activity can reduce the risk of colon cancer, earlier diet and colon cancer studies that did not control for this factor are now being questioned.

- Prostate cancer. As with other cancers, the exact link between dietary fat intake and prostate cancer is not clear.[22] Research shows that there is a consistent link between prostate cancer risk and consumption of animal fats but not other types of fats. The exact mechanism by which animal fats may contribute to prostate cancer has not yet been identified.

Until we know more about the link between diet, especially fat, and cancer, the American Institute for Cancer Research recommends the following diet and lifestyle changes to prevent cancer:[22]

- Maintain a healthy body weight.
- Be physically active for at least 30 minutes a day.
- Avoid sugary drinks and limit consumption of energy-dense foods (foods high in sugar and fat).
- Eat a variety of fruits, vegetables, whole grains, and legumes.
- Limit consumption of red meats, such as beef, pork, and lamb, and avoid processed meats.
- Limit alcohol intake to 2 drinks/day for men and 1 drink/day for women.
- Limit consumption of salty foods and foods processed with salt.
- Don't use supplements to protect against cancer.

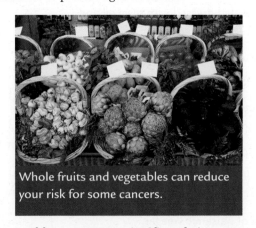

Whole fruits and vegetables can reduce your risk for some cancers.

RECAP *The types of fats we eat can significantly impact our health and risk of disease. Saturated and trans fatty acids increase our risk of heart disease, whereas omega-3 fatty acids can reduce our risk. High levels of LDL-cholesterol and low levels of HDL-cholesterol increase your risk of heart disease. Other risk factors for heart disease include being overweight, being physically inactive, smoking, having high blood pressure, and having diabetes mellitus. Consuming a healthful diet and making certain lifestyle choices will also reduce your risk of some cancers.*

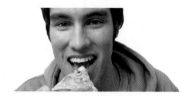

REVIEW QUESTIONS

Circle the correct choice.

1. Cholesterol is
   a. a form of *trans* fatty acid.
   b. a form of saturated fatty acid.
   c. synthesized in the liver and small intestine.
   d. found in leafy green vegetables, flax seeds, and soy.

2. One of the most sensible ways to reduce body fat is to
   a. limit intake of fat to less than 15% of total energy consumed.
   b. exercise regularly.
   c. avoid all consumption of *trans* fatty acids.
   d. restrict total calories to less than 1,200 per day.

3. Micelles assist in the
   a. transport of dietary fat to the wall of the small intestine.
   b. emulsification of dietary fat in the small intestine.
   c. synthesis of cholesterol in the liver.
   d. storage of excess fat in adipose tissue.

4. The risk of heart disease is reduced in people who have high blood levels of
   a. triglycerides.
   b. very-low-density lipoproteins.
   c. low-density lipoproteins.
   d. high-density lipoproteins.

5. Triglycerides with a double carbon bond at one part of the molecule are referred to as
   a. monounsaturated fats.
   b. hydrogenated fats.
   c. saturated fats.
   d. sterols.

6. True or False? The Acceptable Macronutrient Distribution Range (AMDR) for fat is 20% to 35% of total energy.

7. True or False? During exercise, fat cannot be mobilized from adipose tissue for use as energy.

8. True or False? Triglycerides are the same as fatty acids.

9. True or False? *Trans* fatty acids are produced by food manufacturers; they do not occur in nature.

10. True or False? A serving of food labeled *reduced fat* has at least 25% less fat and 25% fewer calories than a full-fat version of the same food.

WEB LINKS

www.americanheart.org
American Heart Association

Learn the best way to help lower your blood cholesterol level. Access the AHA's online cookbook for healthy-heart recipes and cooking methods.

www.caloriecontrol.org
Calorie Control Council

Go to this site to find out more about fat replacers.

www.nhlbi.nih.gov/chd
Live Healthier, Live Longer

Take a cholesterol quiz, and test your heart disease IQ. Create a diet using the Heart Healthy Diet or the TLC Diet online software.

www.nhlbi.nih.gov
National Heart, Lung, and Blood Institute

Learn how a healthful diet can lower your cholesterol levels. Use the online risk assessment tool to estimate your 10-year risk of having a heart attack.

www.cfsan.fda.gov/~dms/transfat.html
Consumer Information on the New *Trans* Fat Labeling Requirements

This page, created by the U.S. Food and Drug Administration, provides information about the required *trans* fat labeling.

www.nih.gov
The National Institutes of Health (NIH)
U.S. Department of Health and Human Services

Search this site to learn more about dietary fats and the DASH Diet (Dietary Approaches to Stop Hypertension).

www.nlm.nih.gov/medlineplus
MEDLINE Plus Health Information

Search for "fats" or "lipids" to obtain additional resources and the latest news on dietary lipids, heart disease, and cholesterol.

www.hsph.harvard.edu/nutritionsource
The Nutrition Source: Knowledge for Healthy Eating
Harvard University's Department of Nutrition

Go to this site and click on "Fats & Cholesterol" to find out how selective fat intake can be part of a healthful diet.

www.ific.org
International Food Information Council Foundation

Access this site to find out more about fats and dietary fat replacers.

TEST YOURSELF ANSWERS

1. False. Although high levels of total blood cholesterol are linked to an increased risk of heart disease, cholesterol is an important component of cell membranes and is essential to human functioning. The body can manufacture cholesterol from components of other nutrients, so we don't need to consume it in our diets. Eating a diet low in saturated fat will also keep intake of dietary cholesterol within recommended levels.

2. True. Fat is our primary source of energy, both at rest and during low-intensity exercise. Fat is also an important fuel source during prolonged exercise.

3. True. Even foods fried in vegetable shortening can be unhealthful because they are higher in *trans* fatty acids. In addition, fried foods are high in fat and energy and can contribute to overweight and obesity.

4. True. Certain essential fatty acids, including EPA and DHA, reduce inflammation, blood clotting, and plasma triglycerides and thereby reduce an individual's risk of a heart attack.

5. False. Cancer develops as a result of a poorly understood interaction between environmental and genetic factors. Researchers are examining the association between high dietary fat consumption and certain cancers, but this research is inconclusive.

NUTRITION LABEL ACTIVITY ANSWERS

1. For the regular Wheat Crackers, the total calories per serving = **150**.

2. The calories from fat per serving = **50**.

3. For the Reduced-Fat Wheat Crackers, the total calories per serving = **130**.

4. The calories from fat per serving = **35**.

REFERENCES

1. Severson, K. 2005. So much for squeaky clean cookies. *New York Times*. March 09, 2005: page D4.
2. U.S. Department of Health and Human Services (DHHS) and the Department of Agriculture (USDA). 2005. *Dietary Guidelines for Americans. Nutrition and Your Health*. Available at www.health.gov/dietaryguidelines/dga2005/report/.
3. Institute of Medicine, Food and Nutrition Board. 2005. *Dietary Reference Intakes for Energy, Carbohydrate, Fiber, Fat, Fatty Acids, Cholesterol, Protein, and Amino Acids (Macronutrients)*. Washington, DC: National Academies Press.
4. American Heart Association (AHA). 2007. Know Your Fats. Available at www.americanheart.org/presenter.jhtml?identifier-532.
5. Kris-Etherton, P. M., W. S. Harris, and L. J. Appel. 2002. Fish consumption, fish oil, omega-3 fatty acids and cardiovascular disease. *Circulation* 106:2747–2757.
6. Jebb, S. A., A. M. Prentice, G. R. Goldberg, P. R. Murgatroyd, A. E. Black, and W. A. Coward. 1996. Changes in macronutrient balance during over- and underfeeding assessed by 12-d continuous whole-body calorimetry. *Am. J. Clin. Nutr.* 64:259–266.
7. Manore, M. M., S. I. Barr, and G. E. Butterfield. 2000. Position of the American Dietetic Association, Dietitians of Canada, and the American College of Sports Medicine: Nutrition and athletic performance. *J. Am. Diet. Assoc.* 100:1543–1556.
8. Lichtenstein, A. H., and L. Van Horn. 1998. Very low fat diets. *Circulation* 98:935–939.
9. Expert Panel on Detection, Evaluation, and Treatment of High Blood Cholesterol in Adults, National Institutes of Health. 2001. Executive Summary of the Third Report of the National Cholesterol Education Program (NCEP) Expert Panel on Detection, Evaluation, and Treatment of High Blood Cholesterol in Adults (Adult Treatment Panel III). *JAMA* 285(19):2486–2509.
10. Allison, D. B., S. K. Egan, L. M. Barraj, C. Caughman, M. Infante, and J. T. Heimbach. 1999. Estimated intakes of *trans* fatty and other fatty acids in the U.S. population. *J. Am. Diet. Assoc.* 99:166–174.
11. Kennedy, E., and D. Bowman. Assessment of the effect of fat-modified foods on dietary quality in adults, 19–50 years, using data from the Continuing Survey of Food Intake by Individuals. *JADA* 2110:101(4):455–460.
12. Melanson, K., and J. Dwyer. 2002. Popular diets for treatment of overweight and obesity. In: Wadden, T. A., and A. J. Stunkard, eds., *Handbook of Obesity Treatment*. New York: Guildford Press, pp. 249–275.
13. National Center for Chronic Disease Prevention and Health Promotion (NCCDPHP). 2002. Chronic Disease Prevention. Chronic Disease Overview. Available at www.cdc.gov/nccdphp/overview.htm.
14. Oomen, C. M., M. C. Ocké, E. J. Feskens, M. A. van Erp-Baart, F. J. Kok, and D. Kromhout. 2001. Association between *trans* fatty acid intake and 10-year risk of coronary heart disease in the Zutphen Elderly Study: A prospective population-based study. *Lancet* 357(9258):746–751.
15. Lichtenstein, A. H., et al. 2006. Diet and lifestyle recommendations revision 2006. A scientific statement from the American Heart Association Nutrition Committee. *Circulation* 114:82–96.
16. Kim, Y. I. 2001. Nutrition and cancer. In: Bowman, B. A., and R. M. Russell, eds., *Present Knowledge in Nutrition,* 8th ed. Washington, DC: International Life Sciences Institute Press.
17. American Institute for Cancer Research (AICR). November, 2007. Guidelines for Cancer Prevention. Available at www.aicr.org. (Accessed January 2008.)
18. Pierce, J. P., et al. 2007. Influence of a diet very high in vegetables, fruit and fiber and low in fat on prognosis following treatment for breast cancer. The Women's Healthy Eating and Living (WHEL) Randomized Trial. *J Am Med Assoc* 298(3):289–298.
19. Prentice, R. L., et al. 2006. Low-fat dietary pattern and risk of invasive breast cancer. The Women's Health Initiative randomized controlled dietary modification trial. *J Am Med Assoc* 295:629–642.
20. Willette, W. C., and M. J. Stamper. 2006. Foundations of a healthy diet. In: Shils, M. E., M. Shike, A. C. Ross, B. Caballero, and R. J. Cousins, Eds., *Modern Nutrition in Health and Disease*, 10th ed. Baltimore, MD: Williams & Wilkins, pp. 1625–1637.
21. Meyerhart, J. A., et al. 2007. Association of dietary patterns with cancer recurrence and survival in patients with stage III colon cancer. *J Am Med Assoc.* 298(7):754–764.
22. American Cancer Society (ACS). June, 2007. What Are the Risk Factors for Prostate Cancer? Available at www.cancer.org. (Accessed January 2008.)

5 Proteins: Crucial Components of All Body Tissues

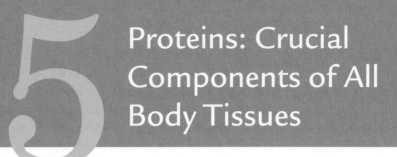

TEST YOURSELF

Are these statements true or false? Circle your guess.

1 Protein is a primary source of energy for our bodies. **TRUE** or **FALSE**

2 We must consume amino acid supplements in order to build muscle tissue. **TRUE** or **FALSE**

3 Any protein eaten in excess is excreted in your urine. **TRUE** or **FALSE**

4 Vegetarian diets are inadequate in protein. **TRUE** or **FALSE**

5 Most people in the United States consume more protein than they need. **TRUE** or **FALSE**

Test Yourself answers can be found at the end of the chapter.

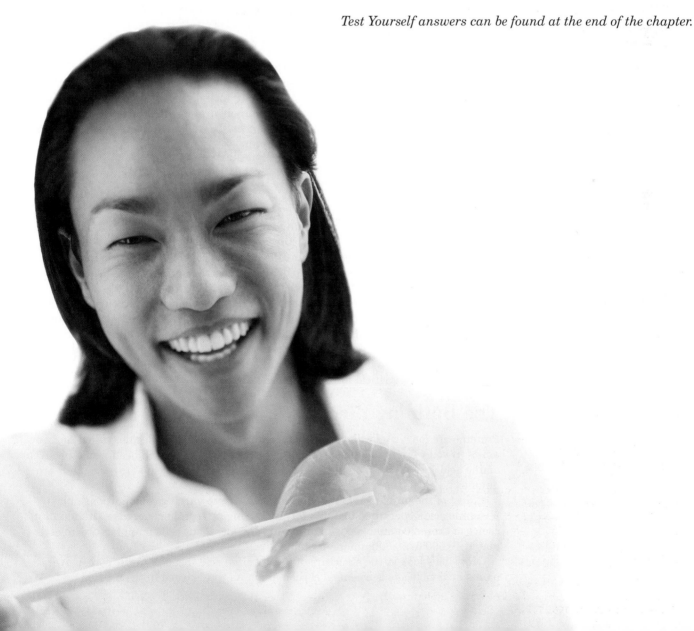

Where I'm starting from ...

How many grams of protein do you think you need to eat each day?

Do you think you get this amount of protein most days?

Yes or NO

How often would you say you go for an entire day without eating meat? (Choose one.)

☐ Every day—I'm a vegetarian.

☐ At least once or twice a week.

☐ Maybe once or twice a month.

☐ Almost never—I don't feel right if I don't eat meat every day.

WHAT DO "MR. UNIVERSE" BILL PEARL, Olympic figure skating champion Surya Bonaly, wrestler "Killer" Kowalski, and hundreds of other athletes have in common? They're all vegetarians! Olympic track icon Carl Lewis states: "I've found that a person does not need protein from meat to be a successful athlete. In fact, my best year of track competition was the first year I ate a vegan diet."[1] Although precise statistics on the number of vegetarian American athletes aren't available, a total of 2.8% of the U.S. population—approximately 5.7 million American adults—are estimated to be vegetarians.[2]

What exactly is a vegetarian anyway? Do you qualify? If so, how do you plan your diet to include sufficient protein, especially if you play competitive sports? Are there real advantages to eating meat, or is plant protein just as good?

It seems as if everybody has an opinion about protein, both how much you should consume and from what sources. In this chapter, we address these and other questions to clarify the importance of protein in the diet and dispel common myths about this crucial nutrient.

What Are Proteins?

Proteins are large, complex molecules found in the cells of all living things. Although proteins are best known as part of our muscle mass, they are in fact critical components of all tissues of the human body, including our bones and blood. In addition, although our bodies prefer to use carbohydrates and fats for energy, proteins do provide energy in certain circumstances. These and many more functions of proteins will be discussed later in this chapter.

How Do Proteins Differ from Carbohydrates and Lipids?

Proteins are one of the three macronutrients and are found in a wide variety of foods. Our bodies are able to manufacture (or *synthesize*) all of the macronutrients. But **DNA,** the genetic material in our cells, dictates the structure only of protein molecules, not of carbohydrates or lipids. We'll explore how our bodies synthesize proteins and the role that DNA plays in this process shortly.

Another key difference between proteins and the other macronutrients lies in their chemical makeup. In addition to the carbon, hydrogen, and oxygen also found in carbohydrates and lipids, proteins contain a special form of nitrogen that our bodies can readily use. When we digest protein-containing plant and animal foods, nitrogen is released for use in many important body processes. Carbohydrates and lipids do not provide this critical form of nitrogen.

The Building Blocks of Proteins Are Amino Acids

Proteins are long, chain-like compounds made up of unique molecules called **amino acids.** If you were to imagine proteins as beaded necklaces, each bead would be an amino acid (FIGURE 5.1). The links that bind the amino acid "beads" to each other are unique chemical bonds called **peptide bonds.**

Most of the proteins in our bodies are made from varying combinations of just 20 amino acids, identified in Table 5.1. By "stringing together" dozens to hundreds of copies of these 20 amino acids in different sequences, our cells manufacture an estimated 10,000 to 50,000 unique proteins.

Now let's look at the structure of these amino acid "beads." At the core of every amino acid molecule is a central carbon atom. As you learned in the previous

---

proteins Large, complex molecules made up of amino acids and found as essential components of all living cells.

DNA A molecule present in the nucleus of all body cells that directs the assembly of amino acids into body proteins.

amino acids Nitrogen-containing molecules that combine to form proteins.

peptide bonds Unique types of chemical bonds in which the amine group of one amino acid binds to the acid group of another in order to manufacture dipeptides and all larger peptide molecules.

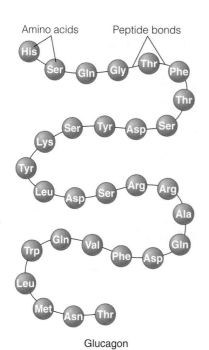

Amino acids · Peptide bonds

His · Ser · Gln · Gly · Thr · Phe · Thr · Ser · Asp · Tyr · Ser · Lys · Tyr · Leu · Asp · Ser · Arg · Arg · Ala · Trp · Gln · Val · Phe · Asp · Gln · Leu · Met · Asn · Thr

Glucagon

FIGURE 5.1 Structure of proteins. Proteins are chains of amino acids linked together by special chemical bonds called peptide bonds. This illustration shows a molecule of glucagon, a protein important in regulating blood glucose level. Notice that glucagon contains sixteen different amino acids. Some of these occur more than once, for a total of 29 amino acids in this protein.

TABLE 5.1 Amino Acids of the Human Body

Essential Amino Acids	Nonessential Amino Acids
These amino acids must be obtained from food.	*These amino acids can be manufactured by the body.*
Histidine	Alanine
Isoleucine	Arginine
Leucine	Asparagine
Lysine	Aspartic acid
Methionine	Cysteine
Phenylalanine	Glutamic acid
Threonine	Glutamine
Tryptophan	Glycine
Valine	Proline
	Serine
	Tyrosine

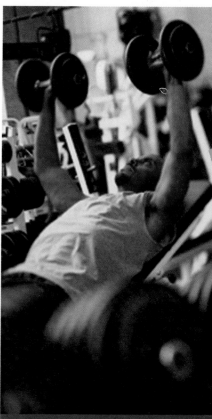

Proteins are an integral part of body tissues, including muscle tissue.

chapter, carbon atoms have four attachment sites. In amino acids, the central carbon's four attachment sites are filled by (**FIGURE 5.2A**):

1. a *hydrogen atom.*
2. an *acid group:* All acid groups in amino acids are identical.
3. an *amine group:* The word *amine* means "nitrogen-containing," and nitrogen is indeed the essential component of the amine portion of the molecule. Like acid groups, all amine groups in amino acids are identical.
4. a *side chain:* This is the portion of the amino acid that makes each unique. As shown in **FIGURE 5.2B**, variations in the structure of the side chain give each amino acid its distinct properties.

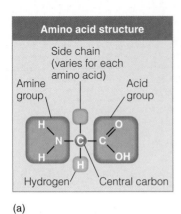

(a)

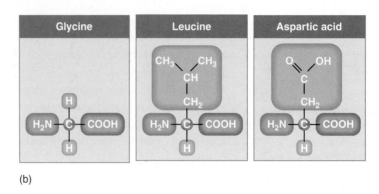

(b)

FIGURE 5.2 Structure of amino acids. (a) All amino acids contain five parts: a central carbon atom, an amine group around the atom that contains nitrogen, an acid group, a hydrogen atom, and a side chain. (b) Only the side chain differs for each of the twenty amino acids, giving each its unique properties.

We Must Obtain Essential Amino Acids from Food

Of the 20 amino acids in our bodies, 9 are classified as essential. This does not mean that they are more important than the 11 nonessential amino acids. Instead, an **essential amino acid** is one that our bodies cannot produce at all or cannot produce in sufficient quantities to meet our physiological needs. Thus, we must obtain essential amino acids from our food. If we do not consume enough of the essential amino acids, we lose our ability to make the proteins and other nitrogen-containing compounds we need.

Our Bodies Can Make Nonessential Amino Acids

Nonessential amino acids are just as important to our bodies as essential amino acids, but our bodies can make them in sufficient quantities, so we do not need to consume them in our diet. We make nonessential amino acids by combining parts of different amino acids and the breakdown products of carbohydrates and fats.

RECAP *Proteins are critical components of all tissues of the human body. Like carbohydrates and lipids, they contain carbon, hydrogen, and oxygen. Unlike the other macronutrients, they also contain nitrogen, and their structure is dictated by DNA. The building blocks of proteins are amino acids. The amine group of the amino acid contains nitrogen. The portion of the amino acid that changes, giving each amino acid its distinct identity, is the side chain. The body cannot make essential amino acids, so we must obtain them from our diet. Our bodies can make nonessential amino acids from parts of other amino acids, carbohydrates, and fats.*

How Are Proteins Made?

Our bodies can synthesize proteins by selecting the needed amino acids from the pool of all amino acids available at any given time. Let's look more closely at how this occurs.

Genes Tell Amino Acids How to Group into Proteins

You are unique because you inherited a unique set of genes from your parents. **Genes** are segments of DNA that carry the instructions for assembling available amino acids into your body's unique proteins. Slight differences in amino acid sequencing lead to slight differences in proteins. These differences in proteins result in the unique physical and physiological characteristics you possess.

essential amino acids   Amino acids not produced by the body that must be obtained from food.

nonessential amino acids   Amino acids that can be manufactured by the body in sufficient quantities and therefore do not need to be consumed regularly in our diet.

gene   Segment of DNA that carries the instructions for assembling available amino acids into a unique protein.

Protein Shape Determines Function

Two amino acids joined together form a *dipeptide,* and three amino acids joined together are called a *tripeptide.* The term *oligopeptide* is used to identify a string of four to nine amino acids. Proteins are made up of *polypeptides*, which are chains of ten or more amino acids linked together by peptide bonds. As a polypeptide chain grows longer, it begins to fold into any of a variety of complex shapes that give proteins their sophisticated structure.

The three-dimensional shape of a protein is critically important because it determines that protein's function in the body. For example, the proteins that form tendons are much longer than they are wide (**FIGURE 5.3A**). Tendons are connective tissues that attach bone to muscle, and their long, rod-like structure provides strong, fibrous connections. In contrast, the proteins that form red blood cells are globular in shape, and they result in the red blood cells being shaped like flattened disks with depressed centers, similar to a microscopic doughnut (**FIGURE 5.3B**). This structure and the flexibility of the proteins in the red blood cells permit them to change shape and flow freely through even the tiniest blood vessels to deliver oxygen and still return to their original shape.

Proteins can uncoil and lose their shape when they are exposed to heat, acids, bases, heavy metals, alcohol, and other damaging substances. The term used to describe this change in the shape of proteins is *denaturation.* When a protein is denatured, its function is lost. Familiar examples of protein denaturation are stiffening of egg whites when they are whipped, the curdling of milk when lemon juice or another acid is added, and the solidifying of eggs as they cook. Denaturation also occurs during protein digestion as a response to body heat and stomach acids.

> RECAP *Amino acids bind together to form proteins. Genes regulate the amino acid sequence, and thus the structure, of all proteins. The shape of a protein determines its function. When a protein is denatured by damaging substances such as heat and acids, it loses its shape and its function.*

Stiffening egg whites denatures some of the proteins within them.

Protein Synthesis Can Be Limited by Missing Amino Acids

For protein synthesis to occur, all essential amino acids must be available to the cell. If this is not the case, the amino acid that is missing or in the smallest supply is

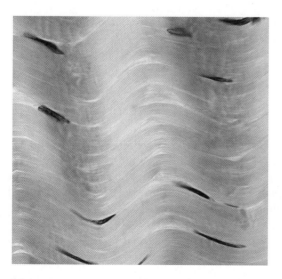

(a)

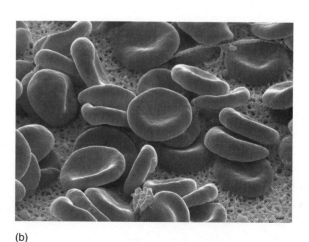

(b)

FIGURE 5.3 Protein shape determines function. (a) The protein in tendons has a long, rod-like structure that provides strong, fibrous connections. (b) The globular shape of the protein in red blood cells contributes to the flexible-disk shape of the cells. This in turn enables their passage through the tiniest blood vessels of the body.

called the **limiting amino acid.** Without the proper combination and quantity of essential amino acids, protein synthesis slows to the point at which proteins cannot be generated. For instance, the protein hemoglobin contains the essential amino acid histidine. If we do not consume enough histidine, our bodies will be unable to make hemoglobin, and we will lose the ability to transport oxygen to our cells. Without oxygen, our cells cannot function and will eventually die.

We can describe proteins as incomplete or complete:

- **Incomplete proteins** do not contain all of the essential amino acids in sufficient quantities to support growth and health. They are also called *low-quality proteins*. Lentils, for example, are an incomplete protein.
- **Complete proteins** have all nine of the essential amino acids. They are also called *high-quality proteins*. These include proteins derived from animal products, such as egg whites, beef, poultry, fish, and dairy products such as milk and cheese. Soybeans also contain all nine essential amino acids and are the only complete vegetable protein.

Protein Synthesis Can Be Enhanced by Mutual Supplementation

Many people believe that we must consume meat or dairy products to obtain complete proteins. Not true! Consider a meal of black beans and rice. Black beans are low in the amino acids methionine and cysteine but have adequate amounts of isoleucine and lysine. Rice is low in isoleucine and lysine but contains sufficient methionine and cysteine. By combining black beans and rice, we create a complete protein source.

Mutual supplementation is the process of combining two or more incomplete protein sources to make a complete protein. The foods involved provide **complementary proteins** that, when combined, provide all nine essential amino acids (FIGURE 5.4). Thus, mutual supplementation is important for people who consume no animal products.

Complementary proteins do not need to be eaten at the same meal. We maintain a free "pool" of amino acids in the blood; these amino acids come from food and sloughed-off cells. When we eat an incomplete protein, its amino acids join those in the free amino acid pool. These free amino acids can then combine to synthesize complete proteins. However, to maximize protein synthesis, it is wise to eat complementary-protein foods during the same day.

> RECAP *For protein synthesis to occur, all nine essential amino acids must be available to the cell. A complete protein provides all nine essential amino acids. Mutual supplementation combines two complementary-protein sources to make a complete protein.*

Why Do We Need to Eat Proteins?

The functions of proteins in the body are so numerous that only a few can be described in detail here. Note that proteins function most effectively when we also consume adequate amounts of energy as carbohydrates and fat. When there is not enough energy available, the body uses proteins as an energy source, limiting their availability for the following functions.

Proteins Contribute to Cell Growth, Repair, and Maintenance

The proteins in our bodies are dynamic, meaning that they are constantly being broken down, repaired, and replaced. When proteins are broken down, many amino acids are recycled into new proteins. Think about all of the new proteins that are

limiting amino acid The essential amino acid that is missing or in the smallest supply in the amino acid pool and is thus responsible for slowing or halting protein synthesis.

incomplete proteins Foods that do not contain all of the essential amino acids in sufficient amounts to support growth and health.

complete proteins Foods that contain all nine essential amino acids.

mutual supplementation The process of combining two or more incomplete protein sources to make a complete protein.

complementary proteins Two or more foods that together contain all nine essential amino acids necessary for a complete protein. It is not necessary to eat complementary proteins at the same meal.

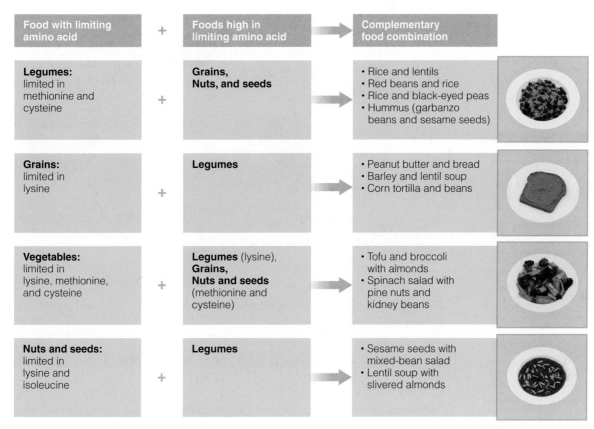

Food with limiting amino acid	+	Foods high in limiting amino acid	→	Complementary food combination
Legumes: limited in methionine and cysteine	+	**Grains, Nuts, and seeds**	→	• Rice and lentils • Red beans and rice • Rice and black-eyed peas • Hummus (garbanzo beans and sesame seeds)
Grains: limited in lysine	+	**Legumes**	→	• Peanut butter and bread • Barley and lentil soup • Corn tortilla and beans
Vegetables: limited in lysine, methionine, and cysteine	+	**Legumes** (lysine), **Grains, Nuts and seeds** (methionine and cysteine)	→	• Tofu and broccoli with almonds • Spinach salad with pine nuts and kidney beans
Nuts and seeds: limited in lysine and isoleucine	+	**Legumes**	→	• Sesame seeds with mixed-bean salad • Lentil soup with slivered almonds

FIGURE 5.4 Complementary food combinations.

needed to allow an embryo to develop and grow into a 9-month-old fetus. In this case, an entirely new human body is being made! In fact, a newborn baby has more than 10 trillion body cells.

Even in the mature adult, our cells are constantly turning over, meaning old cells are broken down and parts are used to create new cells. Our red blood cells live for only 3 to 4 months, and the cells lining our intestinal tract are replaced every 3 to 6 days. In addition, cellular damage that occurs must be repaired in order to maintain our health. The constant turnover of proteins from our diet is essential for such cell growth, repair, and maintenance.

Proteins Act as Enzymes and Hormones

In Chapter 2, we defined *enzymes* as small chemicals, usually proteins, that act on other chemicals to speed up body processes but are not apparently changed during those processes. Enzymes can act to bind substances together or break them apart, and can transform one substance into another (**FIGURE 5.5**). Each cell contains thousands of enzymes that facilitate specific cellular reactions. For example, the enzyme phosphofructokinase (PFK) speeds up the conversion of carbohydrates to energy during physical exercise. Without PFK, we would be unable to generate energy at a fast enough rate to allow us to be physically active.

Also recall from Chapter 2 that *hormones* are substances that act as chemical messengers in the body. They are stored in various glands in the body, which release them in response to changes in the body's environment. They then signal the body's organs and tissues to restore the body to normal conditions. Whereas many hormones are made from lipids (refer to Chapter 4), some are made from amino acids. These include insulin and glucagon, which play a role in regulating blood glucose levels (see Chapter 3), and thyroid hormone, which helps control the rate at which glucose is used for fuel.

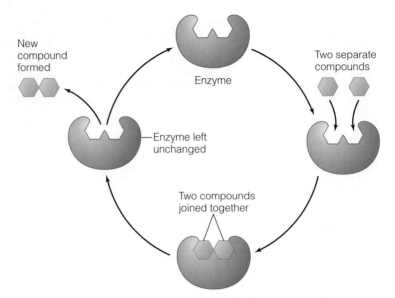

FIGURE 5.5 Proteins act as enzymes. Enzymes facilitate chemical reactions such as joining two compounds together.

Proteins Help Maintain Fluid and Electrolyte Balance

For our bodies to function properly, fluids and *electrolytes* (minerals such as sodium and potassium that are able to carry an electrical charge) must be maintained at healthy levels inside and outside cells and within blood vessels. Proteins help in maintaining fluid and electrolyte balance in two ways:

- They attract fluids. Proteins in the bloodstream, cells, and the spaces surrounding the cells work together to keep both fluids and electrolytes moving across these spaces.

- They move and retain fluids in the proper quantities to help us maintain both fluid balance and blood pressure.

edema A disorder in which fluids build up in the tissue spaces of the body, causing fluid imbalances and a swollen appearance.

transport proteins Protein molecules that help to transport substances throughout the body and across cell membranes.

When protein intake is deficient, the concentration of proteins in the bloodstream is insufficient to draw fluid from the tissues and across the blood vessel walls; fluid then collects in the tissues, causing **edema** (FIGURE 5.6). In addition to being uncomfortable, edema can lead to serious medical problems.

Conduction of nerve signals and contraction of muscles also depends on a proper balance of electrolytes. If protein intake is deficient, we lose our ability to maintain these functions, resulting in potentially fatal changes in the rhythm of the heart. Other consequences of chronically low protein intakes include muscle weakness and spasms, kidney failure, and, if conditions are severe enough, death.

Proteins Transport Nutrients and Other Substances

Proteins play a key role in transporting nutrients and other important substances throughout the body. Some examples of these **transport proteins** include the following:

- Transport proteins located within the cell membrane help maintain fluid and electrolyte balance. These proteins act as pumps to assist in the movement of the electrolytes sodium and potassium into and out of the cell.

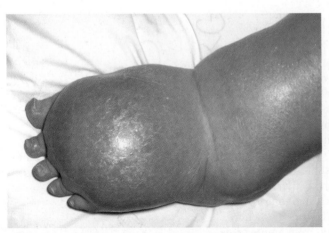

FIGURE 5.6 Edema can result from deficient protein intake. This foot with edema is swollen because of fluid imbalance.

- Transport proteins also carry vitamins and minerals through the bloodstream to the organs and cells that need them. For example, retinol-binding protein is a transport protein that transports fat-soluble vitamin A (also called retinol) in the blood.
- Transport proteins also move glucose from the bloodstream into the cells, where it can be used for energy.

Proteins Help Maintain Acid–Base Balance

The body's cellular processes result in the constant production of acids and bases. *Acids* are substances that contain significant amounts of hydrogen, whereas *bases* are low in hydrogen. Some hydrogen is essential to life, but too much can be harmful to body cells. Thus, the body maintains very tight control over the **pH,** or the level of hydrogen (H), in the blood. Proteins are excellent **buffers,** meaning they help maintain proper acid–base balance. They do this by attracting hydrogen and neutralizing it. Proteins can also release hydrogen when the blood becomes too basic. By buffering acids and bases, proteins help maintain acid–base balance.

Proteins Help Maintain a Strong Immune System

Antibodies are special proteins that help our bodies defend against foreign substances. When bacteria, viruses, toxins, or allergens (substances that cause allergic reactions) enter the body, the immune system produces antibodies that attach to and neutralize the invaders.

Adequate protein is necessary to support the increased production of antibodies that occurs in response to a cold, flu, or allergic reaction. If we do not consume enough protein, our resistance to illnesses and disease is weakened. On the other hand, eating more protein than we need does not improve immune function.

Proteins Serve as an Energy Source

The body's primary energy sources are carbohydrate and fat. So it's not surprising that both these macronutrients have specialized storage forms that can be used for energy—carbohydrate as glycogen and fat as triglycerides. Proteins do not have a specialized storage form for energy. This means that when proteins need to be used for energy, they are taken from the blood and body tissues such as the liver and skeletal muscle.

Adequate intake of carbohydrate and fat spares protein. During times of low carbohydrate and fat intake, the body breaks down proteins, then converts the amino acids into glucose to provide needed energy to the brain. As stated in Chapter 3, this process is called *gluconeogenesis.* In well-nourished people, proteins contribute very little to energy needs. Because we are efficient at recycling amino acids, our protein needs are relatively low as compared to our needs for carbohydrate and fat.

> RECAP *Proteins serve many important functions, including (1) enabling growth, repair, and maintenance of body tissues; (2) acting as enzymes and hormones; (3) maintaining fluid and electrolyte balance; (4) transporting nutrients and other substances; (5) maintaining acid–base balance; (6) making antibodies, which strengthen our immune system; and (7) providing energy when carbohydrate and fat intake are inadequate. Proteins function best when we also consume adequate amounts of carbohydrate and fat.*

What Happens to the Proteins We Eat?

Our bodies do not directly use proteins from the foods we eat to make the proteins we need. Dietary proteins are first digested and broken into smaller particles such as amino acids, dipeptides, and tripeptides, so that they can pass through the intestinal

pH   Stands for percentage of hydrogen. It is a measure of the acidity—or level of hydrogen—of any solution, including human blood.

buffers   Proteins that help maintain proper acid–base balance by attaching to, or releasing, hydrogen ions as conditions change in the body.

antibodies   Defensive proteins of the immune system. Their production is prompted by the presence of bacteria, viruses, toxins, or allergens.

lining cells. In this section, we will review how proteins are digested and absorbed. As you read about each step in this process, refer to FIGURE 5.7 for a visual tour through the digestive system.

Stomach Acids and Pepsin Begin to Break Down Proteins

As shown in step 1 in Figure 5.7, the mechanical digestion of proteins in food occurs through chewing, crushing, and moistening the food with saliva. These actions ease swallowing and increase the surface area for more efficient digestion further down the digestive tract. There is no chemical digestive action on proteins in the mouth.

When proteins reach the stomach, they are broken apart by *hydrochloric acid* (Figure 5.7, step 2). Hydrochloric acid denatures the strands of protein, and converts the inactive enzyme, *pepsinogen,* into its active form, **pepsin.** Although pepsin is a protein, it is not denatured by the acid in the stomach because it has evolved to work optimally in an acidic environment. Pepsin begins breaking proteins into single amino acids and smaller polypeptides that then travel to the small intestine for further digestion.

Enzymes in the Small Intestine Finish Breaking Proteins into Single Amino Acids

In the small intestine, the polypeptides encounter enzymes called **proteases** that digest them into single amino acids, dipeptides, and tripeptides (Figure 5.7, step 3). The cells in the wall of the small intestine then absorb these molecules. Enzymes in the intestinal cells complete digestion by breaking the dipeptides and tripeptides into single amino acids. The amino acids are then transported into the bloodstream to the liver and on to cells throughout our bodies as needed (Figure 5.7, step 4).

Digestibility Affects Protein Quality

As discussed earlier, the number of essential amino acids in a protein affects its quality. Higher-quality-protein foods contain more of the essential amino acids

pepsin   An enzyme in the stomach that begins the breakdown of proteins into shorter polypeptide chains and single amino acids.

proteases   Enzymes that continue the breakdown of polypeptides in the small intestine.

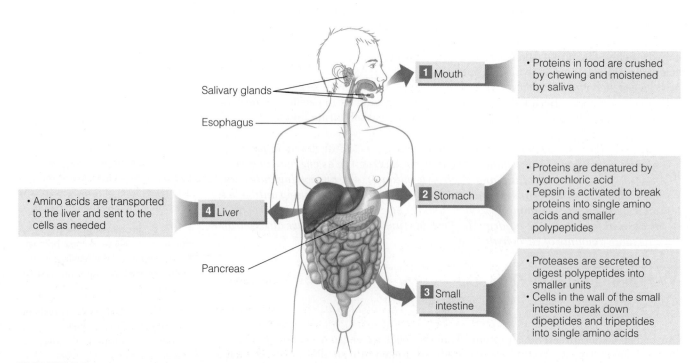

FIGURE 5.7   The process of protein digestion.

needed to build proteins. Another factor to consider when determining protein quality is *digestibility,* or how efficiently our bodies can digest and absorb a protein. Animal foods and legumes, including soy products, have high digestibility, and we absorb almost all of their proteins. Grains and many vegetable proteins are less digestible.

> RECAP *In the stomach, hydrochloric acid denatures proteins and pepsin breaks proteins into single amino acids and smaller polypeptides. In the small intestine, proteases break down polypeptides. Enzymes in the cells in the wall of the small intestine break the remaining peptide fragments into single amino acids, which are then transported to the liver for distribution to the body.*

How Much Protein Should We Eat?

Consuming adequate protein is a major concern for many people. In fact, one of the most common concerns among athletes is that their diets are deficient in protein (see the Nutrition Myth or Fact? box on page 140 for a discussion of this topic). In developed nations, this concern about dietary protein is generally unnecessary, as we can easily consume the protein our bodies need by eating an adequate amount of various foods. In contrast, people in developing nations are at risk for protein deficiency. A severe protein deficit in children, called *kwashiorkor,* commonly develops when a toddler is weaned from breast milk and fed a diet inadequate in protein and high in diluted starches. *Marasmus* is a disease resulting from severe deficits of all of the energy nutrients, as during times of famine. These and other hunger-related diseases are discussed in detail in Chapter 12.

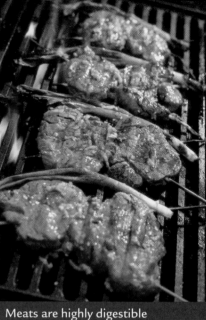

Meats are highly digestible sources of dietary protein.

Recommended Dietary Allowance (RDA) for Protein

How much protein should we eat? Table 5.2 lists the daily recommendations for protein intake for sedentary adults and for athletes. It also provides a calculation for converting the recommendation, which is stated in grams per kilogram of body

TABLE 5.2 Recommended Protein Intakes

Group	Recommended Protein Intake (g/kg body weight/day)*
Most adults[†]	0.8
Nonvegetarian endurance athletes[‡]	1.2 to 1.4
Nonvegetarian strength athletes[‡]	1.6 to 1.7
Vegetarian endurance athletes[‡]	1.3 to 1.5
Vegetarian strength athletes[‡]	1.7 to 1.8

*To convert body weight to kilograms, divide weight in pounds by 2.2.

Weight (lb) ÷ 2.2 = Weight (kg). For example, 150 lb ÷ 2.2 = 68 kg.

Weight (kg) × recommended protein intake = protein intake (grams per day). For example, for a nonathlete, 68 kg × 0.8 = 54.4 grams per day.

Sources: [†]Food and Nutrition Board, Institute of Medicine. 2002. *Dietary Reference Intakes for Energy, Carbohydrate, Fiber, Fat, Fatty Acids, Cholesterol, Protein, and Amino Acids (Macronutrients)*, pp. 465–608. Washington, DC: National Academies Press.

[‡]American College of Sports Medicine, American Dietetic Association, and Dietitians of Canada. 2001. Joint Position Statement. Nutrition and athletic performance. *Med. Sci. Sports Exerc.* 32:2130-2145.

NUTRITION MYTH OR FACT?

Do Athletes Need More Protein Than Inactive People?

At one time, it was believed that the Recommended Dietary Allowance (RDA) for protein, which is 0.8 g/kg body weight, was sufficient for both inactive people and athletes. Recent studies, however, show that the protein needs of athletes are higher.

Athletes need more protein for several reasons:

● Regular exercise increases the transport of oxygen to body tissues, requiring changes in the oxygen-carrying capacity of the blood. To carry more oxygen, we need to produce more of the protein that carries oxygen in the blood (i.e., hemoglobin, which is a protein).

● During intense exercise, we use a small amount of protein directly for energy.

● We also use protein to make glucose to prevent hypoglycemia (low blood sugar) during exercise.

● Regular exercise stimulates tissue growth and causes tissue damage, which must be repaired by additional proteins.

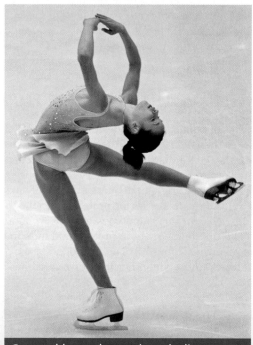

Some athletes who persistently diet are at risk of low protein intake.

As a result of these increased demands for protein, strength athletes (such as weightlifters) need 1.8 to 2 times more protein than the current RDA, and endurance athletes (such as distance runners) need 1.5 to 1.75 times more protein.[3]

Does this mean that, if you are an athlete, you should add more protein to your diet? Not necessarily. Contrary to popular belief, most Americans, including athletes, already consume more than twice the RDA for protein. Thus, they are already more than fulfilling their protein needs. In fact, eating more protein or taking amino acid supplements does not cause muscles to become bigger or stronger. Only regular strength training can achieve these goals. For healthy individuals, evidence does not support eating more than two times the RDA for protein to increase strength, build muscle, or improve athletic performance. By eating a balanced diet and consuming a variety of foods, athletes can easily meet their protein requirements.

weight, into total grams of protein per day. If you are sedentary and weigh 140 lb, you need about 50 g of protein a day. If you're an athlete who weighs 140 lb, you need about 75 to 108 g. Protein needs are higher for children, adolescents, and pregnant/lactating women because more protein is needed during times of growth and development (refer to Chapter 11).

When you consider that a small serving (3 oz) of ground beef or canned tuna provides about 22 to 24 g of protein and a glass of low-fat milk another 8 g, you can see how easy it is to meet this recommendation. In fact, it shouldn't surprise you to learn that most Americans eat 1.5 to 2 times their RDA for protein without any effort! To find out how much protein you eat, use Appendix A, diet analysis software, or log on to the USDA's MyPyramid Tracker.

The recommended percentage of energy that should come from protein is 12% to 20% of your total daily energy intake. Many high-protein, low-carbohydrate diets recommend that a much greater percentage of our daily diet be derived from protein, but as we discuss next, excessive protein intake has some health costs.

RECAP *The RDA for protein for most nonactive, nonpregnant, nonlactating, nonvegetarian adults is 0.8 g per kg body weight. Children, pregnant women, nursing mothers, vegetarians, and athletes need slightly more. Most people who eat enough energy and carbohydrates have no problem meeting their RDA for protein.*

Too Much Dietary Protein Can Be Harmful

High protein intake may increase the risk of health problems. Three health conditions that have received particular attention include heart disease, bone loss, and kidney disease.

High Protein Intake Is Associated with High Cholesterol

High-protein diets composed of predominantly animal sources are associated with higher blood cholesterol levels. This is probably due to the saturated fat in animal products, which is known to increase blood cholesterol levels and the risk of heart disease. Vegetarians have been shown to have a greatly reduced risk of heart disease.[4,5]

High Protein Intake May Contribute to Bone Loss

How might a high-protein diet lead to bone loss? Animal foods contain more of the sulfur amino acids (methionine and cysteine). Metabolizing these amino acids makes the blood more acidic, and calcium, the main mineral component of bone, is pulled from the bone into the blood to buffer these acids. Although eating more protein can cause you to excrete more calcium, it is very controversial whether high protein intakes actually cause bone loss. We do know that eating too little protein causes bone loss and that adequate intakes of animal and soy protein have been shown to protect bone in middle-aged and older women.[6,7] There does not appear to be enough direct evidence at this time to show that higher protein intakes cause bone loss in healthy people.

NUTRI-CASE LIZ

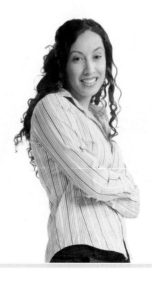

"One of my dancer friends, Silvie, was always a little pudgy, but now she's tighter than I've ever seen her. Yesterday, even our teacher commented on how great she looks! After class, I asked her secret and she said she's been on a high-protein diet for 2 months. She said it's pretty easy to stick to—you just have to avoid starches like bread and pasta—oh, and most sweets, too, though you can still have ice cream. She said she never feels hungry anymore, that the meat and eggs and cheese keep her feeling full. I'm thinking to myself, heck, I'm hungry all the time. So I asked her to bring me her book about the diet so I can try it for myself."

One issue that has been a major controversy for many years is the use of high-protein diets for weight loss. Popular diets such as the Atkins Diet, the Zone Diet, and the Sugar Busters diet support the use of high-protein or low-carbohydrate meals to achieve weight loss. The Highlight on High-Protein Diets features a detailed discussion of this controversial topic. After reading it, what do you think of Liz's idea of trying the diet? Would your opinion change if you learned that her father suffered a heart attack last year at age 49? Why or why not?

HIGHLIGHT

High-Protein Diets: Are They the Key to Weight Loss?

The promotional photo shows an enticing plate of fried eggs and sausage, or a juicy steak on the grill. If you're a meat-eater and want to lose weight, chances are you've at least flirted with the idea of following a high-protein diet. Do these diets help people lose weight and maintain the weight loss, and do they improve our health or harm us?

Supporters of high-protein diets propose that our high-simple-carbohydrate diet (including potatoes, white bread, pasta, and refined sugars) has caused the alarming rise in obesity in the United States in the past few decades. They claim that high-protein diets such as the Atkins Diet result in substantial weight loss. They also say that, despite the high saturated-fat content of animal sources of protein, meat-based high-protein diets do not cause unhealthful changes in blood cholesterol.

Are there any research studies to support these claims? Recently, the results of a few randomized controlled trials studying high-protein diets have been published. These studies have begun to shed some light on the effects of such diets on weight loss and blood lipid levels in obese individuals. Samaha et al. placed participants on either the Atkins Diet or a low-fat diet plan recommended by the American Heart Association.[8] Participants consuming the Atkins Diet lost considerably more weight than people on the low-fat diet over the first 6 months, but weight loss between the two groups was no longer different after 1 year.[9] More significant, people consuming the Atkins Diet had lower triglyceride levels and had less of a decrease in HDL-cholesterol (the "good cholesterol") than people eating the low-

fat diet. In another study conducted over a 1-year period using similar diet plans, the results were quite similar.[10] A recent review of all of the published studies of high-protein, low-carbohydrate diets resulted in the conclusion that there is not enough data currently to make recommendations for or against their use.[11] The authors of this review state that the weight loss that occurs with these diets appears to be more associated with a decreased energy intake and longer diet duration and is not necessarily due to the reduced carbohydrate content of the diet.

Detractors of the Atkins Diet contend that the U.S. population is substantially overweight because we eat too many calories, not because we eat too much carbohydrate or too much fat specifically. Nutrition experts have long agreed that the key to weight loss is eating less energy than you expend. If you eat more energy than you expend, you will gain weight. Thus, any type of diet that contains fewer kilocalories than the person expends will result in weight loss.

Detractors also point out that high-protein, low-carbohydrate diets work, at least in the short term, by causing loss of body *fluids,* not of body *fat.* Reducing carbohydrate intake causes the body to break down its stored carbohydrate (or glycogen) in the liver and muscle; this is necessary to maintain blood glucose levels and provide energy to the brain. As water is stored along with glycogen, using stored carbohydrate for energy results in the loss of water from the body, which registers on the scale as rapid weight loss.

Additionally, a number of potential health risks are associated with eating a diet that is both low in carbohydrate and high in fat. These risks have prevented many nutrition experts from endorsing the Atkins Diet. Some of these health risks include the following:

- Low blood glucose levels leading to low energy levels, diminished cognitive functioning, and elevated ketones. Despite this concern, there is no evidence that following the Atkins Diet has resulted in any serious disability.

- Increased risk of heart disease because high-protein diets that rely on animal sources of protein are typically high in saturated fat. It is well established that eating a diet high in saturated fat increases a person's LDL cholesterol, which in turn increases the risk for heart disease. Nevertheless, the research cited here appears to suggest that high-protein diets do not cause unhealthful changes in blood lipids.

High-protein diets are a multimillion-dollar industry.

High-Protein Diets: Are They the Key to Weight Loss? *(continued)*

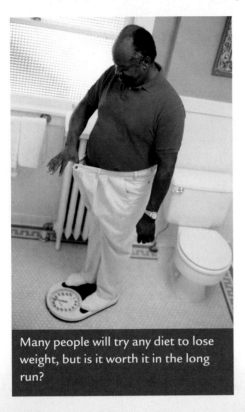

Many people will try any diet to lose weight, but is it worth it in the long run?

● Increased risk of some forms of cancer due to eating a diet that is high in fat and low in fiber. The Atkins Diet recommends few foods that contain fiber and antioxidants, so many nutrition experts are concerned that eating this type of a diet over many years will increase a person's risk for some forms of cancer.

Should you adopt a high-protein diet? This is not an easy question to answer. Each of us must decide on the type of diet to consume based on our own needs, preferences, health risks, and lifestyle. At the present time, there is not enough evidence to prove that the Atkins Diet or other high-protein diets are more effective or healthful than higher-carbohydrate, lower-fat diets. Based on what we currently know, the most sound weight loss plans are those that are moderately reduced in energy intake and contain ample fruits, vegetables, and whole grains, adequate carbohydrate and protein, moderate amounts of total fat, and relatively low amounts of saturated fat. It is also important to choose a food plan that you can follow throughout your lifetime. By researching the benefits and risks of various diet plans, you can make an educated decision about the type of diet that will work best to maintain a healthful weight and muscle mass and provide enough energy and nutrients to maintain your lifestyle and your long-term health.

High Protein Intake Can Be Harmful for People with Kidney Disease

The more protein we eat, the more protein the body has to break down. A waste product of protein digestion is a chemical called *urea:* the kidneys have the job of forming urea when nitrogen is removed from the amine group during amino acid breakdown. A high protein intake can therefore be stressful to kidneys that aren't functioning properly. To reduce stress to their kidneys, people with kidney disease are advised to eat a low-protein diet.

On the other hand, there is no evidence that eating a lot of protein causes kidney disease in healthy people. In fact, one study found that athletes consuming up to 2.8 g of protein per kilogram of body weight per day experienced no reduction in kidney function.[12] Experts agree that eating no more than 2 g of protein per kilogram of body weight each day is safe for healthy people.

People who consume a lot of protein have higher fluid requirements than people who eat an amount closer to their RDA. This is because adequate fluid is needed to flush excess urea from the kidneys. Increased fluid is particularly important for athletes, who need more fluid because of their higher sweat losses (see Chapter 8).

Shopper's Guide: Good Food Sources of Protein

Table 5.3 compares the protein content of a variety of foods. In general, good sources of protein include meats (lean cuts of beef, pork, poultry, seafood), dairy products (low-fat milk-based products and egg whites), soy products, legumes, whole grains, and nuts. A new source of nonmeat protein that is available on the market is *quorn,* a protein product derived from fermented fungus. It is mixed with a variety of other foods to produce various types of meat substitutes.

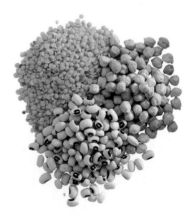

The quality of the protein in some legumes, such as these black-eyed peas, lentils, and garbanzo beans, is almost equal to that of meat.

TABLE 5.3   Protein Content of Commonly Consumed Foods

Food	Serving Size	Protein (g)	Food	Serving Size	Protein (g)
Beef:			*Beans:*		
Ground, lean, baked (15% fat)	3.0 oz	22	Refried	0.5 cup	7
Corned beef, brisket, cooked	3.0 oz	15	Kidney, red	0.5 cup	7.7
Prime rib, broiled (½-in. trim)	3.0 oz	17	Black	0.5 cup	7
Top sirloin, broiled (⅛-in. trim)	3.0 oz	23	Pork and beans, canned	0.5 cup	6.5
Poultry:			*Nuts:*		
Chicken breast, broiled, no skin	3.0 oz	28	Peanuts, dry roasted	1 oz	6.7
Chicken thigh, roasted, no skin	3.0 oz	23	Peanut butter, creamy	2 tbsp.	8
Chicken drumstick, broiled, with skin	3.0 oz	24	Almonds, blanched	1 oz	6
Turkey breast, roasted, Louis Rich	3.0 oz	14	Sunflower seeds	1 oz	5.5
Turkey dark meat, roasted, no skin	3.0 oz	26	Pecan halves	1 oz	2.6
Seafood:			*Cereals, Grains, and Breads:*		
Cod, cooked	3.0 oz	19	Barley, cooked	1 cup	3.6
Salmon, Chinook, baked	3.0 oz	22	Oatmeal, quick instant	1 cup	5.4
Shrimp, steamed	3.0 oz	18	Cheerios	1 cup	3
Oysters, steamed	3.0 oz	16	Corn Bran	1 cup	2
Tuna, in water, drained	3.0 oz	22	Grape Nuts	0.5 cup	6
Pork:			Raisin Bran	1 cup	5
Pork loin chop, broiled	3.0 oz	25	Brown rice, cooked	1 cup	5
Beef ribs, roasted	3.0 oz	19	Whole-wheat bread	1 slice	2.7
Ham, roasted, lean	3.0 oz	20	Rye bread	1 slice	2.7
			Bagel, 3½-in. diameter	1 each	7
Dairy:			*Vegetables:*		
Whole milk (3.3% fat)	8 fl. oz.	7.9	Carrots, raw (7.5 × 1⅛-in.)	1 each	0.7
1% milk	8 fl. oz.	8.5	Asparagus, boiled	6 spears	2
Skim milk	8 fl. oz.	8.8	Green beans, cooked	1 cup	2.4
Low-fat, plain yogurt	8 fl. oz.	13	Broccoli, raw, chopped	1 cup	2.6
American cheese, processed	1 oz	6	Collards, cooked from frozen	1 cup	5
Swiss cheese	1 oz	7.6	Spinach, raw	1 cup	0.9
Cottage cheese, low-fat (2%)	1 cup	28			
Soy Products:					
Tofu	3.3 oz	7			
Tempeh, cooked	3.3 oz	18			
Soy milk beverage	1 cup	11			

Source: Values obtained from U.S. Department of Agriculture (USDA). National Nutrient Database for Standard Reference, Release 20. www.nal.usda.gov/fnic/foodcomp/search. (Accessed February 2008.)

Although most people are aware that meats are an excellent source of protein, many people are surprised to learn that the quality of the protein in some legumes rivals that of meat. As noted earlier, soy is a complete protein, providing all essential amino acids. For more information about the nutrients in soy, claims regarding its health benefits, and ways to enjoy soy, check out the Highlight: What's So Great About Soy? on the next page.

Other legumes include kidney beans, pinto beans, black beans, garbanzo beans (or chickpeas), lentils, green peas, black-eyed peas, and lima beans. In addition to being excellent sources of protein, legumes are also high in fiber, iron, calcium, and many of the B vitamins (although they do not contain vitamin B_{12}). They are also low in saturated fat and have no cholesterol. Because legumes other than soy are deficient in methionine, an essential amino acid, they are often served with grains.

HIGHLIGHT

What's So Great about Soy?

Twenty years ago, if you were able to find a soy-based food in a traditional grocery store in the United States or Canada, it was probably soy milk. Now, it seems there are soy products in almost every aisle, from marinated tofu and tempeh to miso soup to soy-based cheeses, cereals, hot dogs, burgers, frozen dinners, and even tofu ice cream. Why the explosion? What's so great about soy, and should you give it a try?

What Is Soy?

Before we explore the many health claims tied to soy-based foods, let's define some terms. First, all soy-based foods start with soybeans, a staple in many Asian countries. Soybeans provide all essential amino acids and have almost twice as much protein as any other legume (7–10 g of protein in 1 cup of soy milk). Although they also pack from 3 to 10 times as much fat as other beans, almost all of it is unsaturated, and soy has no cholesterol. Soy is also rich in a group of phytochemicals called *isoflavones*. These plant chemicals mimic the effect of the hormone estrogen in the human body. Here are some common varieties of soy-based foods you might find in your local supermarket today:

- *Soy milk* is a beverage produced when soybeans are ground with water. Flavorings are added to make the drink palatable, and many brands of soy milk are fortified with calcium.
- *Tofu* is made from soy milk coagulated to form curds. If the coagulant used is calcium sulfate, the resulting product is high in calcium. Tofu is usually sold in blocks like cheese and is used as a meat substitute. Although many people object to its bland taste and mushy texture, tofu adapts well to many seasonings, and when drained and frozen before cooking, it develops a chewy texture similar to meat. Tofu is also the basis of many processed foods, such as meatless hot dogs and burgers.
- *Tempeh* is a more flavorful and firmer-textured meat substitute made from soybeans fermented with grains. It is often used in stir-fried dishes.
- *Miso* is a paste made from fermented soybeans and grains. It is used sparingly as a base for soups and sauces, as it is very high in sodium.

Soy May Reduce Your Risk of Chronic Disease

Now for the health claims. Proponents say that a diet high in soy protein can reduce your risk for heart disease, certain types of cancer, and osteoporosis (loss of bone density). Let's review the research behind each of these health claims.

Heart Disease

In October 1999, the U.S. Food and Drug Administration (FDA) gave food manufacturers permission to put labels on products high in soy protein stating that a daily diet containing 25 g of soy protein and low in saturated fat and cholesterol may reduce the risk of heart disease.[13] The FDA reviewed 27 relevant clinical studies before concluding that diets providing four servings a day of soy can provoke a modest reduction in blood levels of LDL-cholesterol. The cholesterol-reducing benefits of soy appear to be linked only to soy-based foods, not supplements. The American Heart Association therefore recommends consuming soy milk and tofu as part of a heart-healthy diet.[14]

Cancer Risk

Whereas the cholesterol-reducing benefits of soy seem clear, the claims for soy's effect on cancer risk are controversial. Many studies suggest that soy protects against prostate cancer, which is one of the most common cancers in men.[15] Again, although the isoflavones in soy foods appear to exert the protective effect, researchers recommend eating soy foods, not supplements.

Studies have also suggested that the isoflavones in soy may reduce a woman's risk of breast cancer; however, their findings conflict with those of other studies indicating a possible increased risk. The American Cancer Society explains that the plant estrogens in soy "may have both a protective role and a stimulatory role in breast cancer cell growth depending on several factors, including at what age they're consumed and whether they're consumed as food or as supplement." Several federally funded studies are currently being conducted to further our understanding of the effect of soy on breast cancer risk, but for now, the ACS recommends consuming naturally occurring soy foods as part of a balanced, plant-based diet.[16]

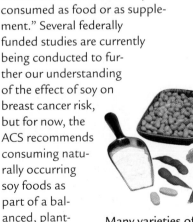

Many varieties of protein-rich soy products are available in supermarkets today.

(continued)

What's So Great about Soy? *(continued)*

Bone Loss

Published studies of the effect of soy on bone density, a particular concern for older women, have also been inconclusive. Whereas some suggest that soy can help keep bones strong, others suggest little benefit. Several new studies investigating the potential link between soy and bone health are currently under way.

Adding Soy to Your Diet

If you decide that you want to try soy, how do you go about it? A first step for many people is to substitute soy milk for cow's milk on its own, or on morning cereal, in smoothies, or in recipes for baked goods. Different brands of soy milk can have very different flavors, so try a few before you decide you don't like the taste.

Here are some other possibilities for adding soy to your diet:[13]

- Try one of the new breakfast cereals made with soy.
- Use soy nut butter (similar to peanut butter), soy deli meats, or soy cheese in sandwiches.
- Try soy sausages, bacon, hot dogs, burgers, ground "beef," and "chicken" patties.
- Toss cubes of prepackaged flavored, baked tofu or tempeh into stir-fried vegetables and serve over Chinese noodles or rice.
- Order soy-based dishes such as spicy bean curd and miso soup at Asian restaurants.
- Eat roasted soy nuts or a soy protein bar for a snack.
- Try soy yogurt and ice cream.

Eating legumes regularly, including foods made from soybeans, may help reduce the risk of heart disease by lowering blood cholesterol levels. Diets high in legumes and soy products are also associated with lower rates of some cancers. If you're not used to eating beans and lentils, the Game Plan on page 147 provides tips for incorporating these nourishing foods into your daily diet.

Fruits, vegetables, and grains are not particularly high in protein; however, these foods provide fiber and many vitamins and minerals and are excellent sources of carbohydrates. Thus, eating fruits, vegetables, and grains can help spare protein for use in building and maintaining our bodies rather than using it for energy.

> RECAP *Eating too much protein may increase your risk for heart disease. Good sources of protein include meats, eggs, dairy products, soy products, legumes, whole grains, and nuts.*

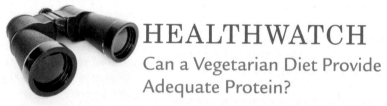

HEALTHWATCH
Can a Vegetarian Diet Provide Adequate Protein?

Vegetarianism is the practice of restricting the diet to food substances of vegetable origin, including fruits, grains, and nuts. To address the question of whether or not a vegetarian diet can provide adequate protein, let's begin with a look at the different types of vegetarian diets.

There Are Many Types of Vegetarian Diets

There are almost as many types of vegetarian diets as there are vegetarians. Some people who consider themselves vegetarians regularly eat fish. Others avoid the flesh of animals but consume eggs, milk, and cheese liberally. Still others strictly avoid all products of animal origin, including milk and eggs and even by-products such as candies and puddings made with gelatin. A type of "vegetarian" diet receiving significant media attention recently is the *flexitarian* diet: flexitarians are

vegetarianism The practice of restricting the diet to food substances of plant origin, including vegetables, fruits, grains, and nuts.

GAME PLAN

Tips for Adding Legumes to Your Daily Diet

They're high in protein and fiber, low in fat, and fill you up with fewer calories than meat sources of protein. What's more, they taste good! Maybe that's why nutrition experts consider legumes an almost perfect food. From main dishes to snacks, here are some simple ways to add legumes to your daily diet. By the way, some people experience uncomfortable intestinal gas after eating legumes. This is produced when bacteria in the colon break down the starches. If you're one of those people, make sure you soak legumes thoroughly, changing the water once or twice, before cooking. You can also try using Beano, an enzyme supplement available in most grocery stores. Taken before meals, it reduces intestinal gas.

Breakfast

❑ Instead of cereal, eggs, or a muffin, microwave a frozen bean burrito for a quick, portable breakfast.

❑ Make your pancakes with soy milk or pour soy milk on your cereal.

❑ If you normally have a side of bacon, ham, or sausage with your eggs, have a side of black beans.

Lunch and Dinner

❑ Try a sandwich made with hummus (a garbanzo bean spread), cucumbers, tomato, avocado, and/or lettuce on whole-wheat bread or in a whole-wheat pocket.

❑ Add garbanzo beans, kidney beans, or fresh peas to tossed salads or make a three-bean salad with kidney beans, green beans, and garbanzo beans.

❑ Make a side dish using legumes, such as peas with pearl onions or succotash (lima beans, corn, and tomatoes).

❑ Make black-bean soup, lentil soup, pea soup, minestrone soup, or a batch of dal (a type of yellow lentil used in Indian cuisine) and serve over brown rice. Top with plain yogurt, a traditional accompaniment in many Asian cuisines.

❑ Make burritos with black or pinto beans instead of shredded meat.

❑ Make a "meatloaf" using cooked, mashed lentils instead of ground beef.

❑ For fast food at home, keep canned beans on hand. Serve over rice with a salad for a complete and hearty meal.

Snacks

❑ Instead of potato chips or pretzels, try one of the new bean chips.

❑ Dip fresh vegetables in bean dip.

❑ Have hummus on wedges of pita bread.

❑ Add roasted soy "nuts" to your trail mix.

❑ Keep frozen tofu desserts such as tofu ice cream in your freezer.

TABLE 5.4 Terms and Definitions of a Vegetarian Diet

Type of Diet	Foods Consumed	Comments
Semivegetarian (also called partial vegetarian or flexitarian)	Vegetables, grains, nuts, fruits, legumes; sometimes seafood, poultry, eggs, and dairy products	Typically exclude or limit red meat; may also avoid other meats.
Pescovegetarian	Similar to a semivegetarian but excludes poultry	*Pesco* means fish, the only animal source of protein in this diet.
Lacto-ovo-vegetarian	Vegetables, grains, nuts, fruits, legumes, dairy products (*lacto*), and eggs (*ovo*)	Excludes animal flesh and seafood; may be deficient in iron and zinc.
Lactovegetarian	Similar to a lacto-ovo-vegetarian but excludes eggs	Relies on milk and cheese for animal sources of protein; may be deficient in iron and zinc.
Ovovegetarian	Vegetables, grains, nuts, fruits, legumes, and eggs	Excludes dairy, flesh, and seafood products; may be deficient in iron and zinc.
Vegan (also called strict vegetarian)	Only plant-based foods (vegetables, grains, nuts, seeds, fruits, legumes)	May not provide adequate vitamin B_{12}, zinc, iron, or calcium.
Macrobiotic diet	Vegan type of diet; becomes progressively more strict until almost all foods are eliminated. At the extreme, only brown rice and small amounts of water or herbal tea are consumed.	Taken to the extreme, can cause malnutrition and death.
Fruitarian	Only raw or dried fruit, seeds, nuts, honey, and vegetable oil	Very restrictive diet; deficient in protein, calcium, zinc, iron, vitamin B_{12}, riboflavin, and other nutrients.

considered semivegetarians who eat mostly plant foods, eggs, and dairy but occasionally eat red meat, poultry, and/or fish.

Table 5.4 identifies the various types of vegetarian diets, ranging from the most inclusive to the most restrictive. Notice that the more restrictive the diet, the more challenging it becomes to achieve an adequate protein intake.

Why Do People become Vegetarians?

When discussing vegetarianism, one of the most often-asked questions is why people would make this food choice. The most common responses are included here.

Religious, Ethical, and Food-Safety Reasons

Some make the choice for religious or spiritual reasons. Several religions prohibit or restrict the consumption of animal flesh; however, generalizations can be misleading. For example, while certain sects within Hinduism forbid the consumption of meat, perusing the menu at an Indian restaurant will reveal that some other Hindus regularly consume small quantities of meat, poultry, and fish. Many Buddhists are vegetarians, as are some Christians, including Seventh-Day Adventists.

Many vegetarians are guided by their personal philosophy to choose vegetarianism. These people feel that it is morally and ethically wrong to consume animals and any products from animals (such as dairy or egg products) because they view the practices in the modern animal industries as inhumane. They may consume milk and eggs but choose to purchase them only from family farms where they believe animals are treated humanely.

There is also a great deal of concern about meat-handling practices, because contaminated meat is allowed into our food supply. For example, in 1982, there was an

HIGHLIGHT

Mad Cow Disease—What's the Beef?

Mad cow disease is a fatal brain disorder caused by a *prion,* which is an abnormal form of protein. Prions cause brain damage by influencing other proteins to take on their abnormal shape. Mad cow disease is also called *bovine spongiform encephalopathy (BSE).* The disease eats away at a cow's brain, leaving it full of sponge-like holes. Eventually, the brain can no longer control vital life functions, and the cow literally "goes mad." Unfortunately, people who eat infected cattle will also be infected. This disease has killed at least 100 people, most of them in Great Britain during a widespread outbreak there in the late 1980s.

Scientists are not certain how the prions are introduced to cattle. They think cattle become infected by eating feed made with the brains and spinal cords of other infected cattle. After exposure, it takes several years for mad cow disease to manifest; thus, scientists speculate that older cattle are more infectious than younger animals. Meat products such as poor-quality sausages and ground meats made using brain and spinal tissue are much more likely to be infected than lean muscle tissue.

The effect of mad cow disease on the European beef market has been staggering, with beef consumption dropping 25% to 70% in certain countries; Great Britain, France, and Germany have been particularly affected. In addition, many countries, including the United States, have banned the import of all cattle, sheep, and goats from Europe. Even cattle that are only potentially infected must be slaughtered. To date, almost 5 million cattle have been destroyed.

Three cases of mad cow disease were found in Canada from 2003 to early 2005. To date, no person eating Canadian beef has developed symptoms suggestive of infection. However, the occurrence of this disease in Canadian cattle

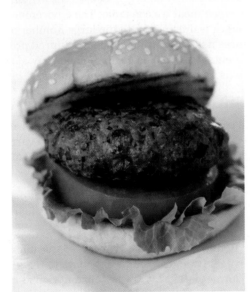

has prompted the United States to temporarily ban the import of Canadian beef. In December 2003, the first case of mad cow disease was reported in the United States, shocking those who believed the food supply to be safe from this disease. This discovery prompted many countries to immediately ban importation of American beef. As a result of this discovery, the federal government and beef industry took aggressive steps to destroy any potentially infected beef and to reassure the public that American beef is safe for consumption. Additional steps taken to protect beef include feeding U.S. cattle high-protein meal made from soybeans and working to ensure that the banning of the use of animal feed made with animal by-products is strictly enforced. In addition, cattle in the United States have for many years been slaughtered at an early age, reducing the likelihood of advanced infection. It is unclear whether, or how long, the ban on Canadian beef will continue.

Should Americans fear our beef supply? The U.S. Department of Agriculture, the Food and Drug Administration, the National Institutes of Health, and the Centers for Disease Control and Prevention are working together to ensure enforcement of the ban related to the use of animal-based feed and to enhance technology that can track signs of the disease and act quickly if it reappears in our food supply. In addition, the U.S. beef industry is highly motivated to comply with safety regulations because reduced beef intake translates into millions of dollars in lost income. Although it is not possible for the United States to be completely immune to mad cow disease, adherence to strict safety standards should minimize our risk and keep our beef safe for human consumption.

outbreak of severe bloody diarrhea that was eventually traced to bacteria in hamburgers served at a fast-food restaurant. Several people became seriously ill and one child died after eating the hamburgers. Another concern surrounding beef is the possibility that it is tainted by the microbes that cause *mad cow disease.* See the Highlight above for a discussion of mad cow disease and its impact on the United States and other countries.

Ecological Reasons

Many people choose vegetarianism because of their concerns about the effect of meat industries on the global environment. They argue that cattle consume large quantities of grain and water, require grazing areas that could be used for plant food production, destroy vulnerable ecosystems including rain forests, and produce wastes that run off into surrounding bodies of water. Meat industry organizations argue that such effects are minor and greatly exaggerated. One area of agreement that has recently emerged focuses the argument not on *whether* we eat meat but on *how much* meat we consume. The environmental damage caused by the raising of livestock is due in part to the large number of animals produced. When a population reduces its consumption of meat, reduced production follows. In addition to the environmental benefits, eating less meat may also reduce our risk for chronic diseases such as heart disease and some cancers.

Health Benefits

Still others practice vegetarianism because of its health benefits. Research over several years has consistently shown that a varied and balanced vegetarian diet can reduce the risk of many chronic diseases. Health benefits include:[17]

- Reduced risk for obesity, type 2 diabetes, high blood pressure, and heart disease, most likely due to the lower saturated-fat content of vegetarian diets.
- Fewer intestinal problems, most likely due to the higher fiber content of vegetarian diets.
- Reduced risk of some cancers, particularly colon cancer.[18] Many components of a vegetarian diet could contribute to reducing cancer risks, including higher fiber, lower dietary fat, lower consumption of **carcinogens** (cancer-causing agents) that are formed when cooking meat, and higher consumption of soy protein, which may have anticancer properties.[19]
- Reduced risk of kidney disease, kidney stones, and gallstones. The lower protein contents of vegetarian diets, plus the higher intake of legumes and vegetables, may be protective against these conditions.

carcinogens   Cancer-causing agents, such as certain pesticides, industrial chemicals, and pollutants.

What Are the Challenges of a Vegetarian Diet?

Although a vegetarian diet can be healthful, it also presents some challenges. With reduced consumption of flesh and dairy products, there is the potential for inadequate intakes of certain nutrients. Table 5.5 lists the nutrients that can be deficient in a vegan type of diet plan and describes good nonanimal sources that can provide these nutrients. Supplementation of these nutrients may be necessary for certain individuals if they cannot consume adequate amounts in their diet.

Can a vegetarian diet provide enough protein? Because high-quality protein sources are quite easy to obtain in developed countries, a well-balanced vegetarian diet can provide adequate protein. In fact, the American Dietetic Association and the Dietitians of Canada endorse an appropriately planned vegetarian diet as healthful, nutritionally adequate, and providing many benefits in reducing and preventing various diseases.[17] As you can see, the emphasis is on a *balanced* and *adequate* vegetarian diet; thus, it is important for vegetarians to consume soy products, eat complementary proteins, and obtain enough energy from other macronutrients to spare protein from being used as an energy source. Although the digestibility of a vegetarian diet is potentially lower than that of an animal-based diet, there is no separate protein recommendation for vegetarians who consume complementary plant proteins.[20]

A Special Food Pyramid Can Help Vegetarians Consume Adequate Nutrients

Vegetarians can use the food pyramid illustrated in FIGURE 5.8 to design a diet that contains adequate levels of all of the necessary nutrients. Figure 5.8 emphasizes the importance of eating whole grains, fruits, vegetables, and legumes at every meal.

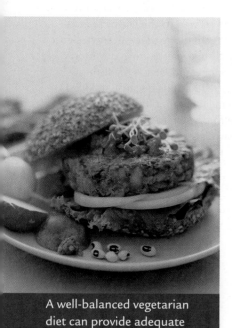

A well-balanced vegetarian diet can provide adequate protein.

TABLE 5.5   Nutrients of Concern in a Vegan Diet

Nutrient	Functions	Non-Meat/Non-Dairy Food Sources
Vitamin B_{12}	Assists with DNA synthesis; protection and growth of nerve fibers	Vitamin B_{12}-fortified cereals, yeast, soy products, and other meat analogs; vitamin B_{12} supplements
Vitamin D	Promotes bone growth	Vitamin D-fortified cereals, margarines, and soy products; adequate exposure to sunlight; supplementation may be necessary for those who do not get adequate exposure to sunlight
Riboflavin (vitamin B_2)	Promotes release of energy; supports normal vision and skin health	Whole and enriched grains, green leafy vegetables, mushrooms, beans, nuts, and seeds
Iron	Assists with oxygen transport; involved in making amino acids and hormones	Whole-grain products, prune juice, dried fruits, beans, nuts, seeds, leafy vegetables such as spinach
Calcium	Maintains bone health; assists with muscle contraction, blood pressure, and nerve transmission	Fortified soy milk and tofu, almonds, dry beans, leafy vegetables, calcium-fortified juices, fortified breakfast cereals
Zinc	Assists with DNA and RNA synthesis, immune function, and growth	Whole-grain products, wheat germ, beans, nuts, and seeds

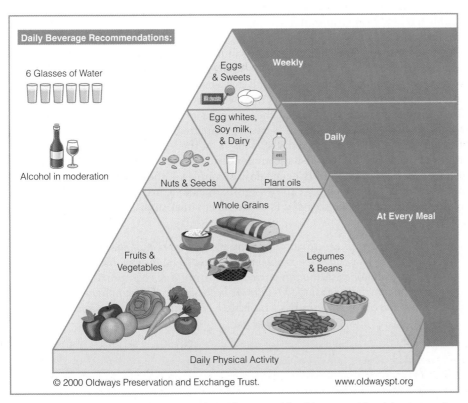

FIGURE 5.8   The Vegetarian Food Guide Pyramid. This pyramid guides general food choices at each meal, daily, and weekly.

NUTRI-CASE THEO

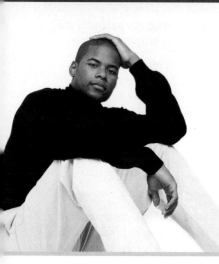

"No way would I ever become a vegetarian! The only way to build up your muscles is to eat meat. I was reading in a bodybuilding magazine last week about some guy who doesn't eat anything from animals, not even milk or eggs, and he looked pretty buff—but I don't believe it. They can do anything to photos these days. Besides, during basketball season, I just crave red meat. If I don't have it, I feel sort of like my batteries don't get charged. It's just not practical for a competitive athlete to go without meat."

What two claims does Theo make here about the role of red meat in his diet? Do you think these claims are valid? Why or why not? What facts might be important to consider about the nature of plant and animal proteins?

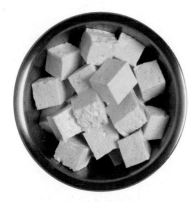

Vegetarians should eat 5 servings of beans, nuts, seeds, eggs, or meat substitutes daily.

Daily foods include nuts and seeds, egg whites, soy milk and dairy products, and plant oils. Weekly choices include eggs and sweets. Although this version provides a helpful illustration of the types of foods recommended for vegetarians, it does not give suggestions for daily number of servings.

Table 5.6 lists food groups and serving recommendations for vegetarians.[21] Notice that there is no separate listing for a group exclusive to milk, yogurt, and cheese. It is recommended that vegetarians should eat 8 or more servings each day of calcium-rich foods, and that these foods can come from any of the calcium-rich foods listed in each food group. Lacto- and lacto-ovo-vegetarians can consume low-fat or nonfat dairy products, while vegans and ovovegetarians can consume calcium-fortified soy or rice milk, yogurt, and cheese products to meet their calcium needs. Another excellent source of calcium is calcium-fortified orange juice. Vegetarians should also consume 5 servings daily of foods from the legumes, nuts, and other protein-rich foods group. It is also recommended that vegetarians consume at least 3 good food sources of vitamin B$_{12}$ each day. Examples of these include 1 cup of fortified soy milk, 1 large egg, ½ cup cow's milk, ¾ cup yogurt, 1 ounce of fortified breakfast cereal, and 1½ ounces of a fortified meat substitute.

> RECAP *A balanced vegetarian diet may reduce the risk of obesity, type 2 diabetes, heart disease, digestive problems, some cancers, kidney disease, kidney stones, and gallstones. Although varied vegetarian diets can provide enough protein, vegetarians who consume no animal products need to supplement their diet with good sources of vitamin B$_{12}$, vitamin D, riboflavin, iron, calcium, and zinc.*

TABLE 5.6 Food Groups and Recommended Serving Sizes for Vegetarians

Food Group	Number of Servings	Foods and Serving Sizes	Calcium-Rich Food Sources
Grains	6	Bread—1 slice Cooked grain or cereal—½ cup Ready-to-eat cereal—1 oz	1 oz calcium-fortified breakfast cereal
Legumes, nuts, and other protein-rich foods	5	Cooked beans, peas, or lentils—½ cup Tofu or tempeh—½ cup Nut or seed butter—2 tbsp. Nuts—¼ cup Meat substitute—1 oz Egg—1 each	Cow's milk or yogurt or fortified soy milk—½ cup Cheese—¾ oz Tempeh or calcium-set tofu—½ cup Almonds—¼ cup Almond butter or sesame tahini—2 tbsp. Cooked soybeans—½ cup Soy nuts—¼ cup
Vegetables	4	Cooked vegetables—½ cup Raw vegetables—1 cup Vegetable juice—½ cup	Bok choy, broccoli, collards, Chinese cabbage, kale, mustard greens, or okra—1 cup cooked or 2 cups raw Fortified tomato juice—½ cup
Fruits	2	Medium fruit—1 each Cut up or cooked fruit—½ cup Fruit juice—½ cup Dried fruit—¼ cup	Fortified fruit juice—½ cup Figs—5 each
Fats	2	Oil, mayonnaise, or soft margarine—1 tsp.	None

Source: Reprinted from *Journal of the American Dietetic Association*, 103(6), Messina et al.: "A New Food Guide for North American Vegetarians." © 2003, with permission from Elsevier.

Where I'm at now ...

At the beginning of this chapter, you estimated how many grams of protein you thought you needed to eat each day. Now jot down how many you really need to eat (use Table 5.2):

How much protein do you actually eat most days? (Use Appendix A, diet analysis software, or log on to the USDA's MyPyramid Tracker to determine your average daily protein intake.)

How are you doing in terms of meeting your daily protein needs? (Choose one.)

☐ I've been eating more protein than I need.

☐ I've been eating less protein than I need.

☐ I've been pretty much on target!

Given what you've learned about plant-based sources of protein, do you plan to make any changes in your choices of meat-based versus vegetarian meals? (Choose one.)

☐ No—I'm already a vegetarian.

☐ No—I'm still more comfortable eating meals that contain meat.

☐ Yes—I feel more comfortable with the idea of eating meatless meals more often.

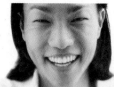

REVIEW QUESTIONS

Circle the correct choice.

1. The process of combining peanut butter and whole-wheat bread to make a complete protein is called
   a. deamination.
   b. vegetarianism.
   c. transamination.
   d. mutual supplementation.

2. Which of the following meals is typical of the vegan diet?
   a. rice, pinto beans, acorn squash, soy butter, and almond milk
   b. veggie dog, bun, and a banana blended with yogurt
   c. raw lean beef and green tea
   d. egg salad on whole-wheat toast, broccoli, carrot sticks, and soy milk

3. Proteins are synthesized following instructions dictated by
   a. enzymes.
   b. DNA.
   c. hormones.
   d. ketones.

4. The portion of an amino acid that contains nitrogen is called the
   a. side chain.
   b. amine group.
   c. acid group.
   d. nitrate cluster.

5. Proteins contain
   a. carbon, oxygen, and nitrogen.
   b. oxygen and hydrogen.
   c. carbon, oxygen, hydrogen, and nitrogen.
   d. carbon, oxygen, and hydrogen.

6. True or False? After leaving the small intestine, amino acids are transported to the liver for distribution throughout the body.

7. True or False? When a protein is denatured, its shape is lost but its function is retained.

8. True or False? All hormones are proteins.

9. True or False? Buffers help the body maintain acid–base balance.

10. True or False? Athletes typically require about three times as much protein as nonactive people.

WEB LINKS

www.eatright.org
American Dietetic Association

Search for vegetarian diets to learn how to plan healthful meat-free meals.

www.aphis.usda.gov
Animal and Plant Health Inspection Service

Select "Hot Issues" or search for "Bovine Spongiform Encephalopathy (BSE)" to learn more about mad cow disease.

www.vrg.org
The Vegetarian Resource Group

Obtain vegetarian and vegan news, recipes, information, and additional links.

www.beef.org
National Cattlemen's Beef Association

An industry Web site providing information about beef production.

www.cdc.gov
Centers for Disease Control and Prevention

Click on the A–Z Index to learn more about *Escherichia coli* and mad cow disease.

www.who.int/nut
World Health Organization Nutrition Site

Visit this site to find out more about the worldwide magnitude of protein-energy malnutrition and the diseases that can result from inadequate intakes of protein, energy-yielding carbohydrates and fats, and various additional nutrients.

www.nlm.nih.gov/medlineplus
MEDLINE Plus Health Information

Search for "sickle cell anemia" and "cystic fibrosis" to obtain additional resources and the latest news about these inherited diseases.

www.nal.usda.gov/fnic
USDA Food and Nutrition Information Center

Click on "Food Composition" on the left navigation bar to find the USDA Nutrient Data Laboratory, a searchable database of nutrient values of foods.

TEST YOURSELF ANSWERS

1. **False.** Although protein can be used for energy in certain circumstances, fats and carbohydrates are the primary sources of energy for our bodies.

2. **False.** There is no evidence that consuming amino acid supplements assists in building muscle tissue. Consuming adequate energy and exercising muscles, specifically using weight training, builds muscle tissue.

3. **False.** Excess protein is broken down and its component parts are either stored as fat or used for energy or tissue building and repair. Only the nitrogen component of protein is excreted in the urine.

4. **False.** Vegetarian diets can meet and even exceed an individual's protein needs, assuming that adequate energy-yielding macronutrients, a variety of protein sources, and complementary protein sources are consumed.

5. **True.** Most people in the United States consume 1.5 to 2 times more protein than they need.

REFERENCES

1. Bennett, J., and C. Lewis. 2001. *Very Vegetarian.* Nashville: Rutledge Hill Press.
2. Vegetarian Resource Group. 2003. *Vegetarian Journal,* Issue 1. Available at www.vrg.org/journal/vj2003issue3/vj2003issue3poll.htm.
3. Lemon, P. W. 2000. Beyond the zone: Protein needs of active individuals. *J. Am. Coll. Nutr.* 19 (5 suppl.):513S–521S.
4. Leitzmann, C. 2005. Vegetarian diets: What are the advantages? *Forum Nutr.* 57:147–156.
5. Szeto, Y. T., T. C. Kwok, and I. F. Benzie. 2004. Effects of a long-term vegetarian diet on biomarkers of antioxidant status and cardiovascular risk. *Nutrition* 20(10):863–866.
6. Munger, R. G., J. R. Cerhan, and B. C.-H. Chiu. 1999. Prospective study of dietary protein intake and risk of hip fracture in postmenopausal women. *Am. J. Clin. Nutr.* 69:147–152.
7. Alekel, D. L., A. St. Germain, C. T. Peterson, K. B. Hanson, J. W. Stewart, and T. Toda. 2000. Isoflavone-rich soy protein isolate attenuates bone loss in the lumbar spine of perimenopausal women. *Am. J. Clin. Nutr.* 72:844–52.
8. Samaha, F. F., N. Iqbal, P. Seshadri, K. L. Chicano, D. A. Daily, J. McGrory, T. Williams, M. Williams, E. J. Gracely, and L. Stern. 2003. A low-carbohydrate as compared with a low-fat diet in severe obesity. *N. Engl. J. Med.* 348:2074–2081.
9. Stern, L., N. Iqbal, P. Seshadri, K. L. Chicano, D. A. Daily, J. McGrory, M. Williams, E. J. Gracely, and F. F. Samaha. 2004. The effects of low-carbohydrate versus conventional weight loss diets in severely obese adults: One-year follow-up of a randomized trial. *Ann. Intern. Med.* 140:778–785.
10. Foster, G. D., H. R. Wyatt, J. O. Hill, B. G. McGuckin, C. Brill, B. S. Mohammed, P. O. Szapary, D. J. Rader, J. S. Edman, and S. Klein. 2003. A randomized trial of a low-carbohydrate diet for obesity. *N. Engl. J. Med.* 348:2082–2090.
11. Bravata, D. M., L. Sanders, J. Huang, H. M. Krumholz, I. Olkin, C. D. Gardner, and D. M. Bravata. 2003. Efficacy and safety of low-carbohydrate diets. A systematic review. *JAMA* 289:1837–1850.
12. Poortmans, J. R., and O. Dellalieux. 2000. Do regular high-protein diets have potential health risks on kidney function in athletes? *Int. J. Sport Nutr.* 10:28–38.
13. Henkel, J. 2000. Soy: Health claims for soy protein, questions about other components. *FDA Consumer Magazine,* May–June. Available at www.fda.gov/fdac/features/2000/300_soy.html.
14. American Heart Association. 2005. Choosing a Heart-Healthy Diet. Available at www.americanheart.org/presenter.jhtml? identifier=353.
15. Kirchheimer, S. 2004. Soy Improves Prostate Cancer Outlook. Available at http://my.webmd.com/content/Article/94/102884.html.
16. American Cancer Society. 2007. Can Phytoestrogens Reduce Breast Cancer Risk and Treat Menopause? Available at www.cancer.org/docroot/MED/content/MED_2_1x_Can_Phytoestrogens_Reduce_Cancer_Risk_and_Treat_Menopause.asp. (Accessed September 12, 2007.)
17. Messina, M., and V. Messina. 1996. *The Dietitian's Guide to Vegetarian Diets.* Gaithersburg, MD: Aspen Publishers.
18. American Dietetic Association; Dietitians of Canada. 2003. Position of the American Dietetic Association and Dietitians of Canada: Vegetarian diets. *J. Am. Diet. Assoc.* 103(6):748–765.
19. Messina, M. J. 1999. Legumes and soybeans: Overview of their nutritional profiles and health effects. *Am. J. Clin. Nutr.* 70 (suppl.):439S–450S.
20. Institute of Medicine, Food and Nutrition Board. 2002. *Dietary Reference Intakes for Energy, Carbohydrate, Fiber, Fat, Fatty Acids, Cholesterol, Protein, and Amino Acids (Macronutrients).* Washington, DC: National Academies Press, pp. 465–608.
21. Messina V., V. Melina, and A. Reed Mangels. 2003. A new food guide for North American vegetarians. *J. Am. Diet. Assoc.* 103(6):771–775.

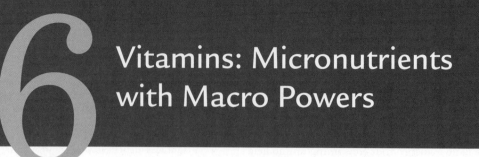

6 Vitamins: Micronutrients with Macro Powers

TEST YOURSELF

Are these statements true or false? Circle your guess.

1 Vitamin D is called the "sunshine vitamin" because our bodies can make it by using energy obtained from sunlight.

TRUE or **FALSE**

2 Taking vitamin C supplements helps prevent colds.

TRUE or **FALSE**

3 The B vitamins are an important source of energy for our bodies.

TRUE or **FALSE**

4 Phytochemicals are a small group of plant chemicals that are believed to cause cancer.

TRUE or **FALSE**

5 Taking a daily multivitamin supplement is a waste of money.

TRUE or **FALSE**

Test Yourself answers can be found at the end of the chapter.

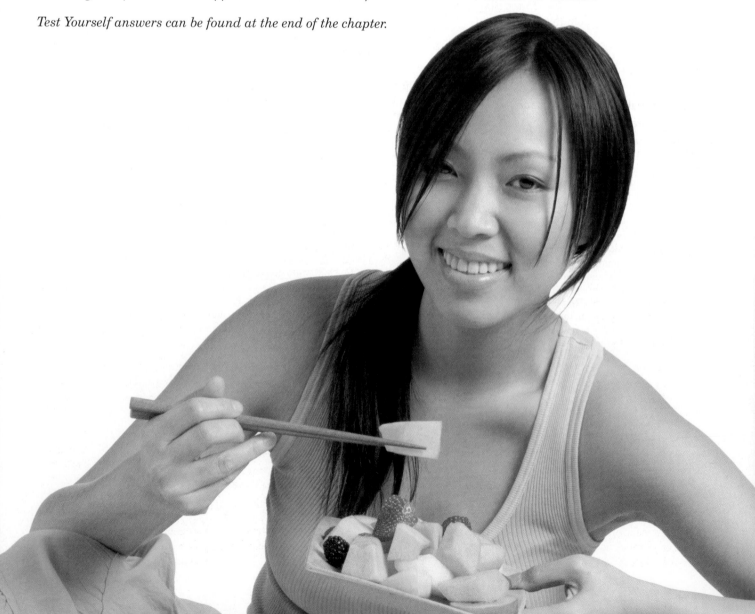

DR. LESLIE BERNSTEIN looked in astonishment at the 80-year-old man in his office. A leading gastroenterologist and professor of medicine at Albert Einstein College of Medicine in New York City, he had admired Pop Katz for years as one of his most healthy patients, a strict vegetarian and athlete who just weeks before had been going on 3-mile runs. Now he could barely stand. He was confused, cried easily, was wandering away from his home, and had lost control of his bladder. Tests showed that he had not had a stroke, did not have a tumor, infection, or Alzheimer disease, and had no evidence of exposure to pesticides or other toxins. A neurologist diagnosed dementia, but Bernstein was unconvinced: How could a man who hadn't been sick for 80 years suddenly become demented? Then it struck him: "The man's been a vegetarian for 38 years. No meat. No fish. No eggs. No milk. He hasn't had any animal protein for decades. He has to be B_{12} deficient!"[1]

Bernstein immediately tested Katz's blood, then gave him an injection of vitamin B_{12}. The blood test confirmed Bernstein's hunch: the level of B_{12} in Katz's blood was too low to detect. The morning after his injection, Katz could sit up without help. Within a week of continuing treatment, he could read, play card games, and hold his own in conversations. Unfortunately, some neurological damage remained, including alterations in his personality and an inability to concentrate. Bernstein notes, "A diet free of animal protein can be healthful and safe, but it should be supplemented periodically with B_{12} by mouth or by injection."[1]

It was not until 1906, when the English biochemist F. G. Hopkins discovered what he called *accessory factors,* that scientists began to appreciate the many critical roles of micronutrients in maintaining human health. Vitamin B_{12}, for instance, was not even isolated until 1948! In this chapter, we explore the roles vitamins play as tissue guardians, antioxidants, and energy generators. But first, let's take a moment to define exactly what vitamins are.

What Are Vitamins?

Vitamins are compounds that contain carbon and are essential in regulating our bodies' processes (FIGURE 6.1). Because our bodies cannot synthesize most vitamins, we must consume them in our diets. Fortunately, most are found in a variety of foods. Vitamins are classified as either fat soluble or water soluble. Here, we discuss the general properties of these two groups.

Fat-Soluble Vitamins Are Stored in the Body

Vitamins A, D, E, and K are **fat-soluble vitamins.** These vitamins are absorbed in our intestines along with dietary fat. They are then transported to the liver or other organs, where they are either used immediately or stored in fatty tissues for later use. Because we are capable of storing fat-soluble vitamins, we do not have to consume the recommended intakes of these nutrients every single day. As long as our diets provide the average amounts recommended over any given time period, we won't develop deficiencies.

Our ability to store fat-soluble vitamins does have a distinct disadvantage. If we consume more of these vitamins than our bodies can use, they can build up to toxic levels in our fatty tissues. Symptoms of toxicity include damage to our hair, skin, bones, eyes, and nervous system. **Megadosing**—that is, taking ten or more times the recommended amount of a nutrient—can even lead to death when it involves the fat-soluble vitamins A and D.

vitamins   Micronutrients that contain carbon and assist us in regulating our bodies' processes. They are classified as water soluble or fat soluble.

fat-soluble vitamins   Vitamins that are not soluble in water but soluble in fat. These include vitamins A, D, E, and K.

megadosing   Taking a dose of a nutrient that is ten or more times greater than the recommended amount.

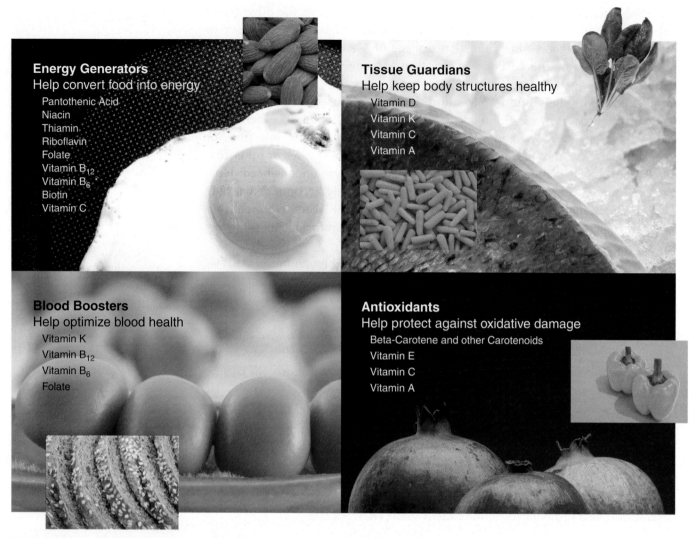

Energy Generators
Help convert food into energy
Pantothenic Acid
Niacin
Thiamin
Riboflavin
Folate
Vitamin B$_{12}$
Vitamin B$_6$
Biotin
Vitamin C

Tissue Guardians
Help keep body structures healthy
Vitamin D
Vitamin K
Vitamin C
Vitamin A

Blood Boosters
Help optimize blood health
Vitamin K
Vitamin B$_{12}$
Vitamin B$_6$
Folate

Antioxidants
Help protect against oxidative damage
Beta-Carotene and other Carotenoids
Vitamin E
Vitamin C
Vitamin A

FIGURE 6.1 The functions of fat-soluble and water-soluble vitamins and related compounds such as beta-carotene and biotin. Good food sources are also shown for each functional group.

Even though we can store fat-soluble vitamins, deficiencies sometimes do occur, especially in people with diseases that prevent the normal absorption of fat and in people who consume very little fat. Using mineral oil as a laxative can result in a significant loss of fat-soluble vitamins in our feces. Deficiencies of fat-soluble vitamins can lead to serious health problems such as night blindness, fragile bones, and even death in the most severe cases.

Fat-soluble vitamins are found in a variety of fat-containing foods. Meats, dairy products, vegetable oils, avocados, nuts, and seeds are all potentially good sources. Table 6.1 identifies major functions and recommended intakes.

Water-Soluble Vitamins Should Be Consumed Daily or Weekly

Vitamin C and the B vitamins (thiamin, riboflavin, niacin, vitamin B$_6$, vitamin B$_{12}$, pantothenic acid, biotin, and folate) are the **water-soluble vitamins.** Because they dissolve in water, these vitamins are readily absorbed through the intestinal wall directly into the bloodstream. They then travel to cells where they are needed.

We cannot store large amounts of water-soluble vitamins, because our kidneys filter out from our bloodstream any that are unneeded. We then excrete them in our urine. Because we do not store large amounts in our tissues, toxicity rarely occurs

water-soluble vitamins Vitamins that are soluble in water. These include vitamin C and the B vitamins.

TABLE 6.1   Fat-Soluble Vitamins

Vitamin Name	Primary Functions	Recommended Intake	Reliable Food Sources
A (retinol, retinal, retinoic acid)	Required for ability of eyes to adjust to changes in light Protects color vision Assists cell differentiation Required for sperm production in men and fertilization in women Contributes to healthy bone Contributes to healthy immune system	RDA: Men = 900 µg Women = 700 µg UL = 3,000 µg/day	Preformed retinol: Beef and chicken liver, egg yolks, milk Carotenoid precursors: spinach, carrots, mango, apricots, cantaloupe, pumpkin, yams
D (cholecalciferol)	Regulates blood calcium levels Maintains bone health Assists cell differentiation	AI (assumes that person does not get adequate sun exposure): Adult aged 19 to 50 y = 5 µg/day Adult aged 50 to 70 y = 10 µg/day Adult aged >70 y = 15 µg/day UL = 50 µg/day	Canned salmon and mackerel, milk, fortified cereals
E (tocopherol)	Protects cell membranes, polyunsaturated fatty acids, and vitamin A from oxidation Protects white blood cells Enhances immune function Improves absorption of vitamin A	RDA: Men = 15 mg/day Women = 15 mg/day UL = 1,000 mg/day	Sunflower seeds, almonds, vegetable oils, fortified cereals
K (phylloquinone, menaquinone, menadione)	Serves as a coenzyme during production of specific proteins that assist in blood coagulation and bone metabolism	AI: Men = 120 µg/day Women = 90 µg/day	Kale, spinach, turnip greens, Brussels sprouts

when we consume these vitamins in our diet. We *can* acquire toxic levels through supplementation, however, if we consume higher amounts than our bodies can eliminate.

A disadvantage of our inability to store large amounts of water-soluble vitamins is that we need to consume them on a daily or weekly basis. If we do not, deficiency symptoms and even disease can result fairly quickly. Fortunately, the water-soluble vitamins are abundant in many foods, including whole grains, fruits, vegetables, meats, and dairy products. Table 6.2 identifies major functions and recommended intakes.

> RECAP *Vitamins are carbon-containing compounds that are essential in regulating a multitude of body processes. Vitamins A, D, E, and K are fat soluble and are present in certain fat-containing foods. We store fat-soluble vitamins in the fatty tissues of our bodies. Water-soluble vitamins include vitamin C and the B vitamins (thiamin, riboflavin, niacin, vitamin B_6, vitamin B_{12}, pantothenic acid, biotin, and folate). Because these vitamins are soluble in water, the body cannot store large amounts and excretes excesses in the urine.*

Tissue Guardians: Vitamins A, D, and K

The fat-soluble vitamins A, D, and K are important for the health of certain body tissues. Vitamin A protects the retina of the eyes, vitamin D is required for healthy bone, and vitamin K guards against blood loss. Let's take a closer look at these three fat-soluble vitamins.

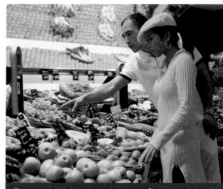

Because we cannot store large amounts of water-soluble vitamins, we need to consume foods that contain them, such as fruits and vegetables, daily.

TABLE 6.2 Water-Soluble Vitamins

Vitamin Name	Primary Functions	Recommended Intake	Reliable Food Sources
Thiamin (vitamin B_1)	Required as enzyme cofactor for carbohydrate and amino acid metabolism	RDA: Men = 1.2 mg/day Women = 1.1 mg/day	Pork, fortified cereals, enriched rice and pasta, peas, tuna, legumes
Riboflavin (vitamin B_2)	Required as enzyme cofactor for carbohydrate and fat metabolism	RDA: Men = 1.3 mg/day Women = 1.1 mg/day	Beef liver, shrimp, milk and dairy foods, fortified cereals, enriched breads and grains
Niacin, nicotinamide, nicotinic acid	Required for carbohydrate and fat metabolism Plays role in DNA replication and repair and cell differentiation	RDA: Men = 16 mg/day Women = 14 mg/day UL = 35 mg/day	Beef liver, most cuts of meat/fish/poultry, fortified cereals, enriched breads and grains, canned tomato products
Pyridoxine, pyridoxal, pyridoxamine (vitamin B_6)	Required as enzyme cofactor for carbohydrate and amino acid metabolism Assists synthesis of blood cells	RDA: Men and women aged 19 to 50 y = 1.3 mg/day Men aged >50 y = 1.7 mg/day Women aged >50 y = 1.5 mg/day UL = 100 mg/day	Chickpeas (garbanzo beans), most cuts of meat/fish/poultry, fortified cereals, white potatoes
Folate (folic acid)	Required as enzyme cofactor for amino acid metabolism Required for DNA synthesis Involved in metabolism of homocysteine	RDA: Men = 400 µg/day Women = 400 µg/day UL = 1,000 µg/day	Fortified cereals, enriched breads and grains, spinach, legumes (lentils, chickpeas, pinto beans), greens (spinach, romaine lettuce), liver
Cobalamin (vitamin B_{12})	Assists with formation of blood Required for healthy nervous system function Involved as enzyme cofactor in metabolism of homocysteine	RDA: Men = 2.4 µg/day Women = 2.4 µg/day	Shellfish, all cuts of meat/fish/poultry, milk and dairy foods, fortified cereals
Pantothenic acid	Assists with fat metabolism	AI: Men = 5 mg/day Women = 5 mg/day	Meat/fish/poultry, shiitake mushrooms, fortified cereals, egg yolk
Biotin	Involved as enzyme cofactor in carbohydrate, fat, and protein metabolism	RDA: Men = 30 µg/day Women = 30 µg/day	Nuts, egg yolk
C (ascorbic acid)	Antioxidant in extracellular fluid and lungs Regenerates oxidized vitamin E Assists with collagen synthesis Enhances immune function Assists in synthesis of hormones, neurotransmitters, and DNA Enhances iron absorption	RDA: Men = 90 mg/day Women = 75 mg/day Smokers = 35 mg more per day than RDA UL = 2,000 mg	Sweet peppers, citrus fruits and juices, broccoli, strawberries, kiwi

Vitamin A Protects Our Sight

Vitamin A is multitalented: its known functions are numerous, and researchers speculate that many are still to be discovered. Most would agree, though, that vitamin A's starring role is in the maintenance of healthy vision. Vitamin A enables us to see images as well as to distinguish different colors. Let's take a closer look at this process.

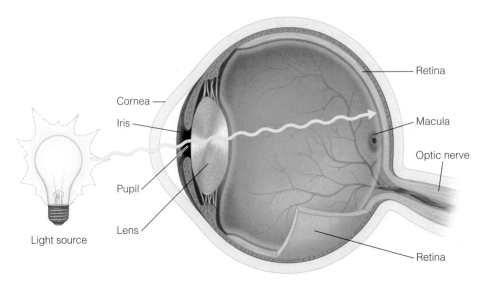

FIGURE 6.2 Vitamin A is necessary to maintain healthy vision. Light enters the eye through the cornea, travels through the lens, and hits the retina located in the back of the eye. The light reacts with the retinal stored in the retina, which allows us to see images.

Light enters our eyes through the cornea, travels through the lens, and then hits the **retina,** a delicate membrane lining the back of the inner eyeball (**FIGURE 6.2**). Indeed, the primary form that vitamin A takes in our bodies is *retinal,* which got its name because it is found in—and integral to—the retina. When light hits the retina, it reacts with the retinal within it. This reaction sparks the transmission of a signal to the brain that is interpreted as a black-and-white image. If the light hitting the retina is bright enough, then retinal can also enable the retina to distinguish the different wavelengths of light as different colors. These processes go on continually, allowing us to perceive moment-by-moment changes in our visual field, such as green and yellow leaves fluttering in the wind.

Our abilities to adjust to dim light and recover from a bright flash of light are also critically dependent on adequate levels of retinal in our eyes. That's why deficiency of vitamin A causes vision disorders, including night blindness, discussed shortly.

How Else Do We Use Vitamin A?

Vitamin A also contributes to **cell differentiation,** the process by which immature cells develop into highly specialized cells that perform unique functions. This process is critical to the development of healthy *epithelial tissues* (the skin and the tissues that line the respiratory and gastrointestinal tract), as well as specialized immune cells called *T lymphocytes,* which help us fight infections.

Vitamin A also:

- helps break down old bone tissue so that new bone can develop,
- is involved in sperm production in men and in fertilization in women, and
- is associated with lower risks of some forms of cancer and heart disease when blood levels of this vitamin are adequate.

Two popular treatments for acne contain derivatives of vitamin A. Retin-A, or tretinoin, is a treatment applied to the skin. Accutane, or isotretinoin, is taken orally. These medications should be used carefully and only under the supervision of a physician. Both medications increase a person's sensitivity to the sun, and it is recommended that exposure to the sun be limited while using them. They also can cause birth defects in infants if used while a woman is pregnant. It is recommended that a woman discontinue use at least 2 years prior to conceiving, and that women of

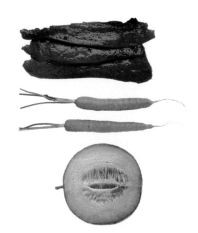

Liver, carrots, and cantaloupe all contain vitamin A.

retina The delicate, light-sensitive membrane lining the inner eyeball and connected to the optic nerve. It contains retinal.

cell differentiation The process by which immature, undifferentiated cells develop into highly specialized functional cells of discrete organs and tissues.

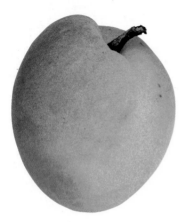

Apricots are high in carotenoids.

childbearing age who are using one of these medications use reliable contraceptives to avoid becoming pregnant. Both medications have also been associated with other toxicity problems in some patients. Interestingly, vitamin A itself has no effect on acne; thus, vitamin A supplements are not recommended in its treatment.

What Is the Role of Beta-Carotene?

Beta-carotene is a water-soluble *provitamin* found in many fruits and vegetables. **Provitamins** are inactive forms of vitamins that the body cannot use until they are converted to their active form. Our bodies convert beta-carotene to an active form of vitamin A called *retinol.* For this reason, beta-carotene is also referred to as a *precursor* of retinol.

Beta-carotene is also classified as a **carotenoid,** one of a group of more than 600 plant pigments that are the basis for the red, orange (think *carrots*), and deep-yellow colors of many fruits and vegetables. (Even dark-green leafy vegetables contain plenty of carotenoids, but the green pigment, chlorophyll, masks their color!) We are just beginning to learn about the many functions of carotenoids in the body and how they influence our health. We do know that carotenoids:

- defend against damage to our cell membranes,
- enhance our immune system,
- protect our skin from the damage caused by the sun's ultraviolet rays, and
- prevent or delay age-related vision impairment.

Carotenoids are also associated with a decreased risk of cardiovascular disease and certain types of cancer. Carotenoids and other beneficial plant chemicals (called *phytochemicals*) are discussed in detail on page 188.

How Much Vitamin A Should We Consume?

Table 6.1 identifies the RDA for vitamin A. Nutrition scientists do not classify beta-carotene and other carotenoids as micronutrients, as they play no known essential roles in our bodies and are not associated with any deficiency symptoms. Thus, no formal DRI for beta-carotene has been determined.

Because the body converts vitamin A and beta-carotene into retinol, you may also see the expression *retinol activity equivalents (RAE)* or *retinol equivalents (RE)* for vitamin A on food labels or dietary supplements. Sometimes, the vitamin A content of foods and supplements is expressed in International Units (IU).

We consume vitamin A from animal foods such as beef liver, chicken liver, eggs, and dairy products. Vitamin A is also available from foods high in beta-carotene and other carotenoids that can be converted to vitamin A. These include dark-green, orange, and deep-yellow fruits and vegetables such as spinach, carrots, mango, and cantaloupe. Common food sources of vitamin A are also identified in FIGURE 6.3.

Vitamin A is highly toxic, and toxicity symptoms develop after consuming only three to four times the RDA. Toxicity rarely results from food sources, but vitamin A supplements are known to have caused severe illness and even death. That's why single-nutrient vitamin A supplements should never be taken unless prescribed by your healthcare provider. Consuming excess vitamin A while pregnant can cause serious birth defects and spontaneous abortion. Other toxicity symptoms include fatigue, loss of appetite, blurred vision, hair loss, skin disorders, bone and joint pain, abdominal pain, nausea, diarrhea, and damage to the liver and nervous system. If caught in time, many of these symptoms are reversible once vitamin A supplementation is stopped. However, permanent damage can occur to the liver, eyes, and other organs. Because liver contains such a high amount of vitamin A, children and pregnant women should not consume liver on a daily or weekly basis.

What happens if we don't consume enough vitamin A? **Night blindness,** the inability to see in dim light, is a major vitamin A–deficiency concern in developing nations. Color blindness and other vision impairments can also occur. If night blindness progresses, it can result in irreversible total blindness due to hardening of the cornea (the transparent membrane covering the front of the eye). This is why it is critical to catch night blindness in its early stages and treat it with either the

---

provitamin An inactive form of a vitamin that the body can convert to an active form. An example is beta-carotene.

carotenoids Fat-soluble plant pigments that the body stores in the liver and adipose tissues. The body is able to convert certain carotenoids to vitamin A.

night blindness A vitamin A–deficiency disorder that results in the loss of the ability to see in dim light.

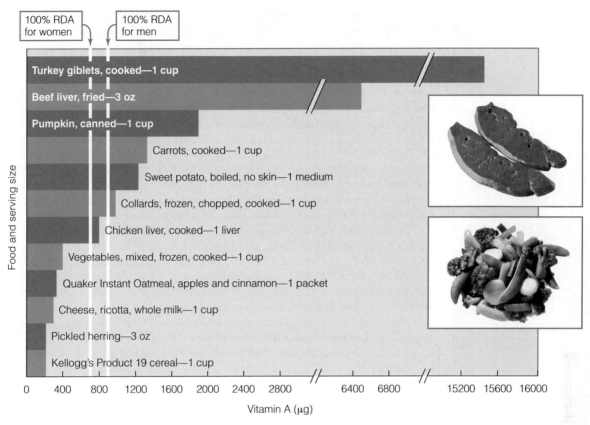

FIGURE 6.3   Common food sources of vitamin A. The RDA for vitamin A is 900 μg per day for men and 700 μg per day for women.

(Data from U.S. Department of Agriculture, Agricultural Research Service. 2007. USDA Nutrient Database for Standard Reference, Release 20. Nutrient Data Laboratory Home Page, www.ars.usda.gov/ba/bhnrc/ndl.)

regular consumption of fruits and vegetables that contain beta-carotene or with vitamin A supplementation.

Other deficiency symptoms include impaired immunity, increased risk of illness and infections, reproductive system disorders, and stunted bone growth. According to the World Health Organization, as many as 250,000 to 500,000 vitamin A–deficient children become blind each year, with half of them dying within 1 year of losing their sight.[2]

Vitamin D Guards Our Bones

Vitamin D is different from other nutrients in that it does not always need to come from the diet. This is because our bodies can synthesize vitamin D using energy from sunlight: when the ultraviolet rays of the sun hit our skin, they react with a cholesterol compound in skin cells. This reaction converts the compound into a precursor of vitamin D, which travels to the liver and then to the kidneys for further conversion into the form of vitamin D our bodies can use.

Vitamin D can be considered not only a nutrient, but also a *hormone* because it is made in one part of the body, yet regulates various activities in other parts of the body. One of its most important functions is to work with other hormones to regulate blood calcium levels. You probably know that calcium is the primary mineral in our bones. According to our body's changing needs for calcium, vitamin D causes more or less calcium to be absorbed from the small intestine and signals the kidneys to excrete more or less in our urine. Vitamin D also assists the process by which calcium is crystallized into bone tissue and assists in cell differentiation.

Table 6.1 identifies the AI for vitamin D. On food and supplement labels, you may see the amount of vitamin D expressed in IU. For conversion purposes, 1 μg of vitamin D is equal to 40 IU of vitamin D, so 5 μg per day = 200 IU.

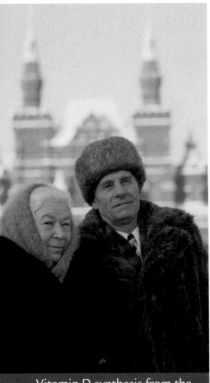

Vitamin D synthesis from the sun is not possible during most of the winter months for people living in high latitudes. Therefore, many people around the world, such as this couple in Russia, need to consume vitamin D in their diets, particularly during the winter.

The AI is based on the assumption that an individual does not get adequate sun exposure. If your exposure to the sun is adequate, then you do not need to consume any vitamin D in your diet. But how do you know whether or not you are getting enough sunshine? Of the many factors that affect our ability to synthesize vitamin D from sunlight, latitude and time of year are most significant. Individuals living in very sunny climates close to the equator, such as the southern United States and Mexico, may synthesize enough vitamin D from the sun to meet their needs throughout the year—as long as they spend a few minutes out of doors each day with at least their arms and face exposed. However, vitamin D synthesis from the sun is not possible in the winter months in Canada and the northern United States, from northern Pennsylvania in the East to northern California in the West. This is because, at northern latitudes during the winter, the sun never rises high enough in the sky to provide the direct sunlight needed. Thus, people living in northern U.S. states and Canada need to consume vitamin D in the winter.

In addition, vitamin D synthesis is decreased in older adults and in people with darkly pigmented skin.[3] These individuals are at increased risk for vitamin D deficiency. Recently a great deal of controversy has been generated regarding the current AI for vitamin D, with a growing number of nutrition experts calling for substantially higher AI values due to the relatively poor vitamin D status of many people of all ages and skin tones around the world.[4-6]

Most foods naturally contain very little vitamin D. Thus, our primary source of vitamin D in the diet is from fortified foods such as milk. As identified in FIGURE 6.4, other common food sources of vitamin D include cod liver oil, fatty fish such as salmon, mackerel, and sardines, and certain fortified cereals. Because plants contain very little vitamin D, vegetarians who consume no dairy products need to obtain their vitamin D from sun exposure, from fortified soy or cereal products, or from supplements.

We cannot get too much vitamin D from sun exposure, as our skin has the ability to limit its production. The only way we can consume too much vitamin D is through supplementation. Toxicity of vitamin D causes the bones to leach calcium into the bloodstream. High blood calcium concentrations cause weakness, loss of appetite, diarrhea, mental confusion, vomiting, and the formation of calcium deposits in soft tissues such as the kidney, liver, and heart.

The primary deficiency associated with inadequate vitamin D is loss of bone mass. Calcium is a key component of bones, but when vitamin D levels are inade-

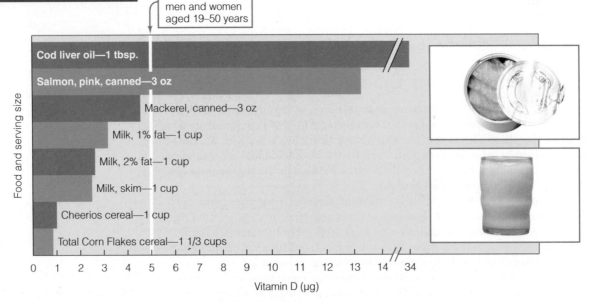

FIGURE 6.4 Common food sources of vitamin D. The AI for vitamin D ranges from 5 to 15 μg/day in adults. (Data from U.S. Department of Agriculture, Agricultural Research Service. 2007. USDA Nutrient Database for Standard Reference, Release 20. Nutrient Data Laboratory Home Page, www.ars.usda.gov/ba/bhnrc/ndl.)

quate, our intestines can only absorb 10% to 15% of the calcium we consume. Vitamin D deficiency disease in children, called **rickets,** causes deformities of the skeleton such as bowed legs and knocked knees (FIGURE 6.5). Rickets was rampant as late as the early 20th century in northern cities of the United States and Europe. In 1921, rickets was considered the most common nutritional disease of children, affecting approximately 75% of infants in New York City.[7] A common folk remedy for rickets, cod liver oil, was widely known to be effective, but it was not until the discovery of vitamin D in the 1930s that the antirickets property of cod liver oil became understood.[8] Rickets still occurs in the United States and throughout the world, especially among dark-skinned toddlers living at northern latitudes who are not fed fatty fish, foods fortified with vitamin D, or supplements.[8] Vitamin D deficiency is also still common among fair-skinned Americans: a recent study found that almost half of white girls aged 9 to 11 years in Maine were deficient in vitamin D at the end of winter, with 17% remaining vitamin D deficient even at the end of summer because they either stayed out of the sun or used sunscreen to protect their skin.[9]

Vitamin D deficiency disease in adults is called **osteomalacia,** a term meaning "soft bones." With osteomalacia, bones become weak and prone to fractures, and the person typically experiences diffuse bone pain. Today, osteomalacia occurs most often in individuals who have diseases that cause intestinal malabsorption of fat, and thus of the fat-soluble vitamins.

Vitamin D deficiency can also contribute to *osteoporosis*, a condition in which the bones are overly porous and prone to fractures (see Chapter 7). Although the symptoms of osteomalacia and osteoporosis are similar, the symptoms of osteomalacia are reversed after treatment with vitamin D, whereas many factors are typically involved in the development and treatment of osteoporosis. Recent evidence suggests that vitamin D deficiency is also associated with an increased risk for some cancers, type 1 diabetes, various forms of arthritis, multiple sclerosis, and infectious diseases such as tuberculosis.[5]

Now that you've read about the "sunshine vitamin," you might be wondering whether or not you should supplement this nutrient, especially if you live in a northern climate. If so, check out the accompanying What About You?: Do You Get Enough Vitamin D?

Vitamin K Protects against Blood Loss

Vitamin K is a fat-soluble vitamin required for blood clotting. It acts as a **coenzyme;** that is, a compound that combines with an inactive enzyme to form an active enzyme. FIGURE 6.6 illustrates how coenzymes work. As a coenzyme, vitamin K assists in the synthesis of a number of proteins involved in the coagulation of blood. Without adequate vitamin K, our blood cannot clot quickly and adequately. This can lead to

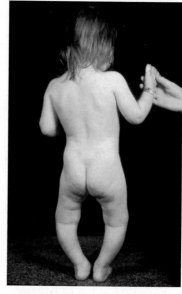

FIGURE 6.5 Vitamin D deficiency in children causes a bone-deforming disease called *rickets.*

rickets Vitamin D–deficiency disease in children. Symptoms include deformities of the skeleton such as bowed legs and knocked knees.

osteomalacia Vitamin D–deficiency disease in adults, in which bones become weak and prone to fractures.

coenzyme A compound that combines with an inactive enzyme to form an active enzyme.

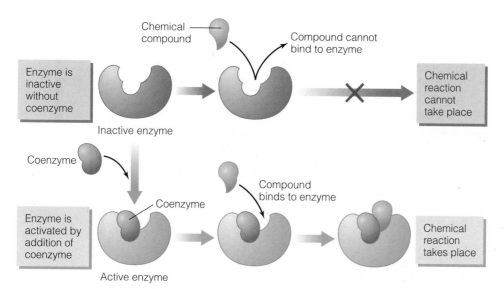

FIGURE 6.6 Coenzymes combine with enzymes to activate them, ensuring that the chemical reactions that depend on these enzymes can occur.

WHAT ABOUT YOU?

Do You Get Enough Vitamin D?

After reading this chapter, you may wonder whether you're getting enough vitamin D to keep your tissues healthy and strong. Take the following simple quiz to find out. For each question, circle Yes or No:

- I live south of 40° latitude (see Figure 6.7 below) and expose my bare arms and face to sunlight (without sunscreen) for at least a few minutes 2 to 3 days per week all year.
  YES or **NO**

- I consume a multivitamin supplement or vitamin D supplement that provides at least 5 μg or 200 IU per day.
  YES or **NO**

- I consume a diet high in fatty fish, fortified milk, and/or fortified cereals that provides at least 5 μg or 200 IU per day.
  YES or **NO**

If you answered **No** to all three of these questions, you are at high risk for vitamin D deficiency. You are probably getting enough vitamin D if you answered **Yes** to at least one of the above questions. Notice, though, that if you rely on sun exposure for your vitamin D, you must make sure that you expose your bare skin to sunlight for an adequate length of time. What's adequate varies for each person: the darker your skin tone, the more time you need in the sun. A general guideline is to expose your skin for a period of time that is one-third the amount of time in which you would get sunburned. This means that if you normally sunburn in 1 hour, you should get 20 minutes of sun two to three times a week. Expose your skin when the sun is high in the sky (generally between the hours of 9 AM and 3 PM). Put on sunscreen only *after* your skin has had its daily dose of sunlight.[3–6]

Remember: If you live in the northern United States or Canada, you cannot get adequate sun exposure to synthesize vitamin D from approximately October through February, no matter how long you might expose your bare skin to the sun. So, if you are not regularly consuming fortified foods, fatty fish, or cod liver oil, you need to supplement vitamin D during those months.

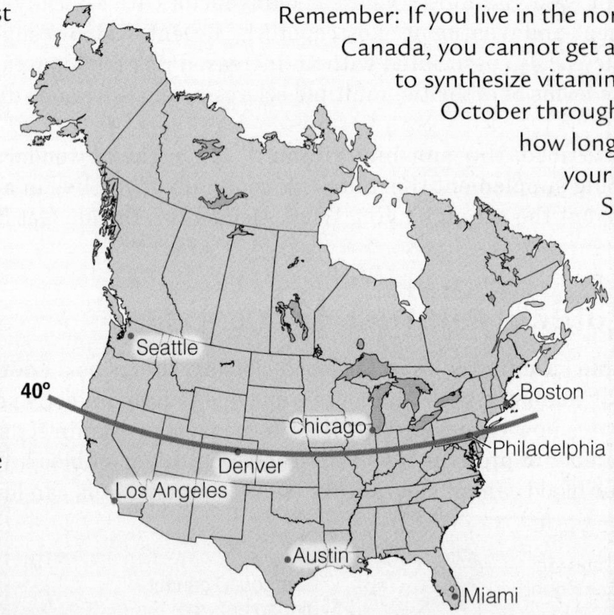

FIGURE 6.7 This map illustrates the geographical location of 40° latitude in the United States. In southern cities below 40° latitude, such as Los Angeles, CA, Austin, TX, and Miami, FL, the sunlight is strong enough to allow for vitamin D synthesis throughout the year. In northern cities above 40° latitude, such as Seattle, WA, Chicago, IL, and Boston, MA, the sunlight is too weak from about mid-October through mid-March to allow for adequate vitamin D synthesis.

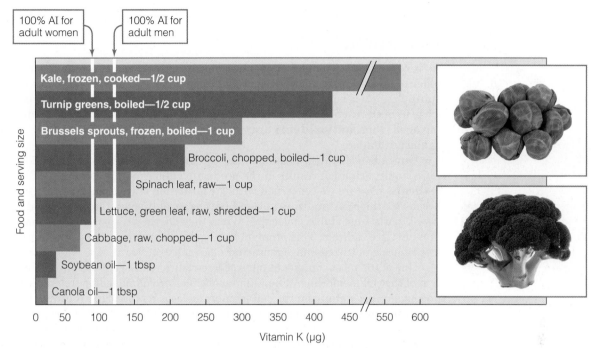

FIGURE 6.8 caption chart labels:

100% AI for adult women
100% AI for adult men

Food and serving size

- Kale, frozen, cooked—1/2 cup
- Turnip greens, boiled—1/2 cup
- Brussels sprouts, frozen, boiled—1 cup
- Broccoli, chopped, boiled—1 cup
- Spinach leaf, raw—1 cup
- Lettuce, green leaf, raw, shredded—1 cup
- Cabbage, raw, chopped—1 cup
- Soybean oil—1 tbsp
- Canola oil—1 tbsp

0   50   100   150   200   250   300   350   400   450   550   600

Vitamin K (µg)

FIGURE 6.8 Common food sources of vitamin K. The AI for vitamin K ranges from 90 µg/day for women to 120 µg/day for men.
(Data from U.S. Department of Agriculture, Agricultural Research Service. 2007. USDA Nutrient Database for Standard Reference, Release 20. Nutrient Data Laboratory Home Page, www.ars.usda.gov/ba/bhnrc/ndl.)

increased bleeding from even minor wounds, as well as internal hemorrhaging. Vitamin K also acts as a coenzyme to facilitate the production of osteocalcin, a protein associated with bone turnover.

Our needs for vitamin K are relatively small, as shown in Table 6.1, but vitamin K is found in few foods. Healthful intestinal bacteria produce vitamin K in the large intestine, providing us with an important nondietary source of vitamin K.

Green leafy vegetables are good sources of vitamin K, including collard greens, spinach, broccoli, Brussels sprouts, and cabbage (FIGURE 6.8). Soybean and canola oils are also good sources.

There are no known side effects associated with consuming large amounts of vitamin K from supplements or from food.[10] People with diseases that cause malabsorption of fat can suffer secondarily from a deficiency of vitamin K. In the United States, physicians typically give newborns an injection of vitamin K at birth, as they lack the intestinal bacteria necessary to produce this nutrient.

RECAP *Vitamin A and its precursor, beta-carotene, are essential for healthy vision, cell differentiation, bone growth, and immune and reproductive function. Single-nutrient supplementation with vitamin A can lead to life-threatening toxicity. Vitamin D regulates blood calcium levels and maintains bone health. Unless we have adequate sun exposure, we need to consume vitamin D in foods or supplements. Vitamin K is essential for blood clotting.*

The Mighty Antioxidants: Vitamins E and C

Fitness and health magazines, supplement companies, and even food manufacturers tout the benefits of antioxidants. But what exactly does this term mean, and why are antioxidant micronutrients important to our health?

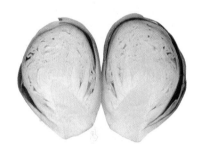

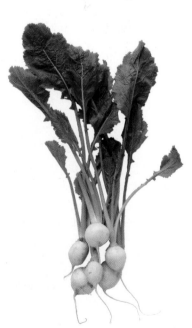

Green leafy vegetables, including Brussels sprouts and turnip greens, are good sources of vitamin K.

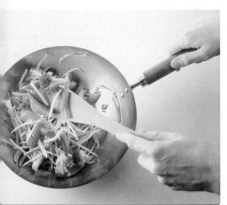

Antioxidant vitamins, found in many fresh vegetables, stabilize free radicals.

What Are Antioxidants, and How Do Our Bodies Use Them?

As we discussed in Chapter 2, chemical reactions occur continuously in our bodies in order to break down the food we eat and reassemble its smaller molecules into the substances we need to live. Many of these chemical reactions involve the exchange of oxygen. Such reactions are collectively referred to as *oxidation.* "Anti" means "against"; thus, **antioxidants** are vitamins and minerals that protect our cells against oxidation.

Our cells need the protection of antioxidants because, although necessary to our functioning, oxidation results in the production of harmful by-products called **free radicals.** Why are we concerned with the formation of free radicals? Simply put, it is because of their destabilizing power. Like chemical thieves, free radicals attempt to "steal" parts from stable molecules. When they do, they transform those molecules into new free radicals. This prompts a dangerous chain reaction as the generated free radicals in turn damage more and more cells.

One of the most significant sites of free-radical damage is within the lipid portion of the cell membrane. When lipid molecules are damaged by free radicals, they no longer repel water, and the cell membrane loses its integrity. It can no longer regulate the movement of fluids and nutrients into and out of the cell. Free radicals also damage our low-density lipoproteins (LDLs), cell proteins, and DNA. Not surprisingly, oxidation is one of the factors thought to cause our bodies to age. In addition, many diseases are linked to free-radical production, including cancer, heart disease, stroke, diabetes, and others.

Antioxidant vitamins, especially vitamins E and C, work by stabilizing free radicals, thereby halting the chain reaction of cell-membrane injury. When our intake of these vitamins is not sufficient, free-radical damage can be significant. Note that the carotenoids discussed earlier, as well as the mineral selenium, also play roles in antioxidant functioning. In addition, many herbs have a long history of use and of claimed benefits in combating aging and the diseases associated with oxidation, such as hypertension, diabetes, and even cancer. Do herbal supplements promote health and longevity? Are they safe? And exactly what qualifies as an herbal supplement? These questions are explored in the accompanying Highlight: Herbal Supplements: Use with Caution.

Vitamin E Maintains Healthy Cells

About 90% of the vitamin E in our bodies is stored in our adipose (fat) tissues; the rest is found in our cell membranes. In these locations, it protects fatty components of our cells from oxidation. It also protects LDLs, red blood cells, and the cells of our lungs, which are continuously exposed to oxygen from the air we breathe.

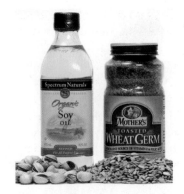

Vegetable oils, nuts, and seeds are good sources of vitamin E.

antioxidant A compound that has the ability to prevent or repair the damage caused by oxidation.

free radical A highly unstable atom with an unpaired electron in its outermost shell.

How Else Do We Use Vitamin E?

In addition to its role as an antioxidant, vitamin E serves other roles essential to human health. It is critical for normal fetal and early-childhood development of nerves and muscles and for neuromuscular function throughout life. It protects white blood cells and other components of the immune system, thereby helping to defend our bodies against infection and disease. Vitamin E also improves the absorption of vitamin A if dietary intake of vitamin A is low.

How Much Vitamin E Should We Consume?

Considering the importance of vitamin E to our health, you might think that you need to consume a huge amount daily. In fact, as you can see in Table 6.1, the RDA for vitamin E for men and women is modest.

HIGHLIGHT

Herbal Supplements: Use with Caution

A common saying in India cautions that "A house without ginger is a sick house." Indeed, ginger, garlic, echinacea, and many other herbs have been used by different cultures throughout the world for centuries to promote health and ward off disease. It is clear that some herbs are effective medicines, but for what disorders, in what forms, and at what dosages? It is equally clear that some herbs promoted as medicines are not effective and that still others are not safe. Here, we discuss the benefits and potential threats of a few of the most commonly used herbs and provide tips for evaluating the effectiveness and safety of any herb you might consider using.

The National Center for Complementary and Alternative Medicine (NCCAM) defines an *herb* (also called a *botanical*) as a plant or plant part used for its scent, flavor, and/or therapeutic properties.[11] In its consumer fact sheet on herbal supplements, NCCAM provides the following points you should consider for your safety before you use herbs:

1. Just because an herbal supplement is labeled "natural" does not mean it is safe or without any harmful effects. Several herbs are known to cause serious health problems.

2. Herbal supplements can act the same way as drugs. Therefore, they can cause medical problems if not used correctly or if taken in large amounts. In some cases, people have experienced negative effects even though they followed the instructions on a supplement label.

3. Women who are pregnant or nursing should be especially cautious about using herbal supplements. This caution also applies to treating children with herbal supplements.

4. It is important to consult your healthcare provider before using an herbal supplement, especially if you are taking any medications. Some herbal supplements are known to interact with medications in ways that cause health problems.

5. If you use herbal supplements, it is best to do so under the guidance of a healthcare professional who has been trained in herbal medicines.

6. In the United States, herbal supplements are regulated by the U.S. Food and Drug Administration (FDA) as foods. This means that they do not have to meet the same standards as drugs for proof of safety, effectiveness, and what the FDA calls Good Manufacturing Practices.

7. The active ingredients in many herbs and herbal supplements are not known. There may be dozens, even hundreds, of unknown compounds in an herbal supplement.

8. Published analyses of herbal supplements have found differences between what's listed on the label and what's in the bottle. This means you may be taking less—or more—of the supplement than what the label indicates. Also, the words *standardized, certified,* or *verified* on a product label are no guarantee of product quality, as in the United States these terms have no legal definition for supplements.

9. Some herbal supplements have been found to be contaminated with metals, unlabeled prescription drugs, microorganisms, or other substances.

10. The federal government has taken legal action against a number of companies that sell and promote herbal supplements on the Internet because they have been shown to contain incorrect or deceptive statements. It is important to evaluate the claims made for supplements prior to using them.[12]

The following herbs are only a few of those promoted to prevent or treat disease. The list is far from exhaustive: The National Institutes of Health estimates that there are currently more than 1,500 herbal products stocked in American stores.[13]

● **Echinacea.** Commonly called "purple coneflower," echinacea has traditionally been recommended for everything from colds to cancer. *Cautions:* Echinacea is not known to have any serious adverse effects, although there have been reports of skin rash and insomnia among some users.[13]

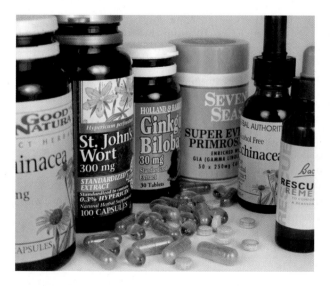

(continued)

Herbal Supplements: Use with Caution *(continued)*

- **Garlic.** Used for centuries worldwide as an antimicrobial, garlic also reduces blood cholesterol and helps prevent heart disease. *Cautions:* Excessive consumption of garlic capsules can cause gastrointestinal discomfort.

- **Ginger.** Ginger is a tropical plant, the underground stem of which (commonly referred to as the root) is used for cooking and medicinal purposes. It is most commonly used to prevent or treat nausea, stomach aches, colds, and flu. Few side effects are reported with ginger when used in small doses. *Cautions*: Gas, bloating, heartburn, and nausea have been reported with powdered ginger.[14]

- **Goldenseal.** The root of the goldenseal plant is traditionally used to treat wounds, ulcers, digestive problems, and infections. One of its active components has antimicrobial properties and may be effective in preventing the growth of cancer cells. *Cautions:* A component of goldenseal has been shown to induce labor in pregnant women. Chronic use may inhibit B-vitamin absorption. Also, goldenseal can cause convulsions, paralysis, respiratory failure, and even death at very high doses.[13]

- **Grape seed extract.** This compound, which is obtained from the extracted, dried seeds of grapes, is promoted as an antioxidant. *Cautions:* Note that the astringent flavor of grape seed extract makes it highly unlikely that it will be

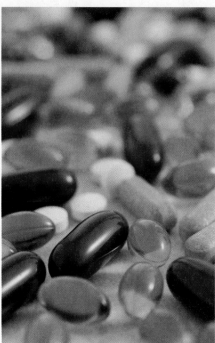

taken in excessive amounts, and the U.S. Food and Drug Administration designates it as safe.[15]

- **Hawthorn.** Medicinal extracts of the leaves and flowers of this shrub have been used for many years for the treatment of hypertension and other heart and circulatory problems. *Cautions:* No significant adverse side effects have been noted when used in clinically recommended dosages; however, hawthorn interacts with several prescription drugs and should only be used in consultation with your healthcare provider.

- **Psyllium.** A common ingredient in over-the-counter laxatives, this seed softens and lubricates stools and may reduce the risk of colon cancer. *Cautions:* Gastrointestinal discomfort may occur if consumed in excessive amounts.

If you are considering trying an herbal supplement for medicinal purposes, the following organizations provide reliable information. For Web addresses, see the Web Links at the end of this chapter:

- Centers for Disease Control and Prevention (CDC)
- U.S. Food and Drug Administration (FDA)
- National Center for Complementary and Alternative Medicine (NCCAM)
- Office of Dietary Supplements (ODS)

Vitamin E is widespread in foods (FIGURE 6.9). Much of the vitamin E that we consume comes from vegetable oils and the products made from them. Safflower oil, sunflower oil, canola oil, and soybean oil are good sources. Nuts, seeds, some vegetables, wheat germ, and soybeans also contribute vitamin E to our diet. Cereals are often fortified with vitamin E, and other grain products contribute modest amounts. Animal and dairy products are poor sources of vitamin E.

Vitamin E is destroyed by exposure to oxygen, metals, ultraviolet light, and heat. Although vegetable oils contain vitamin E, heating these oils destroys vitamin E. Thus, foods that are deep-fried and processed contain little vitamin E. This includes most fast foods and convenience foods.

Vitamin E toxicities and deficiencies are uncommon. One result of significant vitamin E deficiency is a rupturing of red blood cells that leads to *anemia,* a condition in which our red blood cells cannot carry and transport enough oxygen to our tissues. Anemia in turn causes fatigue, weakness, and a diminished ability to perform physical and mental work. Other symptoms of vitamin E deficiency include loss of muscle coordination and reflexes, impaired vision and speech, and reduced immune function.

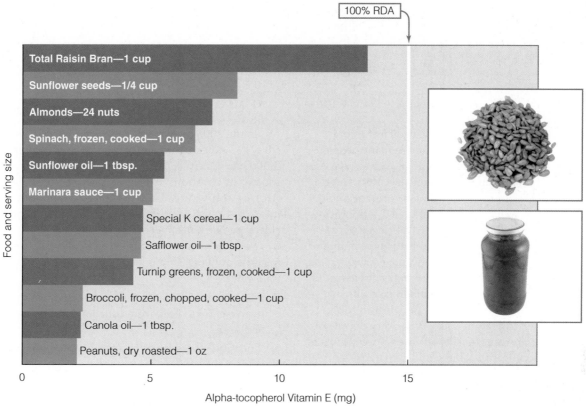

100% RDA

Alpha-tocopherol Vitamin E (mg)

Food and serving size:
- Total Raisin Bran—1 cup
- Sunflower seeds—1/4 cup
- Almonds—24 nuts
- Spinach, frozen, cooked—1 cup
- Sunflower oil—1 tbsp.
- Marinara sauce—1 cup
- Special K cereal—1 cup
- Safflower oil—1 tbsp.
- Turnip greens, frozen, cooked—1 cup
- Broccoli, frozen, chopped, cooked—1 cup
- Canola oil—1 tbsp.
- Peanuts, dry roasted—1 oz

FIGURE 6.9 Common food sources of vitamin E. The RDA for vitamin E is 15 mg per day.
(Data from U.S. Department of Agriculture, Agricultural Research Service. 2007. USDA Nutrient Database for Standard Reference, Release 20. Nutrient Data Laboratory Home Page, www.ars.usda.gov/ba/bhnrc/ndl.)

Vitamin C Protect Cells and Tissues

Vitamin C is also known as *ascorbic acid.* Like vitamin E, vitamin C is a potent antioxidant, but because it is water soluble, it primarily acts within the fluid outside of cells. There, it binds with free radicals, keeping them from destroying cell membranes. It plays a key role in defending our lung tissues from the damage caused by ozone, cigarette smoke, and other airborne pollutants. Indeed, smoking increases a person's need for vitamin C to combat oxidative damage to the lungs. In the stomach, vitamin C reduces the formation of *nitrosamines,* cancer-causing agents found in foods such as cured and processed meats. Vitamin C also regenerates vitamin E after it has been oxidized, enabling vitamin E to "get back to work."

How Else Do We Use Vitamin C?

Another important role of vitamin C is to synthesize **collagen,** a component of bone, teeth, skin, tendons, and blood vessels. Without adequate vitamin C, the body cannot form collagen; thus, bones become brittle, blood vessels leak, wounds fail to heal, and teeth fall out. These symptoms characterize the disease called *scurvy,* which centuries ago was responsible for more than half of the deaths that occurred at sea. During long sea voyages, the crew ate all of the fruits and vegetables early in the trip. These foods are high in vitamin C. Later in the voyage, only grain and animal products were available. These foods do not provide vitamin C. In 1740 in England, Dr. James Lind discovered that consumption of citrus fruits could prevent scurvy. Thus, British sailors were given rations of lime juice, earning them the nickname "limeys."

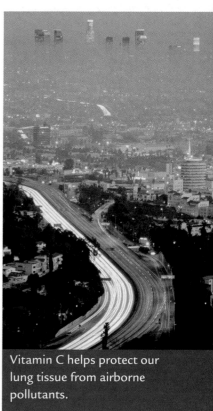

Vitamin C helps protect our lung tissue from airborne pollutants.

collagen   A protein found in all connective tissues in our bodies.

NUTRITION MYTH OR FACT?

Can Vitamin C Prevent the Common Cold?

What do you do when you feel a cold coming on? If you are like many people, you drink a lot of orange juice or take vitamin C supplements to ward it off. But do these approaches really help prevent a cold?

It is well known that vitamin C is important for a healthy immune system. Deficiency of vitamin C can seriously weaken the ability of immune cells to detect and destroy invading microbes, increasing our susceptibility to many diseases and illnesses, including the common cold. It's not surprising, then, that many people turn to vitamin C supplements to prevent colds. When they do, they find their local drug store stocking at least a dozen forms of vitamin C, from lozenges to tablets, and even packets of powder to mix with water into a cold-fighting cocktail. But do these products work?

Unfortunately, it appears they do not. Several large-scale, controlled studies involving children and adults have yielded no conclusive data that large doses of vitamin C prevent colds.[16] Two analyses of the dozens of existing studies of vitamin C and the common cold found that people taking vitamin C experienced as many colds as people who took a placebo.[17,18] The amount of vitamin C taken in these studies was quite high, up to 2,000 mg per day (more than twenty times the RDA).

In the 2005 review, researchers noted that a single study did indicate that a very large dose of vitamin C— 8,000 mg—taken on the first day of a cold appeared to shorten its duration.[17] However, the tolerable upper limit (UL) for vitamin C is 2,000 mg. Excessive amounts of vitamin C can cause severe diarrhea, a particular danger for elderly people and small children.[16]

So what *can* you do to prevent a cold? The National Institute of Allergy and Infectious Diseases suggests the following:[16]

- Because most cold germs enter the body via the eyes or the nose, try to keep from touching or rubbing your eyes and nose.
- If possible, avoid being close to people who have colds.
- Wash your hands frequently with soap and warm (not hot) water throughout cold season and whenever you have had contact with many people (e.g., throughout the work or school day, when returning home from shopping, etc.). Hand-washing is one of the single most effective ways to keep from getting colds or giving them to others. When water isn't available, use an alcohol-based waterless hand cleanser.
- Cold viruses can live for up to 3 hours on your skin or on objects such as telephones, desks, and so forth. Clean environmental surfaces with a virus-killing disinfectant when feasible.

Consuming a healthful diet that includes fruits and vegetables rich in vitamin C will help you maintain a strong immune system, but vitamin C supplements do not appear to confer cold-fighting superpowers in well-nourished people. So the next time you feel yourself getting a cold, you may want to think twice before spending money on extra vitamin C.

Vitamin C assists in the synthesis of other important compounds as well, including DNA, neurotransmitters (chemicals that transmit messages via the nervous system), and various hormones. Vitamin C also enhances our immune response and thus protects us from illness and infection. Indeed, you might have heard that vitamin C supplements can prevent the common cold. See the Nutrition Myth or Fact? box above to find out if this claim is true.

Finally, vitamin C enhances the absorption of iron. It is recommended that people with low iron stores consume vitamin C–rich foods along with iron sources to improve absorption. For people with high iron stores, this practice can lead to iron toxicity.

How Much Vitamin C Should We Consume?

The RDA for vitamin C is listed in Table 6.2. Citrus fruits (such as oranges, lemons, and limes), potatoes, strawberries, tomatoes, kiwi fruit, broccoli, spinach and other leafy greens, cabbage, green and red peppers, and cauliflower are excellent sources (FIGURE 6.10). Because heat and oxygen destroy vitamin C, fresh sources of these foods have the highest content. Cooking foods, especially boiling, leaches them of their vitamin C, which is then lost when we strain them. Forms of cooking that are least likely to compromise the vitamin C content of foods include steaming, microwaving, and stir-frying.

Because vitamin C is water soluble, excess amounts are easily excreted and do not lead to toxicity. Even taking megadoses of vitamin C is not fatally harmful. However, side effects of doses exceeding 2,000 mg per day include nausea, diarrhea, nosebleeds, abdominal cramps, and may increase the risk of kidney stones in some people.[19]

RECAP *Vitamin E protects the fatty portion of our cell membranes from oxidation, enhances immune function, and improves our absorption of vitamin A if dietary intake is low. Vitamin C scavenges free radicals and regenerates vitamin E after it has been oxidized. It is required for the synthesis of collagen and assists in the synthesis of certain hormones, neurotransmitters, and DNA. Vitamin C boosts the absorption of iron.*

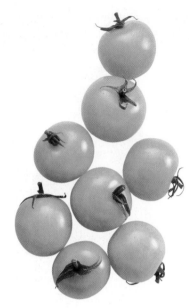

Many fruits, like these yellow tomatoes, are high in vitamin C.

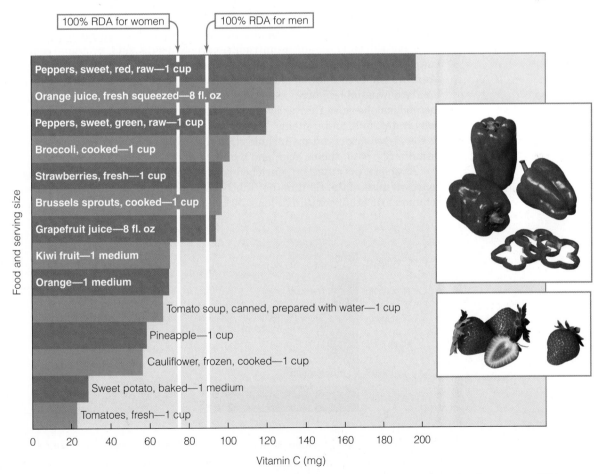

FIGURE 6.10 Common food sources of vitamin C. The RDA for vitamin C is 90 mg per day for men and 75 mg per day for women.
(Data from U.S. Department of Agriculture, Agricultural Research Service. 2007. USDA Nutrient Database for Standard Reference, Release 20. Nutrient Data Laboratory Home Page, www.ars.usda.gov/ba/bhnrc/ndl.)

NUTRI-CASE HANNAH

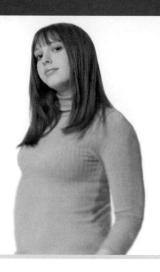

"Since I started college in September, I've had one cold after another. I guess it's being around so many different people every day, plus all the stress. Then a few weeks ago I found this cool orange-tasting vitamin C powder at the health food outlet on campus, and I started mixing it into my orange juice every morning. I guess it's working, because I haven't had a cold since I started using it, but this morning I woke up with stomach cramps and diarrhea, so now I guess I have to worry about a stomach flu. I wish there was a vitamin C powder for that!"

Given what you've learned about the effects of vitamin C supplementation, do you think it is possible that Hannah's vitamin C regimen is doing her more harm than good? Explain.

The Energy Generators: B-Complex Vitamins

Contrary to popular belief, vitamins and minerals do not contain energy (kilocalories). Only the macronutrients (carbohydrates, fats, proteins) contain energy. However, vitamins and minerals do assist the body in *generating* energy. **Metabolism** is the sum of all the chemical and physical processes by which the body breaks down and builds up molecules. The B vitamins play a critical role in energy metabolism, because they assist the chemical reactions that release energy from carbohydrates, fats, and proteins. This group of water-soluble vitamins, also referred to as the *B-complex vitamins,* includes thiamin, riboflavin, vitamin B_6, niacin, folate, vitamin B_{12}, pantothenic acid, and biotin.

As shown in **FIGURE 6.11**, enriched ready-to-eat cereals are a consistently good source of most of the B vitamins. Table 6.2 on page 160 identifies some other common foods that contain at least 50% of the DRI for select B vitamins.

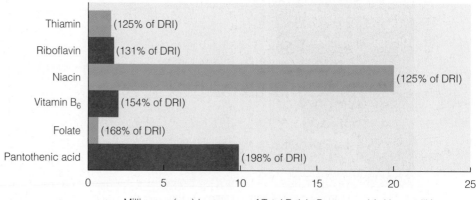

metabolism The sum of all the chemical and physical processes by which the body breaks down and builds up molecules.

FIGURE 6.11   Many enriched ready-to-eat cereals, like the one in this example, are a consistently good source of B-complex vitamins.
(Data from U.S. Department of Agriculture, Agricultural Research Service. 2007. USDA Nutrient Database for Standard Reference, Release 20. Nutrient Data Laboratory Home Page, www.ars.usda.gov/ba/bhnrc/ndl.)

How Do Our Bodies Use B-Vitamins to Produce Energy?

B vitamins help us access the energy in the food we eat by acting as coenzymes. Recall that a coenzyme is a molecule that combines with an enzyme to activate it and help it do its job (see Figure 6.7). Without the B vitamins working as coenzymes, we would be unable to produce the energy necessary to keep us alive.

For instance, thiamin combines with another enzyme to assist in the breakdown of glucose. Riboflavin is a part of two coenzymes that help break down glucose and fatty acids. The specific functions of each B vitamin are described in detail next. Their DRIs are identified in Table 6.2 on page 160.

In addition to the B vitamins and a vitamin-like substance called choline, the minerals iodine, chromium, manganese, copper, and sulfur are also involved in energy metabolism. Minerals are discussed in Chapter 7.

Thiamin (Vitamin B_1) Helps Metabolize Glucose

Thiamin was the first B vitamin discovered, hence its designation as vitamin B_1. Thiamin is part of a coenzyme that plays a critical role in the breakdown of glucose for energy. It also acts as a coenzyme in the metabolism of a few amino acids. Thiamin is also used in producing DNA and plays a role in the synthesis of neurotransmitters.

Good food sources of thiamin include enriched cereals and grains, whole-grain products, ready-to-eat cereals, and ham and other pork products (FIGURE 6.12). There are no known adverse effects from consuming excess amounts of thiamin.

Thiamin-deficiency disease is called **beriberi.** In this disease, the body's inability to metabolize energy leads to muscle wasting and nerve damage; in

beriberi A disease caused by thiamin deficiency.

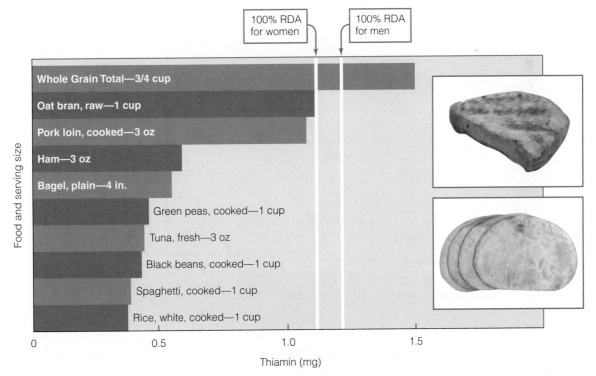

FIGURE 6.12 Common food sources of thiamin. The RDA for thiamin is 1.2 mg/d for men and 1.1 mg/d for women 19 years and older.

(Data from U.S. Department of Agriculture, Agricultural Research Service. 2007. USDA Nutrient Database for Standard Reference, Release 20. Nutrient Data Laboratory Home Page, www.ars.usda.gov/ba/bhnrc/ndl.)

later stages, patients may be unable to move at all. The heart muscle may also be affected, and the patient may die of heart failure. Beriberi is seen in countries in which unenriched, processed grains are a primary food source; for instance, beriberi was widespread in China when rice was processed and refined. Beriberi is also seen in people with heavy alcohol consumption and limited food intake.

Riboflavin (Vitamin B₂) Helps Break Down Carbohydrates and Fats

Riboflavin is an important component of coenzymes that break down carbohydrates and fats. It is also a part of an antioxidant enzyme that helps our cells defend against oxidative damage.

Flavins are yellow pigments, and, indeed, riboflavin is found in egg yolks. Milk is another good source of riboflavin. Because riboflavin is destroyed when it is exposed to light, milk is stored in opaque containers. Other good food sources of riboflavin include yogurt, enriched bread and grain products, ready-to-eat cereals, and organ meats (FIGURE 6.13).

There are no known adverse effects from consuming excess amounts of riboflavin. Riboflavin deficiency is referred to as **ariboflavinosis.** Symptoms of ariboflavinosis include sore throat, swelling of the mucous membranes in the mouth and throat, lips that are dry and scaly, a purple-colored tongue, and inflamed, irritated patches on the skin. Severe riboflavin deficiency can impair the metabolism of vitamin B₆.

ariboflavinosis   A condition caused by riboflavin deficiency.

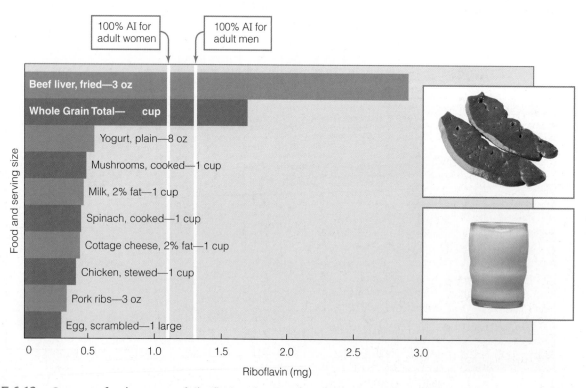

FIGURE 6.13   Common food sources of riboflavin. The RDA for riboflavin is 1.3 mg/d for men and 1.1 mg/d for women 19 years and older.

(Data from U.S. Department of Agriculture, Agricultural Research Service. 2007. USDA Nutrient Database for Standard Reference, Release 20. Nutrient Data Laboratory Home Page, www.ars.usda.gov/ba/bhnrc/ndl.)

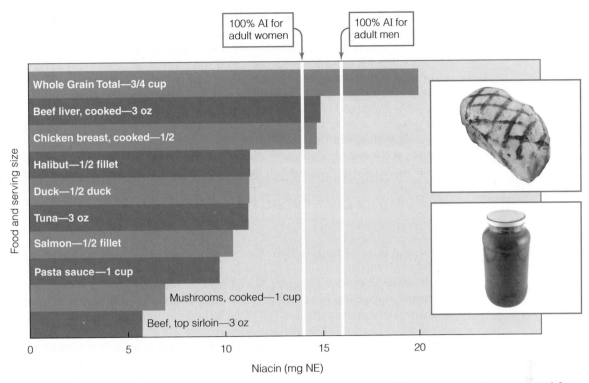

FIGURE 6.14 Common food sources of niacin. The RDA for niacin is 16 mg NE/d for men and 14 mg NE/d for women 19 years and older.
(Data from U.S. Department of Agriculture, Agricultural Research Service. 2007. USDA Nutrient Database for Standard Reference, Release 20. Nutrient Data Laboratory Home Page, www.ars.usda.gov/ba/bhnrc/ndl.)

Niacin Helps Produce Energy and Build and Repair DNA

As a coenzyme, niacin assists in the metabolism of carbohydrates and fatty acids and thus is essential in helping our bodies derive the energy from these foods. Niacin also plays an important role in DNA replication and repair and in the process of cell differentiation. Good food sources include meat, fish, poultry, enriched grain products, and tomato paste (FIGURE 6.14).

pellagra A disease that results from severe niacin deficiency.

Megadoses of niacin have been shown to reduce LDL-cholesterol and raise HDL-cholesterol; therefore, some physicians prescribe a pharmacologic form of niacin for patients with unhealthful blood lipid levels. It is typically prescribed in a time-release preparation to prevent an uncomfortable side effect called *flushing,* which is defined as burning, tingling, and itching sensations accompanied by a reddened flush primarily on the face, arms, and chest. Unfortunately, some prescription forms of niacin can cause liver damage. Niacin toxicity can also cause glucose intolerance, blurred vision, and edema of the eyes.

Pellagra results from severe niacin deficiency. It is characterized by a skin rash, diarrhea, mental impairment, and in severe cases, death (FIGURE 6.15). Pellagra commonly occurred in the southern United States and parts of Europe in the early 20th century but was thought to be caused by infection. In 1914, a physician named

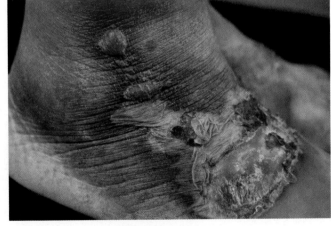

FIGURE 6.15 Pellagra is often characterized by a scaly skin rash.

Dr. Joseph Goldberger began studying the disease. He noticed that it struck only impoverished people who ate a limited, corn-based diet. Goldberger began conducting experiments to test his theory that pellagra was caused by a nutrient deficiency and eventually hit upon brewer's yeast as a cure. Although Goldberger lived until 1937, he died without knowing why brewer's yeast worked. Shortly after Goldberger's death, scientists finally identified niacin and discovered its importance to human health. They quickly determined that corn is low in niacin as well as the amino acid tryptophan, a precursor for niacin, and that brewer's yeast is rich in niacin.

At the present time, pellagra is rarely seen in industrialized countries, except in cases of chronic alcoholism. Worldwide, outbreaks of pellagra still occasionally occur, especially among refugees and during emergencies in developing countries.[7]

Vitamin B_6 (Pyridoxine) Helps Manufacture Nonessential Amino Acids

You can think of vitamin B_6 as the "protein vitamin" because it is needed for more than 100 enzymes involved in protein metabolism.[20] Without adequate vitamin B_6, all amino acids become essential and must be consumed in our diet, as our bodies cannot make them in sufficient quantities. Vitamin B_6 also assists in the synthesis of hemoglobin, a component of red blood cells that transports oxygen, and it helps to maintain blood glucose within a normal range. In addition, vitamin B_6 is needed for the synthesis of neurotransmitters that enable nerve cells to communicate.

Good food sources of vitamin B_6 include enriched ready-to-eat cereals, beef liver, fish, poultry, garbanzo beans, and fortified soy-based meat substitutes (FIGURE 6.16). White potatoes and other starchy vegetables are also good sources.

Vitamin B_6 supplements have been used to treat conditions such as premenstrual syndrome (PMS) and carpal tunnel syndrome. Unfortunately, clinical trials have failed to support any significant benefit of B_6 supplements for these

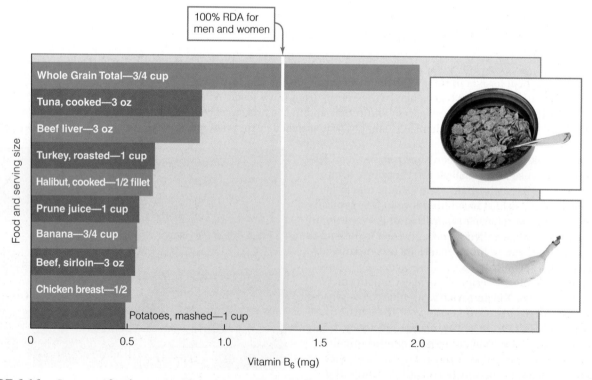

FIGURE 6.16 Common food sources of vitamin B_6. The RDA for vitamin B_6 is 1.3 mg/d for men and women aged 19 to 50 years.

(Data from U.S. Department of Agriculture, Agricultural Research Service. 2007. USDA Nutrient Database for Standard Reference, Release 20. Nutrient Data Laboratory Home Page, www.ars.usda.gov/ba/bhnrc/ndl.)

conditions.[20] What's more, supplementing with B_6 can result in nerve damage to the arms and legs: in one study, 23 of 58 women taking daily vitamin B_6 supplements for PMS had nerve damage.[20]

Vitamin B_6 deficiency is rare in the United States except among people who chronically abuse alcohol and children taking the asthma drug theophylline, which decreases body stores of vitamin B_6. Deficiency symptoms include anemia, convulsions, depression, confusion, and inflamed, irritated patches on the skin. A deficiency of vitamin B_6 may also increase the level of the amino acid **homocysteine** in the blood. High homocysteine levels may damage coronary arteries or promote the formation of clotted arteries, increasing the risk of a heart attack or stroke.[20]

Folate Is Critical during the Earliest Weeks of Pregnancy

All women of childbearing age need to consume adequate folate. This is because folate, which promotes DNA synthesis and cell division, is a critical nutrient during the first few weeks of pregnancy—typically before a woman even knows she is pregnant—when the combined sperm-egg cell is multiplying rapidly to form the primitive tissues of the human body. When folate intake is inadequate in the first weeks of pregnancy, the fetus can develop a *neural tube defect,* a malformation affecting the spinal cord that can cause neurologic problems and impaired movement. Neural tube defects are discussed in detail in Chapter 11.

In everyone, folate is essential for healthy blood. Without sufficient folate, the red blood cells become unable to carry sufficient oxygen to all our body cells, and we become weak and exhausted. This condition is called *macrocytic anemia.* Folate is also important in amino acid metabolism. Like B_6 deficiency, folate deficiency can cause too high a level of the amino acid homocysteine in the blood, a risk factor for heart disease and stroke.

Because of its critical role during the first few weeks of pregnancy, and the fact that many women of childbearing age do not consume adequate amounts, folate has been added to ready-to-eat cereals and bread products. Thus, these two foods are among the primary sources of folate in the United States. Other good food sources include liver, spinach, lentils, oatmeal, asparagus, and romaine lettuce (FIGURE 6.17).

Toxicity can occur when taking supplemental folate. One especially frustrating problem with folate toxicity is that it can mask a simultaneous vitamin B_{12} deficiency. As you saw in the chapter-opening case, a delay in diagnosis of B_{12} deficiency can permanently damage the nervous system. There do not appear to be any clear symptoms of folate toxicity independent from its interaction with vitamin B_{12} deficiency.

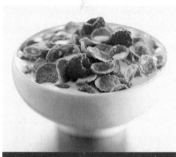

Because of its critical role in the first few weeks of pregnancy, folate is added to all ready-to-eat cereals.

Vitamin B_{12} (Cobalamin) Maintains Healthy Nerves and Blood

In the chapter-opening scenario, you saw the effects of vitamin B_{12} deficiency on Mr. Katz's nervous system. His nerve function deteriorated because adequate levels of vitamin B_{12} are necessary to maintain the sheath that coats nerve fibers. When this sheath is damaged or absent, nerves fire inappropriately, causing numerous physical and cognitive problems. Vitamin B_{12} is also part of coenzymes that assist with formation of blood.

In addition, as with folate and vitamin B_6, adequate levels of vitamin B_{12} are necessary to break down the amino acid homocysteine. When vitamin B_{12} consumption is inadequate, homocysteine levels—and your risk for heart disease or stroke—rise.

Vitamin B_{12} is found only in dairy products, meats, and poultry, so individuals consuming a vegan diet need to eat foods that are fortified with vitamin B_{12} or take vitamin B_{12} supplements or injections (FIGURE 6.18). As we age, our sources of vitamin B_{12} may need to change. Individuals younger than 51 years are generally able to meet the RDA for vitamin B_{12} by consuming it in foods. However, it is estimated that about 10% to 30% of adults older than 50 years have a condition referred to as **atrophic gastritis** that results in low stomach acid secretion.[21] Because stomach

homocysteine An amino acid that requires adequate levels of folate, vitamin B_6, and vitamin B_{12} for its metabolism. High levels of homocysteine in the blood are associated with an increased risk for vascular diseases such as cardiovascular disease.

atrophic gastritis A condition that results in low stomach acid secretion; estimated to occur in about 10% to 30% of adults older than 50 years of age.

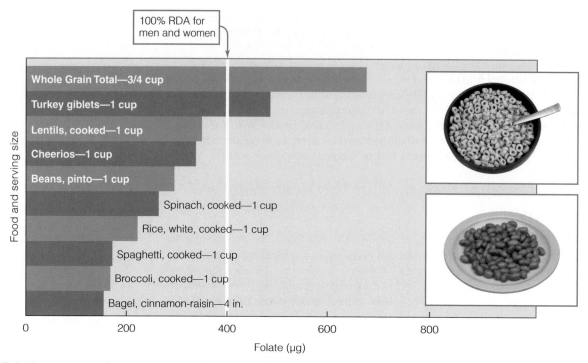

FIGURE 6.17 Common food sources of folate and folic acid. The RDA for folate is 400 μg/d for men and women.
(Data from U.S. Department of Agriculture, Agricultural Research Service. 2007. USDA Nutrient Database for Standard Reference, Release 20. Nutrient Data Laboratory Home Page, www.ars.usda.gov/ba/bhnrc/ndl.)

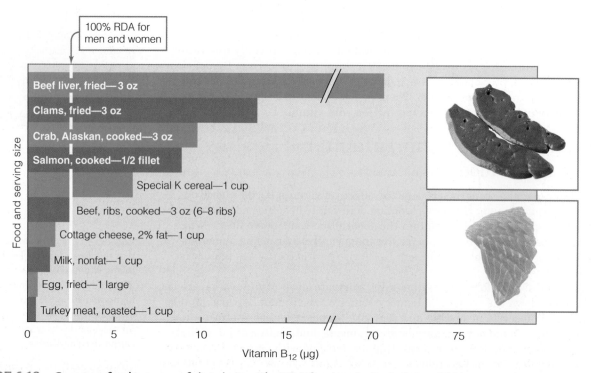

FIGURE 6.18 Common food sources of vitamin B_{12}. The RDA for vitamin B_{12} is 2.4 μg/d for men and women.
(Data from U.S. Department of Agriculture, Agricultural Research Service. 2007. USDA Nutrient Database for Standard Reference, Release 20. Nutrient Data Laboratory Home Page, www.ars.usda.gov/ba/bhnrc/ndl.)

acid separates food-bound vitamin B_{12} from dietary proteins, if the acid content of the stomach is inadequate, then the body cannot free up enough vitamin B_{12} from food sources alone. Since atrophic gastritis is estimated to affect almost one-third of the older adult population, it is recommended that people older than 50 years of age consume foods fortified with vitamin B_{12}, take a vitamin B_{12}–containing supplement, or have periodic B_{12} injections.

Vitamin B_{12} deficiency causes diminished energy and exercise tolerance, fatigue, shortness of breath, and the neurological symptoms described in the chapter-opening scenario. One of the primary causes of vitamin B_{12} deficiency is a condition called *pernicious anemia.* People with pernicious anemia lack adequate amounts of a protein secreted by the stomach that helps vitamin B_{12} to be absorbed into the bloodstream. There are no known adverse effects from consuming excess amounts of vitamin B_{12}.

Pantothenic Acid Assists in Building and Breaking Down Fatty Acids

Pantothenic acid is a component of coenzymes that assist with the metabolism of fatty acids. It is also critical for building new fatty acids.

The prefix *pan-* means "widespread," and indeed pantothenic acid is found in a wide variety of foods, from beef, chicken, organ meats, and egg yolk to potatoes, tomato products, and whole grains. There are no known adverse effects from consuming excess amounts of pantothenic acid. Deficiencies of pantothenic acid are very rare.

Biotin Helps Metabolize All Macronutrients

Biotin is a component of coenzymes that help the body to break down all of the macronutrients. It also plays an important role in gluconeogenesis.

The biotin content has been determined for very few foods, and these values are not reported in food composition tables or dietary analysis programs. Biotin appears to be widespread in foods. There are no known adverse effects from consuming excess amounts, and biotin deficiencies are rare.

Choline Is a Vitamin-Like Substance Found in Many Foods

The carbon-containing compound choline, although not classified as a vitamin, is typically grouped with the B vitamins because of its role in assisting homocysteine metabolism. Choline also accelerates the synthesis and release of *acetylcholine,* a neurotransmitter involved in movement and other functions. It is also necessary for healthy cell membranes, and it plays an important role in the transport and metabolism of fats and cholesterol.

Choline has an AI of 550 mg per day for men ages 19 and older and an AI of 425 mg per day for women ages 19 and older. The choline content of foods is not typically reported in nutrient databases. However, we do know that choline is widespread in foods, especially milk, liver, eggs, and peanuts. Inadequate intakes of choline can eventually lead to liver damage. Excessive intake of supplemental choline results in various toxicity symptoms, including a fishy body odor, vomiting, sweating, diarrhea, and low blood pressure. The UL for choline for adults 19 years of age and older is 3.5 g/day.

RECAP *Water-soluble B vitamins include thiamin, riboflavin, niacin, pyridoxine (vitamin B_6), folate, cobalamin (vitamin B_{12}), pantothenic acid, and biotin. Acting as coenzymes, the B vitamins assist in breaking down food to produce energy. They are commonly found in enriched breads and cereals, meats, dairy products, and some fruits and vegetables. B-vitamin toxicity is rare unless a*

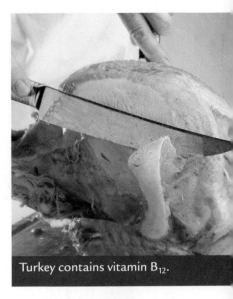
Turkey contains vitamin B_{12}.

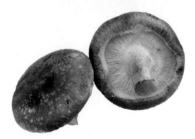
Shiitake mushrooms contain pantothenic acid.

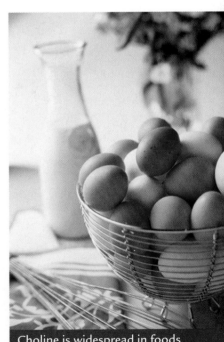
Choline is widespread in foods and can be found in eggs and milk.

person consumes large doses in supplements. B-vitamin deficiencies are not commonly seen except in individuals with another health problem such as alcohol abuse. The exceptions are folate deficiency during early pregnancy, which can lead to neural tube defects in the developing fetus, and vitamin B_{12} deficiency, which leads to anemia and nervous system damage and is sometimes seen in older adults with atrophic gastritis and people consuming a vegan diet. Choline is a carbon-containing compound that assists in homocysteine metabolism.

NUTRI-CASE LIZ

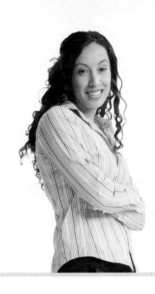

" Ever since my dance company folded after Christmas, I've been feeling exhausted. I know I should start auditioning for other companies, but it just seems too overwhelming right now. I'm cranky and spaced-out, and the least little thing makes me cry. Besides, I'm too fat to audition anywhere these days: because I'm so tired, I've been skipping dance class. When I was still in bed at 11 o'clock this morning, my roommate told me I needed to start taking some B vitamins. She says that they give you energy. Maybe I'll ask her to drive me down to the health food store to buy some. It's only a mile away, but I don't think I have the energy to walk."

Is Liz's roommate correct when she asserts that B vitamins "give you energy"? Considering what you've learned about Liz elsewhere in this book, do you think it is likely that she'd benefit from taking B-vitamin supplements? Why or why not? What other concerns does her situation raise, and what additional advice might you give her?

HEALTHWATCH
Do Antioxidants Protect against Cancer?

Beta-carotene and the antioxidant vitamins E and C protect our cell membranes, proteins, lipoproteins, and DNA from damage by free radicals, so does that mean they protect us against cancer? Before we answer that question, let's take a closer look at precisely what cancer is and how it spreads. **Cancer** is actually a group of diseases that are all characterized by cells that grow "out of control." By this we mean that cancer cells reproduce spontaneously and independently and don't stay within the boundaries of the tissue or organ where they grow. Instead, they aggressively invade tissues and organs far away from those in which they originally formed.

Most forms of cancer result in one or more **tumors,** which are masses of immature cells that have no useful function. Although the word "tumor" sounds frightening, it is important to note that not every tumor is *malignant,* or cancerous. Many are *benign* (not harmful) and are made up of cells that will not spread widely.

FIGURE 6.19 shows how changes to normal cells prompt a series of other changes that can progress into cancer. There are three primary steps of cancer development: initiation, promotion, and progression. These occur as follows:

1. ***Initiation:*** The initiation of cancer occurs when a cell's DNA is *mutated* (or changed). This mutation, which can be caused by a variety of factors, including exposure to a virus, toxic chemical, or other agent, causes permanent changes in the cell. Substances such as toxic chemicals that prompt such cellular mutations are called *carcinogens*.

cancer   A group of diseases characterized by cells that reproduce spontaneously and independently and may invade other tissues and organs.

tumor   Any newly formed mass of undifferentiated cells.

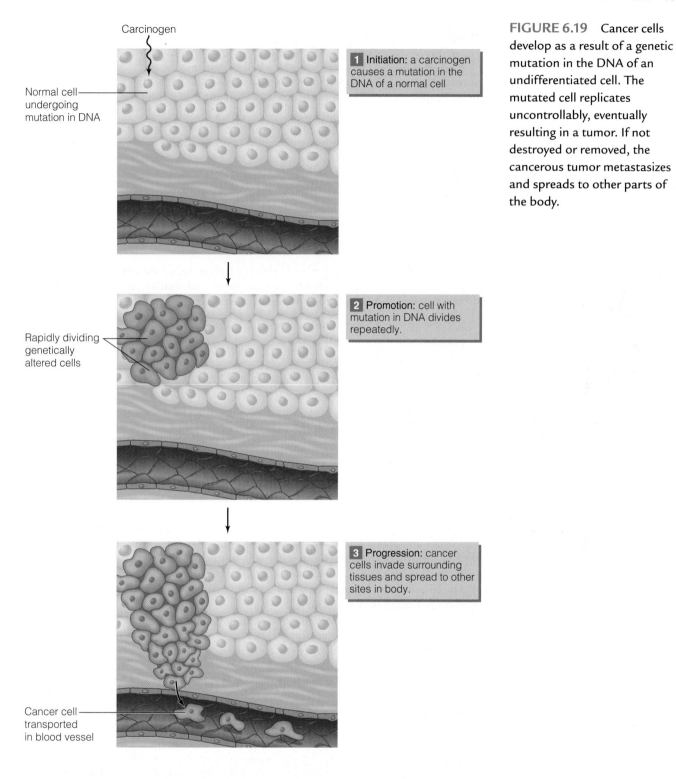

Carcinogen

Normal cell undergoing mutation in DNA

1 Initiation: a carcinogen causes a mutation in the DNA of a normal cell

Rapidly dividing genetically altered cells

2 Promotion: cell with mutation in DNA divides repeatedly.

3 Progression: cancer cells invade surrounding tissues and spread to other sites in body.

Cancer cell transported in blood vessel

FIGURE 6.19 Cancer cells develop as a result of a genetic mutation in the DNA of an undifferentiated cell. The mutated cell replicates uncontrollably, eventually resulting in a tumor. If not destroyed or removed, the cancerous tumor metastasizes and spreads to other parts of the body.

2. ***Promotion:*** During this phase, the mutated cell repeatedly divides. The mutated DNA is locked into each new cell's genetic instructions. These cells also continue to divide uninhibited.

3. ***Progression:*** During this phase, the cancerous cells grow out of control and invade surrounding tissues. These cells then *metastasize* (spread) to other sites of the body. In the early stages of progression, the immune system can sometimes detect these cancerous cells and destroy them. However, if the cells continue to grow, they develop into malignant tumors, and cancer results.

Genetic, Lifestyle, and Environmental Factors Can Increase Our Risk for Cancer

Cancer is the second leading cause of death across all age groups combined in the United States, and researchers estimate that about half of all men and one-third of all women will develop cancer during their lifetimes. But what causes cancer? Are you and your loved ones at risk? The answer depends on several factors, including your family history of cancer, your exposure to environmental agents, and various lifestyle choices. These are discussed, along with several practical steps you can take to reduce your risk of cancer, in the accompanying Game Plan: Simple Steps to Reduce Your Risk of Cancer.

Antioxidants Play a Role in Preventing Cancer and Other Diseases

There is a large and growing body of evidence that antioxidants play an important role in preventing cancer, heart disease, and stroke, as well as certain other diseases. How do they do this? Some proposed mechanisms include:

- Enhancing the immune system, which assists in the destruction and removal of precancerous cells from the body.
- Inhibiting the growth of cancer cells and tumors.
- Preventing oxidative damage to the cells' DNA by seeking out and stabilizing free radicals.
- Reducing inflammation in our blood vessel walls and protecting against the formation and release of blood clots that can cause heart attack and stroke.

Eating whole foods high in antioxidant nutrients such as vitamins E, C, and beta-carotene—especially fruits and vegetables—is shown to be associated with decreased cancer risk.[22] Additional studies show that populations eating diets low in antioxidant nutrients have a higher risk for cancer. Other studies show that people who eat more fruits and vegetables have a significantly reduced risk of heart disease and stroke.[23,24] These studies show a strong *association* between diet and disease risk, but they do not prove cause and effect. Nutrition experts agree that there are important interactions between antioxidant nutrients and other substances in foods, such as fiber and phytochemicals (discussed next), which work together to reduce the risk for many diseases.

The benefit of consuming antioxidants in supplement form is not at all clear. Some studies suggest that antioxidant supplements may reduce cancer or heart disease risk, but others are inconclusive or even show increased risk. For example, the Preventive Services Task Force of the U.S. Agency for Healthcare Research and Quality finds that there is insufficient evidence to recommend either for or against the use of supplements of vitamins A, C, or E, or antioxidant combinations, for the prevention of cancer or cardiovascular disease.[25] A Finnish study found that vitamin E supplementation was not protective against lung cancer but may have a beneficial impact on prostate cancer, whereas another study found no evidence that people taking vitamin E supplements reduced their risk of cancer over those taking a placebo.[12] The World Cancer Research Fund and American Institute for Cancer Research confirm that at the present time, dietary supplements cannot be recommended for cancer prevention in the general population and that nutritional needs should be met through diet alone.[26]

How can there be such conflicting evidence on the effectiveness of supplements? The human body is very complex, as is the development and progression of chronic disease. People differ substantially in their susceptibility for disease and in their response to protective factors. In any research study, it is impossible to control all factors that may influence the risk for disease, and many unknown factors can affect study outcomes. Still, manufacturers continue to produce products, from pills to fortified waters, that provide supplemental vitamins. Are such products worth their cost? Refer to the Highlight box on pages 186–187 to gain a better understanding of situations that may warrant vitamin supplementation.

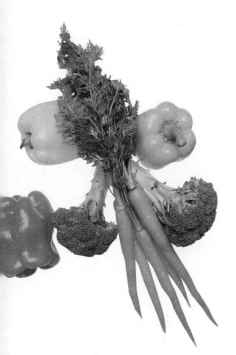

Eating more fruits and vegetables high in antioxidants has been associated with reduced cancer risk.

GAME PLAN
Simple Steps to Reduce Your Risk of Cancer

Cancer often seems to strike apparently healthy people "out of the blue." Because genetic and certain environmental factors are beyond an individual's control, you may be wondering what, if anything, you can do to reduce your risk. Here are some answers:

Nutritional Factors

❑ Eat a variety of colorful fruits and vegetables daily, as these foods are rich in antioxidant nutrients and phytochemicals.

❑ Choose whole grains in preference to refined grains.

❑ Limit your consumption of saturated and *trans* fats. Some studies suggest that diets high in saturated fat could increase our risk of some cancers.

❑ Limit your consumption of red meats, especially those high in fat and processed.

❑ Limit your consumption of nitrates and nitrites. These chemicals are found in cured meats such as sausage, ham, bacon, and many lunch meats. They are known carcinogens.

❑ If you eat meat, avoid cooking methods that require high temperatures, such as broiling, frying, and barbecuing. High-temperature cooking methods prompt the development of carcinogens called *heterocyclic amines* that do not form when meat is cooked more slowly at lower temperatures, such as by roasting or baking.

❑ Maintain a healthful weight. Obesity appears to increase the risk of certain cancers. The exact link between obesity and increased cancer risk is not clear but may be due to hormonal changes that occur with having excess body fat.

Lifestyle Factors

❑ If you smoke cigarettes or cigars or use smokeless tobacco, stop. It is an established fact that these behaviors significantly increase the risk for many forms of cancer. More than forty compounds identified in tobacco and tobacco smoke are known carcinogens.

❑ If you drink alcoholic beverages, limit consumption. Alcohol use is linked with an increased risk of many types of cancer. Alcohol may impair the cell's ability to repair damaged DNA, increasing the possibility of cancer initiation.

❑ Limit your sun exposure and avoid sunburn. Skin cancer is the most common form of cancer in the United States. Most cases are linked to excessive exposure to the ultraviolet (UV) rays of the sun, which can damage the DNA of skin cells. After a few minutes of sun exposure during midday (from about 9 AM to 3 PM) to build up your vitamin D stores, apply sunscreen.

❑ Limit your exposure to environmental and occupational carcinogens. These include such things as second-hand cigarette and cigar smoke and pollutants in the air, the food and water supply, and the workplace.

❑ Adopt a physically active lifestyle. Studies conducted over the past 10 years have shown a possible link between lower cancer risk and higher levels of physical activity. Specifically, the American Cancer Society recommends that you engage in at least moderate activity for 30 minutes or more on 5 or more days of the week.[27]

Source: Some data from American Cancer Society. *Cancer Prevention.* Available at www.cancer.org.

HIGHLIGHT

Pills, Waters, Sodas, Bars . . . Do We Really Need All These Vitamins?

On her way home from work, Judy stops at the grocery store to pick up a frozen dinner and a six-pack of diet soda. In the beverage aisle, she notices a display promoting her favorite soda—but the packaging says, "Now fortified with essential vitamins!" She reads the label and finds that a can of the soda provides 15% of the Daily Value for niacin and vitamins B_6 and B_{12}. Judy hesitates. The soda costs a little more than the version she has always bought before, and she's not even sure what these particular vitamins do. But still, she wonders . . . Maybe it's worth it. Maybe she *does* need some extra vitamins . . .

Although Judy doesn't know it, her confusion reflects an ongoing debate between food manufacturers and consumer advocates about the promotion of what are called *functional foods*. Simply put, a functional food is any food that has been manipulated in order to enhance its role in a healthful diet. Also called *nutraceuticals*, functional foods contain nutrients and/or other substances that provide a health benefit beyond what is provided by the same food in its traditional form. Plain diet soda is not a functional food, but soda with added vitamins is. And although the added nutrient is not always a vitamin—calcium-fortified juices and soy milks also qualify, as do yogurts with specialized strains of bacteria, and many other enhanced foods— vitamin-fortified products do make up a substantial proportion of the functional food market. A stroll through your local grocery store will probably reveal vitamin-enhanced bottled waters, juices, sodas, energy bars, breakfast cereals, breads . . . not to mention several shelves of single-nutrient

and multivitamin pills. So have you ever stopped and asked yourself: Do we really *need* all these vitamins?

Americans spend almost $21.3 billion dollars each year on dietary supplements alone.[28] Is this money always wasted, or do some people really benefit from taking their vitamins in supplements and fortified foods? Let's start to answer this question with a look at how these products are regulated in the United States.

Multivitamin Supplements and Functional Foods Are Not Strictly Regulated

Multivitamin supplements come in many forms, including pills, capsule, liquids, and powders. They are categorized by the FDA within the general group of foods, not drugs. The same is true for functional foods: as long as all ingredients are recognized as safe for consumption, the food is allowed on the market. This means that the regulation of such products is much less rigorous than for drugs. As an informed consumer, you should know that:

- Supplements and functional foods do not need approval from the FDA before they are marketed.
- The manufacturer is responsible for determining that the product is safe; the FDA does not test it for safety prior to marketing.
- In particular, supplement companies do not have to provide the FDA with any evidence that their supplements are safe, unless the company is marketing a new dietary ingredient that was not sold in the United States prior to 1994.
- There are currently no federal guidelines on practices to ensure the purity, quality, safety, and composition of supplements.
- There are no rules to limit the serving size or amount of a nutrient in any supplement or functional food.
- Once a supplement or functional food is marketed, it is the responsibility of the FDA to prove a product is unsafe before the product can be removed from the market.

Despite these limitations in regulations, manufacturers are required to follow certain labeling guidelines. Federal advertising regulations require that any advertising on the label must be truthful and not misleading and that advertisers must have adequate substantiation of all product claims before disseminating the ad. Any products not meeting these labeling and advertising guidelines can be removed from the market. The FDA is currently considering a new regulatory system by which any product bearing health claims would be subject to FDA oversight. But until such a system is in effect, consumers are on their own.

Even eggs can be fortified with omega-3s and vitamin E and turned into functional foods! It is unclear whether they are better for us, but there's no question that they are more expensive.

Pills, Waters, Sodas, Bars . . . Do We Really Need All These Vitamins? *(continued)*

Extra Vitamins Can Be Helpful or Harmful

It is not always easy to determine who should take multi-vitamin supplements and/or consume vitamin-fortified foods. Our nutritional needs change throughout our life span, and some of us may need to take supplements at certain times for various conditions. For instance, people at risk for osteoporosis may benefit from taking vitamin D supplements if their sun exposure is inadequate. Certainly strict vegetarians (vegans) need to supplement their diet with vitamin B_{12}. Thousands of vitamin supplements and vitamin-fortified foods are sold, and it is impossible to discuss here all of the various situations in which these products may be helpful. So to keep our discussion brief, let's focus on describing the most obvious situations in which people may or may not benefit from vitamin supplementation.

Who Might Benefit from Taking Micronutrient Supplements?

Foods contain a diverse combination of compounds that are critical to our health and cannot be packaged in a pill. Thus, supplements are not substitutes for whole foods. However, certain groups of people do benefit from taking supplements. Some examples of widely recommended vitamin or mineral supplements include:

- A single dose of vitamin K for newborns at birth
- Vitamin D supplements for breastfed infants from birth to age 6 months, and iron-fortified cereal for breastfed infants 6 months of age and older
- Fluoride supplements for children not drinking fluoridated water
- Multivitamin/multimineral supplements for people on prolonged energy-restricted diets and for people with HIV/AIDS or other wasting diseases
- Calcium and vitamin D supplements for people at risk for low bone mass
- Vitamin B_{12} supplements for elderly people or vegans

If you identify with one or more of these groups, you should analyze your diet to determine whether or not you actually need supplements. In addition, it is always a good idea to check with your healthcare provider or a registered dietitian (RD) before taking any supplements.

When Can Taking a Vitamin or Mineral Supplement Be Harmful?

Fortified foods typically contain from 10% to 50% of the DRI for any micronutrients they contain. Even if you eat a breakfast cereal providing 100% of the Daily Value for a certain micronu-trient, plus later in the day you eat an energy bar providing 50% of the Daily Value for the same micronutrient, you're unlikely to reach toxic levels unless you are also consuming supplements. Instances in which taking vitamin and mineral supplements is unnecessary or potentially harmful include:

1. Providing fluoride supplements to children who already drink fluoridated water.
2. Taking supplements in the belief that they will cure a disease such as cancer, diabetes, or heart disease.
3. Taking supplements without checking with your health-care provider to determine their reaction with medications you are taking.
4. Taking beta-carotene supplements if you are a smoker. Evidence suggests that beta-carotene supplementation may increase the risk of cancer in smokers.[26]
5. Taking vitamins and minerals in an attempt to improve physical appearance, athletic performance, or energy level. There is no evidence that vitamin and mineral supplements enhance appearance, athletic performance, or energy level in healthy adults who consume a varied diet with adequate energy.
6. Taking supplements in excess of the tolerable upper limit (UL), unless your healthcare provider prescribes them for a diagnosed medical condition. Taking amounts of the fat-soluble vitamin A above the UL can quickly lead to toxicity. In addition, excessive supplementation of some B vitamins can lead to liver damage or nerve damage, and megadoses of vitamin C can cause severe diarrhea and other symptoms.

As advised by the American Dietetic Association, the ideal nutritional strategy for optimizing health is to eat a healthful diet that contains a variety of foods.[29] If you determine that you still do need to supplement and/or consume micronutrient-fortified foods, make sure that together the sources don't provide more than 100% of the recommended levels of any nutrients these products contain. Avoid taking single-nutrient supplements unless advised by your healthcare practitioner.

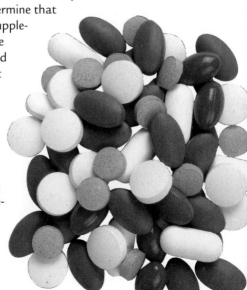

Phytochemicals Appear to Reduce Our Risk of Cancer and Other Diseases

Phytochemicals are naturally occurring chemicals in plants (*phyto-* means "plant"), such as the plant pigments that give fruits and vegetables their rich colors. Many research studies suggest that phytochemicals, working together with other nutrients and fiber in plant-based foods, slow the aging process and reduce the risk for certain forms of cancer, heart disease, stroke, vision impairment, and other diseases. Phytochemicals are found in abundance in fruits, vegetables, whole grains, legumes, seeds, soy products, garlic, onion, and green and black teas. FIGURE 6.20 lists many of the phytochemicals that are specifically linked to cancer prevention and identifies their food sources.

Phytochemicals exhibit clear cancer-prevention properties under laboratory conditions. However, we do not know the specific phytochemical content of most foods, and an ideal phytochemical intake in humans has not yet been determined. That said, a growing body of research suggests that the following phytochemicals do play a role in reducing the risk of some forms of cancer:[23]

- lycopene (found in tomato products, red peppers, pink grapefruit, and watermelon)
- organosulfur compounds (found in garlic, onions, and cruciferous vegetables)
- flavonoids (found in many fruits and vegetables, garlic, green and black teas, and red wine)
- phytoestrogens (found in whole grains, vegetables, and soy products)

Phytochemicals are thought to slow aging and reduce our risk for various diseases in part by moderating the damage done by free radicals. Some also seem to prevent blood clots from forming or to reduce inflammation in the walls of our blood vessels. Some appear able to reduce the ability of bacteria to cling to our tissues, and some may enhance the body's ability to destroy cancer cells or slow or stop their growth.[30] Precisely how phytochemicals perform these functions in conjunction with other nutrients is the subject of current research, as is the question of whether consuming phytochemicals in supplement form is also protective.

Given the many benefits of phytochemicals, you're probably wondering how to be sure you're getting all you need each day. Check out the Game Plan on pages 190–191 for information on how many servings you need, preparation guidelines, and tips for phytochemically charged meals and snacks.

RECAP *Cancer is a group of diseases in which genetically mutated cells grow out of control. Tobacco use, sun exposure, nutritional factors, radiation and chemical exposures, and low physical activity levels are related to a higher risk for some cancers. Eating foods high in antioxidants is associated with lower rates of cancer. Phytochemicals are substances in plants that, together with other nutrients and fiber in plant-based foods, appear to reduce our risk for cancer and heart disease.*

phytochemicals Chemicals found in plants (*phyto-* is from the Greek word for "plant"), such as pigments and other substances, that may reduce our risk for diseases such as cancer and heart disease.

Phytochemical	Health Claims	Food Source	
Carotenoids: alpha-carotene, beta-carotene, lutein, lycopene, zeaxanthin, etc.	Diets with foods rich in these phytochemicals may reduce the risk of cardiovascular disease, certain cancers (e.g., prostate), and age-related eye diseases (cataracts, macular degeneration).	Red, orange, and deep-green vegetables and fruits such as carrots, cantaloupe, sweet potatoes, apricots, kale, spinach, pumpkin, and tomatoes	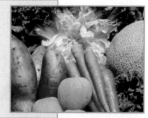
Flavonoids:[1] flavones, flavonols (e.g., quercetin), catechins (e.g., epigallocatechin gallate or EGCG), anthocyanidins, isoflavonoids, etc.	Diets with foods rich in these phytochemicals are associated with lower risk of cardiovascular disease and cancer, possibly because of reduced inflammation, blood clotting, and blood pressure, and increased detoxification of carcinogens or reduction in replication of cancerous cells.	Berries, black and green tea, chocolate, purple grapes and juice, citrus fruits, olives, soybeans and soy products (soy milk, tofu, soy flour, textured vegetable protein), flaxseed, whole wheat	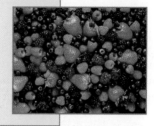
Phenolic acids:[1] ellagic acid, ferulic acid, caffeic acid, curcumin, etc.	Similar benefits as flavonoids.	Coffee beans, fruits (apples, pears, berries, grapes, oranges, prunes, strawberries), potatoes, mustard, oats, soy	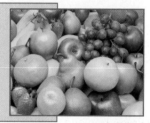
Phytoestrogens:[2] genistein, diadzein, lignans	Foods rich in these phytochemicals may provide benefits to bones and reduce the risk of cardiovascular disease and cancers of reproductive tissues (e.g., breast, prostate).	Soybeans and soy products (soy milk, tofu, soy flour, textured vegetable protein), flaxseed, whole grains	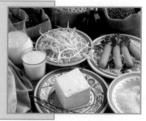
Organosulfur compounds: allylic sulfur compounds, indoles, isothiocyanates, etc.	Foods rich in these phytochemicals may protect against a wide variety of cancers.	Garlic, leeks, onions, chives, cruciferous vegetables (broccoli, cabbage, cauliflower), horseradish, mustard greens	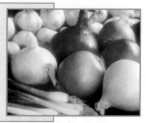

[1] Flavonoids, phenolic acids, and stilbenes are three groups of phytochemicals called phenolics. Flavonoids and phenolic acids are the most abundant phenolics in our diet.
[2] Phytoestrogens include phytochemicals that have mild or anti-estrogenic action in our body. They are grouped together based on this similarity in biologic function, but they also can be classified into other phytochemical groups, such as isoflavanoids.

FIGURE 6.20   Health claims and food sources of phytochemicals.

GAME PLAN

Tips for Increasing Your Phytochemical Intake

As we explained, phytochemicals (pronounced "fight-o-chemicals") help your body to fight chronic disease. So it makes sense to include an appropriate variety of them in your daily diet. But what's appropriate for you? And how can you select and prepare them in ways that work for your busy lifestyle?

Start by reviewing Figure 6.20, which identifies the largest groups of phytochemicals. Because most of these are plant pigments, and many fruits and vegetables contain several different types, you can be sure you are getting a wide variety if you eat 5 to 12 servings of brightly colored fruits and vegetables every day.

Next check out the Fruits & Veggies—More Matters health initiative, which was created by the Centers for Disease Control and Prevention and the Produce for Better Health Foundation to demonstrate that eating more fruits and vegetables can fit in with your busy schedule and help keep you healthy. The initiative offers cooking advice, nutrition information, and shopping and storage tips, and all this and more can be found at www.fruitsandveggiesmorematters.org.

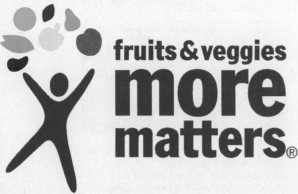

The goal is to eat at least 5 servings of colorful fruits and vegetables each day to help fight cancer, heart disease, and the effects of aging. Here are only a few examples of the wide variety of foods in each group:

❑ Blue-purple foods include eggplant, red onions, purple cabbage, cherries, blackberries, blueberries, raspberries, red grapes, and plums.

❑ Green foods include avocados, broccoli, Brussels sprouts, chives, cabbage, collard greens, green peppers, kale, Swiss chard, leaf lettuces, spinach, and kiwifruit.

❑ White foods include cauliflower, bok choy, white turnips, mushrooms, garlic, onions, leeks, scallions, and bananas.

❑ Yellow-orange foods include carrots, corn, yellow peppers, pumpkin, butternut and other winter squashes, sweet potatoes, cantaloupe, apricots, oranges, papaya, and mangoes.

❑ Red foods include tomatoes, red peppers, apples, strawberries, pink grapefruit, and watermelon.

When Shopping

❑ Build a rainbow in your shopping cart. That way, you'll have on hand several colorful choices to incorporate into meals and snacks each day.

❑ Because fruits and vegetables are perishable, purchase only an amount of fresh produce that you know you can consume within a few days. Nutrient losses increase with each day of storage.

❑ Purchase some less-perishable forms of fruits and vegetables, such as dried fruits, 100% fruit and vegetable juices, soups, canned fruits and vegetables (check for no-sugar and no-sodium added), and frozen vegetables.

In the Kitchen

❑ Wash fresh fruits and vegetables thoroughly, except for berries, which should be washed immediately before eating to discourage spoilage.

GAME PLAN Tips for Increasing Your Phytochemical Intake *(continued)*

❑ Store tomatoes, garlic, and bananas at room temperature.

❑ Store unripened avocados, pears, and other fruits in a lightly closed paper bag until ripe. Then consume or refrigerate.

❑ Store potatoes and onions in a cool, dark location such as a cellar or cool cupboard.

❑ Nutrients become depleted when exposed to air, so peel and cut fruits and vegetables only when you are ready to eat them. Many fruits and vegetables have edible peels that contain important nutrients and fiber, so wash them and eat them unpeeled when possible.

❑ To reduce nutrient loss in cooking water, eat vegetables raw, or zap coarsely chopped vegetables in the microwave for 2–4 minutes with approximately 1 tablespoon of water. Alternatively, stir-fry them in a small amount of oil, or steam them in a basket over simmering water. Always cook vegetables for as short a time as necessary to make them palatable.

❑ Store leftovers in an airtight container in the refrigerator. If you don't plan to eat the leftovers within a few days, freeze them.

❑ Top your breakfast cereal with sliced banana, berries, or raisins or other dried fruits.

❑ Make a quick fruit salad with one can of mandarin orange slices, one can of pineapple chunks, a sliced banana, a chopped apple, and some berries, grapes, or raisins. Serve with yogurt.

❑ Add fresh vegetables to salads, soups, homemade pizza, and pasta.

❑ Add dark-green leaf lettuce, tomato, and onion to sandwiches, or make a veggie sandwich using avocado slices in place of meat.

❑ Next time you're at a barbecue, grill fruits or vegetables on skewers.

❑ For homemade salsa, combine chopped tomatoes, avocado, red onions, cilantro (or coriander), and lime juice.

❑ For shared meals, try a veggie-burrito buffet: set out a plate of warmed corn or whole-wheat tortillas with bowls of warm black or pinto beans, chopped tomatoes, chopped avocado, chopped black olives, minced onion or scallions, and plain yogurt or nonfat sour cream. Invite your friends to assemble their own!

❑ Make gazpacho! In a blender, combine 1–3 cups tomato juice, chunks of green pepper, red onion, a cucumber with seeds removed (no need to peel), the juice of one lime, a garlic clove, a splash each of red wine vinegar and olive oil, a half teaspoon each of basil and cumin, and salt and pepper to taste. Seed and dice 2–3 fresh tomatoes and add to blended ingredients. Chill for several hours. Serve very cold.

On the Run

❑ Buy ready-to-eat vegetables such as baby carrots, cherry tomatoes, and celery sticks, or take a minute to wash and slice a red pepper or broccoli crowns. Toss some in a zip-lock bag to take to school or work.

❑ Throw a single-serving container of unsweetened applesauce, mandarin orange slices, pineapple chunks, or other fruit into your backpack for an afternoon snack. Don't forget the spoon!

❑ Make up small bags of fresh or dried fruits (grapes, raisins, apricots, cherries, prunes, figs, dates, banana chips, etc.) with nuts to take along.

❑ Pack a banana, apple, plum, orange, or other fruit you can eat whole.

❑ Store some juice boxes in your freezer to take along. A frozen juice box will remain cold for several hours.

Source: Some suggestions from Centers for Disease Control and Prevention (CDC) and Produce for Better Health Foundation, available at www.fruitsandveggiesmatter.gov and www.fruitsandveggiesmorematters.org; and Phytochemical Information Center available at www.pbhfoundation.org.

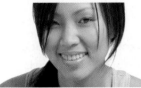
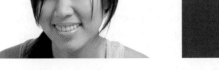

REVIEW QUESTIONS

Circle the correct choice.

1. The B vitamins include:
   a. niacin, folate, and selenium.
   b. thiamin, pantothenic acid, and biotin.
   c. beta-carotene, riboflavin, and pyridoxine.
   d. cobalamin, choline, and chromium.

2. Which of the following is a characteristic of vitamin E?
   a. enhances the absorption of iron
   b. can be manufactured from beta-carotene
   c. is a coenzyme involved in the metabolism of carbo-hydrates and fats
   d. is destroyed by exposure to high heat

3. Which of the following are known carcinogens?
   a. phytochemicals
   b. antioxidants
   c. carotenoids
   d. nitrates

4. Taking daily megadoses of which of the following nutrients may cause death?
   a. vitamin A
   b. vitamin C
   c. vitamin E
   d. riboflavin

5. The vitamin most closely associated with blood clotting is
   a. vitamin A.
   b. vitamin K.
   c. niacin.
   d. vitamin B$_{12}$.

6. True or False? The best way for a woman to reduce her risk of having a baby with a neural tube defect is to begin taking a folate supplement as soon as she learns she is pregnant.

7. True or False? The body absorbs vitamin D from sunlight.

8. True or False? Free-radical formation can occur as a result of normal cellular metabolism.

9. True or False? Pregnant women are advised to consume plentiful quantities of beef liver.

10. True or False? High blood levels of the amino acid homocysteine are associated with an increased risk of heart disease.

WEB LINKS

www.nlm.nih.gov/medlineplus
MEDLINE Plus Health Information

Search for rickets or osteomalacia to learn more about these vitamin D–deficiency diseases.

www.cdc.gov
Centers for Disease Control and Prevention

Visit this site to learn about deficiencies and toxicities of individual nutrients, including neural tube defects. Search under the key phrase "5 a day" for tips on how to increase your consumption of fruits and vegetables.

www.fruitsandveggiesmorematters.org
Fruits & Veggies—More Matters

This health initiative, created by the Centers for Disease Control and Prevention (CDC) and the Produce for Better Health Foundation, promotes eating more fruits and vegetables and provides tips and advice to show that buying, preparing, and eating produce can fit in with your busy schedule and help to keep you healthy.

www.cancer.org
The American Cancer Society (ACS)

Get ACS recommendations for nutrition and physical activity for cancer prevention.

www.cancer.gov
The National Cancer Institute

Learn more about the nutritional factors that can influence your risk for cancer.

www.cfsan.fda.gov/list.html
Center for Food Safety and Applied Nutrition

Select "Dietary Supplements" on the pull-down menu for more information on how to make informed decisions and evaluate information related to dietary supplements.

www.nal.usda.gov/fnic
USDA Food and Nutrition Information Center (FNIC)

Click on the "Dietary Supplements" button to obtain information on vitamin and mineral supplements, including consumer reports and industry regulations.

http://nccam.nih.gov
National Center for Complementary and Alternative Medicine

Visit this site for information on the safety of vitamin, mineral, and herbal supplements and other complementary and alternative therapies, including current consumer alerts and advisories.

http://dietary-supplements.info.nih.gov
Office of Dietary Supplements

Go to this site to obtain current research results and reliable information about dietary supplements.

www.ars.usda.gov/ba/bhnrc/ndl
Nutrient Data Laboratory Home Page

Click on "Search" and then "Nutrient Lists" to find reports listing food sources for selected nutrients.

http://www.bbc.co.uk/health/
BBC Health

Search for vitamins or minerals for further information, signs of deficiency, therapeutic uses, and food sources.

TEST YOURSELF ANSWERS

1. **True.** Our bodies can use energy from sunlight to convert a cholesterol compound in our skin into vitamin D.

2. **False.** Extensive research on vitamin C and colds does not support the theory that taking vitamin C supplements reduces our risk of catching a cold.

3. **False.** B-complex vitamins do not directly provide energy for our bodies. However, they enable our bodies to generate energy from carbohydrates, fats, and proteins.

4. **False.** Phytochemicals are chemicals that occur naturally in plants and appear to reduce our risk for heart disease, some forms of cancer, and certain other diseases.

5. **True and false!** For an individual who consumes a varied diet that provides adequate energy and nutrients, this statement is true. However, many people do not consume a varied diet that provides adequate levels of micronutrients, and others have health issues that increase their requirements or affect their ability to absorb micronutrients from food. For these individuals, a daily multivitamin supplement is not a waste of money—it's a wise investment in their health.

REFERENCES

1. Bernstein, L. 2000. Dementia without a cause: Lack of vitamin B_{12} can cause dementia. *Discover.* Feb. 21 (02).
2. World Health Organization (WHO). 2008. Micronutrient Deficiencies. Vitamin A Deficiency. Available at www.who.int/nutrition/topics/vad/en/.
3. Lim, H. W., B. A. Gilchrest, K. D. Cooper, H. A. Bischoff-Ferrari, D. S. Rigel, W. H. Cyr, S. Miller, et al. 2005. Sunlight, tanning booths, and vitamin D. *J. Am. Acad. Dermatol.* 52:868–876.
4. Heaney, R. P. 2005. The vitamin D requirement in health and disease. *J. Steroid Biochem. Molec. Biol.* 97:13–19.
5. Heaney, R. P. 2007. The case for improving vitamin D status. *J. Steroid Biochem. Molec. Biol.* 103:635–641.
6. Holick, M. F. 2006. Resurrection of vitamin D deficiency and rickets. *J. Clin. Invest.* 116:2062–2072.
7. CDC. 1999. Achievements in public health, 1900–1999: Safer and healthier foods. *Morbidity and Mortality Weekly Report (MMWR)* 48(40):905–913. Available at www.cdc.gov/mmwr/preview/mmwrhtml/mm4840a1.htm.
8. Rajakumar, K. 2003. Vitamin D, cod-liver oil, sunlight, and rickets: A historical perspective. *Pediatrics* 112(2):e132– e135. Available at http://pediatrics.aappublications.org/cgi/content/full/112/2/e132.
9. Sullivan, S. S., C. J. Rosen, W. A. Halteman, T. C. Chen, and M. F. Holick. 2005. Adolescent girls in Maine are at risk for vitamin D insufficiency. *J. Am. Diet. Assoc.* 105:971–974.
10. Institute of Medicine, Food and Nutrition Board. 2001. *Dietary Reference Intakes for Vitamin A, Vitamin K, Arsenic, Boron, Chromium, Copper, Iodine, Iron, Manganese, Molybdenum, Nickel, Silicon, Vanadium, and Zinc.* Washington, DC: National Academy Press.
11. National Center for Complementary and Alternative Medicine. 2004. Herbal Supplements: Consider Safety, Too. Available at http://nccam.nih.gov/health/supplement-safety.
12. National Center for Complementary and Alternative Medicine. 2005. Consumer Advisory: Vitamin E Supplements. Available at http://nccam.nih.gov/health/alters/vitamine/vitamine.htm.
13. Environmental Health Perspectives. 1999. NIEHS News: Medicinal herbs: NTP extracts the facts. *Environ. Health Perspect.* 107(12). Available at http://ehp.niehs.nih.gov/docs/1999/107–12/niehsnews.html.
14. National Center for Complementary and Alternative Medicine (NCCAM). 2006. Herbs at a Glance. Ginger. Available at http://nccam.nih.gov/health/ginger.
15. Food and Drug Administration (FDA). 2003. Agency Response Letter GRAS Notice No. GRN 000124. U.S. Food and Drug Administration. Available at http://www.cfsan.fda.gov/~rdb/opa-g124.html.
16. National Institute of Allergy and Infectious Diseases. December 2004. *The Common Cold.* Available at www.niaid.nih.gov/factsheets/cold.htm.
17. United Press International (UPI). *Vitamin C Fails to Prevent Colds.* Tuesday, June 28, 2005. United Press International. Available at www.nlm.nih.gov/medlineplus/print/news/fullstory-25487.html.
18. Hemila, H. 1997. Vitamin C intake and susceptibility to the common cold. *Br. J. Nutr.* 77:59–72.
19. Massey, L. K., M. Liebman, and S. A. Kynast-Gales. 2005. Ascorbate increases human oxaluria and kidney stone risk. *J. Nutr.* 135:1673–1677.
20. Office of Dietary Supplements (ODS). 2005. Dietary Supplement Fact Sheet: Vitamin B_6. Available at http://ods.od.nih.gov/factsheets/vitaminb6.assumption.

21. Institute of Medicine, Food and Nutrition Board. 1998. *Dietary Reference Intakes for Thiamin, Riboflavin, Niacin, Vitamin B₆, Folate, Vitamin B₁₂, Pantothenic Acid, Biotin, and Choline.* Washington, DC: National Academy Press.

22. Greenwald, P., C. K. Clifford, and J. A. Milner. 2001. Diet and cancer prevention. *Eur. J. Cancer* 37:948–965.

23. Joshipura, K. J., F. B. Hu, J. E. Manson, M. J. Stampfer, E. B. Rimm, F. E. Speizer, et al. 2001. The effect of fruit and vegetable intake on risk for coronary heart disease. *Ann. Intern. Med.* 134:1106–1114.

24. Liu, S., I.-M. Lee, U. Ajani, S. R. Cole, J. E. Buring, and J. E. Manson. 2001. Intake of vegetables rich in carotenoids and risk of coronary heart disease in men: The Physicians' Health Study. *Int. J. Epidemiol.* 30:130–135.

25. Agency for Healthcare Research and Quality (AHRQ), U.S. Preventive Services Task Force (USPSTF). 2003. Routine Vitamin Supplementation to Prevent Cancer and Cardiovascular Disease. Available at www.ahrq.gov/clinic/3rduspstf/vitamins/vitaminsrr.htm.

26. World Cancer Research Fund/American Institute for Cancer Research. 2007. *Food, Nutrition, Physical Activity, and the Prevention of Cancer: A Global Perspective.* Washington, DC: AICR.

27. American Cancer Society. 2002. *Cancer Prevention.* Available at www.cancer.org.

28. Nutrition Business Journal. 2006. *NBJ's Supplement Business Report 2006.* ©Penton Media, Inc.

29. American Dietetic Association. 2001. Position of the American Dietetic Association: Food fortification and dietary supplements. *J. Am. Diet. Assoc.* 101:115–125.

30. Phytochemical Information Center. 2005. 5 a Day. Eat Your Colors, Get Your Phytochemicals. Available at www.5aday.com/html/phytochem/colors.php.

TEST YOURSELF

Are these statements true or false? Circle your guess.

1 Chromium supplements are consistently effective in reducing body fat and enhancing muscle mass.　　**TRUE** or **FALSE**

2 Sodium is unhealthful, and we should avoid consuming it in our diets.　　**TRUE** or **FALSE**

3 Iron deficiency is the most common nutrient deficiency in the world.　　**TRUE** or **FALSE**

4 Osteoporosis, or "porous bones," is a disease that only affects elderly women.　　**TRUE** or **FALSE**

5 Cigarette smoking increases a person's risk for osteoporosis.　　**TRUE** or **FALSE**

Test Yourself answers can be found at the end of the chapter.

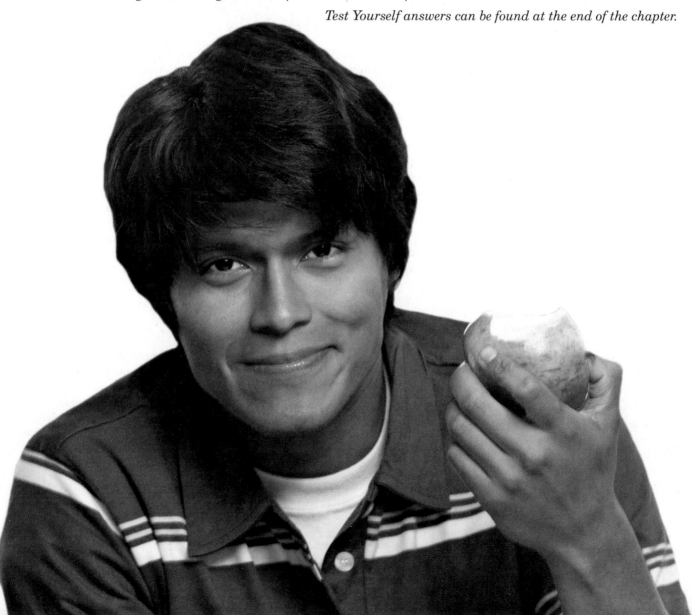

Where I'm starting from...

Do you eat meat, poultry, and/or fish?

Yes or NO

If NO, name some iron-rich foods you do eat:

Do you drink milk?

Yes or NO

If NO, name some calcium-rich foods you do eat or drink:

A S A YOUNG WOMAN, ERIKA GOODMAN leapt across the stage in leading roles with the Joffrey Ballet, one of the premier dance companies in the world. But at the age of 59, she died after falling in her Manhattan apartment. Goodman had a disease called *osteoporosis,* which means "porous bones." As you might suspect, the less dense the bone, the more likely it is to break; indeed, osteoporosis can cause bones to break during even minor weight-bearing activities, such as carrying groceries. In advanced cases, bones in the hip and spine fracture spontaneously, merely from the effort of holding the body erect.

In this chapter, we discuss the minerals that form our bones and explore how mineral deficiencies lead to bone disease. We also explain how minerals called *electrolytes* provide the electrical charge that enables our bodies to dance, work, think . . . indeed, to perform any conscious or unconscious activity. Still other minerals work with the B vitamins to metabolize food into energy, and some help transport oxygen within our blood. As you can see, minerals are absolutely indispensable to our functioning (FIGURE 7.1). Before we discuss individual minerals, let's pause to explore exactly what minerals are.

What Are Minerals?

Minerals are solid, crystalline substances that do not contain carbon and are not broken down during digestion. In fact, they can't be created or destroyed by any natural means, including heat, cold, light, chemicals, or mechanical force. Minerals exist not only in foods, but also in our environment: the zinc in meats is the same as the zinc in the earth's crust.

One of the most important properties of minerals is their ability to carry an electrical charge. Like magnets, minerals with opposite electrical charges bond tightly together to form durable compounds, for instance, in our bones. The electrical charge of minerals also attracts water, so the minerals inside our cells help them retain the amount of water they need to function. And in both our cells and tissues, the electrical charges of various minerals stimulate our nerves to fire and our muscles to contract.

Minerals are classified according to the amounts we need in our diet and according to how much of the mineral is found in our bodies. The two categories of minerals in our diets and bodies are the major minerals and the trace minerals.

Major Minerals Are Required in Amounts Greater Than 100 mg per Day

Major minerals earned their name from the fact that we need to consume at least 100 mg of each per day in our diets. In addition, the total amount of each major mineral present in the body is at least 5 g (or 5,000 mg). For instance, the major mineral calcium is a primary component of our bones. In addition to calcium, the major minerals include sodium, potassium, phosphorus, magnesium, sulfur, and chloride. Table 7.1 identifies the primary functions, recommended intakes, and food sources of these minerals.

Trace Minerals Are Required in Amounts Less Than 100 mg per Day

Trace minerals are those we need to consume in amounts less than 100 mg per day. The total amount of any trace mineral in the body is less than 5 g (or 5,000 mg). The trace minerals include selenium, fluoride, iodine, chromium, manganese, iron, zinc,

minerals Solid, crystalline substances that do not contain carbon and are not changed by natural processes, including digestion.

major minerals Minerals we need to consume in amounts of at least 100 mg per day and of which the total amount present in the body is at least 5 g (or 5,000 mg).

trace minerals Minerals we need to consume in amounts less than 100 mg per day and of which the total amount present in the body is less than 5 g (or 5,000 mg).

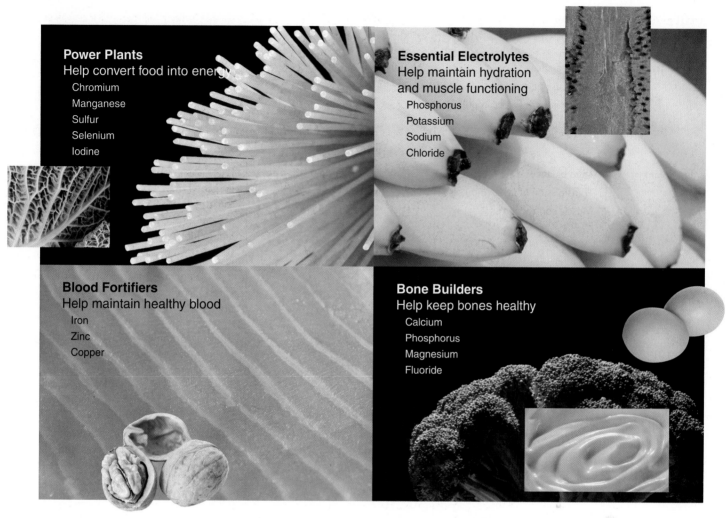

Power Plants
Help convert food into energy
Chromium
Manganese
Sulfur
Selenium
Iodine

Essential Electrolytes
Help maintain hydration
and muscle functioning
Phosphorus
Potassium
Sodium
Chloride

Blood Fortifiers
Help maintain healthy blood
Iron
Zinc
Copper

Bone Builders
Help keep bones healthy
Calcium
Phosphorus
Magnesium
Fluoride

FIGURE 7.1 The functions of the major and trace minerals. Good food sources are also shown for each functional group.

and copper. Table 7.2 on page 199 identifies major functions, recommended intakes, and food sources of these minerals.

Most Ultra-Trace Minerals Are of Uncertain Status

A number of **ultra-trace minerals** are found in our bodies, including boron, molybdenum, nickel, silicon, and others. They are classified as "ultra-trace" because researchers estimate that we have a dietary requirement of less than 1 mg/kg body weight for these minerals.[1] Of those just listed, only molybdenum is considered essential for human health.[1] This mineral is important for key enzymes within the body, and has an RDA of 45 µg/day for adults 19 to 70 years of age. Rich sources of molybdenum are legumes, grains, and nuts.[1] Many other ultra-trace minerals are thought to be important for health, but their exact role in the body is still not clear, and they have no DRI.

> RECAP *Minerals are solid, crystalline substances that do not contain carbon and are not changed by any natural means. We need to consume at least 100 mg per day of the major minerals, which include sodium, potassium, calcium, phosphorus, magnesium, sulfur, and chloride. We need to consume less than 100 mg per day of the trace minerals, which include selenium, fluoride, iodine, chromium, manganese, iron, zinc, and copper. Ultra-trace minerals are required in amounts lower than 1 mg / kg of body weight per day.*

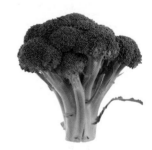

Many different foods provide minerals. Broccoli, for example, is a good source of calcium.

ultra-trace minerals Minerals we need to consume in amounts less than 1 mg/kg body weight per day.

TABLE 7.1 Major Minerals

Mineral Name	Primary Functions	Recommended Intake	Good Food Sources
Sodium	Fluid balance Acid–base balance Transmission of nerve impulses Muscle contraction	AI: Adults = 1.5 g/day (1,500 mg/day)	Table salt as sodium chloride. Processed foods, such as saltine crackers, pickles, chips, canned soups, salted nuts, and processed meats, where sodium chloride or another sodium additive has been added.
Potassium	Fluid balance Transmission of nerve impulses Muscle contraction	AI: Adults = 4.7 g/day (4,700 mg/day)	Fruits, such as bananas, oranges, grapefruit, dates, plums, and tomatoes and vegetables, such as potatoes, spinach, and beans (soy, lima, white, pinto).
Phosphorus	Fluid balance Bone formation Component of ATP, which provides energy for our bodies	RDA: Adults = 700 mg/day	Fish (e.g., halibut, salmon, walleye, tuna), dairy (e.g., milk, yogurt, ricotta cheese), grains and cereals (e.g., oat bran, barley, bulgur, enriched flours)
Chloride	Fluid balance Transmission of nerve impulses Component of stomach acid (HCl) Antibacterial	AI: Adults = 2.3 g/day (2,300 mg/day)	Consumed primarily as table salt (sodium chloride) and in processed foods where sodium chloride has been added.
Calcium	Primary component of bone Acid–base balance Transmission of nerve impulses Muscle contraction	AI: Adults aged 19 to 50 y = 1,000 mg/day Adults aged >50 y = 1,200 mg/day UL 2,500 mg	Regular and fortified dairy products such as milk, yogurt, milkshakes, and cheese, fortified juices, fish with bones (e.g., sardines or salmon), broccoli, kale, and collard greens.
Magnesium	Component of bone Muscle contraction Assists more than 300 enzyme systems	RDA: Men aged 19 to 30 y = 400 mg/day Men aged >30 y = 420 mg/day Women aged 19 to 30 y = 310 mg/day Women aged >30 y = 320 mg/day UL = 350 mg/day	Oysters, beef, pork, chicken, turkey, tuna, lobster, shrimp, salmon, milk, yogurt, whole-grain cereals (oatmeal, shredded wheat, all-bran, buckwheat and wheat flour, and fortified cereals), almonds, walnuts, sunflower seeds, and beans (e.g., lima, white, black, soy, navy).
Sulfur	Component of certain B vitamins and amino acids Acid–base balance Detoxification in liver	No DRI	Sulfur is found in protein sources of food.

Essential Electrolytes: Sodium, Potassium, Chloride, and Phosphorus

electrolyte A substance that dissociates in solution into positively and negatively charged ions and is thus capable of carrying an electric current.

ion Any electrically charged particle.

Recall from Chapter 2 that the interior of body cells contains fluid, and that many cells anchored together in a fluid bath make up our tissues. Dissolved in these cellular and tissue fluids are four major minerals: sodium, potassium, chloride, and phosphorus. There, these minerals are referred to as **electrolytes,** because they form charged particles called **ions,** which carry an electrical current. This electricity is

TABLE 7.2 Trace Minerals

Mineral Name	Primary Functions	Recommended Intake	Good Food Sources
Selenium	Required for carbohydrate and fat metabolism	RDA: Adults = 55 µg/day; UL = 400 µg/day	Brazil nuts, chicken and turkey, seafood (oysters, crab, herring, sardines, clams, tuna, halibut), pork, and grains (whole-wheat flour, barley and enriched grains).
Fluoride	Development and maintenance of healthy teeth and bones	RDA: Men = 4 mg/day; Women = 3 mg/day; UL: 2.2 mg/day for children aged 4 to 8 y; children > 8 y = 10 mg/day	Water that is naturally high in fluoride or to which fluoride has been added; fortified toothpaste and mouthwash.
Iodine	Synthesis of thyroid hormones Temperature regulation Reproduction and growth	RDA: Adults = 150 µg/day UL = 1,100 µg/day	Seafood (shrimp, tuna, lobster, seaweed), dairy products such as milk and yogurt, salt fortified with iodine.
Chromium	Glucose transport Metabolism of DNA and RNA Immune function and growth	AI: Men aged 19 to 50 y = 35 µg/day Men aged >50 y = 30 µg/day Women aged 19 to 50 y = 25µg/day Women aged >50 y = 20µg/day	Mushrooms, oysters, white wine, and apples.
Manganese	Assists many enzyme systems Synthesis of protein found in bone and cartilage	AI: Men = 2.3 mg/day; Women = 1.8 mg/day; UL = 11 mg/day for adults	Whole-grain products (oat bran, whole-wheat flour, bulgur, barley), nuts (pine nuts, hazelnuts, chestnuts, pecans), tea, pineapple, raspberries, beans, and vegetables (okra, spinach).
Iron	Component of hemoglobin in blood cells Component of myoglobin in muscle cells Assists many enzyme systems	RDA: Adult men = 8 mg/day Women aged 19 to 50 y = 18 mg/day Women aged >50 y = 8 mg/day	Clams, chicken, turkey, fish, and ham. Whole grains, fortified cereals, and beans also provide iron, but this plant-based iron is less absorbable.
Zinc	Assists more than 100 enzyme systems Immune system function Growth and sexual maturation Gene regulation	RDA: Men 11 mg/day Women = 8 mg/day UL = 40 mg/day	Meat and seafood, such as beef, pork, chicken, turkey, oysters, tuna, and lobster. Fortified cereals can also be good food sources of zinc.
Copper	Assists many enzyme systems Iron transport	RDA: Adults = 900 µg/day; UL = 10 mg/day	Organ meats, seafood (oysters, lobster, crab), whole-grain breads and cereals, chocolate, nuts and seeds.

the "spark" that stimulates nerves to transmit messages and causes muscles to contract and relax, so electrolytes are critical to nerve and muscle functioning. Serious electrolyte disturbances can impair the electrical stimulation of these tissues and lead to seizures and cardiac arrest.

Electrolytes are also critical to maintaining our fluid balance; that is, they keep our cells from becoming swollen with too much fluid or dehydrated from too little. Two qualities help electrolytes work together to control fluid balance: First, they all strongly attract water. Second, they are not able to move freely from one side of the cell membrane to the other. Instead, potassium and phosphate tend to remain inside our cells, and sodium and chloride tend to remain outside, in the tissue spaces. Although none of the electrolytes can move freely across the cell membrane, water

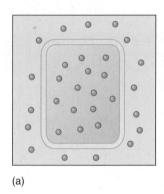
(a)

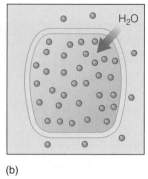
(b)

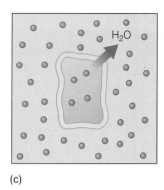
(c)

FIGURE 7.2 The health of the body's cells depends on maintaining the proper balance of fluids and electrolytes on either side of the cell membrane. (a) The concentration of electrolytes is the same on either side of the cell membrane. (b) The concentration of electrolytes is much greater inside the cell, drawing water into the cell and making it swell. (c) The concentration of electrolytes is much greater outside the cell, drawing water out of the cell and making it shrink.

can. Thus, the equal attraction for water of the electrolytes on either side of the cell membrane keeps our bodies in fluid balance (**FIGURE 7.2**).

When our electrolytes go out of balance, body fluids soon go out of balance as well. For instance, imagine a shipwrecked sailor in a lifeboat. With no fresh water to drink, he drinks seawater, which is of course high in sodium. This heavy load of sodium remains in the tissue spaces outside of his cells, where it strongly attracts water. Because the level of electrolytes inside the cells has not been increased, there is now a much greater concentration of electrolytes outside the cells. This higher concentration of electrolytes pulls water out of the cells into the tissue spaces (see Figure 7.2c). This leaves the cells dehydrated. The sailor's body then excretes the salty tissue fluid as urine, decreasing the total amount of water in his body. If the sailor continues to drink seawater, he will become so dehydrated that he will die.

Similarly, food poisoning, eating disorders, and other illnesses involving repeated vomiting and diarrhea can threaten the delicate balance of fluid inside and outside of our cells. With diarrhea or vomiting, the body loses a great deal of fluid from the intestinal tract and the tissue spaces outside of the cells. This heavy fluid loss causes the electrolyte concentration outside the cells to become very high. In response, a great deal of the interior fluid of the cells flows out. The resulting fluid and electrolyte imbalance alters the flow of electrical impulses through the heart, causing an irregular heart rate that can lead to death if left untreated.

The recommended intakes of the electrolytes and other major minerals are identified in Table 7.1.

> RECAP *The major minerals sodium, potassium, chloride, and phosphorus are called electrolytes, because when they dissolve in water, they form electrically charged particles called ions, which can carry an electrical current. Electrolytes assist in nerve transmission, muscle contraction and relaxation, and regulation of fluid balance. Repeated diarrhea or vomiting can threaten fluid balance.*

Sodium Is Part of Table Salt

Many people equate sodium with table salt, but in truth, those crystals in your salt shaker are made up of both sodium and chloride. Over the past 20 years, researchers have linked high sodium intake to an increased risk for high blood pressure. Because of this link, many people have come to believe that sodium is harmful to the body. This simply is not true: sodium is an essential nutrient that the body needs to survive. We'll explore the link between sodium and high blood pressure shortly.

Many popular snack foods are high in sodium.

Why Do We Need Sodium?

Sodium is a major mineral with many functions. As discussed, it helps cells maintain proper fluid balance. It also helps regulate blood pressure and acid–base balance. Along with the other electrolytes, sodium assists with the transmission of nerve signals and aids in muscle contraction and relaxation. Finally, sodium assists in the absorption of certain nutrients, such as glucose.

In addition to its functions in the body, sodium in table salt enhances the flavor of foods. It is also a powerful antimicrobial: for thousands of years, it has been used to preserve meats and other foods from spoilage.

How Much Sodium Should We Consume?

Virtually all of the sodium we consume in our diets is absorbed by the body. To give you a sense of how little sodium we need each day, consider that the AI (1,500 mg) is a little more than half a teaspoon! Most people in the United States greatly exceed this amount, consuming between 3,000 and 6,000 mg of sodium per day.

Sodium is found naturally in many foods, and processed foods typically contain added sodium. Try to guess which of the following foods contains the most sodium: 1 cup of tomato juice, 1 oz of potato chips, or four saltine crackers. Now look at Table 7.3 to find the answer. Are you surprised to discover that of all of these food items, the tomato juice has the most sodium? Lots of processed foods, such as lunchmeats, canned soups and beans, vegetable juices, and prepackaged rice and pasta dishes, are very high in sodium, as are many snack foods and fast foods, not to mention many dishes served in college cafeterias!

Excessive sodium intake can contribute to high blood pressure, clinically known as *hypertension*. This disorder, which is characterized by above-average blood pressure readings, increases the risk for heart disease, stroke, and kidney disease. Normally our body can make adjustments to compensate for a high sodium diet because the kidneys excrete the excess sodium in the urine. But in some individuals, the body is unable to make adjustments to compensate for a high sodium intake and blood pressure increases.

Hypertension is more common in people who consume high-sodium diets, but whether high-sodium diets can actually *cause* hypertension is the subject of some controversy. Research into hypertension funded by the National Institutes of Health (NIH) has led to the development of the DASH diet, an eating plan shown to reduce hypertension. DASH stands for "Dietary Approaches to Stop Hypertension" and includes recommendations for consuming 8 to 10 servings of fruits and vegetables daily, as well as limiting dietary sodium; for example, the lowest-sodium version of the DASH diet recommends 1,500 mg of sodium per day. The DASH diet has been

TABLE 7.3   High-Sodium Foods and Lower-Sodium Alternatives

High-Sodium Food	Sodium (mg)	Lower-Sodium Food	Sodium (mg)
Dill pickle (1 large, 4 in.)	1,181	Low-sodium dill pickle (1 large, 4 in.)	12
Ham, cured, roasted (3 oz)	1,128	Pork, loin roast (3 oz)	48
Corn beef (3 oz)	1,110	Beef chuck roast, cooked (3 oz)	40
Tomato juice, regular (one cup)	680	Tomato juice, lower sodium (1 cup)	141
Tomato sauce, canned (1/2 cup)	642	Fresh tomato (1 medium)	6
Canned cream corn (1 cup)	730	Cooked corn, fresh (1 large ear), boiled	0
Tomato soup, canned (1 cup)	675	Low-sodium tomato soup, canned (1 cup)	60
Potato chips, salted (1 oz)	149	Baked potato, unsalted (1 med)	17
Saltine crackers (4 each)	256	Saltine crackers, unsalted (4 each)	92

Source: U.S. Department of Agriculture, Agricultural Research Service. 2007. USDA Nutrient Database for Standard Reference, Release 20. Nutrient Data Laboratory Home Page. Available at www.ars.usda.gov/nutrientdata. Accessed February 2008.

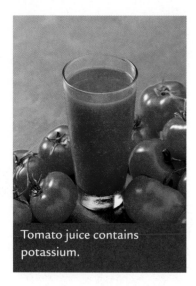

Tomato juice contains potassium.

shown to significantly reduce blood pressure, with the greatest reductions in people following the lowest-sodium version.[2] For more information on the DASH diet, visit the National Institutes of Health Web site at www.nih.gov.

Also controversial is the effect of high sodium intake on bone loss. In some people, consuming too much sodium causes the body to increase its excretion of calcium in the urine. This in turn may increase these people's risk for bone loss; however, the extent to which excess sodium intake affects bone health is unclear.[3] We do know that consuming excessive sodium causes water retention (bloating), as water is pulled from inside the cells into the tissue spaces to dilute the sodium.

Because dietary sodium intake is so high in the United States, deficiencies are extremely rare, except in individuals who sweat heavily or consume little or no sodium in the diet. Nevertheless, certain conditions can cause dangerously low blood sodium levels, called *hyponatremia*. Severe diarrhea, vomiting, or excessive prolonged sweating can result in hyponatremia, and infants can develop it if fed overly diluted formula. It can also occur in people who drink large volumes of water during intense exercise and fail to replace sodium. Symptoms include headaches, dizziness, fatigue, nausea, vomiting, and muscle cramps. If hyponatremia is left untreated, it can lead to seizures, coma, and death. Chapter 8 discusses hyponatremia in more detail.

If you're interested in reducing your sodium intake, what's the best way to start? Check out the accompanying Game Plan: Tips for Sparing the Salt.

Potassium Helps Maintain Healthful Blood Pressure

The major mineral potassium is a component of all living cells and is found in both plants and animals. About 85% of dietary potassium is absorbed, and as with sodium, the kidneys work to regulate its level in our blood. Most excretion of potassium occurs in the urine, with some excretion also in the feces.

Potassium is a primary electrolyte within our cells, where it balances the sodium outside the cell membrane to maintain proper fluid balance. Like sodium, potassium plays a major role in regulating the contraction of muscles and transmission of nerve impulses, and it assists in maintaining blood pressure. In contrast to a high-sodium diet, eating a diet high in potassium actually helps maintain a lower blood pressure.

The best sources of potassium include fresh foods, particularly fresh fruits and vegetables (FIGURE 7.3). Processing foods generally increases their sodium and

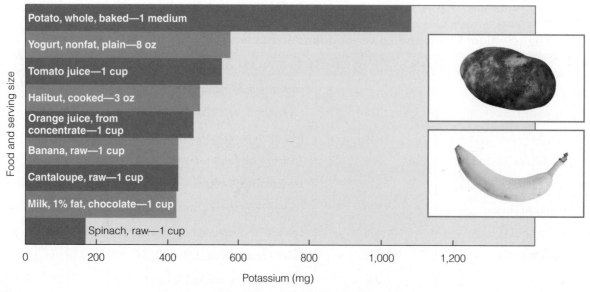

FIGURE 7.3 Common food sources of potassium. The AI for potassium is 4.7 g/day. (Data from U.S. Department of Agriculture, Agricultural Research Service. 2007. USDA Nutrient Database for Standard Reference, Release 20. Nutrient Data Laboratory Home Page. www.ars.usda.gov/nutrientdata.)

GAME PLAN
Tips for Sparing the Salt

If you've decided to try to reduce your intake of sodium, you're probably thinking that the first step is to hide the salt shaker. You're right—limiting the salt you add to foods *is* important! You can train your taste buds to prefer less salt by gradually reducing the amount you use over a period of several weeks to months. If you try this, you might be surprised at how quickly chips, soups, and other foods you once enjoyed start to taste much too salty.

Still, the majority of the sodium in our diet comes from processed food; in other words, from salt that you might not even realize is there. So the next step in reducing your sodium consumption is to shop for fresh whole foods and cook them with less salt. Here are some tips to get you started.

When Shopping

Next time you stock up on processed foods, keep the following shopping tips in mind:

❑ Look for the words "low sodium" on the label, and a sodium amount no higher than 200 mg per serving on the Nutrition Facts panel.

❑ When possible, choose low-sodium alternatives to the following high-sodium foods:

- canned beans, soups, gravies, pasta sauces, soy sauce, other sauces, vegetables, and vegetable juices
- packaged pasta dishes, rice dishes, and potato dishes
- frozen entrees, frozen dinners, frozen pizza, and other frozen meals
- smoked meats and fish
- cheese
- pickles, olives, three-bean salad, salad dressing
- snack foods, such as crackers, cookies, potato chips, pretzels, popcorn, and salted nuts

When Cooking

❑ When you have time for a home-cooked meal, take these steps to limit your sodium intake:

❑ Challenge yourself to use primarily fresh ingredients. For instance, try preparing pasta with fresh tomatoes, instead of prepared pasta sauce.

❑ When using canned beans, rinse them with cold water before heating.

❑ Experiment with salt substitutes.

❑ Substitute herbs or spices for salt. The American Dietetic Association identifies the following as particularly useful in low-sodium cooking:[4]

- **Basil:** fish, lamb, salads, soups, and sauces
- **Cayenne pepper:** soups, casserole, cheese sauces, baked egg dishes, barbequed poultry, and lean meats
- **Cinnamon:** pork, breads, sweet potatoes, squash
- **Cumin:** chili, stews, and beans
- **Curry:** meat, chicken, and fish dishes, and rice
  Dill: fish, chicken, vegetables, potatoes, salads, and pasta
- **Garlic:** lean meats, fish, poultry, soups, salads, vegetables, pasta dishes
- **Lemon or lime juice:** fish, poultry, salads, vegetables, sauces
- **Mint:** salads, potatoes, bulgur, beans
- **Rosemary:** chicken, fish, sauces, stuffing, potatoes, peas
- **Tarragon:** chicken, soups

❑ Add ginger or chilies to a stir-fry.

❑ Use cooking wine for meat, poultry, or fish.

❑ Avoid using the "salt" version of any spice, such as garlic salt.

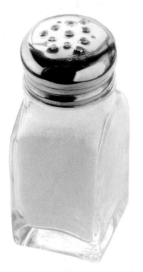

Almost all chloride is consumed through table salt.

decreases their potassium. You can boost your potassium intake and reduce your sodium intake by avoiding processed foods and eating more fresh fruits, vegetables, and whole grains. Most salt substitutes are made from potassium chloride, and these products contain relatively high amounts of potassium.

People with healthy kidneys are able to excrete excess potassium effectively, so toxicity in healthy people is rare. Because potassium is widespread in many foods, a dietary potassium deficiency is also rare. However, potassium deficiency is not uncommon among people who have serious medical disorders, including kidney disease. Extreme dehydration, vomiting, and diarrhea can also cause deficiency, as can abuse of alcohol or laxatives, and use of certain types of diuretics (medications that increase the body's excretion of fluid). Symptoms of potassium deficiency include confusion, loss of appetite, and muscle weakness. Severe deficiency results in fatal changes in heart rate; many deaths attributed to extreme dehydration or to an eating disorder are caused by abnormal heart rhythms due to potassium deficiency.

Chloride Assists Fluid Balance, Digestion, and Nerve Function

Chloride is a major mineral that we obtain almost exclusively from consuming sodium chloride, or table salt. It should not be confused with *chlorine,* which is a poisonous gas used to kill bacteria and other germs in our water supply.

Coupled with sodium in the fluid outside our cells, chloride assists with the maintenance of fluid balance. Chloride is also a part of hydrochloric acid in the stomach, which aids in digesting food (see Chapter 2). Chloride also works with our white blood cells during an immune response to help kill bacteria, and it assists in the transmission of nerve impulses.

Although our primary dietary source of chloride is the salt in our foods, chloride is also found in some fruits and vegetables. As noted earlier, consuming too much salt over a prolonged period leads to hypertension in salt-sensitive individuals. There is no known toxicity symptom for chloride alone. Deficiency is rare, because of the relatively high dietary salt intake in North America. Even when a person consumes a low-sodium diet, chloride intake is usually adequate. A chloride deficiency can occur, however, during conditions of severe dehydration and frequent vomiting.

Phosphorus Assists Fluid Balance

Phosphorus is pooled with potassium in the fluid inside our cells, where it helps to maintain proper fluid balance. As we discuss later in this chapter, phosphorus also plays a critical role in bone formation. FIGURE 7.4 identifies the phosphorus content of some common foods.

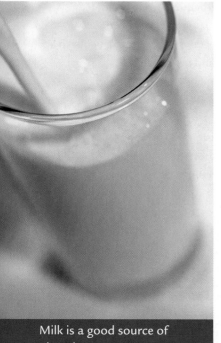

Milk is a good source of phosphorus.

> RECAP *Sodium is a major mineral and is prominent in the fluid outside of cells. Excessive sodium intake has been related to high blood pressure, bloating, and loss of bone density in some studies. Potassium is a major mineral within cells. It helps regulate fluid balance, blood pressure, and neuromuscular function. Chloride is a major mineral pooled together with sodium outside of the cell. It assists with maintaining fluid balance, aids digestion of food, and assists in immunity and neuromuscular function. Phosphorus is another major mineral within our cells. It helps maintain fluid balance and is critical to healthy bones.*

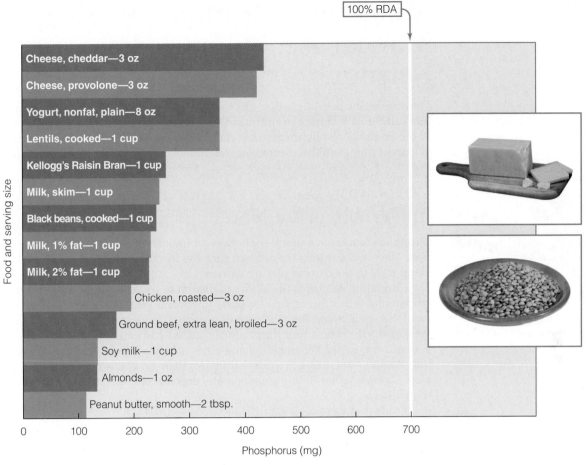

FIGURE 7.4 Common food sources of phosphorus. The AI for phosphorus is 700 mg/day. (Data from U.S. Department of Agriculture, Agricultural Research Service. 2007. USDA Nutrient Database for Standard Reference, Release 20. Nutrient Data Laboratory Home Page. www.ars.usda.gov/nutrientdata.)

NUTRI-CASE JUDY

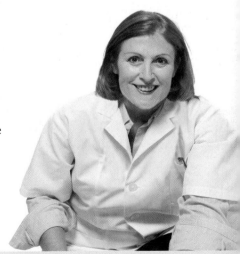

"I've noticed that every time I eat salty foods, I get bloated. With my weight problem, the last thing I need is to retain water. So I've put myself on a strict no-salt diet! I moved the salt shaker to the highest shelf in my kitchen so I won't be tempted to use it, and when I sit down to lunch in the cafeteria at work, the first thing I do is move the salt shaker to another table."

What do you think of Judy's strategy for maintaining a "no-salt diet"? Will the steps she has taken ensure her success, and is her goal wise?

Mineral Power Plants: Chromium, Manganese, Sulfur, Iodine, and Selenium

Many minerals help our bodies use the nutrients in foods by assisting their transport into cells or by helping the enzymes that break down foods into energy. Others assist in the production of hormones that regulate metabolic processes. These minerals are discussed here, and their recommended intakes are listed in Tables 7.1 and 7.2.

Chromium Plays an Important Role in Carbohydrate Metabolism

Chromium is a trace mineral that plays an important role in carbohydrate metabolism. You may be interested to learn that the chromium in our bodies is the same metal used in the chrome plating for cars.

Chromium enhances the ability of insulin to transport glucose from the bloodstream into cells. Chromium also plays important roles in the metabolism of RNA and DNA, in immune function, and in growth. Chromium supplements have been marketed with claims that they reduce body fat and enhance muscle mass. This marketing has targeted bodybuilders and other athletes interested in improving their body composition. Refer to the Nutrition Myth or Fact? box on page 208 to learn more about whether taking supplemental chromium is effective in improving body composition.

Foods that have been identified as good sources of chromium include mushrooms, prunes, dark chocolate, nuts, whole grains, cereals, asparagus, brewer's yeast, some beers, and red wine. There appears to be no toxicity related to consuming chromium in the diet or in supplement form. Chromium deficiency appears to be uncommon in the United States.

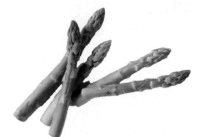

Asparagus is a good dietary source of chromium.

Manganese Assists in Energy Metabolism, Oxidation, and Many Other Processes

A trace mineral, manganese is involved in energy metabolism and in the formation of urea, the primary component of our urine. It also assists in the synthesis of bone tissue and cartilage, a tissue supporting our joints. Manganese also helps protect our bodies from oxidative damage.

Common food sources of manganese are listed in FIGURE 7.5. Manganese toxicity can occur in occupational environments in which people inhale manganese dust and can also result from drinking water high in manganese. Toxicity results in impairment of the neuromuscular system, causing muscle spasms and tremors. Manganese deficiency is rare in humans.

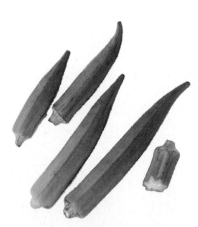

Okra is one of the many foods that contain manganese.

Sulfur Is a Component of Thiamin and Biotin and Helps Stabilize Proteins

Sulfur is a major mineral and a component of the B-vitamins thiamin and biotin. In addition, as part of the amino acids methionine and cysteine, sulfur helps the proteins in our bodies maintain their three-dimensional shapes. The liver requires sulfur to assist in the detoxification of alcohol and various drugs, and sulfur assists us in maintaining acid–base balance.

Our bodies are able to make all the sulfur we need using the amino acids in the protein-containing foods we eat; as a result, we do not need to consume sulfur in the diet, and there is no DRI for sulfur. There are no known toxicity or deficiency symptoms associated with sulfur.

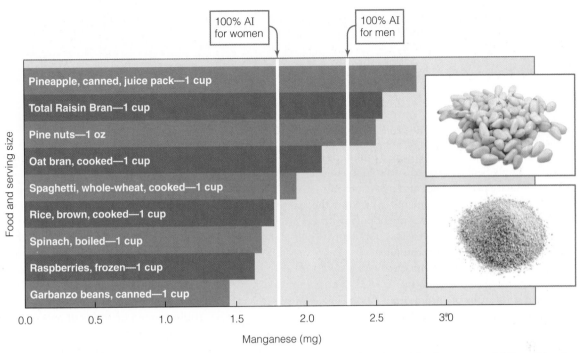

FIGURE 7.5 Common food sources of manganese. The AI for manganese is 2.3 mg/day for men and 1.8 mg/day for women. (Data from U.S. Department of Agriculture, Agricultural Research Service. 2007. USDA National Nutrient Database for Standard Reference, Release 20. www.ars.usda.gov/nutrientdata.)

Iodine Helps Make Thyroid Hormone

Iodine is critical for the synthesis of thyroid hormones. Thyroid hormones are integral to the regulation of body temperature, maintenance of resting metabolic rate, and support of reproduction and growth.

Very few foods naturally contain iodine. Saltwater fish do have high amounts, because marine animals concentrate iodine from seawater. In our foods, iodine is mostly found in the form of iodide. Good sources include iodized salt and breads made with iodized salt, as well as milk and other dairy products. In the United States, iodine has been added to salt since early in the 20th century to combat iodine deficiency resulting from the poor iodine content of soils in this country. Approximately one-half teaspoon of iodized salt meets the entire adult RDA for iodine.

If you consume either too much or too little iodine, your body will stop manufacturing thyroid hormones, leading to *hypothyroidism,* or low levels of thyroid hormones. This causes enlargement of the thyroid gland, called **goiter,** which occurs when the thyroid gland attempts to produce more thyroid hormones (FIGURE 7.6).

Other symptoms of hypothyroidism are decreased body temperature, inability to tolerate cold environmental temperatures, weight gain, fatigue, and sluggishness. If a woman experiences iodine deficiency during pregnancy, her infant has a high risk of being born with a form of mental retardation referred to as **cretinism.** In addition to mental retardation, people with cretinism may suffer from stunted growth, deafness, and muteness.

Selenium Spares Vitamin E and Helps Make Thyroid Hormone

Selenium is a trace mineral found in varying amounts in soil and thus in the foods we eat. The selenium in our bodies is contained in amino acids. Like iodine, selenium is necessary for the production of thyroid hormones. It also works as an antioxidant

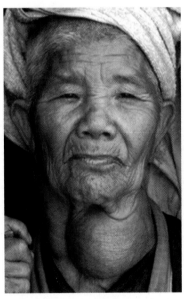

FIGURE 7.6 Goiter, or enlargement of the thyroid gland, occurs with both iodine toxicity and deficiency.

goiter Enlargement of the thyroid gland; can be caused by iodine toxicity or deficiency.

cretinism A form of mental retardation that occurs in individuals whose mothers experienced iodine deficiency during pregnancy.

NUTRITION MYTH OR FACT?

Do Chromium Supplements Enhance Body Composition?

Because athletes are always looking for a competitive edge, there are a multitude of supplements marketed and sold to enhance exercise performance and body composition. Chromium supplements, typically in the form of chromium picolinate, are popular with bodybuilders and weight lifters. This popularity stems from the claims that chromium increases muscle mass and muscle strength and decreases body fat.

An early study of chromium supplementation was promising, in that chromium use in both untrained men and football players was found to decrease body fat and increase muscle mass.[5] These findings caused a surge in popularity of chromium supplements and motivated many scientists across the United States to test the reproducibility of these early findings. The next study of chromium supplementation found no effects of chromium on muscle mass, body fat, or muscle strength.[6]

These contradictory reports led experts to closely examine these two studies and to design more sophisticated studies to assess the effect of chromium on body composition. There were a number of flaws in the methodology of these early studies. One major concern was that the chromium status of the research participants prior to the study was not measured or controlled. It was possible that the participants were deficient in chromium; this deficiency could cause a more positive reaction to chromium than would be expected in people with normal chromium status.

A second major concern was that body composition was measured in these studies using the skinfold technique, in which calipers are used to measure the thickness of the skin and fat at various sites on the body. While this method gives a good general estimate of body fat in young, lean, healthy people, it is not sensitive to small changes in muscle mass. Thus, subsequent studies of chromium used more sophisticated methods of measuring body composition.

The results of research studies conducted over the past 10 years consistently show that chromium supplementation has no effect on muscle mass, body fat, or muscle strength in a variety of groups, including untrained college males and females, obese females, collegiate wrestlers, and older men and women.[7–13] A recent review of 24 studies that examined the effect of 200 to 1,000 µg/d of chromium on body composition found no effect.[14] Despite the overwhelming evidence to the contrary, many supplement companies still claim that chromium supplements enhance strength and muscle mass and reduce body fat. These claims result in millions of dollars of sales of supplements to consumers each year. Armed with this information, you will be able to avoid being fooled by such an expensive nutrition myth.

SOLARAY®
DIETARY SUPPLEMENT
GTF Chromium
200 MCG.
FROM ORGANICALLY BOUND, TRIVALENT CHROMIUM YEAST WITH GLUCOSE TOLERANCE FACTOR
100 CAPSULES

to spare vitamin E and prevent oxidative damage to cell membranes. Its role in preventing heart disease and certain types of cancer is under investigation.

Organ meats and nuts are good sources of selenium. The selenium content of fruits and vegetables depends on the level in the soil in which they are grown. Selenium toxicity is rare.[15] Deficiency is associated with rare forms of heart disease and arthritis. See FIGURE 7.7 for a list of common food sources of selenium.

> RECAP *Chromium enhances the ability of insulin to transport glucose from the bloodstream into cells. Manganese is involved in energy metabolism and in the formation of urea, the primary component of our urine. Sulfur is a major mineral and a component of the B vitamins thiamin and biotin. Iodine and selenium assist in the synthesis of thyroid hormones, and selenium has antioxidant properties.*

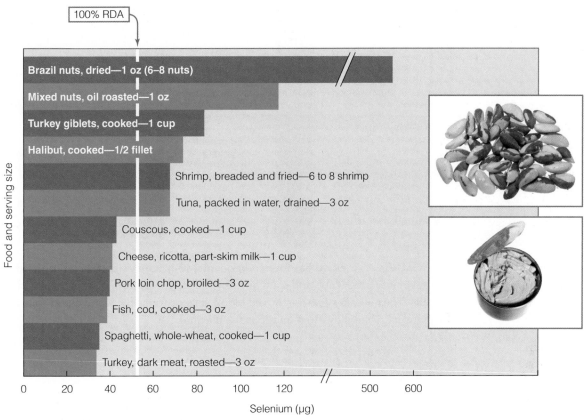

FIGURE 7.7 **Common food sources of selenium. The RDA for selenium is 55 µg per day.** (Data from U.S. Department of Agriculture, Agricultural Research Service. 2007. USDA Nutrient Database for Standard Reference, Release 20. Nutrient Data Laboratory Home Page. www.ars.usda.gov/nutrientdata.)

The Blood Fortifiers: Iron, Zinc, and Copper

Without healthy blood to transport nutrients and oxygen to our cells and to remove cellular wastes, we could not survive. Our health and our ability to perform daily activities are compromised if the quantity and quality of our blood is diminished.

Blood is made up of four components (FIGURE 7.8):

- Red blood cells (*erythrocytes*) are the cells that transport oxygen.
- White blood cells (*leukocytes*) protect us from infection and illness.
- Platelets are cell fragments that assist in the formation of blood clots and help stop bleeding.
- Plasma is the fluid portion of the blood and enables blood to flow easily through the blood vessels.

The nutrients recognized as playing a critical role in maintaining blood health include vitamin K, iron, zinc, and copper. We discussed how vitamin K assists blood clotting in Chapter 6. Here, we focus on the minerals iron, zinc, and copper. Recommended intakes of these minerals are identified in Table 7.2.

Iron Is a Key Component of the Blood Protein Hemoglobin

Iron is a trace mineral that is needed in very small amounts in our diets; nevertheless, it is present in every one of the millions of red blood cells in a single drop of blood.

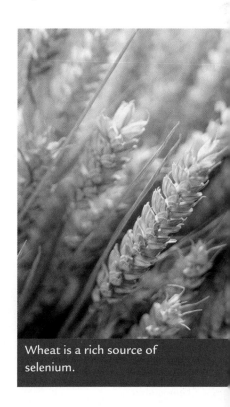

Wheat is a rich source of selenium.

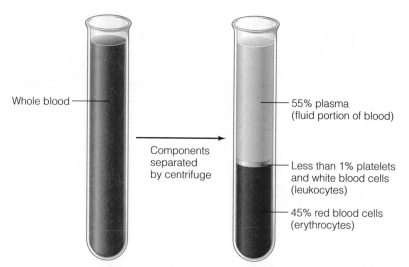

FIGURE 7.8 Blood has four components, which are visible when the blood is drawn into a test tube and spun in a centrifuge. The bottom layer is the red blood cells. The milky layer above the red blood cells contains the white blood cells and the platelets. The yellow fluid on top is the plasma.

Why Do We Need Iron?

Iron is critical to healthy blood because it is a key component of **hemoglobin,** which is the oxygen-carrying protein in our red blood cells. As shown in FIGURE 7.9, the hemoglobin molecule consists of four protein strands studded with four iron-containing **heme** groups. Hemoglobin depends on the iron in its heme groups to carry oxygen. In the bloodstream, iron acts as a shuttle, picking up oxygen from the air we breathe, binding it during its transport in the bloodstream, and then dropping it off again in our tissues.

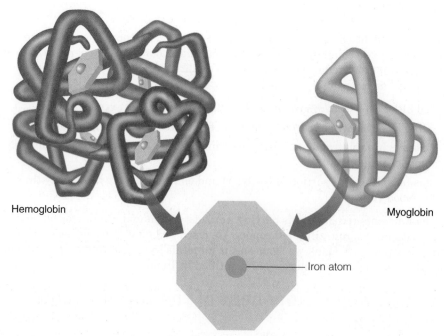

hemoglobin   The oxygen-carrying protein found in our red blood cells; almost two-thirds of all the iron in our bodies is found in hemoglobin.

heme   The iron-containing molecule found in hemoglobin.

FIGURE 7.9 Iron is contained in the heme portion of hemoglobin and myoglobin.

In addition to being a part of hemoglobin, iron is a component of **myoglobin,** an oxygen-binding protein that functions similarly to hemoglobin, but is found in muscle cells. As a part of myoglobin, iron assists in the transport of oxygen into muscle cells, which need oxygen to function.

Finally, iron is found in the body in certain enzymes. As a component of enzymes, it assists energy production from carbohydrates, fats, and protein. Also, iron is part of an antioxidant enzyme system that fights free radicals (discussed in Chapter 6). Interestingly, excessive iron in the body can also promote the production of free radicals.

What Factors Affect Iron Absorption?

The type of iron in the foods you eat is a major factor influencing your iron absorption—and therefore how much you need to eat. Two types of iron are found in foods:

- **Heme iron** is a part of hemoglobin and myoglobin and is found only in animal-based foods such as meat, fish, and poultry. Heme iron is readily absorbed by the body. Thus, animal-based foods are reliable sources of iron.
- **Non-heme iron** is not a part of hemoglobin or myoglobin. It is not easily absorbed by the body. Whereas animal-based foods contain both heme and non-heme iron, all of the iron found in plant-based foods is non-heme iron. This means that plant-based foods are less reliable than animal-based foods as sources of readily absorbed iron.

Two factors enhance the absorption of non-heme iron: Meat, poultry, and fish contain a special factor (called *meat protein factor,* or *MPF*) that enhances the absorption of the non-heme iron in these foods as well as in other foods eaten at the same meal. In addition, consumption of vitamin C (ascorbic acid) can greatly increase the body's absorption of non-heme iron. Thus, the non-heme iron in a bean burrito will be more fully absorbed if the burrito includes chopped tomatoes. Similarly, drinking a glass of orange juice with your breakfast cereal will increase the absorption of the non-heme iron in the cereal. Incidentally, cooking food in a cast-iron pan significantly increases the iron content of the food, as the iron in the pan is absorbed into the food during the cooking process.

Chemicals in certain foods impair iron absorption. These include phytates, which are binding factors found in legumes, rice, and whole grains; and polyphenols, chemicals present in black tea, coffee, and red wine. Soybean protein and calcium also inhibit iron absorption; thus, it is best to avoid drinking soy milk or cow's milk or taking calcium supplements when eating iron-rich foods.

Because of these dietary factors, it is estimated that only about 10% of the iron consumed in a vegan diet is absorbed by the body, while absorption averages 18% for a mixed Western diet.[16] For this reason, iron requirements are 1.8 times higher for vegetarians than for those who eat a mixed diet. This also means that people who eliminate meat, poultry, and fish from their diet are at a higher risk for anemia than those who eat animal-based foods. This risk is compounded for menstruating females; thus, supplementation or careful meal planning in consultation with a registered dietitian is advised.

What Are Iron Needs and Sources?

The iron requirement for young women is higher than for young men because of the iron and blood women lose during menstruation. Pregnancy is also a time of very high iron needs, and the RDA for pregnant women is 27 mg per day. A number of other circumstances significantly affect iron requirements. These are identified in Table 7.4.

Good food sources of heme iron include meats, poultry, and fish, especially clams and oysters. Enriched breakfast cereals and breads and some vegetables and legumes are good sources of non-heme iron. Your body's ability to absorb this non-heme iron can be enhanced by eating these foods with small amounts of meat, fish, or poultry or eating them with vitamin C–rich foods or beverages. FIGURE 7.10 identifies common food sources of iron.

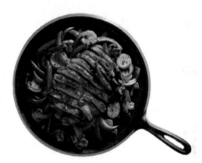

Cooking foods in cast-iron pans significantly increases their iron content.

myoglobin An iron-containing protein similar to hemoglobin, except that it is found in muscle cells.

heme iron Iron that is part of hemoglobin and myoglobin; found only in animal-based foods such as meat, fish, and poultry.

non-heme iron The form of iron that is not a part of hemoglobin or myoglobin; found in animal- and plant-based foods.

TABLE 7.4 Special Circumstances Affecting Iron Status

Circumstances That Improve Iron Status	Circumstances That Diminish Iron Status
Use of oral contraceptives—use of oral contraceptives reduces menstrual blood loss in women. **Breastfeeding**—breastfeeding delays resumption of menstruation in new mothers and so reduces menstrual blood loss. It is therefore an important health measure, especially in developing nations. **Consumption of iron-containing foods and supplements.**	**Use of hormone replacement therapy**—use of hormone replacement therapy in postmenopausal women can cause uterine bleeding, increasing iron requirements. **Eating a vegetarian diet**—vegetarian diets, particularly vegan diets, contain no sources of heme iron or MPF. Due to the low absorbability of non-heme iron, vegetarians have iron requirements that are 1.8 times higher than those of nonvegetarians. **Intestinal parasitic infection**—approximately 1 billion people suffer from intestinal parasite infection. Many of these parasites cause intestinal bleeding and occur in countries in which iron intakes are inadequate. Iron-deficiency anemia is common in people with intestinal parasitic infection. **Blood donation**—blood donors have lower iron stores than nondonors; people who donate frequently, particularly premenopausal women, may require iron supplementation to counter the iron losses that occur with blood donation. **Intense endurance exercise training**—people engaging in intense endurance exercise appear to be at risk for poor iron status due to many factors, including suboptimal iron intake and increased iron loss in sweat and increased fecal losses.

Source: From *Dietary Reference Intakes for Vitamin A, Vitamin K, Arsenic, Boron, Chromium, Copper, Iodine, Iron, Manganese, Molybdenum, Nickel, Silicon, Vanadium, and Zinc.* Reprinted with permission from the National Academies Press. © 2000 by the National Academy of Sciences.

What Happens If We Consume Too Much or Too Little Iron?

Some iron-containing supplements resemble colorful candies, and accidental iron overdose is the most common cause of poisoning deaths in children younger than 6 years of age in the United States.[17] It is important for parents to take the same precautions with dietary supplements as they would with other drugs, keeping them in a locked cabinet or well out of reach of children. Symptoms of iron toxicity include nausea, vomiting, diarrhea, dizziness, confusion, and rapid heart beat. If iron toxicity is not treated quickly, significant damage to the heart, central nervous system, liver, and kidneys can result in death.

Adults who take iron supplements even at prescribed doses commonly experience constipation. Taking vitamin C with the iron supplement not only enhances absorption but also can help reduce constipation.

Iron deficiency is the most common nutrient deficiency in the world. It results in **iron-deficiency anemia,** a disorder in which the red blood cells do not contain enough hemoglobin to deliver to the body's cells and tissues all the oxygen they need. Symptoms include exhaustion, increased risk of infection, and impaired thinking. Severe, chronic iron deficiency can cause premature death. People at particularly high risk include infants and young children, adolescent girls, menstruating women, and pregnant women. Chapter 12 provides more information about the impact of iron deficiency on people around the world.

iron-deficiency anemia
Disorder in which the production of normal, healthy red blood cells decreases and hemoglobin levels are inadequate to fully oxygenate the body's cells and tissues.

RECAP *Iron is a trace mineral that, as part of the hemoglobin protein, transports oxygen in our blood. Meat, fish, and poultry are good sources of heme iron, which is more absorbable than non-heme iron. Iron deficiency is the most common nutrient deficiency in the world.*

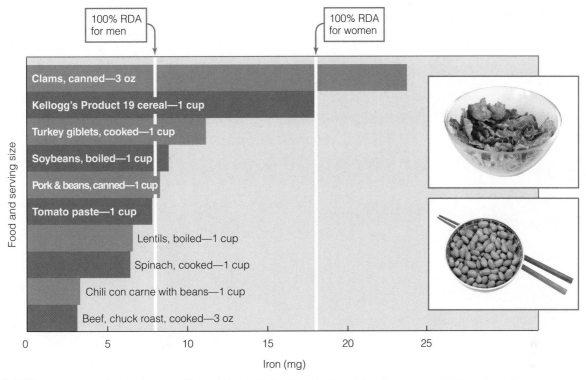

FIGURE 7.10   Common food sources of iron. The RDA for iron is 8 mg/day for men and 18 mg/day for women aged 19 to 50 years.
(Data from U.S. Department of Agriculture, Agricultural Research Service. 2007. USDA Nutrient Database for Standard Reference, Release 20. Nutrient Data Laboratory Home Page. www.ars.usda.gov/nutrientdata.)

Zinc Assists the Work of a Multitude of Different Enzymes

Zinc is a trace mineral that assists the work of approximately 100 different enzymes involved in many different tasks, including metabolism, the production of hemoglobin, and the activation of vitamin A in the retina of the eye. Zinc is also critical for normal growth. In fact, zinc deficiency was discovered in the early 1960s when researchers were trying to determine the cause of severe growth retardation in a group of Middle Eastern men.

Zinc also supports the proper development and functioning of the immune system. This role in immune functioning is behind the development of zinc lozenges, which manufacturers say help fight the common cold. The Nutrition Myth or Fact? box on page 215 explores the question of whether or not these are effective.

As with iron, our need for zinc is relatively small, but our absorption is variable. High non-heme iron intake can inhibit zinc absorption. This is a serious concern for anyone taking iron supplements (which are composed of non-heme iron), but especially for pregnant women, in whom zinc is essential for normal fetal growth. Thus, consultation with a registered dietitian may be advisable. Zinc absorption is also a concern for many vegetarians, whose diets are typically rich in non-heme iron. In addition, vegetarians tend to consume plentiful whole grains and beans: these foods contain phytates and fiber, both of which also inhibit zinc absorption. When whole grains are made into bread using yeast, the yeast produces an enzyme that breaks down the phytates. Thus, the zinc in whole-grain breads is more available for absorption than that found in breakfast cereals. In contrast, high intakes of heme iron appear to have no effect on zinc absorption, and dietary protein, especially animal-based protein, enhances zinc absorption.

Good food sources of zinc include red meats, some seafood, whole-grain breads, and enriched foods. As shown in FIGURE 7.11, zinc is significantly

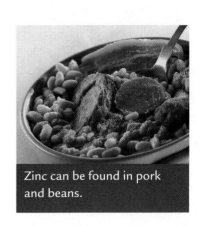

Zinc can be found in pork and beans.

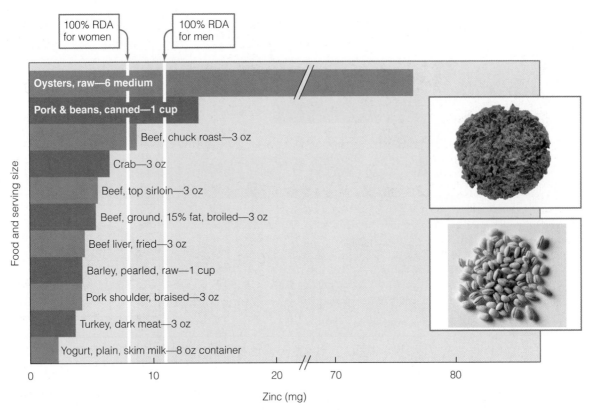

FIGURE 7.11 Common food sources of zinc. The RDA for zinc is 11 mg/day for men and 8 mg/day for women. (Data from U.S. Department of Agriculture, Agricultural Research Service. 2007. USDA Nutrient Database for Standard Reference, Release 20. Nutrient Data Laboratory Home Page. www.ars.usda.gov/nutrientdata.)

more absorbable from animal-based foods; thus, zinc deficiency is a concern for vegetarians.

Eating high amounts of dietary zinc does not appear to lead to toxicity. Zinc toxicity can occur from consuming zinc in supplement form and in fortified foods. Toxicity symptoms include intestinal pain and cramps, nausea, vomiting, loss of appetite, diarrhea, and headaches. Excessive zinc supplementation has also been shown to depress immune function. High intakes of zinc can also reduce the absorption of copper.

In addition to growth retardation, symptoms of zinc deficiency include diarrhea, delayed sexual maturation and impotence, eye and skin lesions, hair loss, and impaired appetite. Because zinc is critical to a healthy immune system, zinc deficiency also results in increased incidence of infections and illnesses.

Copper Helps Transport Iron and Build Tissues

Copper is a component of *ceruloplasmin,* a protein that is critical for the proper transport of iron. If ceruloplasmin levels are inadequate, iron accumulation results and can lead to iron toxicity. Copper also contributes to blood tissue, collagen, and the tissue surrounding nerve fibers. It is part of several enzyme systems and contributes to chemicals called *neurotransmitters* that are important for transmitting nerve signals.

Copper is a trace mineral, and needs are very small. Nevertheless, high intakes of zinc or iron can reduce copper absorption and, subsequently, copper status. Good food sources of copper include organ meats, seafood, nuts, and seeds. Whole-grain foods are also relatively good sources (FIGURE 7.12).

The long-term effects of copper toxicity are not well studied in humans. Copper deficiency is rare.

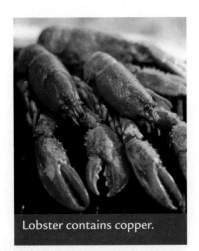

Lobster contains copper.

NUTRITION MYTH OR FACT?

Do Zinc Lozenges Help Fight the Common Cold?

The common cold has plagued human beings since the beginning of time. Children suffer from 6 to 10 colds each year, and adults average 2 to 4 per year. Although colds are typically benign, they result in significant absenteeism from school and work and cause discomfort and stress. It is estimated that more than 200 different viruses can cause a cold, so developing vaccines or treatments for colds is extremely challenging. Nevertheless, researchers continue to attempt to search for a cure for the common cold.

The role of zinc in the health of our immune system is well known. When zinc was specifically shown to inhibit the reproduction of viruses that cause the common cold, some researchers began speculating that taking zinc supplements might reduce the length and severity of colds.[18] Consequently, zinc lozenges were formulated as a means of providing potential relief from cold symptoms. These lozenges are readily found in most drugstores.

Does taking zinc in lozenge form actually reduce the length and severity of a cold? During the past 20 years, numerous research studies have been conducted to try to answer this question. Unfortunately, the results of these studies are inconclusive: about half have found that zinc lozenges do reduce the length and severity of a cold, whereas about half have found that zinc lozenges have no effect on cold symptoms or duration.[19] Some reasons that various studies report different effects of zinc on a cold include:

- **Inability to truly "blind" participants to the treatment.** Because zinc lozenges have a unique taste, it may be difficult to truly "blind" the research participants as to whether they are getting zinc lozenges or a placebo. Knowing which lozenge they are taking could lead participants to report biased results.

- **Self-reported symptoms are subject to inaccuracy.** Many studies had the research participants self-report changes in symptoms, which may be inaccurate and influenced by mood and other emotional factors.

- **Wide variety of viruses that cause a cold.** Because more than 200 viruses can cause a cold, it is highly unlikely that zinc can combat all of these viruses. It is possible that people who do not respond favorably to zinc lozenges are suffering from a cold virus that does not respond to zinc.

- **Differences in zinc formulations and dosages.** The type of zinc formulation and the dosages of zinc consumed by study participants differed across studies, which may determine how quickly the zinc ions are delivered to the tissues in the mouth. These differences most likely contributed to various responses across studies. It is estimated that for zinc to be effective, at least 80 mg of zinc should be consumed each day, and that people should begin using zinc lozenges within 24 to 48 hours of onset of cold symptoms. Also, sweeteners and flavorings found in many zinc lozenges, such as citric acid, sorbitol, and mannitol, may bind the zinc and inhibit its ability to be absorbed into the body, limiting its effectiveness.

Have you ever tried zinc lozenges, and did you find them effective? Even if you only have about a 50% chance of reducing the length and severity of your cold by taking zinc lozenges, next time you feel a cold coming on, will you try them?

One word of caution: if you decide to use zinc lozenges, more is not better. Excessive or prolonged zinc supplementation can depress immune function and cause other mineral imbalances. Check the label of the product you are using, and do not exceed its recommended dosage or duration of use.

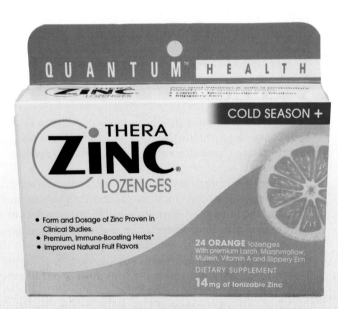

Zinc lozenges come in different formulations and dosages.

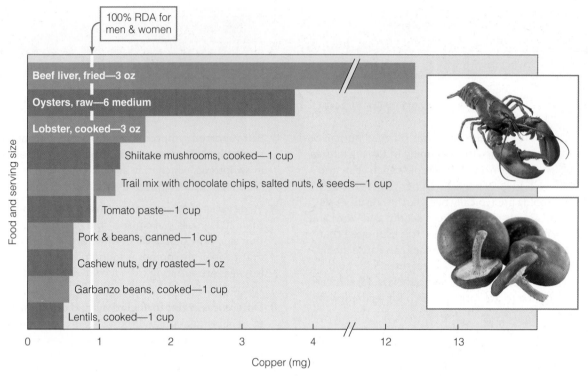

FIGURE 7.12 Common food sources of copper. The RDA for copper is 900 µg/day for men and women.
(Data from U.S. Department of Agriculture, Agricultural Research Service. 2007. USDA Nutrient Database for Standard Reference, Release 20. Nutrient Data Laboratory Home Page. www.ars.usda.gov/nutrientdata.)

> RECAP *Zinc is a trace mineral that is a part of almost 100 enzymes that affect virtually every body system. Zinc plays a critical role in hemoglobin synthesis, physical growth, sexual maturation, and immune function and assists in fighting the oxidative damage caused by free radicals. Copper is a trace mineral that is important in the transport of iron. It also contributes to several tissues and is part of several enzyme systems.*

The Bone Builders: Calcium, Phosphorus, Magnesium, and Fluoride

Contrary to what most people think, our skeleton is not an inactive collection of bones that simply holds the body together. Bones are living organs that contain several tissues, including bone tissue, nerves, cartilage, and connective tissue, with blood vessels supplying vital nutrients.

Bones have many functions. Structurally, they provide physical support and attachments for muscle movement, and they protect our most vulnerable tissues. Think of the hard shell that our skull forms around our delicate brain tissue, or the bony cage of ribs that protects the heart. Bones also act as "mineral banks," storing calcium, phosphorus, magnesium, and fluoride. When these minerals are needed for body processes, bone is broken down so that they can be released into our bloodstream. Also, did you know that most of our blood cells are formed deep within bones?

Given the importance of bones, it is critical we keep them strong. As we discuss shortly, four minerals—calcium, phosphorus, magnesium, and fluoride—help us maintain strong bones. The role of vitamin D in bone health is described in Chapter 6.

Bones Are Made of Minerals and Proteins

We tend to think of bones as totally rigid, but if they were, how could we play basketball or even carry an armload of books up a flight of stairs? Bones need to be both strong and flexible so they can resist the crunching, stretching, and twisting that occur throughout our daily activities. Fortunately, the composition of bone is ideally suited for its complex job. About 65% of bone tissue is made up of an assortment of minerals (mostly calcium and phosphorus) that provide hardness. These minerals form tiny crystals that cluster around *collagen fibers*—protein fibers that provide strength, durability, and flexibility. Collagen fibers are phenomenally strong; they are actually stronger than steel fibers of similar size. They enable bones to bear weight while responding to demands for movement.

If you examine a bone very closely, you will notice two distinct types of tissue (**FIGURE 7.13**): cortical bone and trabecular bone. **Cortical bone,** which is also called *compact bone,* is very dense. It composes approximately 80% of the skeleton. The outer surface of all bones is cortical; in addition, many small bones of the body, such as the bones of the wrists, hands, and feet, are made entirely of cortical bone.

In contrast, **trabecular bone** makes up only 20% of the skeleton. It is found within the ends of the long bones (such as the bones of the arms and legs) and inside the spinal vertebrae, skull, pelvis, and several other bones. Trabecular bone is sometimes referred to as *spongy bone,* because to the naked eye it looks like a sponge. The microscope reveals that trabecular bone is in fact aligned in a precise network of columns that protects the bone from extreme stress. You can think of trabecular bone as the bone's scaffolding.

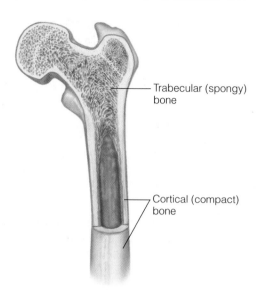

FIGURE 7.13 The structure of bone. Notice the difference in density between the trabecular (spongy) bone and the cortical (compact) bone.

How Do Bones Stay Healthy?

Although the shape and size of bones do not significantly change after puberty, **bone density,** or the strength of bones, continues to develop into early adulthood. *Peak bone density* is the point at which bones are strongest because they are at their highest density. About 90% of a woman's bone density is built by 17 years of age. For men, peak bone density occurs during their 20s. However, male or female, before we reach the age of 30 years, our bones have reached peak density, and by age 40, our bone density begins its irreversible decline.

Just as other body cells die off and are continually replaced, bone mass is regularly recycled. This process, called **remodeling,** involves two steps: the breakdown of existing bone and the formation of new bone (**FIGURE 7.14**). Bone is broken down by cells called **osteoclasts,** which erode the bone surface by secreting enzymes and acids that dig grooves into the bone matrix (see Figure 7.14a). New bone is formed through the action of cells called **osteoblasts,** or "bone builders" (see Figure 7.14b). These cells work to synthesize new bone matrix in the eroded areas.

In young healthy adults, bone building and bone breakdown occur at equal rates, resulting in bone mass being maintained. Around 40 years of age, bone breakdown begins to outpace bone formation, and this imbalance results in a gradual loss in bone density.

Achieving a high peak bone density requires adequate intake of the four minerals discussed in this section, and recommended intakes are identified in Tables 7.1 and 7.2. Adequate protein (see Chapter 5) and vitamins D and K (see Chapter 6) are also essential. In addition to nutrients, healthy bone density requires regular weight-bearing exercise, such as weight lifting, strength training, jumping rope, tennis, jogging and walking, and even doing jumping jacks, all of which appropriately stress the bones and stimulate their growth.

RECAP *Bones are composed of mineral crystals that cluster around collagen fibers. Bone tissue is recycled through a process called* remodeling, *in which osteoclasts break down old bone and osteoblasts lay down new bone.*

cortical bone (compact bone) A dense bone tissue that makes up the outer surface of all bones as well as the entirety of most small bones of the body.

trabecular bone (spongy bone) A porous bone tissue that is found within the ends of the long bones, and inside the spinal vertebrae, flat bones (breastbone, ribs, and most bones of the skull), and bones of the pelvis.

bone density The degree of compactness of bone tissue, reflecting the strength of the bones. *Peak bone density* is the point at which a bone is strongest.

remodeling The two-step process by which bone tissue is recycled; includes the breakdown of existing bone and the formation of new bone.

osteoclasts Cells that break down the surface of bones by secreting enzymes and acids that dig grooves into the bone matrix.

osteoblasts Cells that prompt the formation of new bone matrix by laying down the collagen-containing component of bone that is then mineralized.

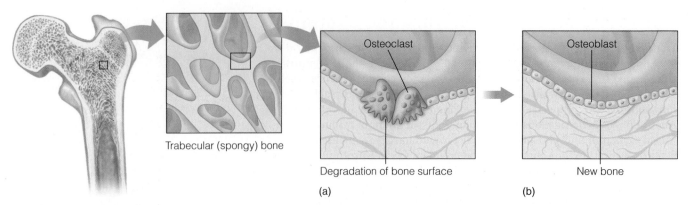

FIGURE 7.14 Bone remodeling involves breakdown and formation. (a) Osteoclasts break down bone, releasing minerals that are then transported to the bloodstream. (b) Osteoblasts work to build new bone by filling the pit formed by the erosion process with new bone.

Calcium Is a Key Component of Our Bones

Calcium is by far the most abundant major mineral in the body, composing about 2% of our entire body weight! Not surprisingly, it plays many critical roles in maintaining overall function and health.

Why Do We Need Calcium?

Calcium has four primary roles in the body. First, it provides structure to the bones and teeth. About 99% of the calcium found in the body is stored in the bones, packed into crystals built up on the collagen foundation. The remaining 1% of calcium in our bodies is found in the blood and soft tissues.

Calcium is alkaline, or basic, and because of this property it plays a critical role in assisting with acid–base balance. If the blood becomes acidic, osteoclasts begin to break down bone. This releases calcium into the bloodstream, making it more alkaline. It's important to consume enough dietary calcium to make sure it balances the calcium taken from the bones.

Calcium is also critical for the normal transmission of nerve impulses. When it flows into nerve cells, it stimulates the release of neurotransmitters, which transfer nerve impulses from one nerve cell to another. Without adequate calcium, the ability of nerves to transmit messages is inhibited. Not surprisingly, when blood calcium levels fall dangerously low, a person can experience seizures.

A fourth role of calcium is to assist in muscle contraction. Contraction of muscles is stimulated when calcium flows into the muscle cell. Muscles relax when calcium is pumped back outside of the muscle cell.

Other roles of calcium include the maintenance of healthy blood pressure, the initiation of blood clotting, and the regulation of various hormones and enzymes. As you can see, calcium is a versatile micronutrient.

How Much Calcium Is Absorbed?

The term **bioavailability** refers to the degree to which the body can absorb and use any given nutrient. Healthy young adults absorb about 30% of the calcium consumed in the diet, whereas older adults may absorb only 25%. This change in calcium absorption with aging explains the higher calcium recommendations for older adults.

The body cannot absorb more than 500 mg of calcium at any one time, and as the amount of calcium in a single meal or supplement goes up, the fraction that is absorbed goes down. Thus, it is important to consume calcium-rich foods throughout the day, rather than relying on a single high-dose supplement.

Dietary factors can also affect the absorption of calcium. Binding factors such as phytates and oxalates occur naturally in some calcium-rich seeds, nuts, grains, and vegetables such as spinach and Swiss chard. Such factors limit calcium absorption.

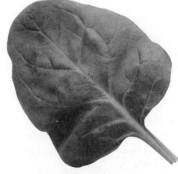

Although spinach contains high levels of calcium, binding factors in the plant prevent much of its absorption.

bioavailability The degree to which our bodies can absorb and use any given nutrient.

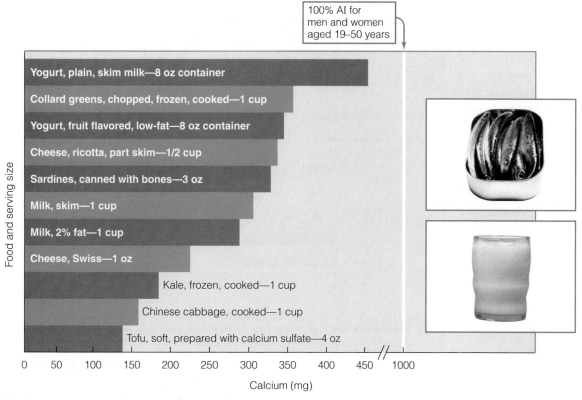

100% AI for men and women aged 19–50 years

Yogurt, plain, skim milk—8 oz container
Collard greens, chopped, frozen, cooked—1 cup
Yogurt, fruit flavored, low-fat—8 oz container
Cheese, ricotta, part skim—1/2 cup
Sardines, canned with bones—3 oz
Milk, skim—1 cup
Milk, 2% fat—1 cup
Cheese, Swiss—1 oz
Kale, frozen, cooked—1 cup
Chinese cabbage, cooked—1 cup
Tofu, soft, prepared with calcium sulfate—4 oz

Food and serving size

0   50   100   150   200   250   300   350   400   450   1000

Calcium (mg)

FIGURE 7.15 Common food sources of calcium. The AI for calcium is 1,000 mg/day for men and women aged 19 to 50. (Data from U.S. Department of Agriculture, Agricultural Research Service. 2007. USDA Nutrient Database for Standard Reference, Release 20. Nutrient Data Laboratory Home Page. www.ars.usda.gov/nutrientdata.)

Additionally, consuming calcium at the same time as iron, zinc, magnesium, or phosphorus has the potential to interfere with the absorption and use of all of these minerals. Finally, because vitamin D is necessary for the absorption of calcium, lack of vitamin D severely limits the bioavailability of calcium.

Dairy products are among the most common and best-absorbed sources of calcium in the U.S. diet. Skim milk, low-fat cheeses, and nonfat yogurt are excellent sources of calcium, and they are low in fat and energy. Cottage cheese is one dairy product that is a relatively poor source of calcium, most of which is lost in processing. Other food sources of absorbable calcium are canned fish with bones (providing you eat the bones) and green leafy vegetables such as kale, turnip greens, collard greens, broccoli, and Chinese cabbage (bok choy). These vegetables contain low levels of oxalates. Many beverages are now available fortified with calcium. For example, you can buy calcium-fortified orange juice, fruit punch, soy milk, and rice milk. Some dairies have even boosted the amount of calcium in their brand of milk. See FIGURE 7.15 for other common food sources of calcium.

How Can You Estimate Your Daily Calcium Intake?

Many people in the United States do not meet the DRI for calcium because they consume very few dairy-based foods and calcium-rich vegetables. At particular risk are menstruating women and girls. There are now quick, simple tools available to assist you in estimating your daily calcium intake. See FIGURE 7.16 for an example of an Internet-based calcium intake tool that Hannah completed to estimate her calcium intake.

What Happens If We Consume Too Much or Too Little Calcium?

In general, consuming extra calcium from food sources does not lead to significant toxicity symptoms in healthy people, because much of the excess calcium is excreted

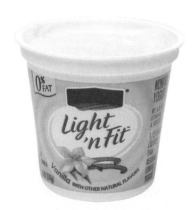

Low- and nonfat yogurts are excellent sources of calcium.

FIGURE 7.16 This graphic illustrates the results of a calcium intake quiz that Hannah completed. As you can see, Hannah did not meet her recommended calcium intake. To try this quiz yourself, go to www.dairycouncilofca.org/Tools/CalciumQuiz/default.aspx. (*Source:* Dairy Council of California. Copyright © 2008 Dairy Council of California. www.dairycouncilofca.org. Reprinted with permission.)

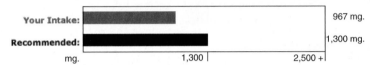

Calcium Quiz (Ca) what's your calcium intake?

Here is what you checked....

Item	No. of Servings	mg/Serving	Total mg
Milk (whole, low-fat or nonfat)	1.00	290	290.00
Cheese (Cheddar/ Monterey Jack types)	1.00	312	312.00
Blended coffee drinks (e.g. lattes, mochas, made with milk)	1.00	250	250.00
Ice cream	1.00	84	84.00
Broccoli	0.50	62	31.00

Hannah, you didn't quite meet your calcium requirement yesterday.

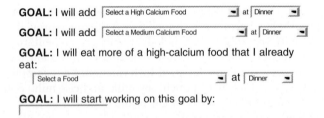

To meet your calcium needs, **you need 333 mg more calcium.** This is equivalent to 1.5 more serving(s) of calcium-rich (300 mg/serving) foods every day. An easy way to make sure you are getting enough calcium is to consume at least 3 servings of dairy foods every day.

Following are some suggestions for eating more calcium-rich foods, and easy ways to work them into your diet. Think about which ones you could do on a regular basis to increase your calcium intake to the recommended level for bone health, weight management and other benefits.

▲ Dip raw vegetables in yogurt
▲ Order a latte or cappuccino instead of your usual cup of morning coffee
▲ Drink a mug of hot cocoa on those chilly afternoons
▲ Eat a bean and cheese burrito for lunch
▲ Add kidney beans in your chili

Try Meals Matter's good source of calcium recipes and quick meals you and your family will enjoy.

Now that you know the number of calcium-rich foods you need to add to your diet and are familiar with some ways to incorporate them into your diet, set a plan to achieve your goal. You can either eat new calcium-rich foods or increase the amount of those that you are already eating.

GOAL: I will add [Select a High Calcium Food ▾] at [Dinner ▾]

GOAL: I will add [Select a Medium Calcium Food ▾] at [Dinner ▾]

GOAL: I will eat more of a high-calcium food that I already eat:
[Select a Food ▾] at [Dinner ▾]

GOAL: I will start working on this goal by:
[   ]

Take one last look at your new goal. Can you picture yourself really carrying it out? If not, what can you do to make it work? Think about the long-term benefits of getting enough calcium such as strengthening your bones, reducing blood pressure, improving weight loss and minimizing your risk of certain cancers. It might also help to tell someone about your plan so they can help support you. Print this page and put it where it will remind you of your plan.

Click here to take the Calcium Quiz again.

in urine and feces. However, excessive intake of calcium from supplements can lead to various mineral imbalances because calcium interferes with the absorption of other minerals, including iron, zinc, and magnesium. It can also cause constipation, as the body attempts to eliminate the excess calcium via the feces. Severe hypercalcemia (excessive calcium in the blood) can lead to death.

There are no short-term symptoms associated with consuming too little calcium. When dietary calcium is low, the body maintains blood calcium levels by taking calcium from the bones. The long-term consequence of inadequate calcium intake is osteoporosis. This disease is discussed in more detail beginning on page 223.

> RECAP *Calcium is the most abundant mineral in the body and a significant component of bones. Bone calcium is used to maintain normal blood calcium if dietary intake is inadequate. Calcium is also necessary for normal nerve and muscle function. Dairy foods, calcium-fortified juices and soy milk, and some dark-green leafy vegetables are excellent sources of calcium.*

Phosphorus Is Part of the Mineral Complex of Bone

As we mentioned earlier in this chapter, the major mineral phosphorus works with potassium inside of our cells to help maintain proper fluid balance. It also plays a critical role in bone formation, as it is a part of the mineral crystals that provide the hardness of bone. About 85% of the body's phosphorus is stored in bones, with the rest stored in soft tissues such as muscles and organs.

Additionally, phosphorus is a primary component of adenosine triphosphate (ATP), the energy molecule. It also helps activate and deactivate enzymes, and is a component of the genetic material in the cells (including both DNA and RNA), cell membranes, and lipoproteins.

Phosphorus is widespread in many foods and is found in high amounts in foods that contain protein (see Figure 7.4 on page 205). Milk, meats, and eggs are good sources. Phosphorus is also found in many processed foods as a food additive, where it enhances smoothness, binding, and moisture retention. In the form of phosphoric acid, it is also a major component of soft drinks. The consumption of soft drinks has been linked by many researchers to poor bone density. The most likely explanation for this link appears to be the *milk-displacement effect;* that is, soft drinks take the place of milk in our diets, depriving us of calcium and vitamin D.[20]

Severely high levels of blood phosphorus can cause muscle spasms and convulsions. Phosphorus deficiencies are rare but can occur in people who abuse alcohol, in premature infants, and in elderly people with poor diets.

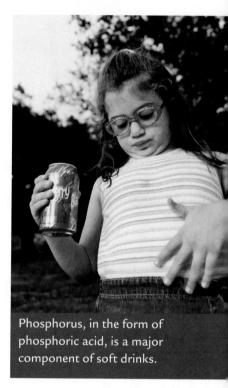

Phosphorus, in the form of phosphoric acid, is a major component of soft drinks.

Magnesium Is Found in Bones and Soft Tissues

Magnesium is a major mineral. About 50% to 60% of the magnesium in the body is found in bones, and the rest is in soft tissues. Magnesium influences the crystallization of bone through its regulation of calcium balance and its interactions with vitamin D and parathyroid hormone.

Magnesium assists more than 300 enzyme systems with roles in the production of ATP, as well as DNA and protein synthesis and repair. Magnesium also supports muscle contraction and blood clotting.

Magnesium is found in green leafy vegetables such as spinach and in whole grains, seeds, and nuts. Other good sources include seafood, beans, and some dairy products (FIGURE 7.17). The magnesium content of drinking water varies considerably: the "harder" the water, the higher its content of magnesium. As you know, dietary fiber is important to our health; however, the ability of the small intestine to absorb magnesium is reduced when we consume a diet that is very high in fiber because it binds with magnesium. Our absorption of magnesium should be sufficient if we consume the recommended amount of fiber each day (19 to 38 g per day depending on life stage and gender).

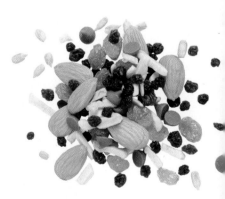

Trail mix with chocolate chips, nuts, and seeds is one common food source of magnesium.

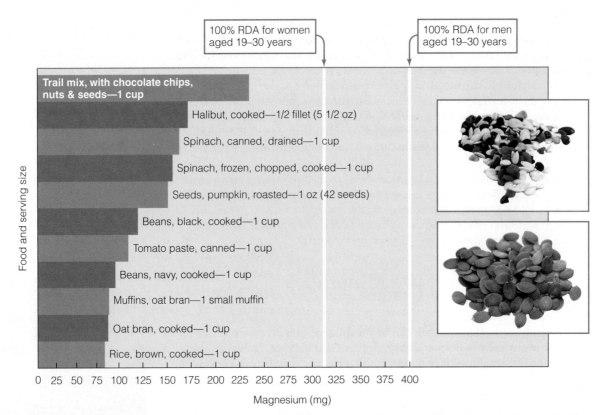

FIGURE 7.17 Common food sources of magnesium. For adult men 19 to 30 years of age, the RDA for magnesium is 400 mg/day; the RDA increases to 420 mg per day for men 31 years of age and older. For adult women 19 to 30 years of age, the RDA for magnesium is 310 mg per day; this value increases to 320 mg per day for women 31 years of age and older.
(Data from U.S. Department of Agriculture, Agricultural Research Service. 2007. USDA Nutrient Database for Standard Reference, Release 20. Nutrient Data Laboratory Home Page. www.ars.usda.gov/nutrientdata.)

Symptoms of magnesium toxicity include diarrhea, nausea, and abdominal cramps. In extreme cases, large supplemental doses can result in acid–base imbalances, massive dehydration, cardiac arrest, and death. Magnesium deficiency causes muscle cramps, spasms or seizures, nausea, weakness, irritability, and confusion. It may result from kidney disease, chronic diarrhea, or chronic alcohol abuse but is uncommon in healthy adults. Considering magnesium's role in bone formation, it is not surprising that long-term magnesium deficiency is associated with osteoporosis.

Fluoride Promotes the Development and Maintenance of Our Teeth and Bones

Fluoride is a trace mineral. About 99% of the fluoride in the body is stored in teeth and bones. During the development of both baby teeth and permanent teeth, fluoride combines with calcium and phosphorus to make teeth more resistant to destruction by acids and bacteria. Thus, teeth that have been treated with fluoride are better protected against dental caries (cavities) than teeth that have not been treated. Fluoride also stimulates new bone growth, and it is currently being researched as a potential treatment for osteoporosis.

The two primary sources of fluoride for people in the United States are fluoridated water and fluoridated dental products such as toothpastes and mouthwashes. Fluoride supplements are available only by prescription, and these are generally given only to children who do not have access to fluoridated water. Tea also contains significant amounts of fluoride independent of whether or not it was made with fluoridated water. There is epidemiological evidence that people who habitually consume tea (for more than 6 years) have significantly higher bone density values than people who are not habitual tea drinkers.[21]

Consuming too much fluoride increases the protein content of tooth enamel, resulting in a condition called **fluorosis.** Because increased protein makes the enamel more porous, the teeth become stained and pitted (FIGURE 7.18). Teeth seem to be at highest risk for fluorosis during the first 8 years of life. Mild fluorosis generally causes white patches on the teeth. Neither mild nor moderate fluorosis appears to impair tooth function.[22]

The primary result of fluoride deficiency is an increased risk for dental caries.[22] Adequate fluoride intake appears necessary at an early age and throughout adult life to reduce the risk for tooth decay. Inadequate fluoride intake may also be associated with lower bone density, but there is not enough research currently available to support the widespread use of fluoride to prevent osteoporosis.

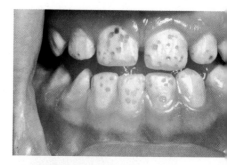

FIGURE 7.18 Consuming too much fluoride causes fluorosis, leading to staining and pitting of the teeth.

RECAP *The major mineral phosphorus helps maintain fluid balance and bone health and is found in many high-protein foods. Magnesium is a major mineral important for bone health, energy production, and muscle function and is found in a wide variety of foods. Fluoride is a trace mineral that supports the health of teeth and bones. Primary sources of fluoride are fluoridated dental products and fluoridated water.*

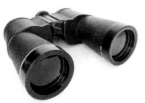

HEALTHWATCH
Are You at Risk for Osteoporosis?

Of the many disorders associated with poor bone health, the most prevalent in the United States is **osteoporosis.** The bone tissue of a person with osteoporosis is more porous and thinner than that of a person with healthy bone. These structural changes weaken the bone, leading to a significantly reduced ability of the bone to bear weight and a high risk for fractures (FIGURE 7.19).

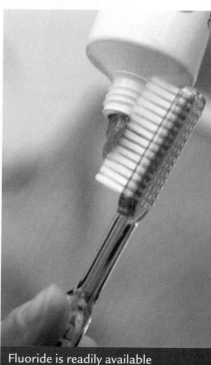

Fluoride is readily available in many communities in the United States through fluoridated water and dental products.

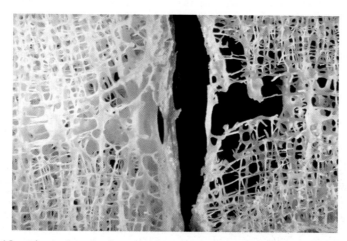

FIGURE 7.19 The trabecular bone within a vertebra of a person with osteoporosis (right) is thinner and more collapsed than the trabecular bone within a vertebra of a healthy person. Notice that the bone tissue on the left is more dense and uniform.

fluorosis A condition marked by staining and pitting of the teeth; caused by an abnormally high intake of fluoride.

osteoporosis A disease characterized by low bone mass and deterioration of bone tissue, leading to increased bone fragility and fracture risk.

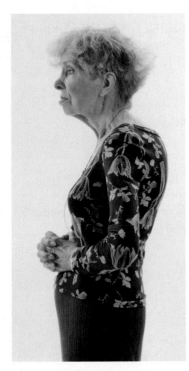

FIGURE 7.20 Gradual compression of the vertebrae in the upper back causes a shortening and rounding of the spine called *kyphosis.*

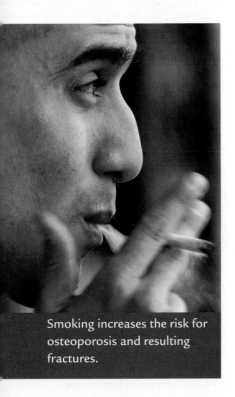

Smoking increases the risk for osteoporosis and resulting fractures.

Osteoporosis is the single most important cause of fractures of the hip and spine in older adults. These fractures are extremely painful and can be debilitating, with many individuals requiring nursing home care. In addition, they cause an increased risk of infection and other illnesses that can lead to premature death, as we saw with the dancer Erika Goodman in our chapter-opening story. In fact, about 24% of older adults who suffer a hip fracture die within 1 year after the fracture occurs.[23] Osteoporosis of the spine also causes a generalized loss of height and can be disfiguring: gradual compression fractures in the vertebrae of the upper back lead to a shortening and rounding of the spine called *kyphosis,* commonly referred to as *dowager's hump* (FIGURE 7.20).

Unfortunately, osteoporosis is a common disease: worldwide, one in three women and one in five men over the age of 50 are affected, and in the United States, more than 10 million people have been diagnosed.[24, 25]

Risk Factors for Osteoporosis

Factors that influence the risk for osteoporosis include:

- **Age.** As discussed previously in this chapter, bone density declines with age. Low bone mass and osteoporosis are therefore significant health concerns for both older men and women. The hormones estrogen in women and testosterone in men play important roles in promoting the deposition of new bone and limiting the activity of osteoclasts. When women go through menopause, estrogen and other reproductive hormones decrease. This decrease makes bone more sensitive to osteoclasts, and a gradual loss of bone mass occurs. Women can lose 20% of their bone mass during the first 5 to 7 years following menopause.[23] Both women and men can suffer from osteoporosis caused by such age-related hormonal changes. In addition, reduced levels of physical activity in older people and a decreased ability to metabolize vitamin D with age exacerbate the hormone-related bone loss.

- **Gender.** Osteoporosis disproportionately affects women: 80% of Americans with osteoporosis are women. This is because women have a lower bone density than men to begin with, and because the decline in estrogen is more significant than the decline in testosterone in men. Also, women live longer than men, and risk increases with age. Secondary factors that are gender-specific include social pressure on girls to be extremely thin, which can lead to amenorrhea (no menstrual period), which reduces the positive impact of estrogen on bone. Extreme dieting is particularly harmful in adolescence, when bone mass is building and adequate consumption of nutrients is critical. In contrast, men experience pressure to "bulk up," typically by lifting weights. This puts healthful stress on the bones, resulting in increased density.

- **Genetics.** Some individuals have a family history of osteoporosis, which increases their risk for this disease. Particularly at risk are Caucasian women of low body weight who have a first-degree relative (mother or sister) with osteoporosis. Asian women are also at high risk.

- **Smoking.** Cigarette smoking is known to decrease bone density because of its effects on hormones that influence bone remodeling; thus, cigarette smoking increases the risk for osteoporosis.

- **Nutrition.** Nutritional factors that appear to affect the risk for osteoporosis include caffeine, sodium, protein, calcium, vitamin D, and fruits and vegetables. Specifically, elderly women who consume high levels of caffeine (more than three cups of coffee per day) have much higher rates of bone loss than women with low intakes.[26] As mentioned earlier, high sodium intake is known to increase the excretion of calcium in the urine, but there is no direct evidence that a high-sodium diet causes osteoporosis. There appears to be an interaction between dietary calcium and protein, in that adequate amounts of each nutrient are needed together to support bone health. Because bones reach peak density when people are young, it is very important that children and adolescents consume a high-quality diet that contains the proper balance of calcium, vitamin D, protein, and other nutrients to allow for optimal bone growth. Also, diets high in fruits and vegetables are associated with improved bone health.[27, 28] This is most likely due to the fact that fruits and vegetables are good sources of nutrients that play a role in bone and collagen health, including magnesium, vitamin C, and vitamin K. Finally, chronic alcohol abuse is detrimental to bone health and is associated with high rates of fractures.

- **Physical activity.** Regular exercise is highly protective against bone loss and osteoporosis. Athletes are consistently shown to have more dense bones than nonathletes, and regular participation in a variety of weight-bearing exercises such as walking, jogging, tennis, and strength training can help increase and maintain bone mass. Exercise causes the muscles to contract and pull on bones; this stresses bone tissue in a healthful way that stimulates increases in bone density. Excessive physical activity can be harmful, however, especially in people who are not eating enough. Research has confirmed this association between poor nutrition, intense physical activity, and bone loss in the *female athlete triad,* a condition discussed in more detail in Chapter 9.

Are you at risk for osteoporosis? Check out the What About You? feature on page 226 to calculate your risk.

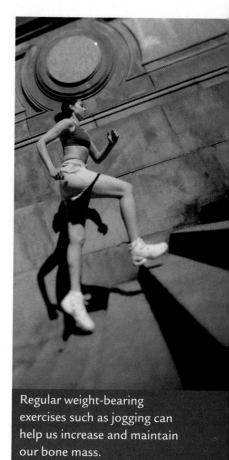

Regular weight-bearing exercises such as jogging can help us increase and maintain our bone mass.

NUTRI-CASE GUSTAVO

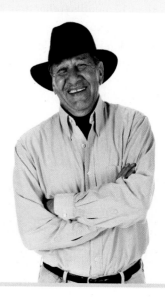

"When my wife, Antonia, broke her hip, I was shocked. You see, the same thing happened to her mother, but she was an old lady by then! Antonia's only 68, and she still seems young and beautiful—at least to me! As soon as she's better, her doctor wants to do some kind of scan to see how thick her bones are. But I don't think she has that disease everyone talks about! She's always watched her weight and keeps active with our kids and grandchildren. It's true she drinks coffee and diet colas, not milk, but that's not enough to make a person's bones fall apart, is it?"

What lifestyle factors increase Antonia's risk for osteoporosis? What risk factors are in her favor? Given what Gustavo has said about his wife's nutrition and lifestyle, do you think he should encourage her to have a bone density scan? Why or why not?

WHAT ABOUT YOU?

Calculate Your Risk for Osteoporosis

One in two women and one in four men will develop osteoporosis in their lifetimes.[23] But if you know you're at risk, you can take the steps identified in this chapter, such as increasing your weight-bearing exercise and making sure you get enough calcium and vitamin D, to maintain the maximum amount of bone mass possible. That's why it's important to assess your risk.

Following is a questionnaire adapted from the National Osteoporosis Foundation to determine your risk for developing osteoporosis. For each question, circle the appropriate answer. The more "yes" answers you have, the greater the likelihood that you're in a higher risk group than the general population.

- Do you have a small, thin bone structure and/or are you Caucasian or Asian?

  YES or NO

- Are you underweight?

  YES or NO

- Have you or a member of your immediate family broken a bone as an adult?

  YES or NO

- If you are female, have your periods stopped for more than 12 months (other than because of pregnancy)?

  YES or NO

- Have you taken high doses of thyroid medications or used glucocorticoids (for example, prednisone, cortisone) for more than 3 months?

  YES or NO

- Do you suffer frequently from diarrhea (caused by such chronic problems as celiac disease or irritable bowel syndrome)?

  YES or NO

- Is your diet low in dairy products and other sources of calcium?

  YES or NO

- Do you lead a sedentary lifestyle (engage in little physical activity most days)?

  YES or NO

- Do you smoke cigarettes?

  YES or NO

- Do you drink more than one alcoholic beverage per day (women) or two alcoholic beverages per day (men)?

  YES or NO

If you answered yes to any of these questions, it does not mean you have osteoporosis.[23] It does, however, suggest that you should discuss the quiz results with your doctor, who will advise you as to whether or not you should take a bone density test.

Source: Some questions taken from the National Osteoporosis Foundation. © 2005. Osteoporosis: Can It Happen to You? Available at www.nof.org. Reprinted by permission.

Treatments for Osteoporosis

Although there is no cure for osteoporosis, a variety of treatments can slow and even reverse bone loss. First, individuals with osteoporosis are encouraged to consume adequate calcium, vitamin D, vitamin K, and other bone-building nutrients and to exercise regularly. Studies have shown that the most effective exercise programs include weight-bearing exercises such as jogging, stair climbing, and resistance training.[29]

In addition, several medications are available that slow or stop bone breakdown but do not affect bone formation. This results in an overall reduction or cessation in the rate of bone loss. The use of *hormone replacement therapy* (HRT) for the prevention of osteoporosis in women is controversial. *HRT* reduces bone loss, increases bone density, and reduces the risk of hip and spinal fractures. However, side effects include breast tenderness, changes in mood, vaginal bleeding, and an increased risk for gallbladder disease. In addition, a recent study found that one type of HRT increases a woman's risk for heart disease, stroke, and breast cancer. Thus, a woman's decision regarding appropriate therapy must weigh the benefits of HRT in reducing fracture risk with the drawbacks of increased risk of other diseases.

RECAP *Osteoporosis increases the risk for fractures and premature death from subsequent illness. Factors that increase the risk for osteoporosis include genetics, being female, being of the Caucasian or Asian race, cigarette smoking, alcohol abuse, sedentary lifestyle, and diets low in calcium and vitamin D. Medications are available for the prevention and treatment of osteoporosis.*

Where I'm at now...

If you don't normally eat meat, poultry, and/or fish, jot down your plan for consuming adequate dietary iron each day:

Now that you've read this chapter, would you say you've been getting enough calcium most days?

Yes or NO

If NO, how do you plan to increase your calcium intake? (Check all that sound good to you):

- ☐ Drink milk or calcium-fortified beverages more often.
- ☐ Put extra milk in my coffee or tea.
- ☐ Eat more yogurt or cheese.
- ☐ Increase my intake of dark-green, leafy vegetables.
- ☐ Choose calcium-fortified cereals and energy bars.
- ☐ Take a calcium supplement.

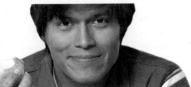

REVIEW QUESTIONS

Circle the correct choice.

1. Which of the following is true of the cell membrane?
   a. It is freely permeable to water and all electrolytes.
   b. It is freely permeable to all electrolytes but not to water.
   c. It is freely permeable to water but not to all electrolytes.
   d. It is impermeable.

2. Which of the following statements about iron is true?
   a. Iron is stored primarily in the heart muscle and skeletal muscles.
   b. Iron is a component of hemoglobin, myoglobin, and certain enzymes.
   c. Iron is a component of red blood cells, white blood cells, platelets, and plasma.
   d. Iron needs are higher for elderly women than for young women.

3. Three important nutrients found in many brands of table salt sold in the United States are:
   a. sodium, chloride, and iodine.
   b. sodium, potassium, and iodine.
   c. sodium, potassium, and chlorine.
   d. sodium, calcium, and magnesium.

4. Which of the following statements about trabecular bone is true?
   a. It accounts for about 80% of the skeleton.
   b. It forms the core of all bones.
   c. It is also called compact bone.
   d. It provides the scaffolding for cortical bone.

5. Calcium is necessary for several body functions, including:
   a. hemoglobin production, nerve transmission, and immune responses.
   b. structure of cartilage, nerve transmission, and muscle contraction.
   c. structure of bone and blood, immune responses, and muscle contraction.
   d. structure of bone, nerve transmission, and muscle contraction.

6. True or False? The process by which bone is formed through the action of osteoblasts and broken down through the action of osteoclasts is called *remodeling*.

7. True or False? Red blood cells contain iron.

8. True or False? There is no DRI for sulfur.

9. True or False? Both zinc deficiency and zinc toxicity are characterized by reduced immune function.

10. True or False? Although osteoporosis can lead to painful and debilitating fractures, it is not associated with an increased risk of premature death.

WEB LINKS

www.iofbonehealth.org

International Osteoporosis Foundation

Find out more about this foundation and its mission to increase awareness and understanding of osteoporosis worldwide.

www.niams.nih.gov/Health%5FInfo/Bone

National Institutes of Health: Osteoporosis and Related Bone Diseases—National Resource Center

Access this site for resources and information on bone diseases, including osteoporosis.

TEST YOURSELF ANSWERS

1. **False.** Research studies have failed to show any consistent effects of chromium supplements on reducing body fat or enhancing muscle mass.

2. **False.** Sodium is a nutrient necessary for health, but we should not consume more than recommended amounts.

3. **True.** Worldwide, iron deficiency is particularly common in infants, children, and women of childbearing age.

4. **False.** Osteoporosis is more common among elderly women, but elderly men are also at increased risk, and some women develop osteoporosis in their middle-adult years. Young women who suffer from an eating disorder and menstrual cycle irregularity, referred to as the *female athlete triad,* also commonly develop osteoporosis.

5. **True.** Cigarette smoking has an unhealthful effect on the hormones that influence the density of our bones. People who smoke have an increased risk for osteoporosis and fractures.

REFERENCES

1. Eckhert, C. D. 2006. Other trace elements. In: Shils, M. E., M. Shike, A. C. Ross, B. Caballero, and R. J. Cousins, Eds. *Modern Nutrition in Health and Disease.* 10th ed. Philadelphia, PA: Lippincott, Williams and Wilkins, pp. 338–350.

2. Sacks, F. M., L. P. Svetkey, W. M. Vollmer, L. J. Appel, G. A. Bray, D. Harsha, E. Obarzanek, P. R. Conlin, E. R. Miller III, D. G. Simons-Morton, N. Karanja, and P.-H. Lin. 2001. Effects on blood pressure of reduced dietary sodium and the Dietary Approaches to Stop Hypertension (DASH) diet. *N Engl J Med* 344:3–10.

3. Cohen, A. J., and F. J. Roe. 2000. Review of risk factors for osteoporosis with particular reference to a possible aetiological role of dietary salt. *Food Chem Toxicol* 38:237–253.

4. American Dietetic Association. 2005. It's National Nutrition Month 2005! Spice up Your Meals and Lower Your Salt Intake. Available at www.eatright.org/Print/PublicMedia_21433.cfm.

5. Evans, G. W. 1989. The effect of chromium picolinate on insulin controlled parameters in humans. *Int J Biosoc Med Res* 11:163–180.

6. Hasten D. L., E. P. Rome, D. B. Franks, and M. Hegsted. 1992. Effects of chromium picolinate on beginning weight training students. *Int J Sports Nutr* 2:343–350.

7. Lukaski, H. C., W. W. Bolonchuk, W. A. Siders, and D. B. Milne. 1996. Chromium supplementation and resistance training: Effects on body composition, strength, and trace element status of men. *Am J Clin Nutr* 63:954–965.

8. Hallmark M. A., T. H. Reynolds, C. A. DeSouza, C. O. Dotson, R. A. Anderson, and M. A. Rogers. 1996. Effects of chromium and resistive training on muscle strength and body composition. *Med Sci Sports Exerc* 28:139–144.

9. Pasman W. J., M. S. Westerterp-Plantenga, and W. H. Saris. 1997. The effectiveness of long-term supplementation of carbohydrate, chromium, fibre and caffeine on weight maintenance. *Int J Obesity Related Metab Disorders* 21:1143–1151.

10. Walker, L. S., M. G. Bemben, D. A. Bemben, and A. W. Knehans. 1998. Chromium picolinate effects on body composition and muscular performance in wrestlers. *Med Sci Sports Exerc* 30:1730–1737.

11. Campbell, W. W., L. J. Joseph, S. L. Davey, D. Cyr-Campbell, R. A. Anderson, and W. J. Evans. 1999. Effects of resistance training and chromium picolinate on body composition and skeletal muscle in older men. *J Appl Physiol* 86:29–39.

12. Volpe, S. L., H. W. Huang, K. Larpadisorn, and I. I. Lesser. 2001. Effect of chromium supplementation and exercise on body composition, resting metabolic rate and selected biochemical parameters in moderately obese women following an exercise program. *J Am Coll Nutr* 20:293–306.

13. Campbell, W. W., L. J. O. Joseph, R. A. Anderson, S. L. Davey, J. Hinton, and W. J. Evans. 2002. Effects of resistive training and chromium picolinate on body composition and skeletal muscle size in older women. *Int J Sports Nutr Ex Metab* 12:125–135.

14. Vincent, J. B. 2003. The potential value and toxicity of chromium picolinate as a nutritional supplement, weight loss agent and muscle development agent. *Sports Med* 33:213–230.

15. Office of Dietary Supplements. 2004. Dietary Supplement Fact Sheet: Selenium. Available at http://ods.od.nih.gov/factsheets/selenium.assumption.

16. Institute of Medicine, Food and Nutrition Board. 2001. *Dietary Reference Intakes for Vitamin A, Vitamin K, Arsenic, Boron, Chromium, Copper, Iodine, Iron, Manganese, Molybdenum, Nickel, Silicon, Vanadium, and Zinc.* Washington, DC: National Academy Press.

17. U.S. Food and Drug Administration. 1997. Preventing iron poisoning in children. *FDA Backgrounder.* Available at www.fda.gov/opacom/backgrounders/ironbg.html. (Accessed January 2004.)

18. Prasad, A. 1996. Zinc: The biology and therapeutics of an ion. *Ann Intern Med* 125:142–143.

19. Jackson J. L., E. Lesho, and C. Peterson. 2000. Zinc and the common cold: A meta-analysis revisited. *J Nutr* 130:1512S–1515S.

20. Heaney, R. P., and K. Rafferty. 2001. Carbonated beverages and urinary calcium excretion. *Am J Clin Nutr* 74:343–347.

21. Wu, C. H., Y. C. Yang, W. J. Yao, F. H. Lu, J. S. Wu, and C. J. Chang. 2002. Epidemiological evidence of increased bone mineral density in habitual tea drinkers. *Arch Intern Med* 162:1001–1006.

22. Institute of Medicine, Food and Nutrition Board. 1997. *Dietary Reference Intakes for Calcium, Phosphorus, Magnesium, Vitamin D, and Fluoride.* Washington, DC: National Academy Press.

23. National Osteoporosis Foundation (NOF). 2007. Fast Facts. Available at www.nof.org/osteoporosis/diseasefacts.htm.

24. International Osteoporosis Foundation. 2004. By 2020, One in Two Americans over Age 50 Will Be at Risk for Fractures from Osteoporosis or Low Bone Mass. Press release issued by the Office of the U.S. Surgeon General, Thursday, October 14, 2004. Available at www.osteofound.org/press_centre/pr_2004_10_14.html.

25. International Osteoporosis Foundation. 2005. The Facts About Osteoporosis and Its Impact. Available at www.osteofound.org/press_centre/fact_sheet.html.

26. Rapuri, P. B., J. C. Gallagher, H. K. Kinyamu, and K. L. Ryschon. 2001. Caffeine intake increases the rate of bone loss in elderly women and interacts with vitamin D receptor genotypes. *Am J Clin Nutr* 74:694–700.

27. Tucker, K. L., M. T. Hannan, H. Chen, L. A. Cupples, P. W. F. Wilson, and D. P. Kiel. 1999. Potassium, magnesium, and fruit and vegetable intakes are associated with greater bone mineral density in elderly men and women. *Am J Clin Nutr* 69:727–736.

28. Tucker, K. L., H. Chen, M. T. Hannan, L. A. Cupples, P. W. F. Wilson, D. Felson, and D. P. Kiel. 2002. Bone mineral density and dietary patterns in older adults: The Framingham Osteoporosis Study. *Am J Clin Nutr* 76:245–252.

29. South-Pal, J. E. 2001. Osteoporosis: Part II. Nonpharmacologic and pharmacologic treatment. *Am Fam Physician* 63:1121–1128.

TEST YOURSELF

Are these statements true or false? Circle your guess.

1 About 50% to 70% of our body weight is made up of water. **TRUE** or **FALSE**

2 Drinking until we are no longer thirsty ensures that we are properly hydrated. **TRUE** or **FALSE**

3 Although persistent vomiting is uncomfortable, it does not have any long-term adverse health effects. **TRUE** or **FALSE**

4 Alcohol consumption is the leading cause of death among people under the age of 21. **TRUE** or **FALSE**

5 Carbonated alcoholic beverages are absorbed more rapidly than noncarbonated varieties. **TRUE** or **FALSE**

Test Yourself answers can be found at the end of the chapter.

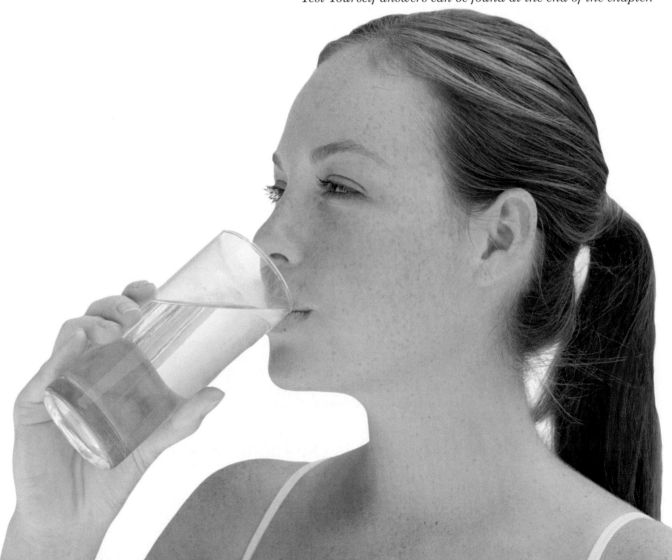

fluid A substance composed of molecules that move past one another freely. Fluids are characterized by their ability to conform to the shape of whatever container holds them.

N APRIL 2002, CYNTHIA LUCERO, a healthy 28-year-old woman who had just completed her doctoral dissertation, was running the Boston Marathon. Although not a professional athlete, Cynthia was running in her second marathon and had trained carefully. While her parents, who had traveled from Ecuador, waited at the finish line, friends in the crowd watched as Cynthia steadily completed mile after mile, taking in fluids as she progressed through the course. They described her as looking strong until she began to jog up Heartbreak Hill, about 6 miles from the finish. At her last fluid stop, she drank copiously. A few minutes later, she began visibly to falter. One of her friends ran to her side and asked if she was okay. Cynthia replied that she felt dehydrated and rubber-legged, then she fell to the pavement. She was rushed to nearby Brigham and Women's Hospital, but by the time she got there, she was in an irreversible coma. The official cause of her death was hyponatremia, a word meaning "inadequate sodium in the blood." Hyponatremia commonly results from a problem called *water intoxication* discussed later in this chapter. According to a study involving the 488 runners in that 2002 Boston Marathon, 13% had hyponatremia by the end of the race, and hyponatremia continues to cause illness and death in runners, triathletes, and even hikers.[1]

What is hyponatremia, and how does it differ from dehydration? Are you at risk for either condition? Do sports beverages confer any protection against these fluid imbalances? If at the start of football practice on a hot, humid afternoon, a friend confided to you that he had been on a drinking binge the night before and had vomited twice that morning, would you urge him to tell his coach? If so, why?

In Chapter 7, we introduced the electrolytes—minerals that help maintain body fluid in balance inside and outside our cells. Here, we explore the role of water and other fluids in keeping the body properly hydrated and take a look at some disorders that can occur when our body fluids are out of balance. We also discuss alcohol, including the benefits of moderate consumption and the problems of alcohol abuse.

What Are Fluids, and What Are Their Functions?

Of course you know that water, orange juice, blood, and urine are all fluids, but what makes them so? A **fluid** is characterized by its ability to move freely and changeably, adapting to the shape of any container that holds it. This might not seem very important, but as you'll learn in this chapter, the fluid within our cells and tissues is critical to the body's ability to function.

Water is the main component of all body fluids. A colorless, odorless, and tasteless liquid, pure water is made up of a precise ratio of hydrogen and oxygen (H_2O). Pure water bonds with other nutrients to produce the milk, juices, mineral water, and thousands of other beverages we drink, and it is a component, in varying amounts, of foods. Essential to life, water is one of the six nutrient groups identified in Chapter 1.

Body Fluid Is the Liquid Portion of Cells and Tissues

Between 50% and 70% of a healthy adult's body weight is water. Think about it: if you weigh 150 lbs, then about 75 to 105 lbs of your body mass isn't solid, but fluid!

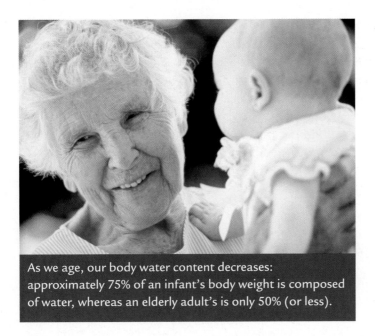

As we age, our body water content decreases: approximately 75% of an infant's body weight is composed of water, whereas an elderly adult's is only 50% (or less).

When we cut a finger, we can see some of this fluid dripping out as blood, but blood alone certainly can't account for 105 lbs! So where is all this fluid hiding?

About two-thirds of the body's fluid, known as *intracellular fluid*, is held within the walls of our cells (FIGURE 8.1). Every cell in the body contains fluid. When cells lose their fluid, they quickly shrink and die. On the other hand, when cells take in too much fluid, they swell and burst apart. This is why appropriate fluid balance—which we'll discuss throughout this chapter—is so critical to life.

The remaining third of the body's fluid, known as *extracellular fluid*, flows outside of the cells (see Figure 8.1). Some of this fluid, known as interstitial fluid (or tissue fluid), flows between the cells that make up a particular tissue, such as the tissue that makes up the liver or the lungs. The rest of the body's extracellular fluid flows within blood vessels or lymphatic vessels. The fluid portion of blood is termed plasma. It transports blood cells within the body's arteries, veins, and capillaries (see Figure 8.1c). The fluid in lymphatic vessels is simply called lymphatic fluid.

Not every tissue in the body contains the same amount of fluid. Lean tissues, such as muscle, are more than 70% fluid, whereas fat tissue is between 10% and 20% fluid. Body fluid also varies according to gender. Males have more lean tissue and thus more body fluid than females. Our percentage of body fluid also decreases as we age, from about 75% in infants to generally less than 50% in older adults. This decrease is related to the loss of lean tissue that occurs as people age.

Fluids Serve Many Critical Functions

Fluids not only quench our thirst; the water they contain performs a number of functions that are critical to support life.

Fluids Dissolve and Transport Substances

As noted earlier, water is an essential nutrient. We can't live without it because it's involved in almost every chemical reaction that occurs in our bodies. It is an excellent **solvent,** which means it is capable of dissolving (i.e., mixing with and breaking apart) a wide variety of substances. Because both the plasma component of blood and the interior of blood cells are mostly water, blood is an excellent vehicle for transporting nutrients and other substances throughout the body. Recall that fats do not dissolve in water. To overcome this chemical incompatibility, fatty substances such as cholesterol and fat-soluble vitamins are either attached to or surrounded by water-soluble proteins so they too can be transported in the blood to the cells.

solvent A substance that is capable of mixing with and breaking apart a variety of compounds. Water is an excellent solvent.

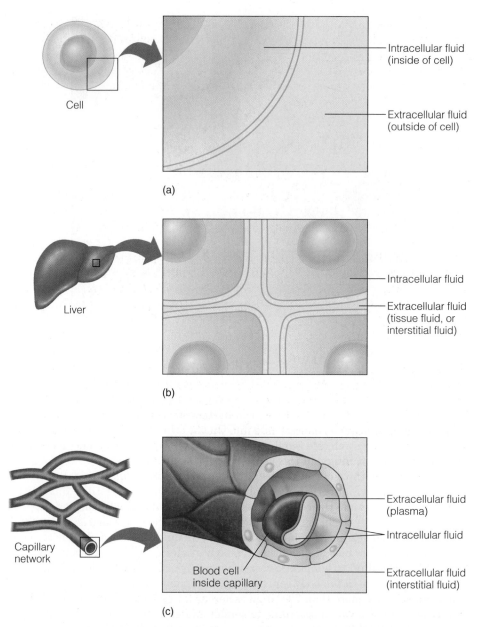

FIGURE 8.1   The components of body fluid. (a) Intracellular fluid is contained within the cells that make up our body tissues. Extracellular fluid is external to cells. (b) Interstitial fluid is external to tissue cells, and (c) plasma is external to blood cells.

The body also uses water to excrete metabolic wastes, excess micronutrients, and other unwanted substances. The kidneys filter these substances from the blood and dilute them with water to create urine, which is stored in the bladder until it flows out of the body via the urethra.

Fluids Account for Blood Volume

Blood volume is the amount of fluid in blood; thus, appropriate fluid levels are essential to maintaining healthful blood volume. When blood volume is low, blood pressure is low. Low blood pressure can cause people to feel tired, lethargic, confused, and dizzy, or even to faint.

In contrast, when the volume of blood rises, it exerts greater pressure against the blood vessel walls. As you learned in Chapter 7, high blood pressure (called

blood volume   The amount of fluid in blood.

hypertension) is an important risk factor for heart disease and stroke. You can't develop hypertension by drinking too much fluid, because your kidneys normally excrete excess fluid in your urine. But if you retain more fluid than your kidneys can excrete, your blood pressure will rise. Recall that excessive sodium consumption can cause fluid retention and hypertension in some salt-sensitive people. Kidney disease can also cause fluid retention.

Fluids Help Maintain Body Temperature

Just as overheating is disastrous to a car engine, a high internal temperature can cause the body to stop functioning. Fluids are vital to the body's ability to maintain its temperature within a safe range.

Two factors account for the cooling power of fluids. First, it takes a lot of external energy to raise the temperature of water. Because the body contains a lot of water, it takes sustained high heat to increase body temperature.

Second, body fluids are our primary coolant. When our temperature rises and our body needs to release heat, it increases the flow of blood from vessels in the warm body core to vessels lying just under the skin. At the same time, the sweat glands secrete more sweat—which is primarily water—from the skin. As this sweat evaporates off of the skin's surface, heat is released into the environment and the skin and underlying blood are cooled (FIGURE 8.2). This cooler blood flows back to the body's core and reduces internal body temperature.

Fluids Protect and Lubricate the Tissues

Fluids protect the organs and tissues from injury. The cerebrospinal fluid that surrounds the brain and spinal column acts as a shock absorber, protecting these vital tissues from damage, and amniotic fluid protects a fetus in a mother's womb.

Body fluids also act as lubricants. Fluid within our joints facilitates smooth joint motion. Fluid covering the lungs allows for their friction-free expansion and retraction within the chest cavity. Tears cleanse and lubricate the eyes. Saliva moistens the food we eat, and the mucus lining the digestive tract facilitates the smooth movement of nutrients.

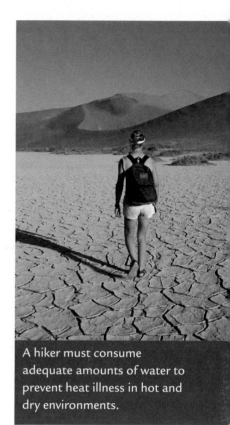

A hiker must consume adequate amounts of water to prevent heat illness in hot and dry environments.

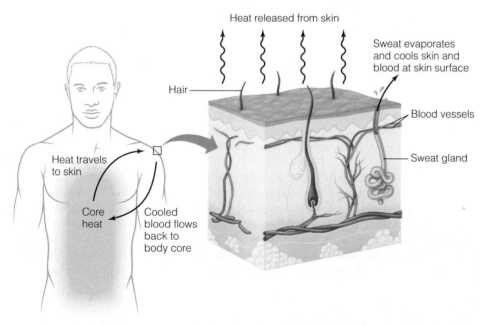

Heat released from skin

Sweat evaporates and cools skin and blood at skin surface

Hair

Blood vessels

Sweat gland

Heat travels to skin

Core heat

Cooled blood flows back to body core

FIGURE 8.2 Evaporative cooling occurs when heat is transported from the body core through the bloodstream to the surface of the skin. When a person sweats, water evaporates into the air and carries away heat. This cools the skin and underlying blood, which then circulates back to the body core, reducing body temperature.

> RECAP *Water is an essential nutrient. Between about 50% and 70% of a healthy adult's body weight is water. About two-thirds of the body's fluid is held within the walls of our cells (intracellular fluid), and the remaining third flows outside of cells (extracellular fluid). Fluids serve many important functions, including dissolving and transporting substances, accounting for blood volume, regulating body temperature, and cushioning and lubricating body tissues.*

How Do Our Bodies Maintain Fluid Balance?

Our bodies maintain a healthy balance of fluid by a series of mechanisms that prompt us to drink and retain fluid when we are dehydrated and to excrete fluid as urine when we consume more than we need.

The Thirst Mechanism Prompts Us to Drink Fluids

Imagine that, at lunch, you ate a ham sandwich and a bag of salted potato chips. Now it's almost time for your afternoon seminar to end, and suddenly you are very thirsty. The last five minutes of class are a torment, and when the instructor ends the session you dash to the nearest drinking fountain. What prompted you to feel so thirsty?

The body's command center for fluid intake is a cluster of nerve cells in the same part of the brain we studied in relation to food intake—that is, the *hypothalamus*. Within the hypothalamus is a group of cells, collectively referred to as the **thirst mechanism,** that causes you to consciously desire fluids. The thirst mechanism prompts us to feel thirsty when it detects either of two conditions:

- *An increased concentration of sodium and other dissolved substances in the blood.* Remember that ham sandwich and those potato chips? Both these foods are salty, and eating them results in high concentrations of sodium in the blood.

- *A decrease in blood volume and blood pressure.* This can occur when we lose fluid during profuse sweating, because of traumatic injury that causes heavy blood loss, or simply when our fluid intake is too low.

Once the hypothalamus detects such changes, it stimulates the release of a hormone that signals the kidneys to reduce urine flow and return more water to the bloodstream. Water is drawn out of the salivary glands in the mouth in an attempt to further dilute the concentration of substances in the blood; this leaves less water available to make saliva and causes the mouth and throat to become dry. Together, these mechanisms help us to retain fluid, prevent a further loss of fluid, and avoid dehydration.

It is unwise to rely solely on the thirst mechanism to indicate when you need to drink. That's because people tend to drink only until they are no longer thirsty, but the amount of fluid they consume may not be enough to achieve fluid balance. This is particularly true when body water is rapidly lost, such as during intense exercise in the heat. Also, in older adults, the thirst mechanism is not as accurate as in younger adults. Because the thirst mechanism has some limitations, it is important that you drink regularly throughout the day, even if you don't feel particularly thirsty.

thirst mechanism A cluster of nerve cells in the hypothalamus that stimulate our conscious desire to drink fluids in response to an increase in the concentration of salt in our blood or a decrease in blood pressure and blood volume.

We Gain Fluids by Consuming Beverages and Foods and through Metabolism

We obtain the water we need each day from three primary sources: beverages, foods, and the production of metabolic water by the body. Of course you know that

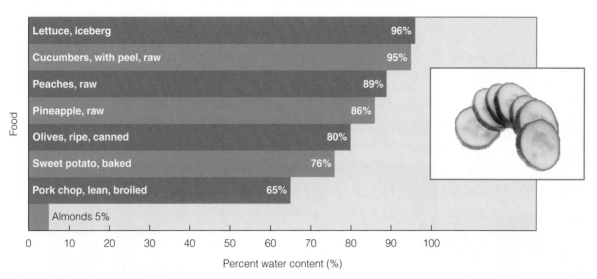

FIGURE 8.3   Water content of different foods. Much of your daily water intake comes from the foods you eat. (Data from U.S. Department of Agriculture, Agricultural Research Service. 2007. USDA National Nutrient Database for Standard Reference, Release 20. Nutrient Data Laboratory Home Page. www.ars.usda.gov/ba/bhnrc/ndl.)

beverages are mostly water, but it isn't as easy to see the water content in foods. For example, iceberg lettuce is about 96% water, and even bacon contains a small amount of water. FIGURE 8.3 shows the water content of commonly consumed foods.

Metabolic water is the water formed from the body's metabolic reactions. In the breakdown of fat, carbohydrate, and protein, water is produced as a by-product. The water that is formed during metabolic reactions contributes about 10% to 14% of the water our bodies need each day.

We Lose Fluids through Urine and Feces, Sweat, Evaporation, and Exhalation

Our kidneys absorb from the bloodstream any water that the body does not need. They then send the fluid, in the form of dilute urine, to the bladder for storage until we urinate. A small amount of water is also lost each day in the feces. However, when someone suffers from severe diarrhea, water loss in the feces can be as high as several liters per day.

We also lose fluid via sweat. Fluid loss in sweat is much higher during physical labor, exercise, and when we are in a hot environment. In fact, some large football players can lose more than 8 liters of fluid per day as sweat![2]

Water is also continuously evaporated from our skin even when we are not obviously sweating. Finally, water is continuously exhaled from the lungs as we breathe.

FIGURE 8.4 shows the estimated amounts and categories of water sources and losses for a woman expending about 2,500 kcal of energy per day. It shows that her fluid losses of 3,000 ml (3 L) per day are matched by her intake of about:

- 2,200 ml (2.2 L) of fluid in beverages
- an additional 500 ml of fluid in foods
- an additional 300 ml of metabolic water

One cup (8 fl oz) of water is equal to 240 ml. Thus, this woman would need to drink about 9 cups of total fluid to meet her needs.

Consumption of **diuretics**—substances that increase fluid loss via the urine—can result in dangerously excessive fluid loss. Some prescription medications have a diuretic effect, and many over-the-counter weight-loss remedies are really just diuretics. Alcohol also has a strong diuretic effect. In the past, it was believed that caffeine-containing beverages such as coffee, tea, and cola acted as diuretics, but

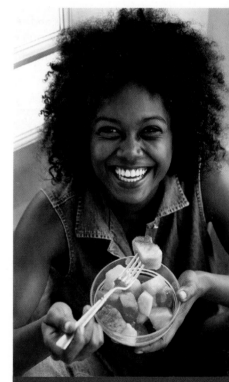

Fruits and vegetables are delicious sources of water.

metabolic water   The water formed as a by-product of our body's metabolic reactions.

diuretic   A substance that increases fluid loss via the urine. Common diuretics include alcohol and some prescription medications for high blood pressure and other disorders.

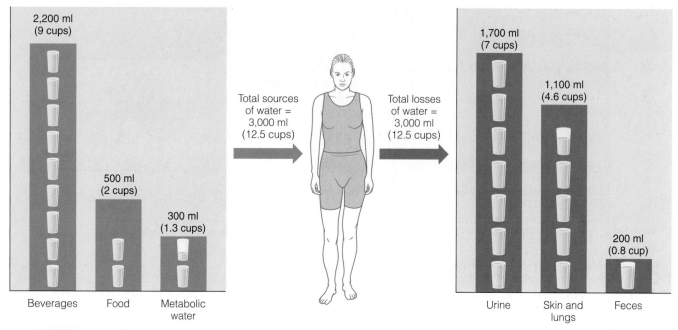

FIGURE 8.4 Amounts and categories of water sources and losses for a woman expending 2,500 kcal per day. Water from metabolism provides 300 ml. The foods she eats provides her with an additional 500 ml. The beverages she drinks, including water, provide the remainder of water she needs, about 2,200 ml. The total of 3,000 ml matches her water losses.

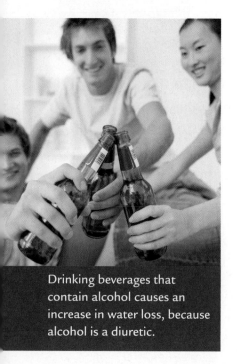

Drinking beverages that contain alcohol causes an increase in water loss, because alcohol is a diuretic.

recent research suggests that caffeinated drinks do not have a significant impact on the hydration status of adults.[3] Although more research needs to be done to verify these findings, it is probably safe to count caffeinated beverages toward your daily fluid requirements. Later in this chapter, we identify ways to determine whether or not you are adequately hydrated.

RECAP *The thirst mechanism prompts us to feel thirsty when it detects an increased concentration of sodium and other dissolved substances in the blood. It is also triggered by low blood volume or blood pressure. A healthy fluid level is maintained in the body by balancing intake with excretion. Primary sources of fluids include water and other beverages, foods, and the production of metabolic water in the body. Fluid losses occur through urine, feces, sweating, evaporation from the skin, and exhalation from the lungs.*

How Much Fluid Should We Drink—and What Kinds?

You need to drink enough fluid every day so that your body can sweat, breathe, and produce urine and feces without drawing water from your cells. But how much is "enough"—for you? The DRI guidelines from the Institute of Medicine recommend that adult males consume approximately 3,000 ml (or 13 cups) of fluids daily from water and other beverages, with an additional 700 ml of water from food. Adult women should consume about 2,200 ml (or 9 cups) of fluid, and an additional 500 ml of water from food.[3] Still, fluid requirements are highly individualized. For example, a male athlete training in a hot environment may need to drink up to 10 L (10,000 ml) of fluid per day, while a petite, sedentary woman who works in a temperature-controlled office building may only require about 2 L (2,000 ml) per day.

Mineral, Fizzy, or Tap: Water Is a Healthful Choice

All beverages provide water, but plain drinking water hydrates your body more efficiently than juices, sodas, and other beverages and does not contribute to weight gain. There are so many types of drinking water available in the United States, how can we distinguish among them? Here's a quick list:

- *Carbonated water* contains carbon dioxide gas. There are two types: in *sparkling water,* the carbon dioxide occurs naturally, whereas in *soda water,* the carbon dioxide is added by the manufacturer. Carbonated water is usually available in several flavors and may or may not contain added sugar.

- *Mineral water* contains 250 to 500 parts per million (ppm) of minerals. While many people enjoy the unique taste of mineral water, a number of brands contain high amounts of sodium so should be avoided by people who are trying to reduce their sodium intake.

- *Distilled water* is processed in such a way that all dissolved minerals are removed; this type of water is often used in steam irons, as it will not clog the iron with mineral buildup.

- *Purified water* has been treated so that all dissolved minerals and contaminants are removed, making this type of water useful in research and medical procedures.

- *Tap water* comes from municipal water systems and is pumped to homes, offices, and public places. It often contains chlorine, which is used as an antimicrobial, and may be fluoridated (see Chapter 7).

- *Well water* is used by many people in rural areas who do not have access to community water supplies. This water can be more pure and better tasting than municipal water, or it can be dangerously high in lead, arsenic, or other impurities. Water-quality testing is important for people who rely on well water for their drinking water.

- *Fortified waters* are canned or bottled waters enriched with certain vitamins, minerals, amino acids, and/or phytochemicals. The labels of some of these products advertise a variety of special health benefits, but most nutrition experts doubt they are worth their higher cost.

One of the major changes in the beverage industry over the past 20 years is the marketing of bottled water. Americans now consume about 26 gallons of bottled water per person per year, making bottled water a $46 billion industry.[4] This meteoric rise in bottled water production and consumption is most likely due to the convenience of drinking bottled water, to the health messages related to drinking more water, and to the public's fears related to the safety of tap water.

This expanded use of bottled water raises two environmental concerns. First, the production of all those water bottles uses huge amounts of energy and resources, and produces industrial wastes. Second, it is estimated that only 10% to 25% of water bottles are currently recycled; thus, landfills are overflowing with discarded water bottles.

Is bottled water safer or more healthful than tap water? Do the environmental concerns related to bottled water use outweigh the health benefits of water consumption? Refer to the Nutrition Myth or Fact? box on bottled water on page 240 to find the answers to these questions.

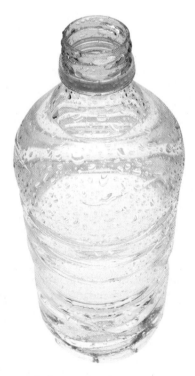

Bottled water has become extremely popular, but how does it compare to tap water?

All Beverages Are Not Created Equal

Many beverages contain several important nutrients in addition to their water content, whereas others provide water and refined sugar but very little else. Low-fat and skim milk are healthful beverage choices, because they contain protein, calcium,

NUTRITION MYTH OR FACT?

Is Bottled Water Safer Than Tap Water?

Bottled water has become increasingly popular during the past 20 years. It is estimated that Americans drink almost 8 billion gallons of bottled water each year.[4,5]

Many people prefer the taste of bottled water to that of tap water. They also feel that bottled water is safer than tap water. Is this true?

The water we drink in the United States generally comes from two sources: surface water and groundwater.

- *Surface water* comes from lakes, rivers, and reservoirs. Common contaminants of surface water include runoff from highways, pesticides, animal wastes, and industrial wastes. Many of the cities across the United States obtain their water from surface-water sources.

Groundwater comes from spaces between underground rock formations called *aquifers*. People who live in rural areas generally pump groundwater from a well as their water source. Hazardous substances leaking from waste sites, dumps, landfills, and oil and gas pipelines can contaminate groundwater. Groundwater can also be contaminated by naturally occurring substances such as arsenic or high levels of iron.

The most common chemical used to treat and purify our water is *chlorine*. Chlorine is effective in killing many contaminants in our water supply. Ozone is also commonly used. Water treatment plants also routinely check our water supplies for hazardous chemicals, minerals, and other contaminants. Because of these efforts, the United States has one of the safest water systems in the world.

The Environmental Protection Agency (EPA) sets and monitors the standards for our municipal water systems. The EPA does not monitor water from private wells, but it publishes recommendations for well owners to help them maintain a safe water supply. Local water regulatory agencies must provide an annual report on specific water contaminants to all households served by that agency.

In contrast, the Food and Drug Administration (FDA) regulates bottled water. It does not require that bottled water meet higher quality standards than public water. As with tap water, bottled water is taken from either surface water or groundwater sources. Bottled water is often treated and filtered differently than tap water, which changes its taste and appearance.

Although bottled water may taste better than tap water, there is no evidence that it is safer to drink. Look closely at the label of your favorite bottled water. If the label states "From a public water source," it has come directly from the tap! Some types of bottled water may contain more minerals than tap water, but there are no other additional nutritional benefits of drinking bottled water. Most bottling plants use an ozone treatment to disinfect water instead of chlorine, and many people feel this process leaves the water tasting better than water treated with chlorine.

Should you spend money on bottled water? The answer depends on personal preference and your source of drinking water. Some people may not have access to safe drinking water where they live, making bottled water the safest alternative water source. If you choose to drink bottled water, look for brands that carry the trademark of the International Bottled Water Association (IBWA). This association follows the regulations of the FDA.

Be wary of vending machines dispensing filtered water where you can fill your own bottles. These machines may not be cleaned and the filters may not be changed on a regular basis, so before using them, contact the vendor to determine how often and how they are serviced. If you get your water from a water cooler, make sure the cooler is cleaned once per month by running one-half gallon of white vinegar through it, then rinsing thoroughly with about 5 gallons of clean water.

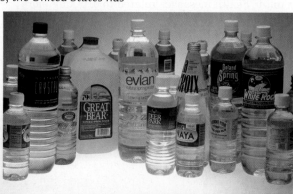

Numerous varieties of drinking water are available to consumers.

If you use a special filtration system at home, be familiar with the contaminants it filters from your water and make sure that you change the filters regularly as recommended by the manufacturer. Be cautious of companies making claims about impurities in your tap water. Verify any tests conducted by a private company with your local water agency. It could save you hundreds or thousands of dollars on an unnecessary or ineffective home purifying system.

For more information on drinking water safety, go to the EPA Web site at www.epa.gov. For information on bottled water, search the FDA Web site at www.fda.gov.

phosphorus, vitamin D, and usually vitamin A. Calcium-fortified soy milk, rice milk, and orange juice are also nutritious options. When purchasing flavored cow's, soy, or rice milks, check the Nutrition Facts Panel for the sugar content. Some brands of chocolate milk, for example, can contain 6 or more teaspoons of refined sugar in a single cup!

Coffee made without cream or non-dairy creamer can be a healthful beverage choice if consumed in moderation. As mentioned earlier, recent research suggests that its caffeine content does not significantly decrease the body's hydration status, and the calcium in coffee drinks made with milk, such as café con leche and café latte, can be significant. Coffee is known to provide several types of phytochemicals that may actually lower risk of certain chronic diseases. Black and green teas also contain phytochemicals with antioxidant properties, and tea with milk provides a small amount of calcium. If you typically add sugar to your coffee or tea, try slowly decreasing the amount you use. You may find that you develop a taste for the slightly bitter flavor of these beverages in their unsweetened state.

Added sugar is also a problem with many juice drinks, flavored waters, and sodas. For example, you might think of cranberry juice cocktail as a healthful beverage, but did you know that one 8-oz serving contains more than 7 teaspoons of sugar? Sweetened flavored waters and sodas can be even higher in sugar, and since many are now packaged in 24-oz bottles, if you drink the whole thing, you can consume up to 20 teaspoons of sugar—that's almost half a cup!

Flavored waters, made with or without added sugars, are widely available, as are so-called "designer" or "enhanced" waters. These beverages are made with added nutrients and herbs that supposedly enhance memory, delay aging, boost energy levels, or strengthen the immune response. The amounts of nutrients used are so low, however, compared to what can be obtained from foods, that they rarely make much of an impact on one's health or well-being.

"Energy drinks" represent another popular beverage option, with over $3 billion in sales in 2006. These products advertise their ability to provide a boost, jump start, buzz, punch, or rocket-powered blast! While attractive to adolescents and young adults, nutrition experts and consumer groups have raised significant concerns.[6] Many of these beverages contain more than three times the amount of caffeine in a comparable serving of cola, and a few contain up to ten times the caffeine in cola. Many also contain guarana seed extract: guarana seeds contain more caffeine than coffee beans, so their "extract" is simply a potent source of additional caffeine. Some also contain taurine, an amino acid associated with muscle contraction. The combined effects of these substances can significantly increase blood pressure and heart rate. Mood swings, insomnia, dizziness, tremors, caffeine dependency, dehydration, and other problems have also been linked to consumption of these beverages.

A final beverage choice is that of a traditional sports beverage, which provides water, electrolytes, and a source of carbohydrate. Because of the potential for fluid and electrolyte imbalances during exercise, some athletes drink sports beverages instead of plain water before, during, and after workouts. Recently, sports beverages have also become popular with recreationally active people and nonathletes. Is it really necessary or helpful for people to consume these beverages? See the Highlight on sports beverages to learn whether they are right for you.

As you can see, American consumers have a wide range of beverage choices available to them. Poor choices can increase total caloric intake and lower daily nutrient intake.[7] Over the past 40 years, the caloric contributions of beverages to total energy intake have almost doubled. In 1965, fewer than 12% of Americans' calories came from beverages; in 2002, that ratio increased to 21% of total calories.[8] Pure drinking water remains calorie and additive free, is highly effective in quenching thirst and maintaining hydration status, and poses no health threat. For most of us, water really is the perfect beverage choice.

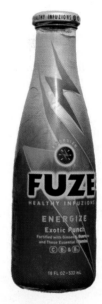

"Energy drinks" are a popular segment of the beverage market, but many contain caffeine and other substances that can cause harmful effects.

HIGHLIGHT

Sports Beverages: Help or Hype?

Once considered specialty drinks used exclusively by elite athletes, sports beverages have become popular everyday choices for both active and nonactive people. The market for these drinks has become so lucrative that many of the large soft drink companies now produce them. This surge in popularity leads us to ask three important questions:

- Do sports beverages benefit athletes?
- Do sports beverages benefit recreationally active people?
- Do nonactive people benefit from consuming sports beverages?

The first question is relatively easy to answer. Sports beverages were originally developed to meet the unique fluid, electrolyte, and carbohydrate needs of competitive athletes. As you learned in this chapter, highly active people need to replenish both fluids and electrolytes to avoid both dehydration and hyponatremia (low blood sodium). Sports beverages can especially benefit athletes who exercise in the heat and are thus at an even greater risk for loss of water and electrolytes through respiration and sweat. The carbohydrates in sports beverages provide critical fuel during relatively intense (more than 60% of maximal effort) exercise bouts lasting more than 1 hour. Thus, competitive athletes are able to exercise longer, maintain a higher intensity, and improve performance times when they drink a sports beverage during exercise.[9]

In addition, sports beverages may help athletes consume more energy than they could by eating solid foods and water alone. Some competitive athletes train or compete for 6 to 8 hours each day on a regular basis. It is virtually impossible for these athletes to consume enough solid foods to support this intense level of exercise.

Do recreationally active or working people benefit from consuming sports beverages? The answer depends on the duration and intensity of exercise, the environmental conditions, and the characteristics of the individual. Here are some situations in which drinking a sports beverage is appropriate:[9]

- Before exercise or manual labor if you are concerned that dehydration might occur, especially if you are already feeling dehydrated prior to starting.
- During exercise or manual labor if you have recently had diarrhea or vomiting.
- During exercise or manual labor in high heat and/or high humidity.
- During exercise or manual labor at high altitude and in cold environments; these conditions increase fluid and electrolyte losses.
- During continuous, vigorous exercise or labor lasting longer than 60 minutes in any climate.
- Between exercise bouts when it is difficult to consume food, such as between multiple soccer matches during a tournament.
- After exercise or manual labor for rapid rehydration.

Recently, sports beverages have become very popular with people who do little or no regular exercise or manual labor. However, there's no evidence that people who don't exercise derive any benefits from consuming sports beverages. Even if they live in a hot climate, they should be able to replenish the fluid and electrolytes they lose during sweating by drinking water and other beverages and eating a normal diet.

The primary negative consequence of drinking sports beverages without exercising is weight gain. Sports beverages contain not only fluid and electrolytes, but also energy. Drinking 12 fl. oz (1.5 cups) of Gatorade adds 90 kcal to a person's daily energy intake. Many inactive people consume two to three times this amount each day, adding 180 to 270 kcal of energy to their diet. With obesity rates at an all-time high, it is important that we attempt to consume only the foods and beverages necessary to support our health. Sports beverages are not designed to be consumed by inactive people, and they do not contribute to their health.

RECAP *Although fluid requirements are highly individualized, adult males require approximately 3.0 L (or 13 cups) of fluids daily and adult females approximately 2.2 L (or 9 cups). All beverages provide water, and some, such as mineral waters, milk, and calcium-fortified beverages, provide other important nutrients as well. Some beverages provide unnecessary and potentially harmful ingredients and should be consumed in limited amounts. Pure water remains the best beverage choice for most people.*

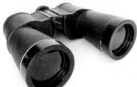

HEALTHWATCH
Can Too Little or Too Much Fluid Intake Be Deadly?

Fluid imbalances can be serious, and even fatal. Dehydration, heat stroke, and hyponatremia are fluid imbalances that produce negative health effects, and each are explained in this section.

Dehydration Is Common with Exercise in Hot Weather

Dehydration is a serious health problem that results when fluid losses exceed fluid intake. It most often occurs as a result of heavy exercise and/or exposure to high environmental temperatures, because loss of body water via sweating and breathing is increased in these circumstances.

Both the elderly and the very young have increased risk for dehydration. The thirst mechanism becomes less sensitive with age, so elderly people can fail to drink adequate amounts of fluid. Older adults also have less body water than younger adults, so fluid imbalances can occur more quickly. On the other hand, because a large proportion of infants' body weight is water, they need to drink a relatively large amount of fluid for their body size. Infants also excrete urine at a higher rate, cannot tell us when they are thirsty, and have a greater ratio of body surface area to body core, causing them to respond more dramatically to heat and cold and to lose more body water than an older child or adult. For these reasons, fluid losses, as with diarrhea or vomiting, must be closely monitored in infants.

Relatively small losses in body water, equal to a 1% to 2% change in body weight, result in symptoms such as thirst, discomfort, and loss of appetite. More severe water losses can cause nausea, flushed skin, and problems with mental concentration. Losses of body water greater than 8% of body weight can result in delirium, coma, and death.

Earlier we discussed the importance of fluid replacement when you are exercising. How can you tell whether you are drinking enough fluid before, during, and after your athletic competitions or exercise sessions? First, you can measure your body weight before and after each session, using the same scale, unclothed or just in your underwear. Whether you've lost 2 oz or 2 lb of body weight during your session, you need to consume enough water and other fluids to regain that weight before you exercise again.

A second method of monitoring your fluid levels is to observe the color of your urine (**FIGURE 8.5**). If you are properly hydrated, your urine should be clear to pale yellow in color, similar to diluted lemonade. Urine that is medium to dark yellow in color, similar to apple juice, indicates inadequate fluid intake. Very dark or brown-colored urine, such as the color of a cola beverage, is a sign of severe dehydration and indicates potential muscle breakdown and kidney damage. People should strive to maintain a urine color that is clear or pale yellow.

How should you replace fluid you've lost during exercise or competition? Start physical activity in a well-hydrated state by slowly drinking water or sport beverages at least 4 hours before the activity. During the session, prevent dehydration by drinking water or sport beverages as needed. A marathon runner may need to drink 400 to 800 ml of a sports beverage per hour during the race; however, a player in a casual tennis match may require much less. Most people can restore fluid and electrolyte balance after activity through normal meals, snacks, and beverages. But if your weight or the color of your urine indicates that you are

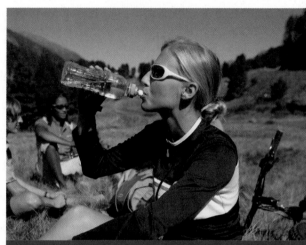

Vigorous exercise causes significant losses of water and electrolytes that must be replenished to optimize performance and health.

dehydration Depletion of body fluid that results when fluid excretion exceeds fluid intake.

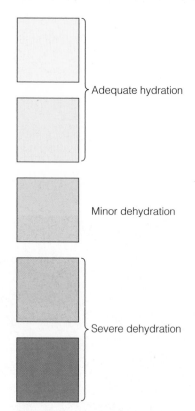

Adequate hydration

Minor dehydration

Severe dehydration

FIGURE 8.5 Urine color chart. Color variations indicate levels of hydration.

significantly dehydrated, one guideline is to drink about 1,500 ml (1.5 L) for each kilogram of body weight lost.[2]

Heat Stroke

Farm workers, construction workers, and others who perform physical labor outdoors in the heat are particularly vulnerable to dangerous fluid loss. So are athletes who train or compete in hot weather. In August 2001, 27-year-old National Football League all-star player Korey Stringer died of complications from **heat stroke** after working out in a hot and humid environment. And in February, 2003, Steve Bechler, a 23-year old pitching prospect with the Baltimore Orioles, died after suffering from heat stroke during a spring training session in Florida. His death may have been complicated by his use of an ephedrine-containing weight-loss drug and by the fact that he was limiting his food and fluid intake in order to lose weight.

Heat stroke occurs when the body cannot release enough heat in sweat to keep the body temperature within a safe range. As noted earlier in this chapter, the body's ability to cool itself via sweating requires that the sweat be able to evaporate: this means that the air around us needs to be somewhat dry. Thus, evaporative cooling is less effective in a humid environment. Body composition also plays a role: Large individuals with a great deal of muscle mass produce a lot of body heat. In addition, people with high levels of body fat, such as Stringer and Bechler, have an extra layer of insulation that makes it difficult to dissipate body heat at rest and during exercise.

Symptoms of heat stroke include a rapid pulse, deep breathing, hot and dry skin, high temperature, and loss of consciousness. And as illustrated in the Korey Stringer and Steve Bechler cases, heat stroke can also be fatal.

You can reduce your risk of heat stroke by maintaining a healthy fluid balance before, during, and after exercise or manual labor. If you are training, competing, or working in a hot environment and begin to feel dizzy, light-headed, disoriented, or nauseated, you should stop immediately. Find a cool place to rest, consume cool beverages such as water or a sports beverage, and ask someone to notify your trainer, coach, or employer that you need assistance.

Water Intoxication

Is it possible to drink too much water? **Water intoxication**, also called *overhydration*, can occur, but it is rare. In nonathletes, it generally occurs only in people with health problems that cause the kidneys to retain too much water. It is more common in endurance athletes such as long-distance runners and triathletes, because kidney function is reduced during intense exercise. When athletes drink too much water and do not replace adequate sodium during a long event, their bodies can retain too much fluid, resulting in a dangerous dilution of blood sodium called *hyponatremia*.

As with Cynthia Lucero, discussed at the beginning of this chapter, hyponatremia can be fatal. Warning signs of hyponatremia include continuing thirst despite fluid intake, nausea, headache, inability to concentrate, and confusion. These symptoms indicate the need for immediate medical assistance.

heat stroke A potentially fatal response to high temperature characterized by failure of the body's heat-regulating mechanisms. Symptoms include rapid pulse, reduced sweating, hot, dry skin, high temperature, headache, weakness, and sudden loss of consciousness. Commonly called *sunstroke*.

water intoxication Dilution of body fluid. It results when water intake or retention is excessive, and can lead to hyponatremia.

> RECAP *Dehydration, heat stroke, and water intoxication can occur when water and electrolyte losses are not balanced with water and electrolyte replacement. These conditions can occur in manual laborers and in athletes training or competing in hot weather, and can be fatal.*

NUTRI-CASE GUSTAVO

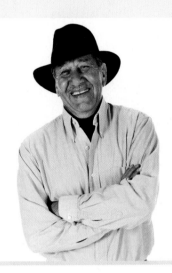

" Something is going on with me this week. Every day at work, I've been feeling weak and like I'm going to be sick to my stomach. It's been really hot, over a hundred degrees out in the fields, but I'm used to that, and besides, I've been drinking lots of water. It's probably just my high blood pressure acting up again."

What do you think might be wrong with Gustavo? If you learned that he was following a low-sodium diet prescribed to manage his high blood pressure, would this information argue for or against your theory, and why? What do you think Gustavo should do differently at work tomorrow?

How Much Alcohol Is Safe to Drink?

Alcohol is the familiar name for a beverage made from fermented fruits, vegetables, and grains. Alcoholic beverages include beer, wine, and distilled spirits such as whiskey. Although alcohol is an energy-rich compound providing 7 kcal/g, it is not considered a nutrient. That's because instead of being essential to our body's functioning, it can significantly impair functioning.

Alcohol Consumption Is Described as Drinks per Day

Alcohol consumption is typically described as *drinks per day*. A **drink** is defined as the amount of a beverage that provides ½ fl. oz of alcohol. Typically, that is equivalent to 1½ oz of distilled spirits (80-proof vodka, gin, whiskey, rum, scotch), 5 oz of wine, or 12 oz of beer or a wine cooler.[10] These amounts are shown in FIGURE 8.6.

Beers, wines, and distilled spirits contain different percentages of alcohol by volume. Beers range from about 3% to 4% alcohol for light beers to 5% or more for regular beers, and as much as 7% for stout beers, malt liquor, and other specialty beers. Wines contain from 7% to 24% alcohol. The alcohol content of distilled spirits is directly related to its **proof**: 100-proof liquor is 50% alcohol, whereas 80-proof liquor is 40% alcohol.

The 2005 *Dietary Guidelines for Americans* advise: "Those who choose to drink alcoholic beverages should do so sensibly and in moderation—defined as the consumption of up to one drink per day for women and up to two drinks per day for men." It is important to understand that these are daily guidelines; a person who abstained from all alcoholic beverages Sunday through Friday but had seven drinks on Saturday night would not be classified as a moderate drinker! The 2005 *Guidelines* also identify specific groups of individuals who should not consume alcohol at all. These include:[11]

- women who are or may become pregnant
- women who are breastfeeding

alcohol A beverage made from fermented fruits, vegetables, or grains and containing the chemical ethanol.

drink The amount of an alcoholic beverage that provides approximately ½ fl. oz of pure ethanol.

proof A measure of the alcohol content of a liquid. For example, 100-proof liquor is 50% alcohol by volume, whereas 80-proof liquor is 40% alcohol by volume.

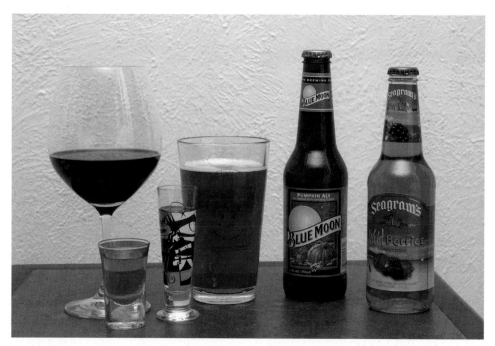

FIGURE 8.6 What does one drink look like? The National Institute on Alcohol Abuse and Alcoholism lists "one drink" as 5 oz of wine, 12 oz of beer or wine cooler, or 1½ oz of distilled spirits.

- people with a history of alcoholism
- people taking medications that interact with alcohol
- people driving, operating machinery, or engaged in other tasks that require attention and coordination

Fewer Than Half of Americans Surveyed Regularly Consume Alcohol

In the United States, self-reports of alcohol consumption by people 18 years and older indicate that fewer than half of those surveyed regularly consume alcohol. About 38% of Americans are lifetime or current abstainers (within previous 12 months), 14% are infrequent alcohol consumers (fewer than 12 drinks over the past 12 months), and 48% are regular alcohol consumers (12 or more drinks over past 12 months).[12]

Alcohol Absorption Rates Vary

Alcohol, which does not require digestion, is absorbed from both the stomach and the intestines. From there, it is transported to the liver, where it is subsequently metabolized or, if consumed in excess, released into the bloodstream and rapidly distributed throughout the body.

The rate at which we absorb alcohol varies. If consumed in the absence of food, alcohol is absorbed from the stomach almost immediately; the consumption of a meal or snack with some fat, protein, and fiber before or with alcohol intake will slow gastric emptying and delay the intestinal absorption of alcohol. Carbonated alcoholic beverages are more rapidly absorbed compared to noncarbonated, thus the infamous intoxicating effect of champagne and sparkling wines. Women often absorb a higher percent of a given intake of alcohol compared to a man of the same size and thus are more susceptible to the behavioral and physiologic effects of alcohol.

In an average, healthy adult, the liver breaks down alcohol at a fairly constant rate, equivalent to approximately one drink per hour. If a person drinks more alcohol than the liver can metabolize over the same period of time, the excess is released back into the bloodstream.

Despite popular theories, there is no practical intervention that will speed up the breakdown of alcohol: it doesn't help to walk around, consume coffee or energy drinks, or use commercial herbal or nutrient supplements. The key to avoiding intoxication is to consume alcohol no more rapidly than about one drink per hour, which allows the liver to break down the alcohol at a rate that equals intake.

As an individual's alcohol intake increases over time, the liver metabolizes alcohol more efficiently and blood alcohol levels rise more slowly. This metabolic tolerance to alcohol explains why people who chronically abuse alcohol must consume increasingly larger amounts before reaching a state of intoxication. Over time, they may need to consume twice as much alcohol as when they first started to drink in order to reach the same state of euphoria.

Of the alcohol we consume, a small amount, typically less than 10%, is excreted through the urine, breath, and sweat. As the blood alcohol concentration increases, so does the level of alcohol in breath vapor; this relationship forms the basis of the common Breathalyzer testing done by law enforcement agencies. It may surprise you to learn that you don't need to drink much alcohol before your driving ability is impaired. For example, certain driving skills are reduced by blood alcohol concentrations (BAC) as low as 0.02%, despite the fact that most states in the United States set the BAC limit at 0.08%.[13] Table 8.1 identifies typical responses of individuals at varying BAC levels.

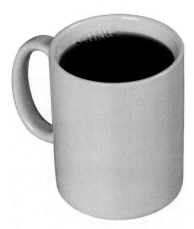

Black coffee will not speed the breakdown of alcohol.

RECAP *Alcohol provides 7 kcal/g but is not a nutrient because it is not essential to body functioning. Alcohol intake is classified in "drinks per day." A drink is defined as the amount of a beverage that provides ½ fl. oz of alcohol. Only about 48% of Americans regularly consume alcohol. Alcohol absorption can be slowed by the consumption of a meal or large snack. The liver breaks down absorbed alcohol at a steady rate of approximately one drink per hour; there is no effective way to speed up this process.*

Moderate Alcohol Consumption Has Health Benefits and Risks

The psychological benefits of moderate alcohol consumption are well-known: it can relieve tension and anxiety while enhancing relaxation and self-confidence. But moderate alcohol consumption has health benefits as well. It has been linked to a reduced risk of cardiovascular disease and certain types of strokes.[14, 15] Alcohol increases levels of protective HDL-cholesterol and reduces the risk of clot formation in the arteries.[16] Although many consumers believe the benefit comes only from the consumption of red wines, recent studies suggest that intakes of white wine, distilled spirits, or even beer have similar effects.[17]

TABLE 8.1 Effects of Blood Alcohol Concentration (BAC) on Brain Activity

Blood Alcohol Concentration (%)	Typical Response
0.02–0.05	Feeling of relaxation, euphoria, relief
0.06–0.10	Impaired judgment, fine motor control, and coordination; loss of normal emotional control; legally drunk in many states (at the upper end of the range)
0.11–0.15	Impaired reflexes and gross motor control; staggered gait; legally drunk in all states; slurred speech
0.16–0.20	Impaired vision; unpredictable behavior; further loss of muscle control
0.21–0.35	Total loss of coordination; in a stupor
0.40 and above	Loss of consciousness; coma; suppression of respiratory response; death

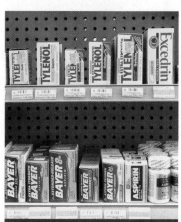

Alcohol can interfere with and increase the risks of using various over-the-counter and prescription medications.

In the elderly, moderate intake of alcohol is thought to stimulate appetite and improve dietary intake.[18] Some, but not all, research suggests that moderate alcohol consumption may lower risk of cognitive impairment and other forms of dementia.[19] As research in this area continues, health care providers will develop a clearer picture of which individuals might benefit from moderate alcohol intake.

Despite these benefits, even moderate drinking can be risky. A person's genetic background, state of health, use of medicines, and age all influence the short- and long-term responses to alcohol intake, even at moderate levels. For example, some studies have reported an increased risk of breast cancer among women consuming even low to moderate levels of alcohol, and others have reported an increase in risk of developing high blood pressure (hypertension) among men consuming as little as two drinks per day.[20] In addition, alcohol consumption interferes with the absorption and utilization of thiamin, folate, and vitamin B_6, increasing your risk of deficiency.

In some drinkers, moderate alcohol intake may increase total energy intake and risk of overweight or obesity; because alcoholic beverages do not trigger the normal satiety response seen with solid foods, most people fail to compensate for the calories by eating less food.[21] In addition, moderate alcohol consumption stimulates appetite over the short term, increasing total energy intake.[21]

Drinking alcohol while taking any one of more than 150 medications can also cause problems.[13, 22] For example, if you are taking antihistamines for an allergy, alcohol will increase their sedative effect, making you extremely drowsy. And you can develop serious liver damage if you are taking large doses of the painkiller acetaminophen (sold in many over-the-counter remedies such as Tylenol), even if you are drinking only moderately.

RECAP *Moderate intake of alcohol is associated with health benefits as well as potential risks. Every individual will have a unique metabolic and behavioral response to a given alcohol exposure and must carefully weigh the pros and cons of alcohol consumption.*

Excessive Alcohol Consumption Leads to Serious Health Problems

Alcohol is a drug. It exerts a narcotic effect on virtually every part of the brain, acting as a sedative and depressant. In varying amounts for different individuals, alcohol suppresses the area of the brain that controls reasoning and judgment, causes blurred vision and slurred speech, and impairs fine and gross motor skills (see Table 8.1). Alcohol also interferes with normal sleep patterns and reduces sexual function.

Excessive alcohol consumption negatively affects not only our physiology, but our mood and behavior as well. Many people who drink to excess experience mood swings, irritability, or intense anger, while others experience sadness or lethargy. Did you know that about 25% of college students report academic consequences of their drinking, such as missing class, falling behind, and getting poor grades?[13] In addition, when alcohol impairs our judgment, it makes us more likely to perform or become the victim of vandalism, physical or sexual assault, and other crimes.[13] And unfortunately, like many drugs, it can be highly addictive.

In the absence of addiction, excessive alcohol consumption is often referred to as *alcohol abuse* or "problem drinking." It's characterized by drinking too *much* or too *often* or *inappropriately* (e.g., when pregnant, just prior to driving a motor vehicle, between classes, or to quell feelings of sadness). Although the legal drinking age in the United States is 21 years, 20% of adolescents report such problem drinking; that is, getting drunk six or more times each year and/or experiencing negative consequences as a result of their drinking. Another 31% of college students also self-report alcohol abuse.[13]

What about you? How much alcohol do you drink, and do you think you should be concerned about it? Check out the What About You? box to help you decide.

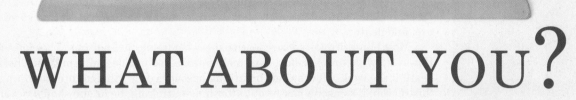

WHAT ABOUT YOU?

Should You Be Concerned about How Much Alcohol You Drink?

As discussed in this chapter, alcohol contributes to societal violence as well as personal illness, disability, and death.

Answering the following questions, provided by the NIAAA, can help you find out if you have a drinking problem[10, 23]. For each question, circle Yes or No.

● Have you ever felt you should cut down on your drinking?
YES or NO

● Have people annoyed you by criticizing your drinking?
YES or NO

● Have you ever felt bad or guilty about your drinking?
YES or NO

● Do you drink alone when you feel angry or sad?
YES or NO

● Has your drinking ever made you late for school or work?
YES or NO

● Have you ever had a drink first thing in the morning to steady your nerves or to get rid of a hangover?
YES or NO

● Do you ever drink after promising yourself you won't?
YES or NO

One "yes" answer suggests a possible alcohol problem. More than one "yes" answer means it is highly likely that a problem exists.

If you think that you might have an alcohol problem, it is important to see a doctor or other healthcare provider right away. They can help you determine if a drinking problem exists and plan the best course of action.[10] If your doctor tells you to cut down on or stop your drinking, these steps from the NIAAA can help you:

1. Write down your reasons for cutting down or stopping, such as complying with drinking-age laws or campus zero-tolerance policies; improving your health or grades; or getting along better with friends.

2. Also write down your goal (e.g., I will stop drinking alcohol as of today, May 18, 2008).

3. To help you achieve your goal, keep a diary listing every time you have a drink, the amount and type, and what circumstances (e.g., peer pressure, loneliness, etc.) prompted you to drink.

4. Make sure there is no alcohol in your dorm room, apartment, car, locker, and so forth. Instead, keep nonalcoholic beverages you enjoy well-stocked wherever you go.

5. Learn how to say NO. You don't have to drink when other people drink. Practice ways to say no politely. For instance, you can tell people that you feel better when you drink less, or that you are watching your weight. Stay away from people who harass you about not drinking.

6. Get support. Tell your family members and trusted friends about your plan to cut down or stop drinking, and ask them to support you in reaching your goal. Or, contact your local chapter of Alcoholics Anonymous, listed in your local phone directory.[10]

Binge Drinking

Binge drinking, the consumption of five or more alcoholic drinks on one occasion, is a common type of alcohol abuse, especially on college campuses. It occurs in approximately 15% of U.S. adults,[24] and young men 18 to 25 years of age report the highest incidence.[25] Many rituals associated with student life, including acceptance into a fraternity or sorority, sports events, and 21st-birthday rituals, involve binge drinking.

The effects of binge drinking range from debilitating to life-threatening. They include reduced motor control, significant disorientation, impaired judgment, memory loss, dehydration, nausea, vomiting, loss of bowel control, and an acute

binge drinking   The consumption of five or more alcoholic drinks on one occasion.

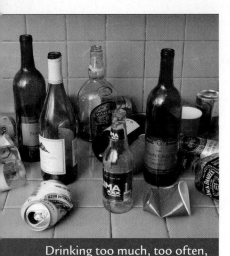

Drinking too much, too often, or inappropriately are signs of alcohol abuse.

headache. Intake that overwhelms the liver's ability to clear the alcohol from the blood results in alcohol poisoning, a potentially fatal consequence of binge drinking. Alcohol poisoning deprives the brain of oxygen. The areas of the brain that regulate breathing and cardiac function shut down, resulting in respiratory and cardiac failure, and death.

Most binge drinkers lose consciousness before alcohol poisoning becomes fatal. However, while unconscious, extremely intoxicated people can vomit and choke to death if the vomit blocks their breathing passages or is inhaled into their lungs. For this reason, if someone passes out after binge drinking, he or she should never be left alone to "sleep it off" but should be monitored for: vomiting; cold, clammy, or bluish skin; and slow or irregular breathing patterns. If these signs are present, emergency healthcare should be sought immediately.

Chronic Alcohol Abuse

Chronic alcohol abuse (excessive intake over a period of several months to years) impairs brain function in other ways. In adolescents and young adults, in whom brain development is ongoing, chronic alcohol abuse may inhibit intellect and abstract reasoning, impair memory, and interfere with goal-oriented behaviors.[26] Even after achieving sobriety, people who have chronically abused alcohol often exhibit ongoing memory and learning problems.

Chronic alcohol abuse can also lead to *alcoholism* (also known as *alcohol dependence*), a disease characterized by the following four symptoms, described by the National Institute on Alcohol Abuse and Alcoholism (NIAAA):[23]

- *Craving:* a strong need, or urge, to drink
- *Loss of control:* not being able to stop drinking once drinking has begun
- *Physical dependence:* withdrawal symptoms, such as nausea, sweating, shakiness, and anxiety after stopping drinking
- *Tolerance:* the need to drink greater amounts of alcohol to get "high"

In addition, chronic alcohol abuse severely damages the liver. As the primary site of alcohol metabolism, the liver is extremely vulnerable to the toxic effects of alcohol. Liver cells are damaged or destroyed during excessive and binge-drinking episodes. If alcohol abuse persists, liver function declines. Alcohol-related **hepatitis** causes anorexia, nausea and vomiting, abdominal pain or tenderness, jaundice, and, on occasion, mental confusion. **Cirrhosis** of the liver is a chronic condition that is characterized by an increase in fibrous tissue and a life-threatening impairment of liver function (FIGURE 8.7). Finally, chronic alcohol abuse is associated with an increased risk of a variety of cancers, including cancer of the mouth, esophagus, and lower gastrointestinal tract.

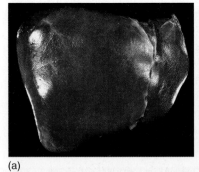
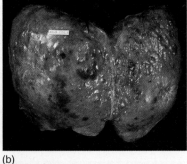

(a)   (b)

FIGURE 8.7 Cirrhosis of the liver, caused by chronic alcohol abuse. (a) A healthy liver. (b) A liver damaged by cirrhosis.

hepatitis Inflammation of the liver; can be caused by a virus or toxic agent such as alcohol.

cirrhosis End-stage liver disease characterized by significant abnormalities in liver structure and function; may lead to complete liver failure.

Alcohol Consumption Also Greatly Increases the Risk of Accidental Death

Alcohol consumption is the leading cause of death for people under the age of 21 and the third leading cause of all deaths in the United States.[23] It has been estimated that as many as 6,000 Americans under the age of 21 die each year from alcohol-related accidents, homicides, and suicides.[23] The risk of falls, drownings, and other potentially fatal accidents also increases with alcohol abuse.

Reading about these problems of alcohol consumption may be prompting you to think about someone you know who abuses or is addicted to alcohol. If so, the accompanying Game Plan has strategies for helping someone with an alcohol problem get treatment.

GAME PLAN

Strategies for Helping Someone with an Alcohol Problem Get Treatment

If you know someone who abuses alcohol by drinking too much, too often, or inappropriately, or who experiences the four symptoms of alcoholism identified by the NIAAA, what should you do? The National Institute on Alcoholism and Alcohol Abuse (NIAAA) suggests the following steps to help someone with an alcohol problem get treatment:[23]

❑ Stop all "cover ups." Family members and friends often make excuses to others to hide the fact that their loved one is drinking. If you've been doing this, stop. It is important that the person experience the full consequences of drinking.

❑ Time your intervention. The best time to talk to the drinker is shortly after an alcohol-related problem has occurred—such as a serious argument or an accident. Choose a time when he or she is sober, both of you are fairly calm, and you have a chance to talk in private.

❑ Be specific. Tell the person that you are worried about his or her drinking. Use examples of the ways in which the drinking has caused problems, including the most recent incident.

❑ State the results. Explain to the person what you will do if he or she doesn't go for help—not to punish the drinker, but to protect yourself from his or her problems. What you say may range from refusing to go with the person to any social activity where alcohol will be served to moving out of shared housing. Do not make any threats you are not prepared to carry out.

❑ Get help. Gather information in advance about treatment options on your campus or in your community. If the person is willing to get help, call immediately for an appointment. Offer to go with the person on the first visit.

❑ Call on a friend. If the person still refuses to get help, ask others to talk with him or her using the steps just described. A friend who is a recovering alcoholic may be particularly persuasive, but any person who is caring and nonjudgmental may help. The intervention of more than one person, more than one time, is often necessary to coax the person to seek help.

❑ Find strength in numbers. If the intervention of individuals one at a time does not persuade the person to seek help, consider joining together to confront the person. This approach should only be tried under the guidance of a healthcare professional who is experienced in this kind of group intervention.

❑ Get support. It is important to remember that you are not alone. Support groups offered on some campuses and in most communities include Al-Anon, which holds regular meetings for adult partners and friends of people with a drinking problem, and Alateen, which is geared to children of alcoholics. These groups help friends and family members understand that they are not responsible for the person's drinking and that they need to take care of themselves, regardless of whether the person chooses to get help.

Where I'm at now...

Now that you've read this chapter, would you say you've been getting enough fluid most days?

Yes or **NO**

What—if anything—do you plan to change about the amounts or kinds of beverages you plan to drink throughout your day?

If you drink alcohol, has reading this chapter caused you to rethink your drinking?

Yes or **NO**

If **Yes**, in what way(s)?

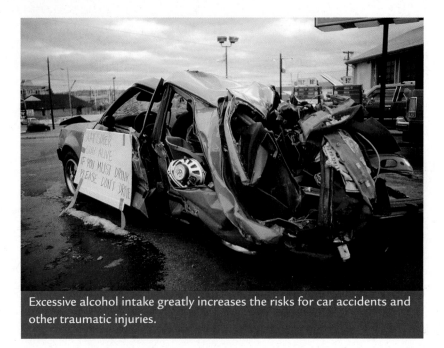

Excessive alcohol intake greatly increases the risks for car accidents and other traumatic injuries.

RECAP *Alcohol abuse (also called problem drinking) occurs when a person drinks too much or too often or inappropriately. Binge-drinking is the consumption of five or more drinks on one occasion. It can cause alcohol poisoning, which can be fatal. Chronic alcohol abuse can result in significant cognitive, emotional, and behavioral deficits, and can lead to alcoholism. It can also severely damage the liver and increase the risk of certain cancers. Alcohol consumption, particularly in underage drinkers, is strongly associated with traumatic death.*

NUTRI-CASE THEO

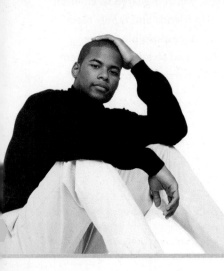

" I was driving home from a post-game party last night when I was pulled over by the police. The officer said I seemed to be driving "erratically" and asked me how many drinks I'd had. I told him I'd only had three beers, and explained that I was pretty tired from the game. Then, just to prove I was fine, I offered to count backwards from a hundred, but I must have sounded sober, because he didn't make me do it. I can't believe he thought I was driving drunk! Still, maybe three beers after a game really is too much."

Do you think it is physically possible that Theo's driving might have been impaired even though he had consumed only three beers? Before you answer, consider that Theo weighs around 170 lb during practice season and that he had just played a long basketball game. What other information would be important to find out to help you answer this question?

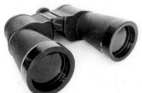

HEALTHWATCH
Fetal Alcohol Syndrome Is Caused by Maternal Consumption of Alcohol

Alcohol is a known *teratogen* (a substance capable of causing birth defects). When a pregnant woman consumes alcohol, it quickly crosses the placenta and accumulates in the fetal bloodstream. The immature fetal liver cannot effectively metabolize alcohol, so it remains in the fetal blood and tissues, where it is associated with a variety of birth defects. These effects are dose-dependent: the more the mother drinks, the greater the potential harm to the fetus. The term **fetal alcohol spectrum disorders (FASD)** is now used to describe the range of consequences that can develop when a fetus is exposed to alcohol.[27] FASD includes fetal alcohol syndrome (FAS), alcohol-related neurodevelopmental disorder (ARND), and alcohol-related birth defects (ARBD). It is estimated that more than 40,000 babies are born each year with some type of FASD, at a cost of up to $6 billion per year.[28]

Fetal alcohol syndrome (FAS) is a condition characterized by malformations of the face, limbs, heart, and nervous system in infants born to mothers who abuse alcohol during pregnancy (**FIGURE 8.8**). In the womb, the fetus with FAS does not grow normally. Newborn and infant mortality is high, and those who survive typically have emotional, behavioral, social, learning, and developmental problems throughout life.

Whereas FAS is usually recognized at birth, due in large part to the characteristic facial features of affected infants, alcohol-related neurodevelopmental disorder (ARND) is a more subtle consequence of maternal alcohol consumption. ARND expresses itself as developmental and behavioral problems (for example, hyperactivity, attention deficit disorder, and impaired learning). Alcohol-related birth defects (ARBD) include abnormalities in the heart, kidney, skeletal system, hearing, and/or vision. Infants and children with ARND and ARBD do not have the characteristic facial features seen in FAS.[27]

Can pregnant women safely consume small amounts of alcohol? Although some pregnant women do have the occasional alcoholic drink with no apparent ill effects, there is no amount of alcohol that is known to be safe. In 2005, the Surgeon General specifically stated that pregnant women should not drink alcohol during pregnancy and pregnant women who had already consumed alcohol during the pregnancy should stop in order to minimize additional risk.[27]

Breastfeeding women should also abstain from alcohol, which rapidly enters breast milk at levels that parallel those in the mother's bloodstream.[29] In addition to inhibiting the mother's milk supply, alcohol can make the baby sleepy, depress the central nervous system, and, over time, slow motor development. During the initial stages of breastfeeding, when the infant nurses nearly around the clock, intake of alcohol should be completely avoided. When feedings become less frequent, an occasional glass of wine or beer is considered safe, as long as there is sufficient time (approximately 2 hours) before the next feeding to allow the alcohol to clear from the breast milk.

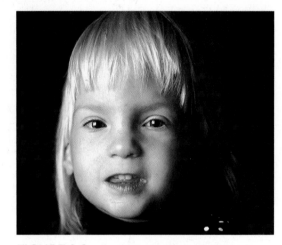

FIGURE 8.8 A child with fetal alcohol syndrome (FAS). The facial features characteristic of children with FAS include a short nose with a low, wide bridge, drooping eyes with an extra skinfold, and a flat, thin upper lip. Behavioral problems and learning disorders are also characteristic. The effects of FAS are irreversible.

fetal alcohol spectrum disorders (FASD) An umbrella term describing the range of effects that can occur in the child of a woman who drinks during her pregnancy. Fetal alcohol syndrome (FAS), alcohol-related neurodevelopmental disorder (ARND), and alcohol-related birth defects (ARBD) are components of FASD.

fetal alcohol syndrome (FAS) Cluster of birth defects in the offspring of a mother who consumed alcohol during pregnancy, including facial deformities, impaired growth, and a spectrum of mild to severe cognitive, emotional, and physical problems.

RECAP *Alcohol is a known teratogen. Fetal alcohol syndrome is a condition characterized by malformations of the face, limbs, heart, and nervous system in infants born to mothers who abuse alcohol during pregnancy. Alcohol-related neurodevelopmental disorder and alcohol-related birth defects can also occur if a woman drinks during her pregnancy. No amount of alcohol during pregnancy is considered safe.*

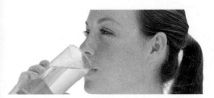

REVIEW QUESTIONS

Circle the correct choice.

1. Which of the following people probably has the greatest percentage of body fluid?
   a. A female adult who is slightly overweight
   b. A male adult who is obese
   c. An elderly male of average weight
   d. A healthy infant of average weight

2. Plasma is one example of
   a. fluid outside our cells.
   b. fluid inside our cells.
   c. an electrolyte.
   d. metabolic water.

3. Pale urine typically indicates
   a. water intoxication.
   b. kidney failure.
   c. adequate hydration.
   d. dehydration.

4. One gram of alcohol provides
   a. 9 kcal of energy.
   b. 8 kcal of energy.
   c. 7 kcal of energy.
   d. varying amounts of energy according to the type of drink (beer, wine, or spirits).

5. Alcohol consumption
   a. is the third leading cause of death in the United States.
   b. is the leading cause of death for Americans under the age of 21.
   c. interferes with the absorption of some B vitamins.
   d. All of the above are true.

6. True or False? Blood volume decreases when the amount of fluid in blood decreases.

7. True or False? A decreased concentration of electrolytes in our blood stimulates the thirst mechanism.

8. True or False? The *Dietary Guidelines for Americans* recommend that people who currently abstain from alcohol begin to drink alcohol in moderation.

9. True or False? Technically speaking, an 8-oz (1-cup, or 250-ml) glass of wine is one drink.

10. True or False? An individual who chronically abuses alcohol requires larger and larger amounts to experience intoxication.

WEB LINKS

www.epa.gov/OW
U.S. Environmental Protection Agency

Go to the EPA's water page for more information about drinking-water quality, standards, and safety.

www.fda.gov
U.S. Food and Drug Administration (FDA)

Search the FDA Web site for information on the safety and quality of bottled water and to learn how it compares to tap water.

www.awwa.org
American Water Works Association

This nonprofit scientific and educational society is dedicated to the improvement of drinking water worldwide. Visit its Web site for everything you've ever wanted to know about drinking water.

www.mayoclinic.com
MayoClinic.com

Search for "hyponatremia" to learn more about this potentially fatal condition.

www.nlm.nih.gov/medlineplus
MEDLINE Plus Health Information

Search for "dehydration" and "heat stroke" to obtain additional resources and the latest news about the dangers of these heat-related illnesses.

www.niaaa.nih.gov
National Institute on Alcohol Abuse and Alcoholism (NIAAA)

Visit this Web site for information on the prevalence, consequences, and treatments of alcohol-related disorders. Professional materials as well as information for family members of alcoholics are available free of charge.

www.ncadd.org
National Council on Alcoholism and Drug Dependence, Inc.

This site provides educational materials and information on alcoholism.

www.collegedrinkingprevention.gov
College Drinking: Changing the Culture

The NIAAA developed this Web site specifically for college students seeking information and advice on the subject of college drinking. Services include self-assessment questionnaires, answers to frequently asked questions, news articles, research, links to support groups, and others.

www.aa.org
Alcoholics Anonymous, Inc.

This Web site provides links to local AA groups and provides information on the AA program.

www.al-anon.alateen.org
Al-Anon Family Group Headquarters, Inc.

This site provides links to local Al-Anon and Alateen groups, which provide support for spouses, children, and other significant adults within the life of an alcoholic.

www.madd.org
Mothers Against Drunk Driving

Links to local chapters, statistics related to drunk driving, and prevention strategies are easily accessed from this Web site.

www.marchofdimes.com
March of Dimes

Information on fetal alcohol syndrome and fetal alcohol effects.

TEST YOURSELF ANSWERS

1. **True.** Between approximately 50% and 70% of our body weight consists of water.

2. **False.** Our thirst mechanism signals that we need to replenish fluids, but it is not sufficient to ensure we are completely hydrated.

3. **False.** Persistent vomiting can lead to long-term health consequences and even death.

4. **True.** According to the National Institute on Alcohol Abuse and Alcoholism, a part of the National Institutes of Health, alcohol consumption is responsible for more deaths of young people annually than any other factor, in part because of its role in motor vehicle accidents, drownings, and homicides.

5. **True.** Carbonated alcoholic beverages such as champagne are absorbed more rapidly than noncarbonated varieties of alcohol.

REFERENCES

1. Almond, C. S. D., et al. 2005. Hyponatremia among runners in the Boston Marathon. *N Engl J Med* 352:1150–1156.
2. Sawka, M. N., L. M. Burke, E. R. Eichner, R. J. Maughan, S. J. Montain, and N. S. Stachenfeld. 2007. American College of Sports Medicine position stand: Exercise and fluid replacement. *Med Sci Sports Exerc* 39(2):377–390.
3. Institute of Medicine. 2004. *Dietary Reference Intakes: Water, Potassium, Sodium, Chloride, and Sulfate.* Washington, DC: The National Academies Press.
4. Wilkins, J. Forgo bottled water and soda to save the planet. *Cornell Chronicle*, August 22, 2007. Available at www.news.cornell.edu/stories/Aug07/bottled.water.sl.html. (Accessed January 2008.)
5. International Bottled Water Association. 2008. Consumers Vote for Bottled Water as Their "Number One" Beverage for a Healthy Lifestyle. Available at www.bottledwater.org/public/2007_releases/2007-06-28_survey.htm. (Accessed January 2008.)
6. Wake Forest University Baptist Medical Center. November 6, 2007. Energy drink "cocktails" lead to increased injury risk, study shows. *ScienceDaily.* Available at www.sciencedaily.com/releases/2007/11/071104191538.html. (Accessed January 2008.)
7. Duffey, K. J., and B. M. Popkin. 2006. Adults with healthier dietary patterns have healthier beverage patterns. *J Nutr* 136:2901–2907.
8. Duffey, K. J., and B. M. Poplin. 2007. Shifts in patterns and consumption of beverages between 1965 and 2002. *Obesity* 15:2739–2747.
9. Manore M., and J. Thompson. 2000. *Sport Nutrition for Health and Performance.* Champaign, IL: Human Kinetics.
10. National Institute on Alcohol Abuse and Alcoholism (NIAAA). 2005a. Alcohol: How to Cut Down on Your Drinking. Available at www.collegedrinkingprevention.gov/facts/cutdrinking.aspx.
11. U.S. Department of Health and Human Services and U.S. Department of Agriculture. 2005. *Dietary Guidelines for Americans.* 6th edition. Washington, DC: U.S. Government Printing Office.
12. National Center for Health Statistics. 2004. *Health, United States, 2004.* Hyattsville, MD: U.S. Department of Health and Human Services.
13. National Institute on Alcohol Abuse and Alcoholism (NIAAA). 2005b. A Snapshot of High-Risk College Drinking Consequences. Available at www.collegedrinkingprevention.gov/facts/snapshot.aspx.
14. Mukamal, K. J., S. E. Chiuve, and E. B. Rimm. 2006. Alcohol consumption and risk for coronary heart disease in men with healthy lifestyles. *Arch Intern Med* 166(19):2145–2150.
15. Kurth, T., S. C. Moore, J. M. Gaziano, C. S. Kase, M. J. Stampfer, K. Berger, and J. E. Buring. 2006. Healthy lifestyle and the risk of stroke in women. *Arch Intern Med* 166:1403–1409.
16. Mukamal, K. J. 2006. The effects of smoking and drinking on cardiovascular disease and risk factors. *Alcohol Research & Health* 29(3):199–202.
17. Mukamal, K. J., H. Chung, N. S. Jenny, L. H. Kuller, W. T. Longstreth, M. A. Mittleman, G. L. Burke, M. Cushman, B. M. Psaty, and D. S. Siscovick. 2006. Alcohol consumption and risk of coronary heart disease in older adults: The cardiovascular health study. *J Am Geriatr Soc* 54:30–37.
18. Byles, J., A. Young, H. Furuya, and L. Parkinson. 2006. A drink to healthy aging: The association between older women's use of alcohol and their health-related quality of life. *J Am Geriatr Soc* 54:1341–1347.
19. Solfrizzi, V., A. D'Introno, A. M. Colacicco, C. Capurso, A. Del Parigi, G. Baldassarre, P. Scapicchio, E. Scafato, M. Amodio, A. Capurso, and F. Panza for the Italian Longitudinal Study on Aging Working Group. 2007. Alcohol consumption, mild cognitive impairment, and progression to dementia. *Neurology* 68:1790–1799.

20. Stranges, S., T. Wu, J. M. Born, et al. 2004. Relationship of alcohol drinking pattern to risk of hypertension. *Hypertension* 44:813–819.

21. Caton, S. J., M. Ball, A. Ahern, and M. M. Hetherington. 2004. Dose-dependent effects of alcohol on appetite and food intake. *Physiol Behav* 81:51–58.

22. National Institute on Aging. September 2005. Alcohol use and abuse. *Age Page.* Available at www.nia.nih.gov/HealthInformation/Publications/alcohol.htm. (Accessed January 2008.)

23. National Institute on Alcohol Abuse and Alcoholism (NIAAA). 2005c. FAQ's on Alcohol Abuse and Alcoholism. Available at www.niaaa.nih.gov/faq.

24. Nelson, D. E., T. S. Naimi, and R. H. E. Wells. Metropolitan-area estimates of binge drinking in the United States. *Am J Public Health* 94:663–671.

25. Naimi, T. S., R. D. Brewer, A. Mokdad, C. Denny, and M. K. Serdula. 2003. Binge drinking among U.S. adults. *JAMA* 289:70–79.

26. Tapert, S.F., L. Caldwell, and C. Burke. 2004/2005. Alcohol and the adolescent brain: Human studies. *Alcohol Research & Health* 28:205–212.

27. U.S. Department of Health and Human Services, Center for Substance Abuse Prevention. 2007a. Preventing FASD: Healthy Women, Healthy Babies. DHHS Publication No. (SMA) 07-4253.

28. U.S. Department of Health and Human Services, Center for Substance Abuse Prevention. 2007b. Fetal Alcohol Spectrum Disorders by the Numbers. DHHS Publication No. (SMA) 06-4236.

29. Ladewig, P. A., M. L. London, and M. R. Davidson. 2006. *Contemporary Maternal-Newborn Care.* 6th edition. Upper Saddle River, NJ: Prentice Hall Health, p. 856.

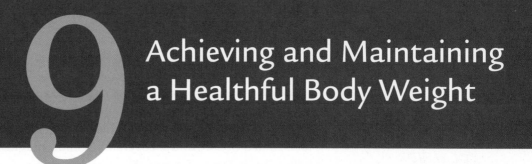

9 Achieving and Maintaining a Healthful Body Weight

TEST YOURSELF

Are these statements true or false? Circle your guess.

1 People who are physically active but overweight should not be considered healthy. **TRUE** or **FALSE**

2 Although a majority of Americans are overweight, only about 10% of Americans are obese. **TRUE** or **FALSE**

3 Being underweight can be just as detrimental to our health as being obese. **TRUE** or **FALSE**

4 Getting your body composition measured at the local fitness club will give you an accurate assessment of your body fat level. **TRUE** or **FALSE**

5 Only females get eating disorders. **TRUE** or **FALSE**

Test Yourself answers can be found at the end of the chapter.

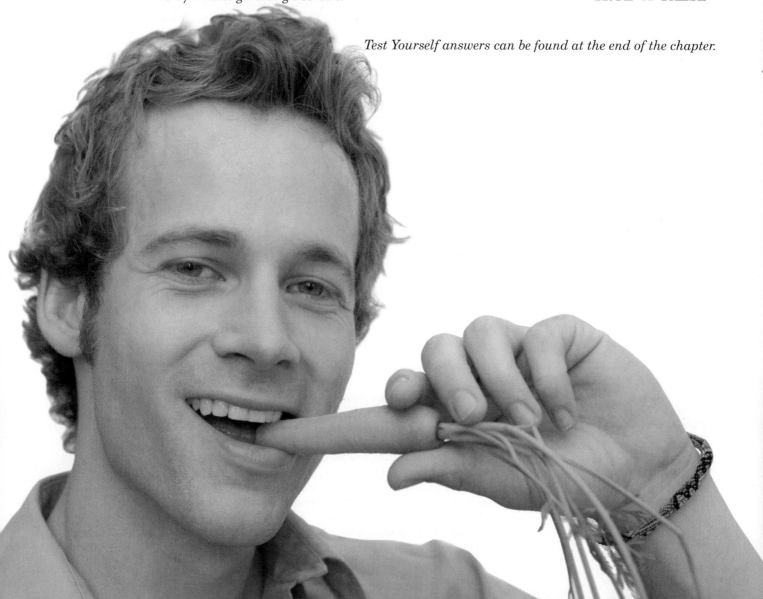

AS A TEENAGER, she won a full athletic scholarship to Syracuse University, where she was honored for her "significant contribution to women's athletics and to the sport of rowing." After graduating, she became a television reporter and anchor for an NBC station in Flagstaff, Arizona. Then she went into modeling, and soon her face smiled out from the covers of fashion magazines, cosmetics ads, even a billboard in Times Square. Now considered a "supermodel," she hosts her own television show, has her own Web site, her own clothing line, and even a collection of dolls. *People* magazine has twice selected her as one of the "50 Most Beautiful People," and *Glamour* magazine named her "Woman of the Year." So who is she? Her name is Emme Aronson . . . and by the way, her average weight is 190 lbs.

Emme describes herself as "very well-proportioned." She focuses not on maintaining a certain weight but instead on keeping healthy and fit. So she eats when she's hungry and works out regularly. Observing that, "We live in a society that is based on the attainment of unrealistic beauty," Emme works hard to get out the message that self-esteem should not be contingent on size. She frequently speaks to young people about body image concerns, and recently published her first children's book, *What Are You Hungry For?*, to encourage children to celebrate their individuality. Characteristically, she says of herself, "I don't know if I'll ever be perfect, but I'm happy with who I am."[1,2]

Are you happy with your weight, shape, body composition, and fitness? If not, what needs to change—your diet, the amount or type of physical activity you do, or maybe just your attitude? How much control do we have over our body weight? To what extent are our sizes and shapes due to genetics? What influence does society—including food advertising—have? And if you decide that you do need to lose weight, what's the best way to do it? In this chapter, we will explore these questions and provide some answers.

What Is a Healthful Body Weight?

As you begin to think about achieving and maintaining a healthful weight, it's important to make sure you understand what a healthful body weight actually means. We can define a healthful weight as all of the following:[3]

- A weight that is appropriate for your age and physical development.
- A weight that is consistent with your genetic background and family history.
- A weight that you can achieve and sustain without severely curtailing your food intake or constantly dieting.
- A weight that is compatible with normal blood pressure, lipid levels, and glucose tolerance.
- A weight that promotes good eating habits and allows you to participate in regular physical activity.
- A weight that is acceptable to you.

As you can see, a healthful weight is not one in which a person must be extremely thin or overly muscular. In addition, there is no one particular body type that can be defined as healthful. Thus, achieving a healthful body weight should not be dictated by the latest fad or current societal expectations of what is acceptable.

Now that we know what a healthful body weight is, let's look at some terms applying to underweight and overweight:

- **Underweight** is defined as having too little body fat to maintain health, causing a person to have a weight for a given height that is below an acceptably defined standard.
- **Overweight** is defined as having a moderate amount of excess body fat, resulting in a person having a weight for a given height that is greater than an accepted standard but is not considered obese.
- **Obesity** is defined as having an amount of excess body fat that adversely affects health, resulting in a person having a weight for a given height that is substantially greater than an accepted standard.
- **Morbid obesity** is defined as having a body weight that exceeds 100% of normal, putting the individual at very high risk for serious health consequences.

In the *Healthwatch* sections at the end of this chapter, we discuss obesity and morbid obesity in more detail, as well as disordered eating. All of these conditions can cause severe, even life-threatening illness.

> RECAP *A healthful body weight is one that is appropriate for your age and physical development; is consistent with your genetic background and family history; can be achieved and sustained without constant dieting; is consistent with normal blood pressure, lipid levels, and glucose tolerance; promotes good eating habits and allows for regular physical activity; and is acceptable to you. Dangerously unhealthful body weights include underweight, obesity, and morbid obesity.*

Is Your Body Weight Healthful?

Try one or more of the following three methods to determine how your current weight might be affecting your health:

- Determine your body mass index.
- Estimate your body composition.
- Assess your fat distribution pattern.

Determine Your Body Mass Index

Body mass index (BMI) is a commonly used comparison of a person's body weight to his or her height. To determine your BMI, plot your weight and height on the graph in FIGURE 9.1. You can calculate your BMI more precisely on the Internet using the BMI calculator found at www.nhlbisupport.com/bmi/. A person with a BMI value less than 18.5 is considered underweight, and a BMI value between 18.5 and 25 is considered desirable. Overweight is defined as a BMI between 25.1 and 29.9; a person is considered obese if his or her BMI value is 30 or higher.

Your BMI is important because it provides an important clue to your overall health. Research studies show that a person's risk for type 2 diabetes, high blood pressure, heart disease, and other diseases largely increases when BMI is above a value of 30. In addition, the mortality rate, or death rate, increases significantly above a value of 30. On the other hand, having a very low BMI, defined as a value below 18.5, is also associated with increased risk of serious health problems and premature death.

Although calculating BMI can be very helpful in estimating disease risk, this method is limited when used with people who have a disproportionately higher muscle mass for a given height. For example, one of Theo's friends, Randy, is a weight lifter. Randy is 5′ 7″ and weighs 200 lb. Using Figure 9.1, you can see that Randy's BMI is over 30, placing him in the high-risk category for many diseases. But is Randy really overweight? To answer that question, an assessment of body composition is necessary.

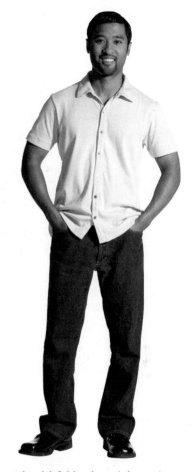

A healthful body weight varies from person to person.

underweight Having too little body fat to maintain health, causing a person to have a weight for a given height that is below an acceptably defined standard.

overweight Having a moderate amount of excess body fat, resulting in a person having a weight for a given height that is greater than an accepted standard but is not considered obese.

obesity Having an excess body fat that adversely affects health, resulting in a person having a weight for a given height that is substantially greater than an accepted standard.

morbid obesity A condition in which a person's body weight exceeds 100% of normal, putting him or her at very high risk for serious health consequences.

body mass index (BMI) A measurement representing the ratio of a person's body weight to his or her height.

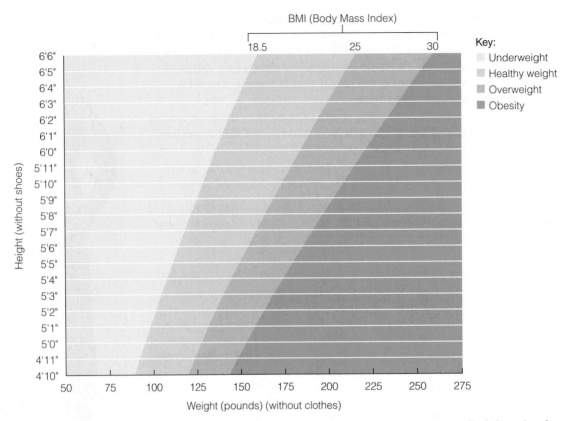

FIGURE 9.1 Measure your body mass index (BMI) using this graph. To determine your BMI, find the value for your height on the left and follow this line to the right until it intersects with the value for your weight on the bottom axis. The area on the graph where these two points intersect is your BMI.

Estimate Your Body Composition

There are many methods available to assess your **body composition**, or the amount of body fat (or *adipose tissue*) and lean body mass (or *lean tissue*) you have. These methods provide only an estimate of your body fat and lean body mass, not an exact percentage of these tissues. Because their margin of error can range from 3% to more than 20%, you should not rely on body composition results as the only indicator of your health status. The following are the most common methods of measuring body composition:

body composition The ratio of a person's body fat to lean body mass.

- *Underwater weighing method.* In underwater weighing, a technician first weighs a person using a traditional scale. Then the person is submerged underwater and weighed again (**FIGURE 9.2**). Because fat floats, the amount of water displaced provides an accurate body composition measurement. This method is not widely available in the United States except in exercise physiology laboratories. If you have access to a laboratory performing underwater weighing, it is worth having the procedure done, because it is considered one of the most accurate. Under the best of circumstances, underwater weighing can estimate body fat within a 2% to 3% margin of error.[4] This means that if your underwater weighing test shows you have 20% body fat, this value could be no lower than 17% nor higher than 23%. The test does not work well with obese people.

- *Skinfold measurements.* Measuring skinfolds involves painlessly "pinching" a fold of skin and its underlying fat at various locations of the body such as the upper arm and waist (**FIGURE 9.3**). The fold is measured using a device called a caliper. This method cannot be used with many obese people, as their skinfolds are too large. Another major drawback of this method is that it relies on a tech-

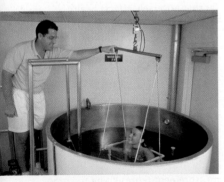

FIGURE 9.2 Underwater weighing.

nician applying the correct one of more than 400 equations developed in research studies. Many places that offer this measurement employ untrained technicians who use only one equation for their entire client base, severely limiting its accuracy. When performed by a skilled technician, skinfold measurement has a margin of error of 3% to 4%.[4]

● *Bioelectrical impedance analysis (BIA).* This method involves sending a very low level of electrical current through a person's body (**FIGURE 9.4**). Because water is a good conductor of electricity, and lean body mass is made up mostly of water, the rate at which the electricity is conducted gives an indication of a person's lean body mass and body fat. One of the challenges of BIA is that the person being measured must have adhered to restrictions on food, alcohol, and exercise prior to the test. Another challenge is that, as with the skinfold method, most BIA technicians use only one equation for all clients. When done under the best of circumstances, BIA can estimate your body fat with an error of 3% to 4%.[4]

● *Bod Pod®.* This machine uses air displacement to measure body composition (**FIGURE 9.5**). The person being measured sits in the large, egg-shaped chamber for about 5 minutes, during which time the machine measures how much air is displaced. The Bod Pod® is expensive and is currently used mostly in research settings. Although this method appears to be fairly accurate, failure to adhere to several important testing criteria can alter findings.[4]

Let's return to Randy, whose BMI is over 30. Is he overweight? Randy trains with weights 4 days per week, rides an exercise bike for about 30 minutes per session three times per week, and does not take drugs, smoke cigarettes, or drink alcohol. Through his local gym, Randy contacted a technician skilled in skinfold measurement. The results indicated that his body fat is 9%. See Table 9.1 for a list of the percent body fat standards that are associated with good health and the absence of chronic disease. According to this table, Randy's body fat values are within the healthful range. Randy is an example of a person whose BMI appears high but who is maintaining a healthful weight.

Assess Your Fat Distribution Pattern

To complete your evaluation of your current body weight, it's important to consider the way fat is distributed throughout your body. This is because your fat distribution pattern is known to affect your risk for various diseases. FIGURE 9.6 shows two types of fat patterning:

● In *apple-shaped fat patterning,* or upper-body obesity, fat is stored mainly around the waist. Apple-shaped patterning is known to significantly increase a

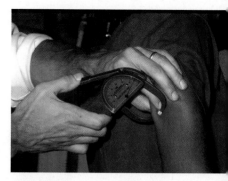

FIGURE 9.3 Skinfold measurement.

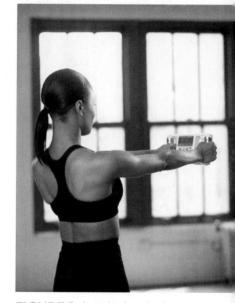

FIGURE 9.4 Bioelectrical impedance analysis (BIA).

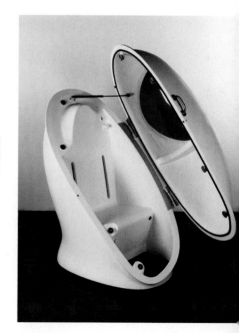

FIGURE 9.5 The Bod Pod®.

TABLE 9.1 Percent Body Fat Standards for Health

| | **Body Fat Levels** | | | | |
	Unhealthfully Low	Low Level of Acceptable	Acceptable	Upper Level of Acceptable	Obesity
Men:					
Young adult	<8	8	13	22	>22
Middle adult	<10	10	18	25	>25
Elderly	<10	10	16	23	>23
Women:					
Young adult	<20	20	28	35	>35
Middle adult	<25	25	32	38	>38
Elderly	<25	25	30	35	>35

Source: Reprinted from Lohman, T. G., L. Houtkooper, and S. B. Going. 1997. Body fat measurement goes high-tech: Not all are created equal. *ACSM's Health Fit. J.* 7:30–35.

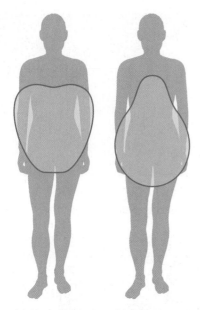

(a) Apple-shaped fat patterning   (b) Pear-shaped fat patterning

FIGURE 9.6 Fat distribution patterns. (a) An apple-shaped fat distribution pattern increases an individual's risk for many chronic diseases. (b) A pear-shaped distribution pattern does not seem to be associated with an increased risk for chronic disease.

person's risk for many chronic diseases, such as type 2 diabetes, heart disease, and high blood pressure. It is thought that this patterning causes problems with the metabolism of fat and carbohydrate, leading to unhealthful changes in blood cholesterol, insulin, glucose, and blood pressure. Men tend to store fat in the apple-shaped pattern.

- In *pear-shaped fat patterning,* or lower-body obesity, fat is stored mainly around the hips and thighs. This pattern does not seem to significantly increase a person's risk for chronic diseases. Premenopausal women tend to store fat in the pear-shaped pattern; postmenopausal women tend to store fat in the apple-shaped pattern.

You can use the following three-step method to determine your type of fat patterning:

1. Ask a friend to measure the circumference of your natural waist; that is, the narrowest part of your torso as observed from the front (FIGURE 9.7a).
2. Now have that friend measure your hip circumference at the maximal width of the buttocks as observed from the side (FIGURE 9.7b).
3. Now divide the waist value by the hip value. This measurement is called your *waist-to-hip ratio.* For example, if your natural waist is 30 in. and your hips are 40 in., then your waist-to-hip ratio is 30 divided by 40, which equals 0.75.

Once you figure out your ratio, how do you interpret it? An increased risk for chronic disease is associated with the following waist-to-hip ratios:

- In men, a ratio higher than 0.90.
- In women, a ratio higher than 0.80.

These ratios suggest an apple-shaped fat distribution pattern. In addition, waist circumference alone can indicate your risk for chronic disease. For males, your risk of chronic disease is increased if your waist circumference is above 40 inches (or 102 cm). For females, your risk is increased above 35 inches (or 88 cm).

> RECAP *Body mass index, body composition, and the fat distribution pattern are tools that can help you evaluate the health impact of your current body weight. None of these methods is completely accurate, but the information they provide may help you to decide whether or not your current weight contributes to your wellness and is acceptable to you.*

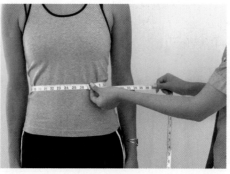
(a)

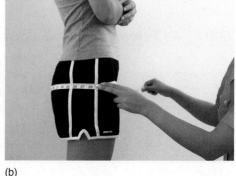
(b)

FIGURE 9.7 Determining your type of fat patterning. (a) Measure the circumference of your natural waist. (b) Measure the circumference of your hips at the maximal width of the buttocks as observed from the side. Dividing the waist value by the hip value gives you your waist-to-hip ratio.

What Makes Us Gain and Lose Weight?

Have you ever wondered why some people are thin and others are overweight, even though they seem to eat about the same diet? If so, you're not alone. For hundreds of years, researchers have puzzled over what makes us gain and lose weight. In this section, we explore some information and current theories that may shed light on this question.

We Gain or Lose Weight When Our Energy Intake and Expenditure Are Out of Balance

Fluctuations in body weight are a result of changes in our **energy intake**, or the food we eat, and our **energy expenditure**, or the amount of energy we expend at rest, as a result of eating, and as a result of the physical activity we do. This relationship between what we eat and what we do is defined by the energy balance equation:

Energy balance occurs when energy intake = energy expenditure

This means that our energy is balanced when we consume the same amount of energy that we expend each day. FIGURE 9.8 shows how our weight changes when we change either side of this equation. From this figure, you can see that in order to lose body weight, we must expend more energy than we consume. In contrast, to gain weight, we must consume more energy than we expend. Finding the proper balance between energy intake and expenditure allows us to maintain a healthful body weight.

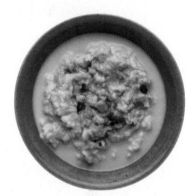

The energy provided by a bowl of oatmeal is derived from its protein, carbohydrate, and fat content.

Energy Intake Is the Food We Eat Each Day

Energy intake is the amount of energy in the food we eat each day. This value includes the carbohydrate, fat, protein, and alcohol that each food contains; vitamins, minerals, and water have no energy value, so they contribute zero kilocalories to our energy intake. Our daily energy intake is expressed as *kilocalories per day* (or *kcal/day*).

You have several options for determining how much energy is in the foods you eat. For packaged foods, read the "Calories" line on the Nutrition Facts Panel, and make sure you adjust the value according to the serving size you eat. For instance, if a serving is listed as half a cup, but you routinely eat a full cup, then you need to double the value. For fresh foods such as fruits, vegetables, meats, and so forth, use the Nutrient Values in Appendix A of this book. Alternatively, to determine how much energy you consumed in one meal or one day, log on to www.MyPyramid.gov and enter the foods into the MyPyramid Plan (see the box on the right side of the home page).

When our total daily energy intake exceeds the amount of energy we expend, we gain weight. An excess intake of approximately 3,500 kcal will result in a gain of 1 lb. Without exercise or other increased physical activity, this gain will likely be fat.

Energy Expenditure Includes More Than Just Physical Activity

Energy expenditure (also known as *energy output*) is the energy the body expends to maintain its basic functions and to perform all levels of movement and activity. We can calculate how much energy we expend in a typical 24-hour period by adding together estimates of the energy we use during rest, as a result of eating food, and as a result of physical activity. These three factors are referred to as our *basal metabolic*

energy intake The amount of food a person eats; in other words, it is the number of kilocalories consumed.

energy expenditure The energy the body expends to maintain its basic functions and to perform all levels of movement and activity.

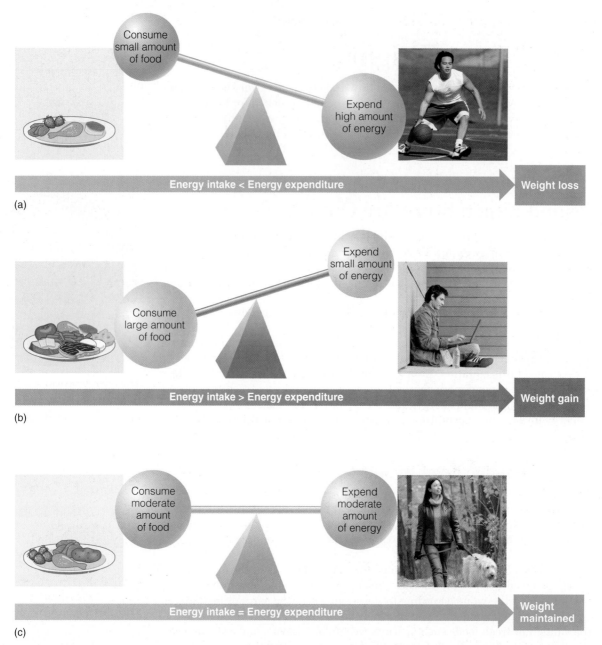

(a)

Energy intake < Energy expenditure — Weight loss

(b)

Energy intake > Energy expenditure — Weight gain

(c)

Energy intake = Energy expenditure — Weight maintained

FIGURE 9.8 Energy balance describes the relationship between the food we eat and the energy we burn each day. (a) Weight loss occurs when food intake is less than energy output. (b) Weight gain occurs when food intake is greater than energy output. (c) We maintain our body weight when food intake equals energy output.

rate (BMR), the *thermic effect of food (TEF),* and the *energy cost of physical activity* (FIGURE 9.9).

Basal Metabolic Rate Is Energy Output at Rest **Basal metabolic rate (BMR)** is the energy we expend just to maintain our bodies' *basal,* or *resting,* functions. These functions include breathing, circulation, maintaining body temperature, synthesis of new cells and tissues, secretion of hormones, and nervous system activity. The majority of our energy output each day (about 60–75%) is a result of our BMR.[5] This means that 60% to 75% of our energy output goes to fuel the basic activities of staying alive, aside from any physical activity.

BMR varies widely among people. The primary influence on our BMR is the amount of lean body mass that we have. People with a higher lean body mass have a higher BMR, because it takes more energy to support lean tissue. Age is another

basal metabolic rate (BMR) The energy the body expends to maintain its fundamental physiologic functions.

TABLE 9.2 Factors Affecting Basal Metabolic Rate (BMR)

Factors That Increase BMR	Factors That Decrease BMR
Higher lean body mass	Lower lean body mass
Greater height (more surface area)	Lower height
Younger age	Older age
Elevated levels of thyroid hormone	Depressed levels of thyroid hormone
Stress	Starvation or fasting
Male gender	Female gender
Pregnancy and lactation	
Certain drugs such as stimulants, caffeine, and tobacco	

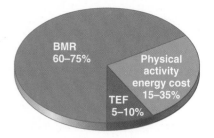

Components of energy expenditure

FIGURE 9.9 The components of energy expenditure include basal metabolic rate (BMR), the thermic effect of food (TEF), and the energy cost of physical activity. BMR accounts for 60% to 75% of our total energy output, whereas TEF and physical activity together account for 25% to 40%.

factor: BMR decreases approximately 3% to 5% per decade after age 30. Much of this change is due to the loss of lean body mass resulting from inactivity. Thus, much of this decrease may be prevented with regular physical activity. Several other factors that can affect a person's BMR are listed in Table 9.2.

How can you estimate your BMR? Begin by converting your current body weight in pounds to kilograms, by dividing pounds by 2.2. For instance, if you weigh 175 lb, your weight in kilograms is 79.5:

$$175 \text{ lb}/2.2 = 79.5 \text{ kg}$$

If you're a male, you can assume that your weight in kilograms roughly matches the kilocalories (kcals) you expend per hour: that is, 79.5 kcals per hour. Thus, your BMR for a 24-hour day is:

$$79.5 \text{ kcals per hour} \times 24 \text{ hours} = 1{,}908$$

Females have less lean body mass on average than males, so their BMR is considered about 90% of the BMR for males of the same weight. Thus, if you're a woman who weighs 175 lb, you'll need to multiply the 1,908 BMR for males by 0.9 to get your final value. Here's the full equation for women:

$$175 \text{ lb}/2.2 = 79.5 \text{ kg}$$

$$79.5 \text{ kcals per hour} \times 24 \text{ hours} = 1{,}908 \text{ BMR for males}$$

$$1{,}908 \times 0.9 = 1{,}717 \text{ BMR for women}$$

The Thermic Effect of Food Is the Energy Expended to Process Food The **thermic effect of food** is the energy we expend to digest, absorb, transport, metabolize, and store the nutrients we eat. The thermic effect of food is equal to about 5% to 10% of the energy content of a meal. Thus, if a meal contains 500 kcal, the thermic effect of processing that meal is about 25 to 50 kcal. Interestingly, our bodies use less energy to digest, transport, and store fat and relatively more to process protein and carbohydrate.

The Energy Cost of Physical Activity Is Highly Variable The **energy cost of physical activity** represents about 15% to 35% of our total energy output each day. This is the energy that we expend due to any movement or work above basal levels. This includes low-intensity activities such as sitting, standing, and walking and higher-intensity activities such as running, skiing, and bicycling. One of the most obvious ways to increase how much energy we expend as a result of physical activity is to do more activities for a longer period of time.

Table 9.3 lists the energy cost of certain activities. As you can see, activities that involve moving our larger muscle groups (or more parts of the body) require more energy. The amount of energy we expend during activities is also affected by our body size. This is why the kilocalories of energy in the third column of Table 9.3 are expressed per pound of body weight.

thermic effect of food The energy expended as a result of processing food consumed.

energy cost of physical activity The energy expended on body movement and muscular work above basal levels.

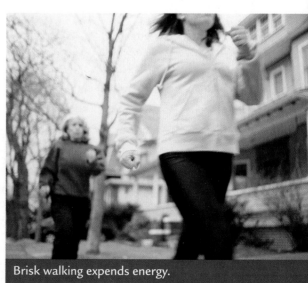

Brisk walking expends energy.

TABLE 9.3   Energy Costs of Various Physical Activities

Activity	Intensity	Kilocalories Used per Pound per Hour
Sitting, quietly watching television	Light	0.48
Sitting, reading	Light	0.62
Sitting, studying including reading or writing	Light	0.86
Cooking or food preparation (standing or sitting)	Light	0.95
Walking, shopping	Light	1.09
Walking, 2 mph (slow pace)	Light	1.2
Cleaning (dusting, straightening up, vacuuming, changing linen, carrying out trash)	Moderate	1.2
Stretching—Hatha yoga	Moderate	1.2
Weight lifting (free weights, Nautilus, or universal type)	Light or moderate	1.42
Bicycling < 10 mph	Leisure (work or pleasure)	1.9
Walking, 4 mph (brisk pace)	Moderate	2.4
Aerobics	Low impact	2.4
Weight lifting (free weights, Nautilus, or universal type)	Vigorous	2.86
Bicycling 12 to 13.9 mph	Moderate	3.82
Running, 5 mph (12 minutes per mile)	Moderate	3.82
Running, 6 mph (10 minutes per mile)	Moderate	4.77
Running, 8.6 mph (7 minutes per mile)	Vigorous	6.68

Source: Ainsworth B. E., W. L. Haskell, M. C. Whitt, M. L. Irwin, A. M. Swartz, S. J. Strath, W. L. O'Brien, D. R. Bassett, Jr., K. H. Schmitz, P. O. Emplaincourt, D. R. Jacobs, Jr., and A. S. Leon. 2000. Compendium of physical activities: An update of activity codes and MET intensities. *Med. Sci. Sports Exerc.* 32: S498–S516.

> RECAP   *The energy balance equation relates food intake to energy expenditure. Eating more energy than you expend causes weight gain, whereas eating less energy than you expend causes weight loss. The three components of this equation are basal metabolic rate, the thermic effect of food, and the energy cost of physical activity.*

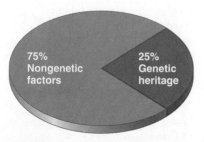

Percent (%) contribution to body fat

FIGURE 9.10   Research indicates that about 25% of our body fat is accounted for by our genetic heritage. However, nongenetic factors such as diet and exercise play a much larger role.

Genetic and Physiologic Factors Affect Our Tendency to Gain or Lose Weight

Our genetic background influences our height, weight, body shape, basal metabolic rate, and other aspects of our physiology (how the body functions). A classic study shows that the body weights of adults who were adopted as children are similar to the weights of their biological parents, not their adoptive parents.[6] FIGURE 9.10 shows that about 25% of our body fat is accounted for by genetic influences. Some proposed theories linking genetics with body weight are the thrifty gene theory, the set-point theory, and the leptin theory.

The Thrifty Gene Theory

The **thrifty gene theory** suggests that some people possess a gene (or genes) that causes them to be energetically thrifty. This means that both at rest and during activity, these people expend less energy than those who do not possess this gene. The proposed purpose of this gene is to protect a person from starving to death during times of extreme food shortages. This theory has been applied to some Native American tribes, as these societies were exposed to centuries of feast and famine. Those with a thrifty metabolism survived when little food was available, and this trait was passed on to future generations. Although an actual thrifty gene (or genes) has not yet been identified, researchers continue to study this explanation as a potential cause of obesity.

If this theory is true, think about how people who possess this thrifty gene might respond to today's environment. Low levels of physical activity, inexpensive food sources that are high in fat and energy, and excessively large serving sizes are the norm in our society. People with a thrifty metabolism would experience more weight gain than those without the gene, and their bodies would be more resistant to weight loss. Theoretically, having thrifty genetics appears advantageous during times of minimal food resources; however, this state could lead to very high levels of obesity in times of plenty.

The Set-Point Theory

The **set-point theory** suggests that our bodies are designed to maintain our weights within a narrow range, or at a "set point." In many cases, our bodies appear to respond in such a way as to maintain our current weights. When we dramatically reduce energy intake (such as with fasting or strict diets), our bodies respond with physiologic changes that cause our BMRs to drop. This causes a significant slowing of our energy output. In addition, being physically active while fasting or strictly dieting is difficult because we just don't have the energy for it. These two mechanisms of energy conservation may contribute to some of the rebound weight gain many dieters experience after they quit dieting. Rebound weight gain can be avoided with exercise, which increases BMR.

In some people, overeating may cause an increase in BMR. This effect is thought to be associated with an increased thermic effect of food as well as an increase in spontaneous movements, or fidgeting. This in turn increases energy output and prevents weight gain. These changes may explain why some people fail to gain as much weight as might be expected from eating excess food.

We don't eat the exact same amount of food each day; some days we overeat, other days we eat less. When you think about how much our daily energy intake fluctuates (about 20% above and below our average monthly intake), our ability to maintain a certain weight over long periods of time suggests that there is some evidence to support the set-point theory.

Can we change our set point? It appears that when we maintain changes in our diet and activity level over a long period of time, our set point does change. Many people do successfully lose weight and maintain that weight loss over long periods of time, largely because they consistently eat a healthful diet and engage in regular physical activity. Thus, the set-point theory does not imply that we cannot maintain weight loss.

The Leptin Theory

Leptin, first discovered in mice, is a hormone that is produced by body fat. Leptin acts to reduce food intake, and it causes a decrease in body weight and body fat. Obese mice were found to have genetic mutations in the *ob* gene, or obesity gene, and these mutations caused overeating, decreased energy output, and extreme obesity in these animals. When the *ob* gene is functioning normally, it produces leptin. When there is a genetic mutation of the *ob* gene, leptin is not secreted in sufficient amounts, food intake increases dramatically, and energy output is reduced.

thrifty gene theory A theory that suggests that some people possess a gene (or genes) that causes them to be energetically thrifty, resulting in them expending less energy at rest and during physical activity.

set-point theory A theory that suggests that the body raises or lowers energy expenditure in response to increased and decreased food intake and physical activity. This action serves to maintain an individual's body weight within a narrow range.

leptin A hormone that is produced by body fat that acts to reduce food intake, and it causes a decrease in body weight and body fat.

A great deal of excitement was generated about how leptin might decrease obesity in humans. Unfortunately, studies have shown that although obese mice respond positively to leptin injections, obese humans tend to have very high amounts of leptin in their bodies and are insensitive to leptin's effects. In truth, we have just begun to learn about leptin and its role in human physiology.

> RECAP *Our genetic background and individual physiology influences our height, weight, body shape, and metabolic rate. The thrifty gene theory suggests that some people possess a thrifty gene, or set of genes, that causes them to expend less energy than people who do not have this gene. The set-point theory suggests that our bodies are designed to maintain weight within a narrow range. Leptin is a hormone produced by body fat that reduces food intake and decreases body weight and fat. The role of leptin in weight regulation and obesity is still under investigation.*

Lifestyle Choices Adopted in Childhood Influence Adult Weight

In addition to genetic factors, the environmental factors present in our childhood can influence our food choices, activity level, and other behaviors as adults and cause us to weigh more or less than others of similar body type. For example, children who are very physically active and eat healthful diets that do not contain a lot of excess fat and sugar are less likely to be overweight or obese as children. In contrast, children who spend most of their time on the computer or watching television and who eat a lot of foods that contain excess fat and sugar are more likely to be overweight or obese as children. When these patterns are carried into adulthood, they can result in adult overweight and obesity. We know that being overweight or obese as a child can be detrimental to our health as we age, as childhood overweight has been shown to significantly increase a person's risk of heart disease and premature death in adulthood.[7]

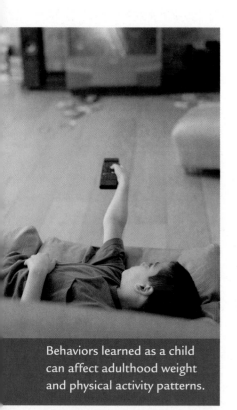

Behaviors learned as a child can affect adulthood weight and physical activity patterns.

Cultural and Economic Factors Affect Food Choices and Body Weight

Both cultural and economic factors can contribute to obesity. As discussed in detail in Chapter 1, cultural factors (including religious beliefs and learned food preferences) affect our food choices and eating patterns. In addition, the customs of many cultures put food at the center of celebrations of festivals and holidays, and overeating is tacitly encouraged. In addition, as both parents now work outside the home in most American families, more people are embracing the "fast-food culture," preferring and almost exclusively choosing highly processed and highly caloric fast foods from restaurants and grocery stores to lower-kilocalorie, home-cooked meals.

Coinciding with these cultural influences on food intake are cultural factors that promote an inactive life. Research with sedentary ethnic minority women in the United States indicates that other common barriers to increasing physical activity include lack of personal motivation, no physically active role models to emulate, acceptance of larger body size, exercise being considered culturally unacceptable, and fear for personal safety in both rural and urban settings.[8,9] In short, cultural factors influence both food consumption and levels of physical activity, and can contribute to weight gain.

Socioeconomic status is known to be related to health status, particularly in developed countries such as the United States: people of lower economic status have higher rates of obesity and related chronic diseases than people of higher socioeconomic status.[10] In addition to the impact of one's income on access to healthcare, economic factors strongly impact our food choices and eating behaviors. It is a common belief that healthful foods are expensive, and that only wealthy people can afford to purchase them. While it is true that certain foods considered more healthful,

NUTRITION MYTH OR FACT?

Does It Cost More to Eat Right?

The shelves of American supermarkets are filled with an abundance of healthful food options: organic meats and produce, exotic fish, out-of-season fresh fruits and vegetables that are flown in from warmer climates, whole-grain breads and cereals, and low-fat and low-sodium options of traditional foods. With all of this choice, it would seem easy for anyone to consume healthful foods throughout the year. But a closer look at the prices of these foods suggests that, for many, they simply are not affordable. This raises the question: Does eating right have to be expensive?

It is a fact that organic foods are more expensive than non-organic options. However, as we'll explore in detail in Chapter 12, there is little evidence indicating that organic foods are actually more healthful choices than non-organic foods. In addition, some of the lowest-cost foods currently available in stores are also some of the most nutritious: these include beans, lentils, and other legumes, seasonal fruits, root vegetables such as potatoes and winter squashes, frozen fruits and vegetables, and cooking oils high in mono- and poly-unsaturated fats. In fact, frozen as well as canned fruits and vegetables are generally just as nutritious as fresh options, and may be more so depending on how long the fresh produce has been transported and stored, and how long it has been sitting on the supermarket shelves. Thus, with some knowledge, skills, and focused attention, people can still eat healthfully on a tight budget.

Here are some more tips to help you save money when shopping for healthful foods:

- Buy whole grains such as cereals, brown rice, and pastas in bulk—they store well for longer periods and provide a good base for meals and snacks.

- Buy frozen vegetables on sale and stock up—these are just as healthful as fresh vegetables, require less preparation, and are many times cheaper.
- If lower-sodium options of canned vegetables are too expensive, buy the less expensive regular option and drain the juice from the vegetables before cooking.
- Consume smaller amounts of leaner meats—by eating less you'll not only save money but reduce your total intake of energy and fat while still providing the nutrients that support good health.
- Choose frozen fish or canned salmon or tuna packed in water as an alternative to fresh fish.
- Avoid frozen or dehydrated prepared meals. These are usually expensive, high in sodium, saturated fats, and energy, and low in fiber and other important nutrients.
- Buy generic or store brands of foods—be careful to check the labels to ensure the foods are similar in nutrient value as the higher-priced options.
- Cut coupons from local newspapers and magazines, and watch the sale circulars so that you can stock up on healthful foods you can store.
- Consider cooking more meals at home; you'll have more control over what goes into your meals and will also be able to cook larger amounts and freeze leftovers for future meals.

As you can see, eating healthfully does not have to be expensive. However, it helps to become a savvy consumer by reading food labels, comparing prices, and gaining the skills and confidence to cook at home. The information shared throughout this text should help you acquire these skills so that you can eat healthfully even on a limited budget!

such as organic foods, imported fruits and vegetables, many fish, and leaner selections of some meats, can be costly, does healthful eating always have to be expensive? Refer to the Nutrition Myth or Fact? box to learn more about whether a healthful diet can also be an affordable diet.

Social Factors Influence Eating Behavior and Physical Activity

Social factors can encourage us to overeat or to choose high-kilocalorie foods. For example, pressure from family members to eat the way they do, choosing the same foods and the same cooking methods, or being told as a child to "clean your plate," can be a significant barrier to weight loss. Like cultural gatherings, family parties,

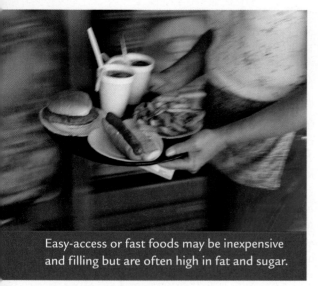

Easy-access or fast foods may be inexpensive and filling but are often high in fat and sugar.

company picnics, a barbecue with friends, and other social occasions can also provide excuses to overeat. Do you eat differently when you attend a birthday party? It's often hard to resist burgers, hot dogs, pizza, potato chips, birthday cake, ice cream, and many other foods that taste great but are relatively high in fat and energy. The pressure to overeat on such occasions is high.

We also have numerous opportunities to overeat because of easy access to foods high in fat and energy throughout our normal daily routine. For instance, how many fast-food venues are on your college campus? How many vending machines do you pass every day?

Furthermore, it probably hasn't escaped you that food manufacturers are producing products in ever-larger serving sizes. For instance, in 2005, the Mars candy company introduced a supersize version of M&M's candy, with each piece about 55% larger than the standard size M&M's. Other supersize examples include the Monster Thickburger from Hardee's restaurant, the Full House XL pizza from Pizza Hut, and the Enormous Omelet Sandwich from Burger King.[11] Serving sizes have become so large that many Americans are suffering from "portion distortion." To test your understanding of a serving size, take the "Portion Distortion" interactive quiz from the National Institutes of Health at http://hp2010.nhlbihin.net/portion.

Even store-bought foods we have traditionally considered healthful, such as peanut butter, yogurt, and milk, are often filled with added sugars and other ingredients that are high in energy. For instance, one national brand of yogurt packs 20 grams of sugar—that's 5 teaspoons—into a small (4.5-oz) serving.

On the other hand, we don't expend much energy preparing our food anymore, as we eat so many ready-to-serve meals and dine out so often. A report from the National Restaurant Association states that the typical American individual buys a snack or meal away from home an average of almost 6 times per week, and annual spending on food away from home is $1,078 per person.[12] College students may go for weeks without eating a single home-cooked meal. Although typically inexpensive, the meals served at many of the diners, fast-food restaurants, and cafeterias favored by students offer large serving sizes high in saturated and *trans* fats, simple sugars, and energy, and low in fiber-rich carbohydrates and omega fatty acids. Is it even possible to eat out healthfully? Absolutely, if you're smart about it! The accompanying Game Plan identifies some tactics for eating smart when eating out.

Similarly, social factors can cause people to be less active. For instance, whereas generations ago most jobs required physical labor, many adults now sit all day working at "desk jobs." For children, cuts in school budgets have meant reductions in physical education programs. At the same time, new educational standards have increased schools' focus on academics and reduced the time for recess. In many schools, the traditional morning recess period has been entirely eliminated. In addition, as people have moved from cities and rural villages into suburbs, they have switched from walking to driving. At home, both children and adults routinely choose sedentary activities such as TV viewing and computer use instead of choosing more physically active pursuits.

A reason many college students give for not exercising is lack of time: attending classes, studying, working a part-time job, and maintaining family and peer relationships may not allow adequate time for scheduled exercise sessions. Other social factors restricting physical activity include living in an unsafe community, watching a lot of television, coping with family or work responsibilities, and living in an area with harsh weather conditions. Many overweight people identify such factors as major barriers to maintaining a healthful body weight, and research seems to confirm their influence.

Several studies have examined the specific influence of television watching on obesity in both children and adults. A study of 11- to 13-year-old schoolchildren found that children who watched more than 2 hours of television per night were more likely to be overweight or obese than children who watched less than 2 hours of television per night. Interestingly, adults who reported an increase in television watching of

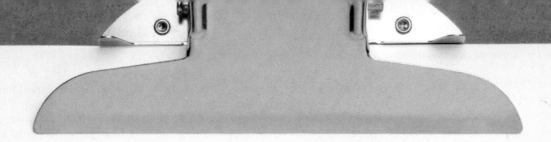

GAME PLAN

Tactics for Eating Smart When Eating Out

During the past 20 years, there has been phenomenal growth in the restaurant industry, particularly in the fast-food market. During this same period, rates of obesity have increased dramatically (see Figure 1.2 on page 4). Figure 9.11 shows two meals from popular fast-food restaurants, McDonald's and Subway. The lunch on the left, a Big Mac hamburger with extra-large French fries and an apple pie, provides 1,429 kilocalories and contains 47% of its total energy as fat. In contrast, the Subway meal of one 6″ cold-cut trio sandwich, a granola bar with chocolate chips, and a medium apple provides 610 kilocalories and contains 31% of its total energy as fat.

The energy provided in the McDonald's lunch is enough to support an entire day's needs for a small, sedentary woman! Similar meals at other fast-food restaurants are also high in kilocalories, total fat, and sodium. This example makes it easier to see how a person could become overweight or obese if consuming meals like this on a regular basis. The lesson? Seemingly small choices, such as what type of fast food to choose for lunch, can make a big difference to your waistline.

Does this mean that eating out—especially fast food—cannot be a part of a healthful diet? Not if you make smart choices. Try one or more of these tactics every time you eat out:

❑ Avoid all-you-can eat buffet-style restaurants.

❑ Choose lower-fat versions of your favorite meals. Even fast-food restaurants typically offer "lite" or lower-fat menu items that you can choose.

❑ Order a healthful appetizer as your entreé.

❑ If a child-size portion is available for your menu choice, order it.

❑ Share your meal with a friend. Many restaurant meals are large enough for two people.

❑ Order any meat item grilled or broiled. Avoid fried foods.

❑ Instead of a hamburger, choose a chicken burger, fish burger, or veggie burger.

❑ Order a meatless dish filled with vegetables and whole grains. Avoid dishes with cream sauces or a lot of cheese.

❑ Order broth-based soups instead of cream-based soups.

❑ Instead of French fries, order a salad, and choose low-fat or nonfat dressing.

❑ Order beverages with few or no kilocalories such as water, tea, or diet drinks, or order skim milk. Also request skim milk in lattés, cappuccinos, and other coffee drinks. Beware of milkshakes! A McDonald's chocolate milkshake provides 422 kilocalories!

❑ Don't feel you have to eat everything you are served. If you're satiated, stop!

❑ Skip dessert or share one dessert with a lot of friends! Another healthful alternative is to order fresh fruit for dessert.

❑ Watch out for those "yogurt parfaits" now offered at several fast-food restaurants. Many are loaded with saturated fat, simple sugars, and kilocalories.

About 1,430 kcal	About 610 kcal
McDonald's Big Mac hamburger French fries, extra large 3 tbsp. ketchup Apple pie 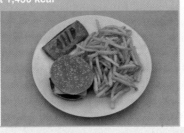	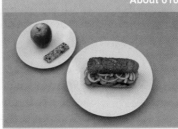 Subway cold cut trio 6" sandwich Granola bar, hard, w/choc. chips, 1 bar (24 g) 1 fresh medium apple

FIGURE 9.11   The energy density of two fast-food meals. The meal on the left is higher in total kilocalories and fat, while the meal on the right is lower in kilocalories and fat and the preferred choice for a person trying to lose weight.

20 hours per week (approximately 3 hours per day) over a 9-year period had a significant increase in waist circumference, indicating significant weight gain.[13]

On the other hand, social pressures to maintain a lean body are great enough to encourage some people to undereat, or to avoid foods they perceive as "bad," especially fats. Our society ridicules, and often ostracizes, overweight people, many of whom even face job discrimination. Media images of waif-like fashion models and men in tight jeans with washboard abdomens and muscular chests encourage many people—especially adolescents and young adults—to skip meals, resort to crash diets, and exercise obsessively. Even some people of normal body weight push themselves to achieve an unrealistic and unattainable weight goal, in the process threatening their health and even their lives (see the *Healthwatch* later in this chapter for consequences of disordered eating).

> RECAP *Our diet and activity patterns as children influence our body weights as adults. Cultural and economic factors also influence body weight through their effects on personal food preferences and financial limitations on food choice. Social factors influencing our weights include ready availability of high-kilocalorie foods, lack of physical activity, and too much television watching. Prejudices against those who are overweight can drive people to use unhealthful methods to achieve an unrealistic body weight.*

How Many Kilocalories Do You Need?

Given everything we've discussed so far, you're probably asking yourself, "How much should I eat?" This question is not always easy to answer, as our energy needs fluctuate from day to day according to our activity level, environmental conditions, and other factors such as the amount and type of food we eat and our intake of caffeine. So how can you make a general estimate of how many kilocalories your body needs per day?

A simple way to estimate your total daily kilocalorie needs is to multiply your BMR by a varying amount according to how active you are. The formula provided below is a simplified version of activity factors measured during a 1919 study of basal metabolism, and these factors are still in use today.[14] As with the formula for BMR, these activity factors do not account for wide variations in body composition such as those that occur in the very old, the very muscular, or the obese. Those who are very muscular typically need more kilocalories than the formula suggests, and the elderly and obese need fewer. The formula is as follows:

- If you do little or no exercise or physical labor, multiply your BMR by 1.2.
- If you participate in moderate exercise or labor 3 to 5 times a week, multiply your BMR by 1.5.
- If you participate in intense exercise or labor 6 to 7 times a week, multiply your BMR by 1.75.

For example, let's say that Rashid is a male student who weighs 160 lb. To calculate his BMR, he divides his weight in pounds by 2.2 to determine his weight in kilograms, then multiplies that number by 24 hours:

$$160 \text{ lb}/2.2 = 72.72 \text{ kg} \times 24 = 1,745$$

Rashid's BMR is 1,745. He does no regular exercise and spends his waking hours pretty much sitting in classes, studying, watching television, working a part-time job at a computer, driving to and from school, and so forth. Let's see how many kilocalories he needs per day to maintain his current weight and level of activity:

$$\text{BMR of } 1,745 \times 1.2 = 2,094 \text{ kcal per day}$$

If Rashid wants to lose weight, he needs to increase his level of physical activity or consume fewer than 2,094 kcal a day. Even if he doesn't want to lose weight, Rashid should begin a program of physical activity, at least 30 minutes a day most days of the week, to increase his wellness. Chapter 10 discusses ways to increase your physical activity.

For a more precise estimate of your kilocalorie needs, you can use Table 9.3 to calculate the actual kilocalories you expend in physical activity on any given day (see page 266). Then add that to your BMR. Precise calculations of energy expenditure are nearly impossible in real life, however. That's because we don't really spend long stretches of time sitting completely still, or performing exactly the same activity at exactly the same pace. For instance, while you were quietly studying for an hour, did you get up and stretch, or go to the bathroom, or rush downstairs to answer the door? Despite its limitations, estimating the energy you use during various activities can give you a general sense of the number of kilocalories you expend on an average day and perhaps provide you with an incentive to increase your physical activity.

RECAP *Accurately determining daily energy needs is difficult due to the limitations of currently available estimation methods. A simple way to estimate daily energy needs is to calculate your BMR and then multiply it by a number reflecting your daily activity level.*

How Can You Achieve and Maintain a Healthful Body Weight?

Achieving and maintaining a healthful body weight involves three primary strategies:

- Gradual changes in energy intake
- Incorporation of regular and appropriate physical activity
- Application of behavior modification techniques

In this section, we first discuss how to reduce your energy intake gradually by setting realistic goals and eating smaller portion sizes. We then discuss ways to incorporate regular physical activity into your daily life. We go on to discuss popular diet plans, which may or may not incorporate the three strategies just listed. We then explain how to design a personalized weight-loss plan that includes all three of these strategies. Finally, we review the use of prescribed medications and dietary supplements in losing weight. To further assist you, guidelines for a sound weight-loss plan are identified in the Game Plan on page 274.

Reduce Your Energy Intake Gradually

A healthful and effective weight-loss plan involves a modest reduction in energy intake. Two ways to help you reduce your energy intake include setting realistic goals and eating smaller portion sizes of foods lower in fat.

Set Realistic Goals

The first key to safe and effective weight loss is setting realistic goals related to how much weight to lose and how quickly (or slowly) to lose it. Although making gradual changes in body weight is frustrating for most people, this slower change is much more effective in maintaining long-term weight loss. Ask yourself the question, "How long did it take me to gain this extra weight?" If you are like most people, your answer is that it took one or more years, not just a few months. A fair expectation for weight loss is similarly gradual: experts recommend a pace of about 0.5 to 2 pounds per week.

Your weight-loss goals should also take into consideration any health-related concerns you may have. After checking with your physician, you may decide initially to set a goal of simply maintaining your current weight and preventing additional weight gain. After your weight has remained stable for several weeks, you might then write down realistic goals for weight loss.

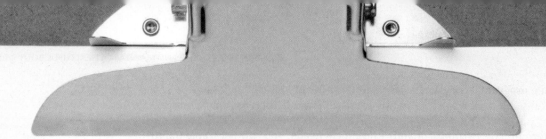

GAME PLAN

Steps toward Sustained Weight Loss

Now that you know how to spot a fad diet, you may be wondering what makes a weight-loss plan sound. That is, what should you do to lose weight and keep it off while staying well nourished and healthy? An expert panel from the National Institutes of Health recommends these steps toward weight loss that lasts.[15]

Dietary Recommendations

❑ Aim for a weight loss of 0.5 to 2 lb per week. Remember that 1 lb of fat is equal to about 3,500 kilocalories.

❑ To achieve this rate of weight loss, reduce your current energy intake by approximately 250 to 1,000 kilocalories a day. A weight-loss plan should never provide less than a total of 1,200 kilocalories a day.

❑ Aim for a total fat intake of 15% to 25% of total energy intake, and choose unsaturated rather than saturated or *trans* fats.

❑ Limit your intake of simple sugars.

❑ Consume 25 to 35 g of fiber a day.

❑ Consume 1,000 to 1,500 mg of calcium a day.

❑ Select leaner cuts of meat (such as the white meat of poultry and extra-lean ground beef) and reduced-fat or skim dairy products.

❑ Select lower-fat food preparation methods (baking, broiling, and grilling instead of frying).

❑ Save high-fat, high-kilocalorie snack foods for occasional special treats.

Steps for Increasing Your Physical Activity

❑ Try to do a minimum of 30 minutes of moderate physical activity most, or preferably all, days of the week. Moderate physical activity includes walking, jogging, riding a bike, roller skating, and so forth.

❑ Ideally, do 45 minutes or more of moderate physical activity at least 5 days per week.

❑ Keep clothes and equipment for physical activity in convenient places.

❑ Move throughout the day, such as by taking stairs, pacing while talking on the phone, doing sit-ups while watching television, and so forth.

❑ Join an exercise class, mall-walking group, running club, yoga group, or any group of people who are physically active.

❑ Use the "buddy" system by exercising with a friend or relative and/or calling this support person when you need an extra boost to stay motivated.

❑ Prioritize exercise by writing it down, along with your classes and other engagements, in your daily planner.

❑ See Chapter 10 for more information on increasing your physical activity.

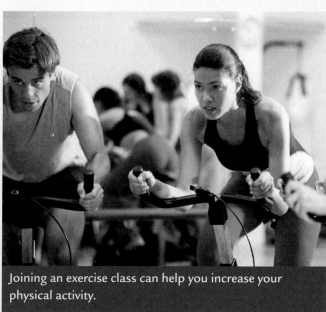

Joining an exercise class can help you increase your physical activity.

Steps for Modifying Your Food-Related Behavior

❑ Eat only at set times in one location. Do not eat while studying, working, driving, watching television, and so forth.

❑ Keep a log of what you eat, when, and why. See the What About You? box in Chapter 1, page 12.

❑ Avoid shopping when you are hungry.

❑ Avoid buying problem foods—that is, foods that you may have difficulty eating in moderate amounts.

❑ Avoid purchasing high-fat, high-sugar food from vending machines and convenience stores.

❑ At fast-food restaurants, choose small portions of foods lower in fat and simple sugars.

❑ Follow the serving sizes indicated in MyPyramid. For a fun way to test your understanding of a serving size, take the "Portion Distortion" interactive quiz from the National Institutes of Health at http://hin.nhlbi.nih.gov/portion/.

❑ Serve your food portions on smaller dishes so they appear larger.

❑ Avoid feelings of deprivation by eating small, regular meals throughout the day.

❑ Whether at home or dining out, share food with others.

❑ Prepare healthful snacks to take along with you so that you won't be tempted by foods from vending machines, fast-food restaurants, and so forth.

❑ Chew food slowly, taking at least 20 minutes to eat a full meal, and stopping at once if you begin to feel full.

❑ Reward yourself for positive behaviors by getting a massage, buying new clothes, or going out to a movie or concert.

❑ Set reasonable goals, and don't punish yourself if you deviate from your plan (and you will—everyone does). Ask others to avoid responding to any slips you make.

Source: Adapted from National Heart, Lung, and Blood Institute Expert Panel, National Institutes of Health. 1998. *Clinical Guidelines on the Identification, Evaluation, and Treatment of Overweight and Obesity in Adults.* Washington, DC: Government Printing Office.

Goals that are more likely to be realistic and achievable share the following characteristics:

- They are specific. Telling yourself, "I will eat less this week" is not helpful because the goal is not specific. An example of a specific goal is, "I will eat only half of my restaurant entrée tonight and take the rest home and eat it tomorrow for lunch."

- They are reasonable. If you are not presently physically active, it would be unreasonable to set a goal of exercising for 30 minutes every day. A more reasonable goal would be to exercise for 15 minutes per day, 3 days per week. Once you've achieved that goal, you can increase the frequency, intensity, and time of exercise according to the improvements in fitness that you have experienced.

- They are measurable. Effective goals are ones you can measure. An example is, "I will lose at least half a pound this week," or "I will substitute drinking water for my regular soft drink at lunch each day this week." Thus, recording your specific, reasonable goals and measuring them will help you to better determine whether you are achieving them.

By monitoring your progress regularly you can determine whether you are meeting your goals or whether you need to revise them based on accomplishments or challenges that arise.

Eat Smaller Portions of Lower-Fat Foods

One of the most challenging issues related to food is understanding what a healthful portion size is, and how to reduce the portion sizes of foods that we eat. As discussed earlier in this chapter, the portion sizes of packaged foods and restaurant meals have expanded considerably over the past 40 years, and many people trying to lose weight find it challenging to understand how much is reasonable to eat. Recent studies indicate that when children and adults are presented with large portions of foods and beverages, they eat more energy overall and do not respond to cues of fullness.[16,17]

In general, two effective weight-loss strategies include: reducing both the portion size and energy density of the foods you consume; and replacing sweetened sodas, milkshakes, and other energy-dense beverages with low-kilocalorie or non-kilocalorie beverages.[17] In addition, the following specific changes can significantly reduce your energy intake:

1. Follow the serving sizes recommended in MyPyramid (page 20). Making this change involves understanding what constitutes a serving size and measuring foods to determine whether they meet or exceed the recommended serving size.

2. Reduce the amount of foods that are high in fat and energy in your daily diet. People trying to lose weight should aim for a total fat intake of 15% to 25% of total energy intake. This goal can be achieved by eliminating extra fats such as butter, margarine, and mayonnaise and high-fat snack foods such as ice cream, doughnuts, and cakes. Save these foods as occasional special treats. Select lower-fat versions of the foods listed in MyPyramid. For example, select leaner cuts of meat (such as the white meat of poultry and extra-lean ground beef) and reduced-fat or skim dairy products. Also, choose baked or broiled foods and avoid fried foods. And don't forget to switch from a sugar-filled beverage to a low-kilocalorie or non-kilocalorie beverage during and between meals.

3. Consume foods that are relatively low in energy density. This includes foods such as salads (with low- or non-kilocalorie dressings), fruits, vegetables, and broth-based soups. These foods are low in energy and high in fiber, water, and nutrients. Because they contain relatively more water and fiber than more energy-dense foods, they can help you feel satiated without having to consume a lot of energy.

Participate in Regular Physical Activity

Recall from Chapter 1 that the *Dietary Guidelines for Americans* emphasize the role of physical activity in maintaining a healthful weight. Why is being physically active so important? Of course we expend extra energy during physical activity, but there's more to it than that, because exercise alone (without a reduction of energy intake) does not result in dramatic decreases in body weight. Instead, one of the most important reasons for being regularly active is that it helps us maintain or increase our lean body mass and our BMR. In contrast, energy restriction alone causes us to lose lean body mass and decrease our BMR. As you've learned, the more lean body mass we have, the more energy we expend—even at rest.

While very few weight-loss studies have documented long-term maintenance of weight loss, those that have find that only people who are regularly active are able to maintain most of their weight loss. The National Weight Control Registry is an ongoing project documenting the habits of people who have lost weight and kept it off. Among the 784 people studied thus far, the average weight loss was 66 pounds, and the group maintained the minimum weight-loss criteria of 30 pounds for more than 5 years.[18] Almost all of the people in the study (89%) reported changing both physical activity and dietary intake to lose weight and maintain weight loss. No one form of exercise seemed to be most effective, but many people reported doing some form of aerobic exercise (such as bicycling, walking, running, aerobic dance, step aerobics, or hiking) and weight lifting for at least 45 minutes most days of the week. In fact, on average, this group expended more than 2,800 kilocalories each week through physical activity!

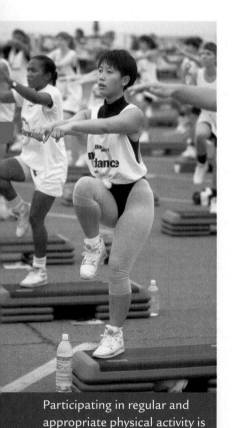

Participating in regular and appropriate physical activity is one of the main components of a weight-change plan.

In addition to expending energy and maintaining lean body mass and BMR, regular physical activity improves cardiovascular and respiratory health, enhances mood, results in a higher quality of sleep, increases self-esteem, and gives us a sense of accomplishment (see Chapter 10 for more benefits of regular physical activity). All of these changes enhance our ability to engage in long-term healthful lifestyle behaviors.

Incorporate Behavioral Modification Strategies into Your Daily Life

Successful weight loss and long-term maintenance of a healthful weight require people to modify their behaviors. Some behavior modifications related specifically to food and physical activity have been discussed in the previous sections. Here are a few more ways to change your behavior to increase your chances of success:

- Eat only at set times in one location. Do not eat while studying, working, driving, watching television, and so forth.

- Keep a log of what you eat, when, and why. Try to identify social or emotional cues that cause you to overeat, such as getting a poor grade on an exam, or feeling lonely. Then strategize about non-food-related ways to cope, such as phoning a sympathetic friend. Use the What About You? box in Chapter 1 on page 12 to assist you in determining how external and internal cues affect your eating behaviors.

- Save high-fat, high-kilocalorie snack foods such as ice cream, donuts, and cakes for occasional special treats.

- Avoid buying problem foods—that is, foods that you may have difficulty eating in moderate amounts.

- Avoid purchasing high-fat, high-sugar foods from vending machines and convenience stores.

- Serve your food portions on smaller dishes so they appear larger.

- Avoid feelings of deprivation by eating small, regular meals throughout the day.

- Whether at home or dining out, share food with others. Refer back to the Game Plan on page 271 for tips on eating smart when eating out.

- Prepare healthful snacks to take along with you so that you won't be tempted by foods from vending machines, fast-food restaurants, and so forth.

- Chew food slowly, taking at least 20 minutes to eat a full meal, and stopping at once if you begin to feel full.

- Always use appropriate utensils.

- Leave food on your plate or store it for the next meal.

If You Decide to Follow a Popular Diet Plan, Choose One Based on the Three Strategies

With the assistance of MyPyramid and the information in this book, you are ready to design your own personalized diet plan. If you'd feel more comfortable following an established plan, however, an unlimited number are available. How can you know whether or not a plan is based on sound dietary principles, and whether its promise of long-term weight loss will prove true for *you*? Look to the three strategies just identified:

- Does the plan promote gradual reductions in energy intake?

- Does it advocate increased physical activity?

- Does it include strategies for modifying your eating and activity-related behaviors?

Reputable diet plans incorporate all of these strategies. Unfortunately, many dieters are drawn to fad diets, which do not.

HIGHLIGHT

The Anatomy of Fad Diets

Fad diets are weight-loss programs that enjoy short-term popularity and are sold based on a marketing gimmick that appeals to the public's desires and fears. In addition, the goal of the person or company designing and marketing the diet is not to improve public health but to make money. How can you tell if the program you are interested in is a fad diet? Here are some pointers to help you:

- The promoters of the diet claim that the program is new, improved, or based on some new discovery; however, no scientific data are available to support these claims.

- The program is touted for its ability to result in rapid weight loss or body-fat loss, usually more than 2 lb per week, and may include the claim that weight loss can be achieved with little or no physical exercise.

- The diet includes special foods and supplements, many of which are expensive and/or difficult to find or can only be purchased from the diet promoter. Common recommendations for these diets include avoiding certain foods, only eating a special combination of certain foods, or including magic foods in the diet that "burn" fat and speed up metabolism.

- The diet may include a rigid menu that must be followed daily or may allow only a few select foods each day.

Alternatively, the diet may focus on one macronutrient group (e.g., protein) and severely restrict the others (e.g., carbohydrate and fat). Variety and balance are discouraged, and certain specific foods (such as all dairy products or all foods made with refined flour) may be entirely forbidden.

- Many fad diets identify certain foods and/or supplements as critical to the success of the diet and usually include claims that these substances can cure or prevent a variety of health ailments or that the diet can stop the aging process.

It is estimated that we currently spend more than $33 billion on fad diets each year.[19] The success of fad diets typically lies in the ability of diet promoters to persuade people that they can lose weight quickly with no significant change in their lifestyle. Fad diets also tend to appeal to goals many people share, such as becoming more attractive or strong, reducing the effects of aging such as wrinkles and loose skin, and enjoying better health. In a world where many people feel they have to meet a certain physical standard to be valued, these types of diets flourish. Unfortunately, the only people who usually benefit from them are their marketers, who can become very wealthy promoting programs that are highly ineffectual.

Avoid Fad Diets

Beware of fad diets! They are simply what their name implies — fads that do not result in long-term, healthful weight changes. To be precise, fad diets are programs that enjoy short-term popularity and are sold based on a marketing gimmick that appeals to the public's desires and fears. Of the hundreds of such diets on the market today, most will "die" within a year, only to be born again as a "new and improved" fad diet. The goal of the person or company designing and marketing a fad diet is to make money. How can you tell if the program you are interested in qualifies as a fad diet? Check out the Highlight on Fad Diets above for some pointers to help you.

Diets Focusing on Macronutrient Composition May or May Not Work for You

A comprehensive review of the currently available evidence shows that achieving a negative energy balance is the major factor in successful weight loss.[20] The macronutrient composition of a diet does not appear to affect the amount of weight lost. In other words, *what* you eat is far less important than *how much* you eat. That said, the three main types of weight-loss diets that have been most seriously and comprehensively researched all encourage increased consumption of one or two macronutrients and reduced consumption of one or two others. Provided here is a brief review of these three main types and their general effects.[20]

Moderate-Fat, High-Carbohydrate, Moderate-Protein Diets   Moderate-fat, high-carbohydrate, moderate-protein diets that are balanced in nutrients typically contain 20% to 30% of total energy intake as fat, 55% to 60% of total energy intake as carbohydrate, and 15% to 20% of energy intake as protein. These diets include Weight Watchers, Jenny Craig, and others that follow the general guidelines of the USDA MyPyramid. All of these diet plans emphasize that weight loss occurs when energy intake is lower than energy expenditure. The goal is gradual weight loss, or about 1 to 2 lb of body weight per week. Typical energy deficits are between 500 and to 1,000 kilocalories/per day. It is recommended that women eat no less than 1,000 to 1,200 kilocalories/day and that men consume no less than 1,200 to 1,400 kilocalories/day. Regular physical activity is encouraged.

To date, these types of low-energy diets have been researched more than any others. There is a substantial amount of high-quality scientific evidence (from randomized controlled trials) that they are effective in decreasing body weight. In addition, the people who lose weight on these diets also decrease their LDL-cholesterol, reduce their blood triglyceride levels, and decrease their blood pressure. The diets are nutritionally adequate if the individual's food choices follow the guidelines of MyPyramid. If the individual's food choices are not varied and balanced, the diets may be low in nutrients such as fiber, zinc, calcium, iron, and vitamin B_{12}. Under these circumstances, supplementation is needed.

High-Fat, Low-Carbohydrate, High-Protein Diets   High-fat, low-carbohydrate, high-protein diets cycle in and out of popularity on a regular basis. By definition, these types of diets generally contain about 55% to 65% of total energy intake as fat, less than 100 g of carbohydrate per day, and the balance of daily energy intake as protein. Examples of these types of diets include Dr. Atkins Diet Revolution, the Carbohydrate Addict's Diet, Life Without Bread, Sugar Busters, and Protein Power. These diets minimize the role of restricting total energy intake on weight loss. They instead advise participants to restrict carbohydrate intake, proposing that carbohydrates are addictive and that they cause significant overeating, insulin surges leading to excessive fat storage, and an overall metabolic imbalance that leads to obesity. The goal is to reduce carbohydrates enough to cause ketosis, which will decrease blood glucose and insulin levels and reduce appetite.

Countless people claim to have lost substantial weight on these types of diets; however, quality scientific studies are just beginning to be conducted. Here is what is currently known based on the limited evidence:

- People do lose weight with high-fat, low-carbohydrate, high-protein diets.

- People who lose weight may also experience positive metabolic changes such as decreased blood lipid levels, decreased blood pressure, and decreased blood glucose and insulin.

- The amount of weight loss and improvements in metabolic health measured with these diets are no greater than those seen with higher-carbohydrate diets.

- Long-term compliance on these diets also appears to be similar to that of other types of diets and may be more affected by psychological factors than by the macronutrient composition of the diet.

It is important to recognize that high-fat, low-carbohydrate, high-protein diets are nutritionally inadequate and require supplementation. In addition, reported side effects of these diets include constipation, diarrhea, ketone breath, headaches, insomnia, nausea, fatigue, and thirst. Thus, these diets must be approached cautiously, especially if you have any health concerns.

Low-Fat and Very-Low-Fat Diets   Low-fat diets contain 11% to 19% of total energy as fat, whereas very-low-fat-diets contain less than 10% of total energy as fat. Both of these types of diets are high in carbohydrate and moderate in protein. Examples include Dr. Dean Ornish's Program for Reversing Heart Disease and the New Pritikin Program. These diets do not focus on total energy intake but emphasize eating foods higher in complex carbohydrates and fiber. The Ornish diet is

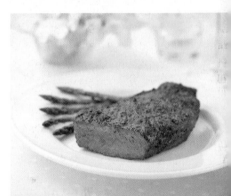

"Low-carb" diets may lead to weight loss but are nutritionally inadequate and can cause negative side effects.

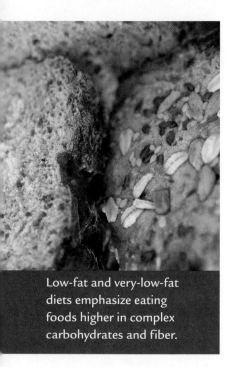

Low-fat and very-low-fat diets emphasize eating foods higher in complex carbohydrates and fiber.

vegetarian, whereas the Pritikin diet allows 3.5 oz of lean meat per day. Consumption of sugar and white flour is very limited. Regular physical activity is a key component of both diets.

These programs were not originally designed for weight loss but rather were developed to decrease or reverse heart disease. They are not popular with consumers, who tend to view them as too restrictive and difficult to follow. Thus, there are limited data on their effects. However, high-quality evidence suggests that people following these diets do lose weight, and some data suggest that these diets may also decrease LDL-cholesterol, blood triglyceride levels, glucose, insulin levels, and blood pressure. Few side effects have been reported in people following these diets; the most common is flatus that typically decreases over time. Low-fat diets are low in vitamin B_{12}, and very-low-fat diets are low in essential fatty acids, vitamins B_{12} and E, and zinc. Thus, supplementation is needed. The diets are not considered safe for people with diabetes who are insulin dependent (either type 1 or type 2) or for people with carbohydrate-malabsorption illnesses.

Weight Loss Can Be Enhanced with Prescribed Medications

The biggest complaint about recommendations for healthful weight loss is that they are too difficult for most people to follow. After trying many different weight-loss programs over several years or even decades, some people look to prescription drugs for help. These drugs typically act as appetite suppressants and may also increase satiety.

Weight-loss medications should be used only with proper supervision from a physician. One reason physician involvement is so critical is that many drugs developed for weight loss have serious side effects. Some have even proven deadly. Fenfluramine (brand name Pondimin), dexfenfluramine (brand name Redux), and a combination of phentermine and fenfluramine (called "phen-fen") are appetite-suppressing drugs that were banned from the market in 1996. Use of the drugs resulted in illness and several deaths and caused an increased risk for heart and lung disease.

Two relatively new prescription weight-loss drugs are available. Sibutramine (brand name Meridia) is an appetite suppressant, and orlistat (brand name Xenical) is a drug that acts to inhibit the absorption of dietary fat from the intestinal tract, which can result in weight loss in some people. The long-term safety and efficacy of these drugs are still being explored.

These medications are justified only for people who are severely obese. That's because the health risks of severe obesity override the risks of the medications. They should only be used while under a physician's supervision so that progress and health risks can be closely monitored. In addition, these drugs are most effective when combined with a program that supports energy restriction, regular exercise, and increasing physical activity throughout the day.

Using Dietary Supplements to Lose Weight Is Controversial

Over-the-counter supplements are also marketed for weight loss. It is important to remember that the Food and Drug Administration (FDA) regulates prescription drugs and over-the-counter medications, but the FDA does not have direct control over dietary supplements. Thus, dangerous or ineffective supplements can be marketed and sold without meeting strict safety guidelines and are unlikely to be pulled from the shelves.

For example, dieter's teas are herbal teas sold over the counter that may be advertised as laxatives or as a weight-loss aid. Their claims for weight loss are based on the erroneous but popular belief that increased bowel movements result in decreased absorption of energy from foods. In truth, laxative-induced diarrhea does not significantly reduce our absorption of energy. These teas contain plant-based laxatives such as senna, aloe, castor oil, and buckthorn, which can cause abdominal cramps, diarrhea, nausea, vomiting, fainting, and/or rebound chronic constipation. At least four deaths have been linked with excessive use of these teas.[21] As a result, the FDA has advised that these products list warnings on the label that include information about their laxative properties and side effects.

In addition, heart problems and deaths have been associated with use of the herb ephedra, a stimulant commonly claimed to promote weight loss.[22] The FDA has banned the manufacture and sale of ephedra in the United States because of its potentially fatal side effects. Ephedra is also banned by international, national, and collegiate sports governing bodies. Some herbal supplement producers still include *ma huang,* the so-called herbal ephedra, in their weight-loss products. Some herbal weight-loss supplements contain a combination of *ma huang,* caffeine, and aspirin. As you can see, using weight-loss supplements can have dangerous consequences.

> **RECAP** *Achieving and maintaining a healthful body weight involves gradual reductions in energy intake, such as by eating smaller portion sizes and limiting dietary fat; incorporating regular physical activity; and applying appropriate behavioral modification techniques. Fad diets do not incorporate these strategies and do not result in long-term, healthful weight change. Diets based on macronutrient composition may promote long-term weight loss, but some have unhealthful side effects. When necessary, drugs can be used to reduce obesity with a doctor's prescription and supervision. Using dietary supplements to lose weight is controversial and can even be dangerous.*

NUTRI-CASE HANNAH

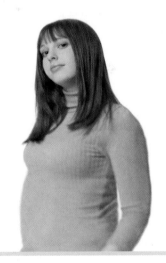

"I wonder what it would be like to be able to look in the mirror and not feel fat. Like my friend Kristi—she's been skinny since we were kids. I'm just the opposite: I've felt bad about my weight ever since I can remember. One of my worst memories is from the YMCA swim camp the summer I was 10 years old. Of course we had to wear a swimsuit, and the other kids picked on me so bad I'll never forget it. One of the boys called me "fatso," and the girls were even meaner, especially when I was changing in the locker room. That was the last year I was in the swim camp, and I've never owned a swimsuit since."

Think back to your own childhood. Were you ever teased for some aspect of yourself that you felt unable to change? How might organizations that work with children, such as schools, YMCAs, scout troops, and church-based groups, increase their leaders' awareness of social stigmatization of overweight children and reduce incidents of teasing, bullying, and other insensitivity?

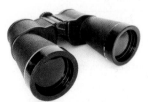

HEALTHWATCH
How Can You Avoid Obesity?

At the beginning of this chapter, we defined obesity as having an amount of excess body fat that adversely affects health, resulting in a person having a weight for a given height that is substantially greater than some accepted standard. People with a BMI between 30 and 39.9 are considered obese. Morbid obesity occurs when a person's body weight exceeds 100% of normal. People who are morbidly obese have a BMI greater than or equal to 40.

Both overweight and obesity are now considered an epidemic in the United States. As shown in Figure 1.2 on page 4, obesity rates have increased more than 50% over the past 20 years. This alarming rise in obesity is a major public health concern because it is linked to many chronic diseases, including heart disease, high blood pressure, type 2 diabetes, some cancers, heartburn, gastroesophageal reflux disease (GERD), sleep apnea, respiratory problems, and osteoarthritis. At least five of the nine leading causes of death in the United States are associated with obesity (FIGURE 9.12).

In addition, it has been estimated that the financial costs associated with obesity total more than $99 billion. These costs affect not just the person with obesity but all of society, as they increase the costs of healthcare and medications, reduce productivity because of days of lost work, and reduce future earnings because of premature death.

What Causes Obesity?

Obesity is known as a **multifactorial disease**, meaning that there are many things that cause it. This makes obesity extremely difficult to treat. Although it is certainly true that obesity, like overweight, is caused by eating more energy than is expended, it is also true that some people are more susceptible to becoming obese than others, and some are more resistant to weight loss and maintaining weight loss. Research on the causes and best treatments of obesity is ongoing, but let's explore some current theories.

Genetic Factors

Because our genetic background influences our height, weight, body shape, and metabolic rate, it also affects our risk for obesity. Some obesity experts point out that, if proven, the existence of a thrifty gene or genes (discussed earlier) would show that obese people have a genetic tendency to expend less energy both at rest and

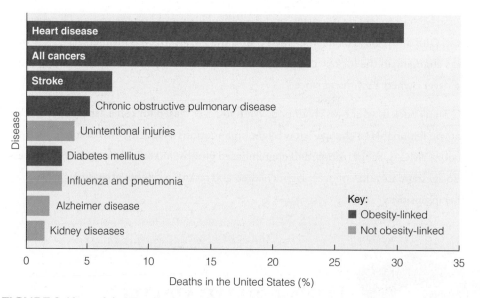

FIGURE 9.12   Of the nine leading causes of death in the United States, obesity is linked to five (see areas shaded in red).

(Adapted from National Center for Chronic Disease Prevention and Health Promotion [NCCDPHP]. 2003. Chronic Disease Prevention. Chronic Disease Overview. Available at www.cdc.gov/nccdphp/overview.htm.)

multifactorial disease   Any disease that may be attributable to one or more of a variety of causes.

during physical activity. Other researchers are working to determine whether the set-point theory can partially explain why many obese people are very resistant to weight loss. As we learn more about genetics, we will gain a greater understanding of the role that our genetic background plays in the development and treatment of obesity.

Childhood Overweight and Obesity Are Linked to Adult Obesity

The prevalence of overweight in children and adolescents is increasing at an alarming rate (FIGURE 9.13). There was a time when having extra "baby fat" was considered good for the child. We assumed that childhood overweight and obesity were temporary, and that the child would "grow out of it." Unfortunately, this is wishful thinking: it has been estimated that overweight adolescents have a 70% chance of becoming overweight or obese adults.[23]

Obesity in childhood has serious health consequences. Many obese children show risk factors for chronic disease while they are young, including elevated blood pressure, high cholesterol levels, and changes in insulin and glucose metabolism that can result in the early onset of type 2 diabetes (formerly known as *adult onset diabetes*). In some communities, children as young as 6 years of age have already been diagnosed with type 2 diabetes.

What factors contribute to obesity in children? Having either one or two overweight parents increases the risk of obesity two to four times.[24] In addition, for young people, it has been suggested that if the child gains a substantial amount of

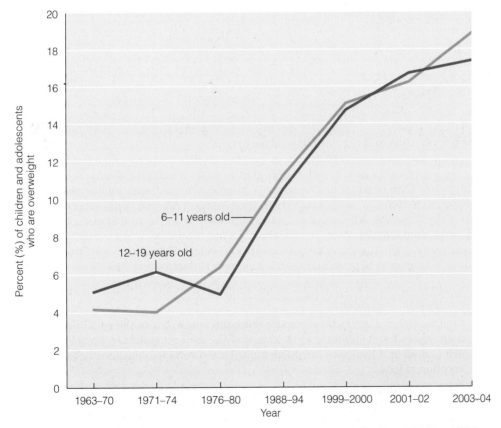

FIGURE 9.13 Increases in childhood and adolescent overweight from 1963 to 2004. (Adapted from Centers for Disease Control and Prevention. National Center for Health Statistics. 2007. Prevalence of Overweight Among Children and Adolescents: United States, 2003–2004. Available at http://www.cdc.gov/nccdphp/dnpa/obesity/childhood/prevalence.htm.)

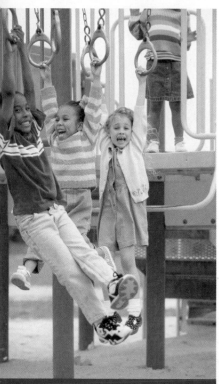

Adequate physical activity is instrumental in preventing childhood obesity.

weight in any one of three critical periods, his or her risk of obesity and related diseases in adulthood will be significantly increased. These periods are

- Gestation and early infancy
- The period of normal weight gain (called *adiposity rebound*) that occurs between 5 and 7 years of age
- Adolescence (or puberty)

An undeniably important contributor to childhood obesity includes low physical activity levels. As we said earlier, this in turn is influenced by certain changes in our society. There was a time when children played outdoors regularly, when physical education was offered daily in school, and when sports were a mainstay of after-school programs. Today, many children cannot play outdoors because of safety concerns or lack of recreational facilities, and few schools offer daily physical education to children. In addition, many popular after-school activities for children today are sedentary in nature, including playing video games, watching television, using the computer, and playing with handheld game toys. As childhood and adolescence are critical times for forming activity habits, the inactivity many young people experience today will likely have a significant impact on their potential for obesity as adults.

How Is Obesity Treated?

The first line of defense in treating obesity is a reduced-energy diet and an increased level of physical activity. The National Institutes of Health recommend that people who are obese work with their healthcare practitioner to design and maintain a low-fat diet (less than 30% of total energy from fat) that has a deficit of 500 to 1,000 kcal/day.[15] They also recommend that people increase their physical activity gradually so that they build up to a program in which they are exercising at least 30 minutes a day, five times a week. The Institute of Medicine concurs that 30 minutes a day, five times a week is the minimum amount of physical activity needed, but up to 60 minutes per day may be necessary for many people to lose weight and to sustain a body weight in the healthy range over the long-term.[25]

As discussed earlier in this chapter, prescription medications are used to treat some cases of obesity. Again, these medications should only be used while under a physician's supervision, and they appear to be most effective when combined with energy restriction and regular physical activity.

For people who are morbidly obese, surgery may be recommended. Generally, surgery is advised in people with a BMI greater than or equal to 40 or people with a BMI greater than or equal to 35 who have other life-threatening conditions such as diabetes, hypertension, or elevated cholesterol levels.[15] Any surgical procedure is more risky for people who are obese, so weight-loss surgery is considered a last resort, to be used only for obese people who have not been able to lose weight by less drastic means. The three most common types of weight-loss surgery performed are gastroplasty, gastric bypass, and gastric banding (FIGURE 9.14):

- *Gastroplasty* involves partitioning or "stapling" a small section of the stomach to reduce total food intake.
- *Gastric bypass surgery* involves attaching the lower part of the small intestine to a greatly reduced stomach, so that most of the food consumed bypasses the stomach and all of it bypasses the duodenum. This results in significantly less absorption of food.
- *Gastric banding* is a relatively new procedure in which stomach size is reduced using a constricting band, thus restricting food intake.

Are surgical procedures successful in reducing obesity? About one-third to one-half of people who receive obesity surgery lose significant amounts of weight and keep this weight off for at least 5 years. The reasons that one-half to two-thirds do not experience long-term success include that some are unable to eat less over time, even with a smaller stomach. For others, staples and gastric bands loosen and stom-

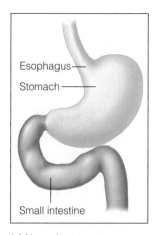

(a) Normal anatomy

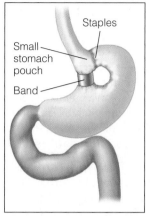

(b) Vertical banded gastroplasty

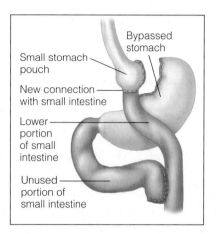

(c) Gastric bypass

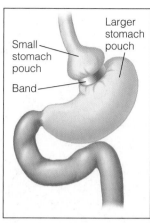

(d) Gastric banding

FIGURE 9.14 Various forms of surgery alter (a) the normal anatomy of the gastrointestinal tract to promote weight loss. Three surgical procedures used to reduce morbid obesity are (b) vertical banded gastroplasty, (c) gastric bypass, and (d) gastric banding.

ach pouches enlarge. Some individuals do not survive the surgery. Although these surgical procedures are extremely risky, those who lose weight, keep it off, and improve their health feel that the eventual benefits are worth the risks.

Liposuction is a cosmetic surgical procedure that removes fat cells from localized areas in the body. It is not recommended or typically used to treat obesity or morbid obesity. The procedure is not without risks; blood clots, skin and nerve damage, adverse drug reactions, pain, and perforation injuries can and do occur as a result of liposuction. It can also result in deformations in the area where the fat is removed. This procedure is not the solution to long-term weight loss, as the millions of fat cells that remain in the body after liposuction enlarge if the person continues to overeat. In addition, although liposuction may reduce the fat content of a localized area, it does not reduce a person's risk for the diseases that are more common among overweight or obese people. Only traditional weight loss with diet and exercise can reduce body fat and the risks for chronic diseases.

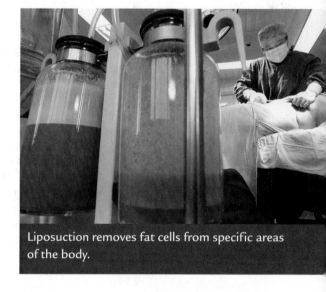

Liposuction removes fat cells from specific areas of the body.

RECAP *Obesity is caused by many factors, including genetics, a history of childhood obesity, overconsumption of kilocalories, and lack of adequate physical activity. Treatments for obesity and morbid obesity include low-energy, low-fat diets in combination with regular physical activity; weight-loss prescription medications; and/or weight-loss surgery.*

What If You Are Underweight?

With so much emphasis in the United States on obesity and weight loss, some find it surprising that many people are trying to gain weight. These include people who are clinically underweight; that is, people with a BMI of less than 18.5. Being underweight can be just as unhealthful as being obese, as underweight increases the risk for infections, osteoporosis, and other diseases, and can even be fatal. In addition, many athletes want to gain weight in order to increase their strength and power for competition.

Eat More Energy Than Expended

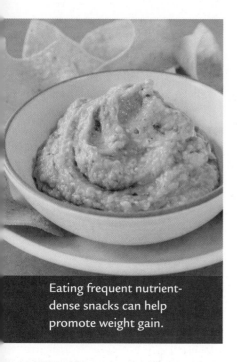

Eating frequent nutrient-dense snacks can help promote weight gain.

To gain weight, people must eat more energy than they expend. Although overeating large amounts of high-saturated-fat foods (such as bacon, sausage, and cheese) can cause weight gain, doing this without exercising is not considered healthful because most of the weight gained is fat, and high-fat diets increase our risks for cardiovascular and other diseases. Unless there are medical reasons to eat a high-fat diet, it is recommended that people trying to gain weight eat a diet that is relatively low in dietary fat (less than 35% of total kilocalories) and relatively high in complex carbohydrates (55% of total kilocalories). Recommendations for weight gain include:

- Eat a diet that includes about 500 to 1,000 kilocalories per day more than is needed to maintain current body weight. Although we don't know exactly how much extra energy is needed to gain 1 lb, estimates range from 3,000 to 3,500 kilocalories. Thus, eating 500 to 1,000 kilocalories per day in excess should result in a gain of 1 to 2 lb of weight each week.

- Eat a diet that contains about 55% of total energy from carbohydrate, 25% to 35% of total energy from fat, and 10% to 20% of total energy from protein.

- Eat frequently, including meals and numerous snacks throughout the day. Many underweight people do not take the time to eat often enough.

- Avoid the use of tobacco products, as they depress appetite and increase metabolic rate, which prevent weight gain. In addition, they increase our risks for lung, mouth, esophageal, and other cancers.

- Exercise regularly, and incorporate weight lifting or some other form of resistance training into your exercise routine. This form of exercise is most effective in increasing muscle mass. Performing aerobic exercise (such as walking, running, bicycling, or swimming) at least 30 minutes a day for 3 days per week will help maintain a healthy cardiovascular system.

The key to gaining weight is to eat frequent meals throughout the day and to select energy-dense foods. When selecting foods that are higher in fat, make sure you select foods higher in polyunsaturated and monounsaturated fats (such as peanut butter, olive and canola oils, and avocados). Smoothies and milkshakes made with low-fat milk or yogurt are another great way to take in a lot of energy. Eating fruit or raw vegetables with peanut butter, hummus, guacamole, or cream cheese and including salad dressings on your salad are other ways to increase the energy density of foods. The biggest challenge to weight gain is setting aside time to eat; by packing a lot of foods to take with you throughout the day, you can enhance your opportunities to eat more.

Avoid Protein Supplements and Steroid Products

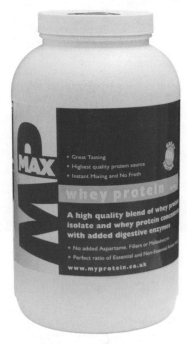

Protein powders or amino acid supplements will not enhance muscle growth or make you stronger.

As with weight loss, there are many products marketed for weight gain. One of the most common claims is that these products are *anabolic;* that is, that they increase muscle mass. These products include amino acid and protein supplements, anabolic **steroids** (manufactured versions of the male hormone testosterone), and androstenedione, a substance that became very popular after baseball player Mark McGwire claimed he used it during the time he was breaking home run records. Do these substances really work?

A growing body of evidence exists to show that amino acid and protein supplements do not enhance muscle gain or result in improvements in strength.[26] Anabolic steroids can increase body weight and muscle mass, but are known to cause major health problems. Although the case of Mark McGwire may seem to suggest that androstenedione is an extremely effective product for building muscle mass, gaining strength, and improving performance, several studies report that this product did not have any benefits.[27–29] Protein supplements and androstenedione are legal to sell in the United States, but these and other potentially anabolic substances are banned by the National Football League, the National Collegiate Athletic Association, and the International Olympic Committee.

The health consequences of using protein supplements are unknown. As just noted, the adverse effects of anabolic steroids are severe. They include unhealthful

steroid Man-made derivatives of testosterone, the male sex hormone.

NUTRI-CASE THEO

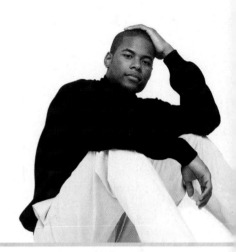

"I'm sick and tired of everybody everywhere complaining about how they can't lose weight even though they're starving themselves and feel hungry all the time. Nobody talks about people like me, who have exactly the opposite problem. I keep super-busy, I'm almost never hungry, and I can't keep weight on! It's especially bad right now because its basketball season: no matter what I do, the pounds peel off! For breakfast this morning, I had bacon and eggs. For lunch, I'll probably eat a couple of ham sandwiches. Then a protein bar after practice, and for dinner, I'll probably go out for burgers with my friends. What more can I do? Don't tell me to eat between meals because, like I said, I'm just not that hungry."

Given what you've learned about energy balance and weight management, what, if any, problems do you perceive with Theo's food intake today? What changes in his food choices might help stimulate his appetite? What else might he do to gain weight?

---

changes in blood cholesterol, mood disturbances (such as anger leading to violence), testicular shrinkage and breast enlargement in men, and irreversible clitoral enlargement in women (see Chapter 10 for a more detailed discussion of anabolic steroid use). Androstenedione causes unhealthful changes in high-density and low-density lipoprotein (HDL and LDL) levels in middle-aged-men, potentially increasing their risk for heart disease.[28] We also know that buying these substances can have a substantial slenderizing effect—on your wallet!

> RECAP *Weight gain can be achieved by eating more and performing weight lifting and aerobic exercise. Protein and amino acid supplements and androstenedione do not increase muscle growth or strength, and their potential side effects are unknown. Anabolic steroid use can increase body weight and muscle mass but is known to cause major health problems.*

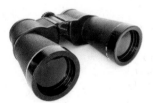

HEALTHWATCH
Disordered Eating: Are You at Risk?

Disordered eating is a general term used to describe a variety of atypical eating behaviors that people use to achieve or maintain a lower body weight. These behaviors may be as simple as going on and off diets or as extreme as refusing to eat any fat. Such behaviors don't usually continue for long enough to make the person seriously ill, nor do they significantly disrupt the person's normal routine.

In contrast, some people restrict their eating so much or for so long that they become dangerously underweight. These people have an **eating disorder**, a psychiatric condition that involves extreme body dissatisfaction and long-term eating patterns that negatively affect body functioning. The two more commonly diagnosed eating disorders are anorexia nervosa and bulimia nervosa. **Anorexia nervosa** is a potentially life-threatening eating disorder that is characterized by self-starvation, which eventually leads to a severe nutrient deficiency. In contrast, **bulimia nervosa** is characterized by recurrent episodes of extreme overeating and compensatory behaviors to prevent weight gain, such as self-induced vomiting, misuse of laxatives, fasting, or excessive exercise. Both disorders will be discussed in more detail shortly.

disordered eating Disordered eating is a general term used to describe a variety of abnormal or atypical eating behaviors that are used to keep or maintain a lower body weight.

eating disorder An eating disorder is a clinically diagnosed psychiatric disorder characterized by severe disturbances in body image and eating behaviors.

anorexia nervosa A serious, potentially life-threatening eating disorder that is characterized by self-starvation, which eventually leads to a deficiency in energy and essential nutrients that are required by the body to function normally.

bulimia nervosa A serious eating disorder characterized by recurrent episodes of binge-eating and recurrent inappropriate compensatory behaviors in order to prevent weight gain, such as self-induced vomiting, fasting, excessive exercise, or misuse of laxatives, diuretics, enemas, or other medications.

WHAT ABOUT YOU?

Are You at Risk for an Eating Disorder?

Take a look at the Eating Issues and Body Image Continuum below (Figure 9.15). Which of the five columns best describes your feelings about food and your body? If you identify with the statements on the left side of the continuum, you probably have few issues with food or body image. Most likely you accept your body size and view food as a normal part of maintaining your health and fueling your daily physical activity.

As you progress to the right side of the continuum, food and body image become bigger issues, with food restriction becoming the norm. If you identify with the statements on the far right, you are probably afraid of eating and dislike your body. If so, you should consult a healthcare professional as soon as possible. The earlier you seek treatment, the more likely you can take ownership of your body and develop a healthful approach to food.

• I am not concerned about what others think regarding what and how much I eat. • When I am upset or depressed I eat whatever I am hungry for without any guilt or shame. • I feel no guilt or shame no matter how much I eat or what I eat. • Food is an important part of my life but only occupies a small part of my time. • I trust my body to tell me what and how much to eat.	• I pay attention to what I eat in order to maintain a healthy body. • I may weigh more than what I like, but I enjoy eating and balance my pleasure with eating with my concern for a healthy body. • I am moderate and flexible in goals for eating well. • I try to follow Dietary Guidelines for healthy eating.	• I think about food a lot. • I feel I don't eat well most of the time. • It's hard for me to enjoy eating with others. • I feel ashamed when I eat more than others or more than what I feel I should be eating. • I am afraid of getting fat. • I wish I could change how much I want to eat and what I am hungry for.	• I have tried diet pills, laxatives, vomiting, or extra time exercising in order to lose or maintain my weight. • I have fasted or avoided eating for long periods of time in order to lose or maintain my weight. • I feel strong when I can restrict how much I eat. • Eating more than I wanted to makes me feel out of control.	• I regularly stuff myself and then exercise, vomit, or use diet pills or laxatives to get rid of the food or calories. • My friends/family tell me I am too thin. • I am terrified of eating fat. • When I let myself eat, I have a hard time controlling the amount of food I eat. • I am afraid to eat in front of others.
FOOD IS NOT AN ISSUE	**CONCERNED WELL**	**FOOD PREOCCUPIED/ OBSESSED**	**DISRUPTIVE EATING PATTERNS**	**EATING DISORDERED**
BODY OWNERSHIP	**BODY ACCEPTANCE**	**BODY PREOCCUPIED/ OBSESSED**	**DISTORTED BODY IMAGE**	**BODY HATE/ DISASSOCIATION**
• Body image is not an issue for me. • My body is beautiful to me. • My feelings about my body are not influenced by society's concept of an ideal body shape. • I know that the significant others in my life will always find me attractive. • I trust my body to find the weight it needs to be at so I can move and feel confident of my physical body.	• I base my body image equally on social norms and my own self-concept. • I pay attention to my body and my appearance because it is important to me, but it only occupies a small part of my day. • I nourish my body so it has the strength and energy to achieve my physical goals. • I am able to assert myself and maintain a healthy body without losing my self-esteem.	• I spend a significant time viewing my body in the mirror. • I spend a significant time comparing my body to others. • I have days when I feel fat. • I am preoccupied with my body. • I accept society's ideal body shape and size as the best body shape and size. • I'd be more attractive if I was thinner, more muscular, etc....	• I spend a significant amount of time exercising and dieting to change my body. • My body shape and size keeps me from dating or finding someone who will treat me the way I want to be treated. • I have considered changing or have changed my body shape and size through surgical means so I can accept myself. • I wish I could change the way I look in the mirror.	• I often feel separated and distant from my body—as if it belongs to someone else. • I hate my body and I often isolate myself from others. • I don't see anything positive or even neutral about my body shape and size. • I don't believe others when they tell me I look okay. • I hate the way I look in the mirror.

FIGURE 9.15 The Eating Issues and Body Image Continuum. The progression from normal eating (far left) to eating disorders (far right) occurs on a continuum.

(*Source*: Smiley, King, and Avey. University of Arizona Campus Health Service. Original Continuum, C. Shisslak. Preventive Medicine and Public Health. Copyright ©1997 Arizona Board of Regents. Used with permission.)

Eating Behaviors Occur on a Continuum

When does normal dieting cross the line into disordered eating? Eating behaviors occur on a *continuum,* a spectrum that can't be divided neatly into parts. An example is a rainbow—where exactly does the red end and the orange begin? Thinking about eating behaviors as a continuum makes it easier to understand how a person could progress from relatively normal eating behaviors to a pattern that is disordered. For instance, let's say that for several years you've skipped breakfast in favor of a mid-morning snack, but now you find yourself avoiding the cafeteria until early after-noon. Is this normal? To answer that question, you'd need to consider your feelings about food and your **body image**—the way you perceive your body.

Take a moment to take the self-test in the accompanying What About You? It will help clarify how you feel about your body and about food and whether or not you're at risk for an eating disorder.

Many Factors Contribute to Disordered Eating Behaviors

The factors that result in the development of disordered eating are very complex, but research indicates that a number of psychological, interpersonal, social, and biological factors may contribute in any particular individual.

Influence of Family

Research suggests that family conditioning, structure, and patterns of interaction can influence the development of an eating disorder. Based on observational studies, compared to families without a member with an eating disorder, families with an anorexic member show more rigidity in their family structure, less clear interpersonal boundaries, and tend to avoid open discussions on topics of disagreement. Conversely, families with a member diagnosed with bulimia nervosa tend to have a less stable family organization and to be less nurturing, more angry, and more disruptive.[30] In addition, childhood physical or sexual abuse can increase the risk of an eating disorder.[31]

Influence of Media

As media saturation has increased over the last century, so has the incidence of eating disorders among white women.[32] Every day, we are confronted with advertisements in which computer-enhanced images of lean, beautiful women promote everything from beer to cars (FIGURE 9.16). Most adult men and women understand

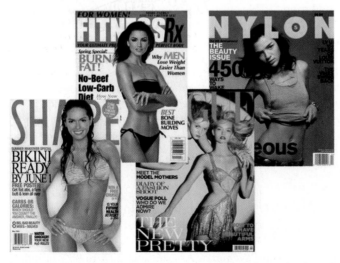

FIGURE 9.16 Photos of celebrities or models are often airbrushed or altered to "enhance" physical appearance. Unfortunately, many people believe that these are accurate portrayals and strive to reach this unrealistic level of physical beauty.

body image A person's perception of his or her body's appearance and functioning.

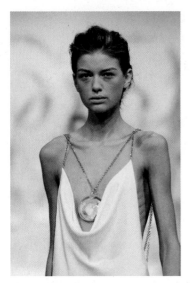

FIGURE 9.17 Until recently, the "in" look among runway models required extreme emaciation, often achieved by self-starvation and/or drug abuse.

that these images are unrealistic, but adolescents, who are still developing a sense of their identity and body image, lack the same ability to distance themselves from what they see.[33] Because body image influences eating behaviors, it is not unlikely that the barrage of media models may be contributing to the increase in eating disorders. However, scientific evidence demonstrating that the media is *causing* increased eating disorders is difficult to obtain.

Influence of Social and Cultural Values

Eating disorders are significantly more common in white females in Western societies than in other women worldwide. This may be due in part to the white Western culture's association of slenderness with health, wealth, and high fashion (FIGURE 9.17). In contrast, until recently, the prevailing view in developing societies has been that excess body fat is desirable as a sign of health and material abundance.

The members of society with whom we most often interact—our family members, friends, classmates, and co-workers—also influence the way we see ourselves. Their comments related to our body weight or shape can be particularly hurtful—enough so to cause some people to start down the path of disordered eating. For example, individuals with bulimia nervosa report that they perceived greater pressure from their peers to be thin than controls, while research shows that peer teasing about weight increases body dissatisfaction and eating disturbances.[34] Thus, our comments to others regarding their weight do count.

Influence of Personality

A number of studies suggest that people with anorexia nervosa exhibit increased rates of obsessive-compulsive behaviors and perfectionism. They also tend to be socially inhibited, compliant, and emotionally restrained.[35] Unfortunately, many studies observe these behaviors only in individuals who are very ill and in a state of starvation, which may affect personality. Thus, it is difficult to determine if personality is the cause or effect of the disorder.

In contrast to people with anorexia nervosa, people with bulimia nervosa tend to be more impulsive, have low self-esteem, and demonstrate an extroverted, erratic personality style that seeks attention and admiration. In these people, negative moods are more likely to cause overeating than food restriction.[35]

Influence of Genetic Factors

Overall, the diagnosis of anorexia nervosa and bulimia nervosa is several times more common in siblings and other blood relatives who also have the diagnosis than in the general population.[36] This observation might imply the existence of an "eating disorder gene"; however, it is difficult to separate the contribution of genetic and environmental factors within families.

RECAP *Eating behaviors occur along a continuum. Disordered eating is a term that describes a variety of atypical eating behaviors that people use to achieve or maintain a lower body weight, whereas an eating disorder is a psychiatric condition that involves extreme body dissatisfaction and long-term eating patterns that negatively affect body functioning. The development of disordered eating behaviors and eating disorders may be influenced by family environment, the media, society, culture, personality, and genetics.*

Anorexia Nervosa Is a Potentially Deadly Eating Disorder

According to the American Psychiatric Association, 90% to 95% of individuals with anorexia nervosa are young girls or women.[36] Approximately 0.5% to 1% of American females develops anorexia, and between 5% and 20% of these will die from complications of the disorder within 10 years of initial diagnosis.[31] These statistics make

HIGHLIGHT

Eating Disorders in Men: Are They Different?

David was tired of being called "fat boy." But the real motivation behind his weight loss was his coach's end-of-season threat: if he didn't lose at least 20 lb, he wouldn't make the soccer team again next year. David couldn't imagine his life without soccer, so he started cutting back on his snacks and running a couple of mornings a week at the gym. He lost 2 lb, but it took him 4 weeks. Discouraged by the slow pace, he eliminated all snacking, put less on his plate at mealtimes, and ran every day, first 2 miles, then 3, then 5. The weight started dropping more dramatically, and he loved the high he got from "running on empty." Four months into his program, he'd lost all 20 lb, and added weight training to his program. By the time the soccer season started, he'd lost 32 lb, and his coach rewarded him with more time on the field. He knew he should slack off on the dieting and exercise now that he was in practice every day, but something made him keep at it. Every time he went to the gym, he saw guys more trim, more buff than he was. And he was determined to become like them. No one was ever going to call him "fat boy" again.

Like many people, you might find it hard to believe that "real men" like David develop eating disorders . . . or if they do, their disorders must be somehow "different," right? To explore this question, let's take a look at what research has revealed about similarities and differences between men and women with eating disorders.

Comparing Men and Women with Eating Disorders

Until about a decade ago, little research was conducted on eating disorders in males. Recently, however, eating disorder experts have begun to examine the gender-differences debate in detail and have discovered that eating disorders in males are largely similar to eating disorders in females. But some differences *do* exist.

Females with eating disorders say they *feel* fat even though they typically are of normal weight or even underweight before they develop the disorder. In contrast, males who develop eating disorders are more likely to have actually *been* overweight or even obese.[37,38] Thus, the male's fear of "getting fat again" is based on reality. In addition, males with disordered eating are less concerned with

actual body weight (i.e., scale weight) than females but are more concerned with body composition (i.e., percentage of muscle mass compared to fat mass).

Whereas dieting itself is a common trigger for eating disorders in both males and females, research suggests that the factors *initiating* the dieting behavior differ.[39] There appear to be four reasons why males diet: to improve athletic performance, to avoid being teased for being fat, to avoid obesity-related illnesses observed in male family members, and to improve a homosexual relationship.[40] Similar factors are rarely reported by women.

The methods that men and women use to achieve weight loss also appear to differ. Males are more likely to use excessive exercise as a means of weight control, whereas females use more passive methods such as severe energy restriction, vomiting, and laxative abuse. These weight-control differences may stem from the societal biases surrounding dieting and male behavior; that is, dieting is considered to be more "acceptable" for women, whereas the overwhelming sociocultural belief is that "real men don't diet."[38]

Reverse Anorexia Nervosa: The New Male Eating Disorder?

Is there an eating disorder unique to men? Recently, some eating disorder experts who work with men have suggested that there is. Observing men who are distressed by the idea that they are not sufficiently lean and muscular, who spend long hours lifting weights, and who follow an extremely restrictive diet, they have defined a disorder called *reverse anorexia nervosa.* (The disorder is also called *muscle dysphoria* or *muscle dysmorphia.*) Men with reverse anorexia nervosa perceive themselves as small and frail even though they are actually quite large and muscular. Thus, like men with true anorexia nervosa, they suffer from a body image distortion, but it is reversed. No matter how "buff" or "chiseled" he becomes, his biology cannot match his idealized body size and shape.[40]

There are other "reversals" in these men compared to men with anorexia and other eating disorders. For instance, men with reverse anorexia nervosa

Men are more likely than women to exercise excessively in an effort to control their weight.

(continued)

Eating Disorders in Men: Are They Different? *(continued)*

frequently abuse performance-enhancing drugs. Additionally, whereas people with anorexia eat little of anything, men with reverse anorexia tend to consume excessive high-protein foods and dietary supplements such as protein powders.

On the other hand, men with reverse anorexia share some characteristics with men and women with other eating disorders. For instance, they too report "feeling fat" and engage in the same behaviors indicating an obsession with appearance (such as looking in the mirror). They also express significant discomfort with the idea of having to expose their bodies to others (for example, take off their clothes in the locker room) and have increased rates of mental illness.[41]

There are some outward indications that someone may be struggling with reverse anorexia nervosa. Not all of them apply to all men with the disorder. If you notice any of these behaviors in a friend or relative, talk about it with him and let him know that help is available.

- Rigid and excessive schedule of weight training.
- Strict adherence to a high-protein, muscle-enhancing diet.
- Use of anabolic steroids, protein powders, or other muscle-enhancing drugs or supplements.
- Poor attendance at work, school, or sports activities because of interference with rigid weight-training schedule.
- Avoidance of social engagements where the person will not be able to follow his strict diet.
- Avoidance of situations in which the person would have to expose his body to others.
- Frequent and critical self-evaluation of body composition.

Do you know anyone who might have reverse anorexia nervosa? If you do, maybe you're wondering how you can tell whether your friend's concern about his body size is extreme or a simple enthusiasm for weight lifting. The warning signs just listed may help. If you think they apply to your friend, talk to him about it. Though reverse anorexia nervosa isn't typically life-threatening, it can certainly cause distress and despair, and therapy—especially participation in an all-male support group—can help.

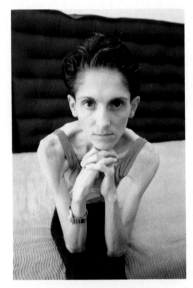

FIGURE 9.18 People with anorexia nervosa experience an extreme drive for thinness, resulting in potentially fatal weight loss.

amenorrhea Amenorrhea is the absence of menstruation. In females who had previously been menstruating, it is defined as the absence of menstrual periods for 3 or more months.

anorexia nervosa the most common and deadly psychiatric disorder diagnosed in women and the leading cause of death in females between the ages of 15 and 24 years.[31] As the statistics indicate, anorexia nervosa also occurs in males, but the prevalence is much lower than in females.[37]

Signs and Symptoms of Anorexia Nervosa

The classic sign of anorexia nervosa is an extremely restrictive eating pattern that leads to self-starvation (FIGURE 9.18). These individuals may fast completely, restrict energy intake to only a few kilocalories per day, or eliminate all but one or two food groups from their diet. They also have an intense fear of weight gain, and even small amounts (for example, 1–2 lb) trigger high stress and anxiety.

In females, **amenorrhea** (no menstrual periods for at least 3 months) is a common feature of anorexia nervosa. It occurs when a young woman consumes insufficient energy to maintain normal body functions. The signs of an eating disorder such as anorexia nervosa may be somewhat different in males. For more information on eating disorders in men, see the Highlight: Eating Disorders in Men: Are They Different? on pages 291–292.

Health Risks of Anorexia Nervosa

Left untreated, anorexia nervosa eventually leads to a deficiency in energy and other nutrients that are required by the body to function normally. The body will then use stored fat and lean tissue (such as organ and muscle tissue) as an energy source to maintain brain tissue and vital body functions. The body will also shut down or reduce nonvital body functions to conserve energy. Electrolyte imbalances can lead to heart failure and death. FIGURE 9.19 highlights many of the health problems that occur in people with anorexia nervosa.

Because the best chances for recovery occur when an individual receives intensive treatment early, it is important to recognize the signs of anorexia nervosa. Use these signs as a guide to help identify those at risk and to encourage them to seek help. Discussing a friend's eating disorder can be difficult. It is important to choose

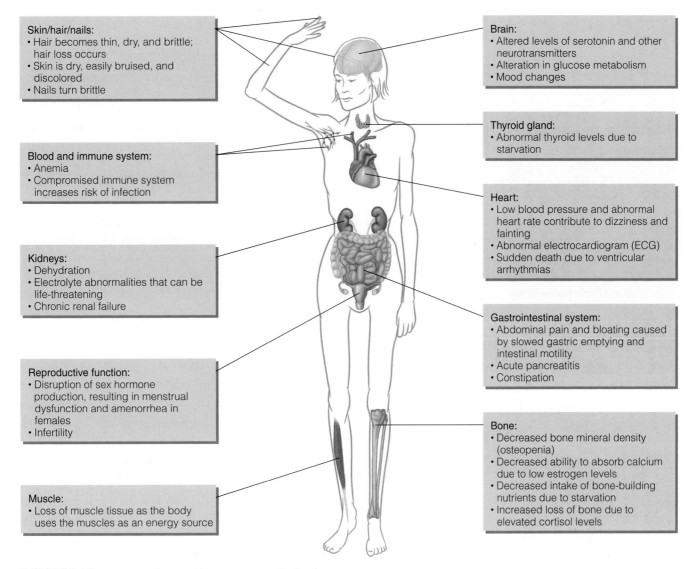

Skin/hair/nails:
- Hair becomes thin, dry, and brittle; hair loss occurs
- Skin is dry, easily bruised, and discolored
- Nails turn brittle

Blood and immune system:
- Anemia
- Compromised immune system increases risk of infection

Kidneys:
- Dehydration
- Electrolyte abnormalities that can be life-threatening
- Chronic renal failure

Reproductive function:
- Disruption of sex hormone production, resulting in menstrual dysfunction and amenorrhea in females
- Infertility

Muscle:
- Loss of muscle tissue as the body uses the muscles as an energy source

Brain:
- Altered levels of serotonin and other neurotransmitters
- Alteration in glucose metabolism
- Mood changes

Thyroid gland:
- Abnormal thyroid levels due to starvation

Heart:
- Low blood pressure and abnormal heart rate contribute to dizziness and fainting
- Abnormal electrocardiogram (ECG)
- Sudden death due to ventricular arrhythmias

Gastrointestinal system:
- Abdominal pain and bloating caused by slowed gastric emptying and intestinal motility
- Acute pancreatitis
- Constipation

Bone:
- Decreased bone mineral density (osteopenia)
- Decreased ability to absorb calcium due to low estrogen levels
- Decreased intake of bone-building nutrients due to starvation
- Increased loss of bone due to elevated cortisol levels

FIGURE 9.19   Impact of anorexia nervosa on the body.

an appropriate time and place to raise your concerns and to listen closely and with great sensitivity to their feelings. The Game Plan on page 295 outlines an approach you might use in talking with a friend or family member who might have an eating disorder.

Bulimia Nervosa Is Characterized by Bingeing and Purging

Bulimia nervosa is an eating disorder characterized by repeated episodes of **binge-eating** followed by some form of **purging**. While binge-eating, the person feels a loss of self-control, including an inability to end the binge once it has started.[42] At the same time, the person feels a sense of euphoria not unlike a drug-induced high. A "binge" is usually defined as a quantity of food that is large for the person and for the amount of time in which it is eaten (**FIGURE 9.20**). For example, a person may eat a dozen brownies with two quarts of ice cream in 30 minutes.

The prevalence of bulimia nervosa is higher than anorexia nervosa and is estimated to affect 1% to 4% of women. Like anorexia nervosa, bulimia nervosa is found predominantly in women: 6 to 10 females are diagnosed for every 1 male. The mortality rate is lower than for anorexia nervosa, with 1% of patients dying within 10 years of diagnosis.[31]

binge-eating   Consumption of a large amount of food in a short period of time, usually accompanied by a feeling of loss of self-control.

purging   An attempt to rid the body of unwanted food by vomiting or other compensatory means, such as excessive exercise, fasting, or laxative abuse.

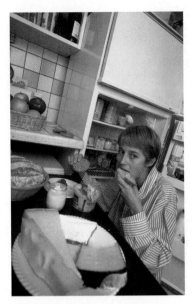

FIGURE 9.20 People with bulimia nervosa can consume relatively large amounts of food in brief periods of time.

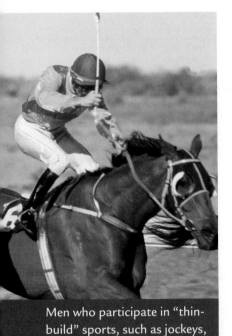

Men who participate in "thin-build" sports, such as jockeys, have a higher risk for bulimia nervosa than men who do not.

binge-eating disorder A disorder characterized by binge-eating an average of twice a week or more, typically without compensatory purging.

Although the prevalence of bulimia nervosa is much higher in women, rates for men are significant in some predominately "thin-build" sports in which participants are encouraged to maintain a low body weight (e.g., horse racing, wrestling, crew, and gymnastics). Individuals in these sports typically do not have all the characteristics of bulimia nervosa, however, and the purging behaviors they practice typically stop once the sport is discontinued.

An individual with bulimia nervosa typically purges after most episodes, but not necessarily on every occasion, and weight gain as a result of binge-eating can be significant. Methods of purging include vomiting, laxative or diuretic abuse, enemas, fasting, or excessive exercise. For example, after a binge, a runner may increase her daily mileage to equal the "calculated" energy content of the binge.

Symptoms of Bulimia Nervosa

In addition to the recurrent and frequent binge eating and purging episodes, the National Institute of Mental Health has identified the following symptoms of bulimia nervosa:

- chronically inflamed and sore throat
- swollen glands in the neck and below the jaw
- worn tooth enamel and increasingly sensitive and decaying teeth as a result of exposure to stomach acids
- gastroesophageal reflux disorder
- intestinal distress and irritation from laxative abuse
- kidney problems from diuretic abuse
- severe dehydration from purging of fluids

Health Risks of Bulimia Nervosa

The destructive behaviors of bulimia nervosa can lead to illness and even death. The most common health consequences associated with bulimia nervosa are:

- Electrolyte imbalance typically caused by dehydration and the loss of potassium and sodium from the body with frequent vomiting. This can lead to irregular heartbeat and even heart failure and death.
- Gastrointestinal problems: inflammation, ulceration, and possible rupture of the esophagus and stomach from frequent bingeing and vomiting. Chronic irregular bowel movements and constipation may result in people with bulimia who chronically abuse laxatives.
- Dental problems: tooth decay and staining from stomach acids released during frequent vomiting.

As with anorexia nervosa, the chance of recovery from bulimia nervosa increases, and the negative effects on health decrease, if the disorder is detected at an early stage. Familiarity with the warning signs of bulimia nervosa can help you identify friends and family members who might be at risk.

Binge-Eating Disorder Can Cause Significant Weight Gain

When was the last time a friend or relative confessed to you about "going on an eating binge"? Most likely, they explained that the behavior followed some sort of stressful event, such as a problem at work, the break-up of a relationship, or a poor grade on an exam. Many people have one or two binge episodes every year or so, in response to stress. But in people with **binge-eating disorder**, the behavior occurs an average of twice a week or more and is not usually followed by purging. This lack of compensation for the binge distinguishes binge-eating disorder from bulimia nervosa and explains why the person tends to gain a lot of weight.

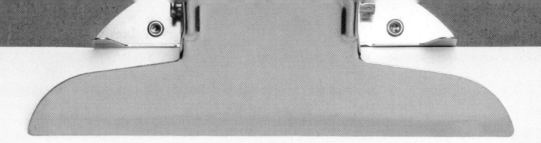

GAME PLAN

Discussing an Eating Disorder with a Friend or Family Member: What Do You Say?

If you are worried about your friend's eating behaviors or attitudes, it is important to express your concerns in a loving and supportive way. It is also necessary to discuss your worries early on, rather than waiting until your friend has endured many of the damaging physical and emotional effects of eating disorders. In a private and relaxed setting, talk to your friend in a calm and caring way about the specific things you have seen or felt that have caused you to worry.

What to Say—Step by Step

❑ **Schedule a time to talk.** Set aside a time for a private, respectful meeting with your friend to discuss your concerns openly and honestly in a caring and supportive way. Make sure you will be some place away from other distractions.

❑ **Communicate your concerns.** Share your memories and knowledge of specific times when you felt concerned about the person's eating or exercise behaviors. Explain that you think these things may indicate that there could be a problem that needs professional attention.

❑ **Ask your friend to explore these concerns** with a counselor, doctor, registered dietitian, or other healthcare professional who is knowledgeable about eating issues. If you feel comfortable doing so, offer to help your friend make an appointment or accompany your friend on their first visit.

❑ **Avoid conflicts or a "battle of the wills" with your friend.** If your friend refuses to acknowledge that there is a problem, restate your feelings and the reasons for them and leave yourself open and available as a supportive listener.

❑ **Avoid placing shame, blame, or guilt** on your friend regarding their actions or attitudes. Do not use accusatory "you" statements such as, "You just need to eat" or "You are acting irresponsibly." Instead use "I" statements such as, "I am concerned about you because you refuse to eat breakfast and lunch" or "It makes me afraid to hear you vomiting."

❑ **Avoid giving simple solutions.** For example, "If you would just stop, everything would be fine!"

❑ **Express your continued support.** Remind your friend or family member that you care and want him or her to be healthy and happy.

After talking with your friend, if you are still concerned with their health and safety, find a trusted adult or medical professional to talk to. This is probably a challenging time for both of you. It could be helpful for you, as well as your friend, to discuss your concerns and seek assistance and support from a professional.

Source: Reprinted with permission from National Eating Disorders Association. 2002. *What Should I Say? Tips for Talking to a Friend Who May be Struggling with an Eating Disorder.* For more information: http://www.nationaleatingdisorders.org.

The prevalence of binge-eating disorder is estimated to be 2% to 3% of the adult population and 8% of the obese population. In contrast to anorexia and bulimia, binge-eating disorder is also common in men. Our current food environment, which offers an abundance of good-tasting, cheap food any time of the day, makes it difficult for people with binge-eating disorder to avoid food triggers.

As you would expect, the increased energy intake associated with binge-eating significantly increases a person's risk of being overweight or obese. In addition, the types of foods individuals typically consume during a binge episode are high in fat and sugar, which can increase blood lipids. Finally, the stress associated with binge-eating can have psychological consequences, such as low self-esteem, avoidance of social contact, depression, and negative thoughts related to body size.

The Female Athlete Triad Consists of Three Disorders

The **female athlete triad** is a term used to describe a serious syndrome that consists of three medical disorders seen in some female athletes: disordered eating, menstrual dysfunction such as amenorrhea, and osteoporosis (FIGURE 9.21). Sports that emphasize leanness or a thin body build may place a young girl or a woman at risk for the female athlete triad. These include figure skating, gymnastics, diving, and others. Classical ballet dancers are also at increased risk for the disorder.

Active women experience the general social and cultural demands placed on women to be thin, as well as pressure from their coach, teammates, judges, and/or spectators to meet weight standards or body-size expectations for their sport. Failure to meet these standards can result in severe consequences such as being cut from the team, losing an athletic scholarship, or decreased participation with the team.

female athlete triad   A serious syndrome that consists of three medical disorders seen in some female athletes: disordered eating, amenorrhea, and osteoporosis.

NUTRI-CASE LIZ

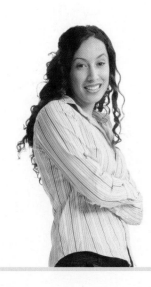

"I used to dance with a really cool modern company, where everybody looked sort of healthy and 'real.' No waifs! When they folded after Christmas, I was really bummed, but this spring, I'm planning to audition for the City Ballet. My best friend dances with them, and she told me that they won't even look at anybody over 100 pounds. So I've had to put myself on a pretty strict diet. Most days, I come in under 1,200 calories, though some days I cheat and then I feel so out of control. Last week, my dance teacher stopped me after class and asked me whether or not I was menstruating. I thought that was a pretty weird question, so I just said sure, but then when I thought about it, I realized that I've been so focused and stressed out lately that I really don't know! The audition is only a week away, so I'm going on a juice fast this weekend. I've just got to make it into the City Ballet!"

What factors increase Liz's risk for the female athlete triad? If you were to explain to her about osteoporosis, stress fractures, and increased injuries, do you think that this might change her disordered eating behaviors? Why or why not? What, if anything, do you think Liz's dance teacher should do? Why is intervention even necessary, since the audition is only a week away?

FIGURE 9.21 The female athlete triad is a syndrome composed of three coexisting disorders: disordered eating, menstrual dysfunction such as amenorrhea, and osteoporosis.

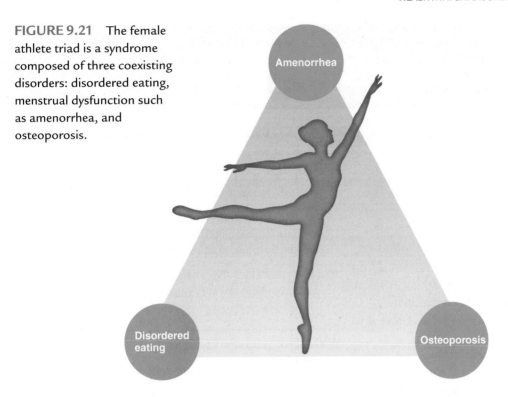

As the pressure to be thin mounts, active women may engage in disordered eating behaviors. Energy restriction combined with high levels of physical activity can disrupt the menstrual cycle and result in amenorrhea. Female athletes with menstrual dysfunction also typically have reduced levels of the reproductive hormones estrogen and progesterone. When estrogen levels in the body are low, it is difficult for bone to retain calcium, and gradual loss of bone mass occurs. Thus, many female athletes develop premature bone loss (osteoporosis) and are at increased risk for fractures.

Treatment for Disordered Eating Requires a Multidisciplinary Approach

As with any health problem, prevention is the best treatment for disordered eating. People having trouble with eating and body image issues need help to deal with these issues before they develop into something more serious.

Treating anyone with disordered eating requires a multidisciplinary approach. In addition to a physician and psychologist, a nutritionist, the person's coach (if an athlete), and family members and friends all must work together. Patients who are severely underweight, display signs of malnutrition, are medically unstable, or are suicidal may require immediate hospitalization. Conversely, patients who are underweight but are still medically stable may enter an outpatient program designed to meet their specific needs. Some outpatient programs are extremely intensive, requiring patients to come in each day for treatment, whereas others are less rigorous, requiring only weekly visits for meetings with a psychiatrist or eating disorder specialist.

RECAP *Anorexia nervosa is a life-threatening disorder in which the person refuses to maintain a minimally normal body weight. Bulimia nervosa is characterized by binge-eating followed by purging. In contrast, in binge-eating disorder, no purging typically occurs, and significant weight gain is likely. The female athlete triad is a syndrome consisting of three distinct disorders: disordered eating, menstrual dysfunction such as amenorrhea, and osteoporosis. Treatment of eating disorders requires a multidisciplinary approach; severely malnourished patients require hospitalization as a life-saving measure.*

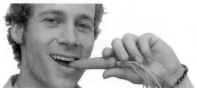

REVIEW QUESTIONS

Circle the correct choice.

1. The ratio of a person's body weight to height is represented as his or her:
   a. body composition.
   b. basal metabolic rate.
   c. bioelectrical impedance.
   d. body mass index.

2. The body's total daily energy expenditure includes:
   a. basal metabolic rate, thermal effect of food, and effect of physical activity.
   b. basal metabolic rate, movement, temperature regulation, and sleeping.
   c. effect of physical activity, standing, and sleeping.
   d. body mass index, thermal effect of food, and effect of physical activity.

3. All people gain weight when they:
   a. eat a high-fat diet (>35% fat).
   b. take in more energy than they expend.
   c. fail to exercise.
   d. take in less energy than they expend.

4. The set-point theory proposes that:
   a. obese people have a gene not found in slender people that regulates their weight so that it always hovers near a given set point.
   b. obese people have a gene that causes them to be energetically thrifty.
   c. all people have a genetic set point for their body weight.
   d. all people have a hormone that regulates their weight so that it always hovers near a given set point.

5. The components of the female athlete triad are
   a. disordered eating, diarrhea, and osteoarthritis.
   b. anorexia nervosa, menstrual dysfunction, and fractures.
   c. anorexia nervosa, irregular periods, and osteoporosis.
   d. disordered eating, menstrual dysfunction, and osteoporosis.

6. True or False? Pear-shaped fat patterning is known to increase a person's risk for many chronic diseases, including diabetes and heart disease.

7. True or False? One lb of fat is equal to about 3,500 kilocalories.

8. True or False? People with binge-eating disorder typically purge to compensate for the binge.

9. True or False? Recommendations for weight gain include avoiding both aerobic and resistance exercise for the duration of the weight-gain program.

10. True or False? The risks of gastric surgery in people who are obese are very high.

WEB LINKS

www.nhlbisupport.com/bmi
National Heart, Lung, and Blood Institute BMI Calculator

Calculate your body mass index (BMI) on the Internet.

www.ftc.gov
Federal Trade Commission

Roll over "Consumer Protection" and then click on "Consumer Information." The "Diet Health and Fitness" section provides information on how to avoid false weight-loss claims.

www.consumer.gov/weightloss
Partnership for Healthy Weight Management

Visit this site to learn about successful strategies for achieving and maintaining a healthful body weight.

www.eatright.org
American Dietetic Association

Go to this site to learn more about fad diets.

www.oa.org
Overeaters Anonymous

Visit this site to learn about ways to reduce compulsive overeating.

www2.niddk.nih.gov/HealthEducation/HealthNutrit
National Institute of Diabetes and Digestive and Kidney Disease

Find out more about appropriate weight loss and control.

http://hp2010.nhlbihin.net/portion
National Institutes of Health Portion Distortion Site

Visit this site and take the interactive "Portion Distortion" quiz to challenge your understanding of portion sizes. For instance, how does a standard restaurant cup of coffee compare to a coffee mocha from a national-chain coffeehouse? Find out, and then guess how long you'd have to walk to burn off that mocha!

www.sne.org
Society for Nutrition Education

Click on "Resources and Relationships" and then "Weight Realities Resources" for additional resources related to positive attitudes about body image and healthful alternatives to dieting.

www.obesity.org
American Obesity Association

A comprehensive site on overweight and obesity.

www.harriscentermgh.org
Harris Center, Massachusetts General Hospital

This site provides information about current eating disorder research, as well as sections on understanding eating disorders and resources for those with eating disorders.

www.nimh.nih.gov
National Institute of Mental Health (NIMH) Office of Communications and Public Liaison

Search this site for "disordered eating" or "eating disorders" to find numerous articles on the subject.

www.anad.org
National Association of Anorexia Nervosa and Associated Disorders

Visit this site for information and resources about eating disorders.

www.anred.com
Anorexia Nervosa and Related Eating Disorders, Inc.

Provides information and resources related to anorexia nervosa, bulimia nervosa, binge-eating disorder, and other less well-known eating disorders.

www.nationaleatingdisorders.org
National Eating Disorders Association

This site is dedicated to expanding public understanding of eating disorders and promoting access to treatment for those affected and support for their families.

TEST YOURSELF ANSWERS

1. **False.** Health can be defined in many ways. An individual who is overweight, but who exercises regularly and has no additional risk factors for various diseases (e.g., unhealthful blood lipid levels, smoking, etc.), is considered a healthy person.

2. **False.** According to the Centers for Disease Control and Prevention, in 2003, all 50 states in the United States had obesity rates of at least 15% to 19%, and 35 states had obesity rates of at least 20%.

3. **True.** Being underweight increases our risk for illness and premature death and in many cases can be just as unhealthful as being obese.

4. **False.** Body composition assessments can help give us a general idea of our body fat levels, but most methods are not extremely accurate.

5. **False.** Males also are diagnosed with eating disorders, but the incidence is much lower than for females.

REFERENCES

1. Emme. 2008. Bio profile; books. Available at http://emmestyle.com. (Accessed March 2008.)
2. PBS. 2004. Beyond the scale. *Healthweek.* Available at www.pbs.org/healthweek/featurep3_428.htm. (Accessed February 2004.)
3. Manore, M. M., and J. Thompson. 2000. *Sport Nutrition for Health and Performance.* Champaign, IL: Human Kinetics.
4. Heyward, V. H., and D. R. Wagner. 2004. *Applied Body Composition Assessment.* 2nd ed. Champaign, IL: Human Kinetics.
5. Ravussin, E., S. Lillioja, T. E. Anderson, L. Christin, and C. Bogardus. 1986. Determinants of 24-hour energy expenditure in man: Methods and results using a respiratory chamber. *J. Clin. Invest.* 78:1568–1578.
6. Stunkard A. J., T. I. A. Sørensen, C. Hanis, T. W. Teasdale, R. Chakraborty, W. J. Schull, and F. Schulsinger. 1986. An adoption study of human obesity. *N. Engl. J. Med.* 314:193–198.
7. Gunnell, D. J., S. J. Frankel, K. Nanchahal, T. J. Peters, and G. Davey Smith. 1998. Childhood obesity and adult cardiovascular mortality: A 57-y follow-up study based on the Boyd Orr cohort. *Am. J. Clin. Nutr.* 67:1111–1118.
8. Eyler, A. E., D. Matson-Koffman, D. Rohm-Young, S. Wilcox, J. Wilbur, J. L. Thompson, B. Sanderson, and K. R. Evenson. 2003. Quantitative study of correlates of physical activity in women from diverse racial/ethnic groups: The Women's Cardiovacular Health Network Project. *Am. J. Prev. Med.* 25(3Si):93–103.
9. Eyler, A. E., D. Matson-Koffman, J. R. Vest, K. R. Evenson, B. Sanderson, J. L. Thompson, J. Wilbur, S. Wilcox, and D. Rohm-Young. 2002. Environmental, policy, and cultural factors related to physical activity in a diverse sample of women: The Women's Cardiovascular Health Network Project—Summary and Discussion. *Women and Health.* 36:123–134.
10. Pickett, K. E., S. Kelly, E. Brunner, T. Lobstein, and R. G. Wilkinson. 2005. Wider income gaps, wider waistbands? An ecological study of obesity and income inequality. *J. Epidemiol. Community Health* 59:670–674.
11. Elliott, S. 2005. Calories? Hah! Munch some mega M&M's. *The New York Times,* Friday, August 5, p. C5.
12. National Restaurant Association. 2007. Restaurant Industry to Continue to Be Major Driver in Nation's Economy Through Sales, Employment Growth in 2008. Available at www.restaurant.org/pressroom/pressrelease.cfm?ID=1535. (Accessed March 2008.)
13. Koh-Banerjee, P., N. F. Chu, D. Spiegelman, B. Rosner, G. Colditz, W. Willett, and E. Rimm. 2003. Prospective study of the association of changes in dietary intake, physical activity, alcohol consumption, and smoking with 9-y gain in waist circumference among 16,587 U.S. men. *Am. J. Clin. Nutr.* 78:719–27.
14. Harris, J., and F. Benedict. 1919. *A Biometric Study of Basal Metabolism in Man.* Washington DC: Carnegie Institute of Washington.

15. Ello-Martin, J. A., J. H. Ledikwe, and B. J. Rolls. 2005. The influence of food portion size and energy density on energy intake: Implications for weight management. *Am. J. Clin. Nutr.* 82(suppl.):236S–241S.

16. Flood, J. E., L. S. Roe, and B. J. Rolls. 2006. The effect of increased beverage portion size on energy intake at a meal. *J. Am. Diet. Assoc.* 106:1984–1990.

17. Klem, M. L., R. R. Wing, M. T. McGuire, H. M. Seagle, and J. O. Hill. 1997. A descriptive study of individuals successful at long-term maintenance of substantial weight loss. *Am. J. Clin. Nutr.* 66: 239–246.

18. American Dietetic Association. 2001. Send Fad Diets down the Drain. Available at www.eatright.org.

19. Freedman, M. R., J. King, and E. Kennedy. 2001. Popular diets: a scientific review. *Obes. Res.* 9(suppl. 1):1S–40S.

20. National Institutes of Health. National Heart, Lung, and Blood Institute. 1998. Clinical Guidelines on the Identification, Evaluation, and Treatment of Overweight and Obesity in Adults. Executive Summary. Available at www.nhlbi.nih.gov/guidelines/obesity/ob_exsum.pdf.

21. Food and Drug Administration (FDA). 1997. Dieter's Brews Makes Tea Time a Dangerous Affair. Available at www.pueblo.gsa.gov/cic_text/health/teatime/597_tea.html.

22. Food and Drug Administration (FDA). 2005. Sales of supplements containing ephedrine alkaloids (ephedra) prohibited. Available at www.fda.gov/oc/initiatives/ephedra/february2004/.

23. Torgan, C. 2002. Childhood Obesity on the Rise. The NIH Word on Health. Available at www.nih.gov/news/WordonHealth/jun2002/childhoodobesity.htm.

24. Dietz, W. H. 1994. Critical periods in childhood for the development of obesity. *Am. J. Clin. Nutr.* 59:955–959.

25. Institute of Medicine. Food and Nutrition Board. 2002. *Dietary Reference Intakes for Energy, Carbohydrate, Fiber, Fat, Fatty Acids, Cholesterol, Protein, and Amino Acids (Macronutrients).* Washington, DC: The National Academies Press.

26. Kreider, R. B., V. Miriel, and E. Bertun. 1993. Amino acid supplementation and exercise performance. *Sports Med.* 16:190–209.

27. Joyner, M. J. 2000. Over-the-counter supplements and strength training. *Exerc. Sport Sci. Rev.* 28:2–3.

28. Broeder, C. E., J. Quindry, K. Brittingham, et al. 2000. The Andro Project: Physiological and hormonal influences of androstenedione supplementation in men 35- to 65-years-old participating in a high-intensiy resistance training program. *Arch. Int. Med.* 160:3093–3104.

29. Brown, G. A., M. D. Vukovich, T. A. Reifenrath, et al. 2000. Effects of anabolic precursors on serum testosterone concentra-tions and adaptations to resistance training in young men. *Int. J. Sport Nutr. Ex. Metab.* 10:340–359.

30. Vandereycken, W. 2002. Families of patients with eating disorders. In Fairburn, D. G., and K. D. Brownell, eds. *Eating Disorders and Obesity: A Comprehensive Handbook.* 2nd ed. New York Guilford Press, pp. 215–220.

31. Patrick, L. 2002. Eating disorders: A review of the literature with emphasis on medical complication and clinical nutrition. *Altern. Med. Rev.* 7(3):184–202.

32. Striegel-Moore R. H., and L. Smolak. 2002. Gender, ethnicity, and eating disorders. In Fairburn, D. G., and K. D. Brownell, eds. *Eating Disorders and Obesity: A Comprehensive Handbook.* 2nd ed. New York: Guilford Press, pp. 251–255.

33. Steinberg, L. 2002. *Adolescence.* 6th ed. New York: McGraw-Hill.

34. Stice, E. 2002. Sociocultural influences on body image and eating disturbances. In Fairburn, D. G., and K. D. Brownell, eds. *Eating Disorders and Obesity: A Comprehensive Handbook.* 2nd ed. New York: Guilford Press, pp. 103–107.

35. Wonderlich, S. A. 2002. Personality and eating disorders. In Fairburn, D. G., and K. D. Brownell, eds. *Eating Disorders and Obesity: A Comprehensive Handbook.* 2nd ed. New York: Guilford Press, pp. 204–209.

36. American Psychiatric Association. 1994. *Diagnostic and Statistical Manual of Mental Disorders* (DSM-IV). 4th ed. Washington DC: American Psychiatric Association.

37. Robb, A. S., and M. J. Dadson. 2002. Eating disorders in males. *Child Adolesc. Psychiatric. Clin. N. Am.* 11:399–418.

38. Beals, K. A. 2004. *Disordered Eating in Athletes: A Comprehensive Guide for Health Professionals.* Champaign, IL: Human Kinetics Publishers.

39. Andersen A. E. 1992. Eating disorders in male athletes: A special case? In Brownell K. D., J. Rodin, and J. H. Wilmore, eds. *Eating, Body Weight and Performance in Athletes: Disorders of Modern Society.* Philadelphia: Lea and Febiger, pp. 172–188.

40. Andersen, A. E. 2001. Eating disorders in males: Gender divergence management. *Currents* 2(2). University of Iowa Health Care. Available at www.uihealthcare.com/news/currents/vol2issue2/eatingdisordersinmen.html.

41. Pope H. G., K. A. Phillips, and R. Olivardia. *The Adonis Complex: The Secret Crisis of Male Body Obsession.* New York: The Free Press. 2000.

42. Garfinkel, P. E. 2002. Classification and diagnosis of eating disorders. In Fairburn D. G., and K. D. Brownell, eds. *Eating Disorders and Obesity: A Comprehensive Handbook.* 2nd ed. New York: Guilford Press, pp. 155–161.

TEST YOURSELF

Are these statements true or false? Circle your guess.

1 Almost half of all Americans report being inactive. **TRUE** or **FALSE**

2 Moderate physical activity, such as walking, housework, or gardening, does not yield significant health benefits. **TRUE** or **FALSE**

3 Eating extra protein helps us to build muscle. **TRUE** or **FALSE**

4 Most ergogenic aids are ineffective, and some can be dangerous. **TRUE** or **FALSE**

5 Carbohydrate loading before a 1,500-meter run can improve performance. **TRUE** or **FALSE**

Test Yourself answers can be found at the end of the chapter.

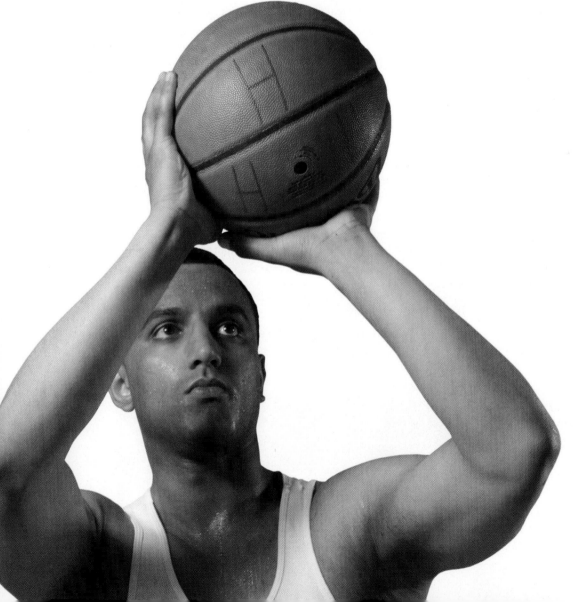

Where I'm starting from...

Would you like to increase your current level of physical activity?

Yes or **No**

If you answered **Yes**, why? (Choose as many as you want):

❑ I'd like to lose weight.

❑ I want to improve my health.

❑ I want to feel stronger and more fit.

❑ I'd like to join a sports team or compete in an athletic event.

❑ I want to sleep better and feel less stressed out.

❑ Other:

physical activity Any movement produced by muscles that increases energy expenditure; includes occupational, household, leisure-time, and transportation activities.

exercise A subcategory of leisure-time physical activity; any activity that is purposeful, planned, and structured.

physical fitness The ability to carry out daily tasks with vigor and alertness, without undue fatigue, and with ample energy to enjoy leisure-time pursuits and meet unforeseen emergencies.

aerobic exercise Exercise that involves the repetitive movement of large muscle groups, increasing the body's use of oxygen and promoting cardiovascular health.

I N JUNE 2007, Bill Finch of North Carolina won two gold medals in track and field at the National Senior Olympics. In the 800-meter dash, he clocked 6:34.25, and in the 1,500-meter dash, he made 13:07.12. If his performance times don't impress you, perhaps they will when you consider his age: at the time Finch gave these winning performances, he was 95 years old!

There's no doubt about it: regular physical activity dramatically improves our strength, stamina, health, and longevity. But what qualifies as "regular physical activity"? In other words, how much do we need to do to reap the benefits? And if we do become more active, does our diet have to change, too?

A nourishing diet and regular physical activity are like teammates, interacting in a variety of ways to improve our strength and stamina and increase our resistance to many chronic diseases and acute illnesses. In this chapter, we define physical activity, identify its many benefits, and discuss the nutrients needed to maintain an active life.

Why Engage in Physical Activity?

The term **physical activity** describes any movement produced by muscles that increases energy expenditure. Different categories of physical activity include occupational, household, leisure time, and transportation.[1] **Exercise** is considered a subcategory of leisure-time physical activity and refers to activity that is purposeful, planned, and structured.[2]

Physical Activity Increases Our Fitness

A lot of people are looking for a "magic pill" that will help them maintain weight loss, reduce their risk of diseases, make them feel better, and improve their quality of sleep. Although many people are not aware of it, regular physical activity is this "magic pill." That's because it promotes **physical fitness:** the ability to carry out daily tasks with vigor and alertness, without undue fatigue, and with ample energy to enjoy leisure-time pursuits and meet unforeseen emergencies.[1]

The components of physical fitness are identified in Table 10.1.[3] Notice that this table includes three types of exercise: aerobic exercise, resistance training, and stretching:

● **Aerobic exercise** involves the repetitive movement of large muscle groups, which increases the body's use of oxygen and promotes cardiovascular health. In

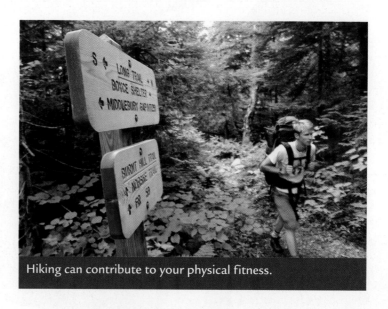

Hiking can contribute to your physical fitness.

TABLE 10.1 The Components of Fitness

Fitness Component	Examples of Activities One Can Do to Achieve Fitness in Each Component
Cardiorespiratory	Aerobic-type activities such as walking, running, swimming, cross-country skiing
Musculoskeletal fitness:	Resistance training, weight lifting, calisthenics, sit-ups, push-ups
Muscular strength	Weight lifting or related activities using heavier weights with few repetitions
Muscular endurance	Weight lifting or related activities using lighter weights with greater number of repetitions
Flexibility	Stretching exercises, yoga
Body composition	Aerobic exercise and resistance training can help optimize body composition

your daily life, you get aerobic exercise when you walk to school, work, or a bus stop or take the stairs to a third-floor classroom.

- **Resistance training** is a form of exercise in which our muscles work against resistance, such as against handheld weights. Carrying grocery bags or books and moving heavy objects are everyday activities that make our muscles work against resistance.
- **Stretching** exercises are those that increase flexibility, as they involve lengthening muscles using slow, controlled movements. You can perform stretching exercises even while you're sitting in a classroom listening to a lecture by flexing, extending, and rotating your neck, limbs, and extremities.

Physical Activity Reduces Our Risk for Chronic Disease

In addition to contributing to our fitness, physical activity can reduce our risk for certain diseases. Specifically, the health benefits of physical activity include:

- *Reduces our risks for, and complications of, heart disease, stroke, and high blood pressure:* Regular physical activity increases high-density lipoprotein (HDL) cholesterol (the "good" cholesterol) and lowers triglycerides in the blood, improves the strength of the heart, helps maintain healthy blood pressure, and limits the progression of atherosclerosis (or hardening of the arteries).
- *Reduces our risk for obesity:* Regular physical activity maintains lean body mass and promotes more healthful levels of body fat, may help in appetite control, and increases energy expenditure and the use of fat as an energy source.
- *Reduces our risk for type 2 diabetes:* Regular physical activity enhances the action of insulin, which improves the cells' uptake of glucose from the blood, and can improve blood glucose control in people with diabetes, which in turn reduces the risk for, or delays the onset of, diabetes-related complications.
- *May reduce our risk for colon cancer:* Although the exact role that physical activity may play in reducing colon cancer risk is still unknown, we do know that regular physical activity enhances gastric motility, which reduces transit time of potential cancer-causing agents through the gut.
- *Reduces our risk for osteoporosis:* Regular physical activity, especially weight-bearing exercise, increases bone density and enhances muscular strength and flexibility, thereby reducing the likelihood of falls and the incidence of fractures and other injuries when falls occur.

resistance training Exercise in which our muscles act against resistance.

stretching Exercise in which muscles are gently lengthened using slow, controlled movements.

Regular physical activity is also known to improve our sleep patterns, reduce our risk for upper respiratory infections by improving immune function, and reduce anxiety and mental stress. It also can be effective in treating mild and moderate depression.

Most Americans Are Inactive

Until quite recently, humans were very physically active. This was not by choice, but because their survival depended upon it. Prior to the industrial age, humans expended a considerable amount of energy each day foraging and hunting for food, planting and harvesting food, preparing food once it was acquired, and securing shelter. In addition, their diet was composed primarily of small amounts of lean meats and naturally grown vegetables and fruits. This lifestyle pattern contrasts considerably with today's lifestyles, which are characterized by sedentary jobs, easy access to an overabundance of energy-dense foods, and few opportunities or little interest in expending energy through occupational or recreational activities.

Given these changes, it isn't surprising that most people find the "magic pill" of regular physical activity difficult to swallow. Despite the plethora of benefits derived from being regularly active, most people in the United States are physically inactive. The Centers for Disease Control and Prevention report that over half of all U.S. adults do not do enough physical activity to meet national health recommendations, and almost 16% of adults in the United States admit to doing no leisure-time physical activity at all (FIGURE 10.1).[4] These statistics mirror the reported increases in obesity, heart disease, and type 2 diabetes in industrialized countries.

This trend toward inadequate physical activity levels is also occurring in young people. Only 17% of middle and junior high schools and only 2% of senior high schools require daily physical activity for all students.[5] Low rates of voluntary participation in physical education (PE) compound this problem, as less than 30% of high school students participate in daily PE. Because our habits related to eating and physical activity are formed early in life, it is imperative that we provide opportunities for children and adolescents to engage in regular, enjoyable physical activity. An active lifestyle during childhood increases the likelihood of a healthier life as an adult.

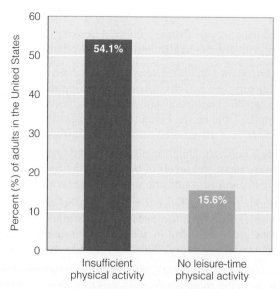

FIGURE 10.1 Rates of physical inactivity in the United States. Over 50% of the U.S. population does not do enough physical activity to meet national health recommendations, and almost 16% report doing no leisure-time physical activity. (From Centers for Disease Control and Prevention [CDC]. 2005. Adult participation in recommended levels of physical activity—United States, 2001 and 2003. *Morbid. Mortal. Wkly. Rep.* 54[47]:1208–1212.)

RECAP *Physical activity is any movement produced by muscles that increases energy expenditure. Physical fitness is the ability to carry out daily tasks with vigor and alertness, without undue fatigue, and with ample energy to enjoy leisure-time pursuits and meet unforeseen emergencies. Physical activity provides a multitude of health benefits, including reducing our risks for obesity and many chronic diseases and relieving anxiety and stress. Despite the many health benefits of physical activity, most people in the United States, including many children, are inactive.*

What Is a Sound Fitness Program?

There are several widely recognized qualities of a sound fitness program, as well as guidelines to help you design one that is right for you. These are explored in this section.

A Sound Fitness Program Meets Your Personal Goals

A fitness program may be ideal for someone else, but that doesn't necessarily mean it is right for you. Before you design or evaluate any program, you need to know what you intend to get from it; in other words, you need to define your personal fitness goals. Do you want to prevent osteoporosis, diabetes, or another chronic disease that runs in your family? Do you want to lose excess body fat? Do you simply want to increase your energy and stamina? Or do you intend to compete in athletic events? Each of these scenarios would require a very different fitness program. This concept is referred to as the *specificity principle:* specific actions yield specific results.

Training is generally defined as activity leading to skilled behavior. Training is very specific to any given activity or goal. For example, if you want to train for athletic competition, a traditional approach that includes planned, purposive exercise sessions under the guidance of a trainer or coach would probably be most beneficial. If you want to achieve cardiorespiratory fitness, you would likely be advised to participate in an aerobics class at least 3 times a week, or jog for at least 20 minutes 3 times a week.

In contrast, if your goal were simply to maintain your overall health, you might do better to follow the 1996 report of the Surgeon General on achieving health through regular physical activity.[1] This report emphasizes that significant health benefits, such as reducing your risk for certain chronic diseases, can be achieved by participating in a moderate amount of physical activity (such as 30 minutes of gardening, housework, brisk walking, or bike riding) on most, if not all, days of the week. The 2005 *Dietary Guidelines for Americans* also recommend engaging in at least 30 minutes of moderate physical activity most days of the week. If 30 minutes at one time seems daunting, note that health benefits occur even when the time spent performing the physical activities is cumulative (for example, brisk walking for 10 minutes 3 times a day). Although these guidelines are appropriate for achieving health benefits, they are not necessarily of sufficient intensity and duration to improve physical fitness.

A Sound Fitness Program Is Fun and Includes Variety

One of the most important goals for everyone is fun; unless you enjoy being active, you may find it very difficult to maintain your physical fitness. What activities do you consider fun? If you enjoy the outdoors, hiking, camping, fishing, and rock climbing are potential activities for you. If you would rather exercise with friends on your lunch break, walking, climbing stairs, jogging, roller-blading, or bicycle riding may be more appropriate. Or you may find it more enjoyable to stay indoors and use the programs and equipment at your local fitness club . . . or purchase your own treadmill and free weights to use at home.

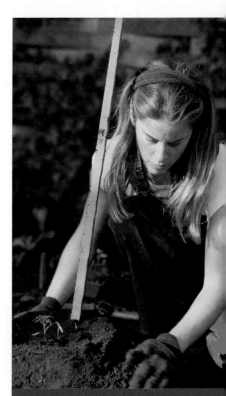

Moderate physical activity, such as gardening, helps maintain overall health.

Variety is critical to maintaining your fitness. Although some people enjoy doing similar activities day after day, most of us get bored with the same fitness routine. Incorporating a variety of activities into your fitness program will help maintain your interest and increase your enjoyment while at the same time promoting the different types of fitness identified in Table 10.1.

Variety can be achieved by:

- combining aerobic exercise, resistance training, and stretching;
- combining indoor and outdoor activities throughout the week;
- taking different routes when you walk or jog each day;
- watching a movie, reading a book, or listening to music while you ride a stationary bicycle or walk on a treadmill;
- participating in different activities each week such as walking, dancing, bicycling, yoga, weight lifting, swimming, hiking, and gardening.

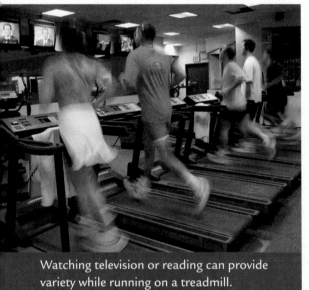

Watching television or reading can provide variety while running on a treadmill.

This "smorgasbord" of activities can increase your fitness without leading to monotony and boredom.

Fortunately, a fun and useful tool has been developed to help you increase the variety of your physical activity choices (FIGURE 10.2). The **Physical Activity Pyramid** makes recommendations for the type and amount of activity to perform weekly to increase your fitness. The bottom of the pyramid describes activities that should be done every day, including walking more, taking the stairs instead of the elevator, and working in your garden. Aerobic activities such as bicycling and brisk walking and recreational activities such as soccer, tennis, and basketball should be done 3 to 5 times each week, for at least 20 or 30 minutes. Flexibility, strength, and leisure activities should be done 2 to 3 times a week. The top of the pyramid emphasizes things we should do less of, including watching TV and playing computer games. By following the Physical Activity Pyramid, we can gradually increase our cardiorespiratory fitness, muscular strength and endurance, flexibility, bone density, and muscle mass and decrease our body fat.

RECAP *A sound fitness program must meet your personal fitness goals, such as reducing your risks for disease or preparing for competition in athletic events. It should also be fun and include activities you enjoy. Variety and consistency are important to help you maintain interest and achieve physical fitness in all components.*

Physical Activity Pyramid A pyramid similar to the previous USDA Food Guide Pyramid that makes recommendations for the type and amount of activity that should be done weekly to increase physical activity levels.

overload principle Placing an extra physical demand on your body in order to improve your fitness level.

FIT principle The principle used to achieve an appropriate overload for physical training. Stands for frequency, intensity, and time of activity.

A Sound Fitness Program Appropriately Overloads the Body

In order to improve your fitness level, you must place an extra physical demand on your body. This is referred to as the **overload principle.** A word of caution is in order here: *the overload principle does not advocate subjecting your body to inappropriately high stress,* because this can lead to exhaustion and injuries. In contrast, an appropriate overload on various body systems will result in healthy improvements in fitness.

To achieve an appropriate overload, you should consider three factors, collectively known as the **FIT principle:**

- Frequency
- Intensity
- Time of activity

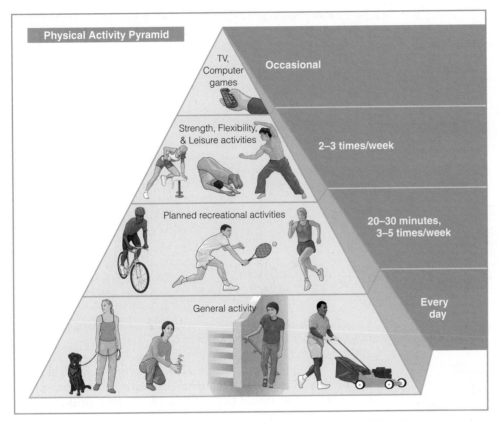

FIGURE 10.2 You can use this Physical Activity Pyramid as a guide to increase your level of physical activity.
(From Corbin, C. B., and R. D. Pangrazi. 1998. Physical Activity Pyramid rebuffs peak experience. *ACSM Health Fitness J.* 2[1]. Copyright © 1998.)

You can use the FIT principle to design either a general physical fitness program or a performance-based exercise program. **FIGURE 10.3** shows how the FIT principle can be applied to a cardiorespiratory and muscular fitness program.

Let's consider each of the FIT principle's three factors in more detail.

Frequency

Frequency refers to the number of activity sessions per week. Depending on your goals for fitness or health, the frequency of your activities will vary. To achieve cardiorespiratory fitness, working out 3 to 5 days a week appears optimal. On the other hand, working out more than 5 days a week does not cause significant gains in fitness but can substantially increase your risk for injury. In contrast, only 2 to 3 days a week are needed to achieve muscular fitness and 2 to 4 for flexibility. For achieving general health-related goals, we should do some type of activity (aerobic, resistance, or stretching) every day.

Intensity

Intensity refers to the amount of effort expended in an activity or, to put it another way, how difficult the activity is to perform. We can describe the intensity of activity as low, moderate, or vigorous:

- **Low-intensity activities** are those that cause very mild increases in breathing, sweating, and heart rate.
- **Moderate-intensity activities** cause moderate increases in breathing, sweating, and heart rate. For instance, you can carry on a conversation, but not continuously.
- **Vigorous-intensity activities** produce significant increases in breathing, sweating, and heart rate, so that talking is difficult.

frequency Refers to the number of activity sessions per week you perform.

intensity Refers to the amount of effort expended during the activity, or how difficult the activity is to perform.

low-intensity activities Activities that cause very mild increases in breathing, sweating, and heart rate.

moderate-intensity activities Activities that cause noticeable increases in breathing, sweating, and heart rate.

vigorous-intensity activities Activities that produce significant increases in breathing, sweating, and heart rate; talking is difficult when exercising at a vigorous intensity.

	Frequency	Intensity	Time
Cardiorespiratory fitness	3–5 days per week	64%–90% maximal heart rate	At least 20 consecutive minutes
Muscular fitness	2–3 days per week	70%–85% maximal weight you can lift	1–3 sets of 8–12 lifts* for each set *A minimum of 8–10 exercises involving the major muscle groups such as arms, shoulders, chest, abdomen, back, hips, and legs is recommended.
Flexibility	2–4 days per week	Stretching through full range of motion	2–4 repetitions per stretch* *Hold each stretch for 15–30 seconds.

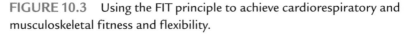

FIGURE 10.3   Using the FIT principle to achieve cardiorespiratory and musculoskeletal fitness and flexibility.

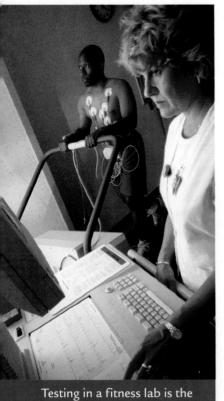

Testing in a fitness lab is the most accurate way to determine maximal heart rate.

For achieving health-related goals, even low-intensity activities can provide significant benefits. For achieving physical fitness goals, you can calculate the range of exercise intensity that is appropriate for you by estimating your **maximal heart rate,** which is the rate at which your heart beats during maximal-intensity exercise. FIGURE 10.4 shows an example of a heart rate training chart. For achieving and maintaining physical fitness, your heart rate during exercise should be between 64% and 90% of your maximal heart rate. If you've been inactive for a long time, you may want to exercise at the lower end of the range, at least for a few weeks. If you're more physically fit or are striving for a more rapid improvement in fitness, you may choose to exercise at the higher end of the range. **Athletes,** people trained to compete in sports, generally train at a higher intensity, around 80% to 95% of their maximum heart rate. So what is your maximal heart rate and training range? To find out, try the easy calculation in the What About You? box on page 310.

Although the calculation *220 − age* has been used extensively for years to predict maximal heart rate, it is not intended to accurately represent everyone's true maximal heart rate or to be used as the standard of aerobic training intensity. The most accurate way to determine your own maximal heart rate is to complete a maximal exercise test in a fitness laboratory; however, this test is not commonly available and can be very expensive. So most people continue to rely on the *220 − age* calculation to give them a general idea of their aerobic training range.

Time of Activity

Time of activity refers to how long each session lasts. To achieve general health, you can do multiple short bouts of activity that add up to 30 minutes each day. However, to achieve higher levels of fitness, it is important that the activities be done for at least 20 to 30 consecutive minutes.

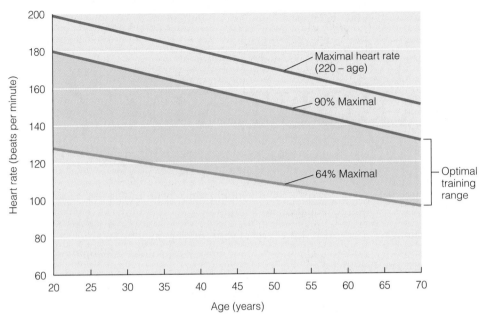

FIGURE 10.4 This heart rate training chart can be used to estimate your aerobic exercise intensity. The top line indicates the predicted maximal heart rate value for a person's age (220 – age). The shaded area represents the heart rate values that fall between 64% and 90% of maximal heart rate, which is the range generally recommended to achieve aerobic fitness.

Table 10.2 compares the guidelines for achieving health to those for achieving physical fitness. The guidelines you follow will depend on your personal goals. These recommendations apply to people of all ages, and following either set will allow you to improve and maintain your health. People with heart disease, high blood pressure, diabetes, osteoporosis, or arthritis should get approval to exercise from their healthcare practitioner prior to starting a fitness program. In addition, a medical evaluation should be conducted before starting an exercise program for an apparently healthy, but currently inactive man 40 years or older or woman 50 years or older.

A Sound Fitness Plan Includes Warm-Up and Cool-Down Periods

To properly prepare for and recover from an exercise session, warm-up and cool-down activities should be performed. **Warm-up,** also called preliminary exercise,

maximal heart rate The rate at which your heart beats during maximal-intensity exercise.

athlete Any person trained to compete in sports.

time of activity How long each exercise session lasts, not including warm-up and cool-down periods.

warm-up Also called preliminary exercise; includes activities that prepare you for an exercise session, including stretching, calisthenics, and movements specific to the exercise you are about to engage in.

TABLE 10.2 Physical Activity Guidelines for Achieving Health Versus Physical Fitness

	Health	Physical Fitness
Frequency	Daily	2–5 days per week (3–5 days for cardiorespiratory fitness, 2–3 days for muscular fitness and flexibility)
Intensity	Any level	64%–90% of maximal heart rate
Time	Accumulation of a minimum of 30 minutes each day	20–60 minutes of continuous or intermittent activity
Type	Any activity	Aerobic-type activities, resistance exercises to enhance muscular strength and endurance, and flexibility exercises

Source: Data from American College of Sports Medicine (ACSM). 2006. ACSM's Guidelines for Exercise Testing and Prescription. 7th ed. Philadelphia: Lippincott Williams and Wilkins; and U.S. Department of Health and Human Services. 1996. *Physical Activity and Health: A Report of the Surgeon General.* Atlanta, GA: U.S. Department of Health and Human Services, Centers for Disease Control and Prevention, National Center for Chronic Disease Prevention and Health Promotion.

WHAT ABOUT YOU?

What's Your Maximal Heart Rate and Training Range?

You can estimate your maximal heart rate by using the following easy calculation:

>your maximal heart rate = 220 minus your age

Let's say you are 20 years old:

>your maximal heart rate = 220 − 20 = 200 beats per minute (bpm)

Now let's calculate your training range. As we said in the text, for nonathletes this number is 64% to 90% of your maximal heart rate. If you want to work out at the lower end of your range, you should multiply your maximal heart rate by 64%. If your maximal heart rate is 200, then your equation is

>lower end of your training range = 200 bpm × 0.64 = 128 bpm

If you want to work out at the higher end of your range, you should multiply your maximal heart rate by 90%:

>higher end of your training range = 200 bpm × 0.90 = 180 bpm

Thus, your training range is between 128 and 180 bpm.

includes general activities such as gentle aerobics, calisthenics, and then stretching followed by specific activities that prepare you for the actual activity, such as jogging or swinging a golf club. Your warm-up should be brief (5 to 10 minutes), gradual, and sufficient to increase muscle and body temperature but should not cause fatigue or deplete energy stores.

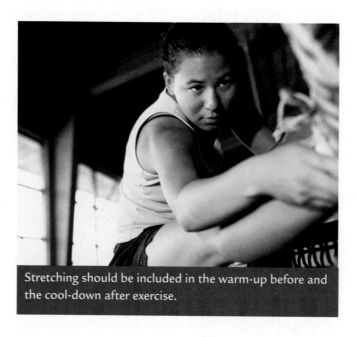

Stretching should be included in the warm-up before and the cool-down after exercise.

Warming up prior to exercise is important, as it properly prepares your muscles for exertion by increasing blood flow and body temperature. It enhances the body's flexibility and may also help to prepare you psychologically for the exercise session or athletic event.

Cool-down activities are done after the exercise session is completed. Similar to the warm-up, the cool-down should be gradual and allow your body to slowly recover. Your cool-down should include some of the same activities you performed during the exercise session, but at a low intensity, and you should allow ample time for stretching. Cooling down after exercise assists in the prevention of injury and may help reduce muscle soreness.

Now that you know the benefits of regular physical activity and the characteristics of a sound fitness plan, how do you get started? If you haven't been active until now, it's important to set realistic goals you can achieve in a short period of time. For instance, "I want to perform at least 30 minutes of physical activity each day on at least 5 days next week." For tips on incorporating physical activity into your daily life, check out the Game Plan on page 312.

cool-down Activities done after an exercise session is completed. Should be gradual and allow your body to slowly recover from exercise.

NUTRI-CASE JUDY

"I can't remember a time in my life when I wasn't trying to lose weight. But nothing ever works, and when I go off a diet, I always end up fatter than I started out! These last couple of years I'd sort of given up, but last week I had my annual check-up and my doctor confirmed what I already knew—I'm obese! The doctor also said my weight is contributing to my high blood sugar, and that my blood pressure is high, too. As a nurse's aide, I see every day the health problems caused by obesity. Still, knowing how bad it is doesn't help me to lose the weight and keep it off. So we talked about some "slow and steady" strategies for losing weight: I promised I'd do a better job of watching my diet, take my medications as prescribed, and start working out at the new fitness center here at the hospital. I checked it out on my lunch break today, and I guess it's okay. They have a couple of treadmills and stationary bikes right in front of a big TV so you can watch the soaps while you work out. Still, I'm not really sure what I'm supposed to do or how many times a week or for how long. I mean, if I only had to lose 5 pounds that would be easy. But I've got to lose 50! And I only get half an hour for lunch!"

Imagine that you were a trainer at the Valley Hospital employee fitness center, and Judy told you about her weight-loss and health goals. Applying the FIT principle, recommend an initial physical activity program that can get Judy started on improving her health that includes an appropriate:

- number of times per 5-day work week
- intensity
- duration of activity
- variety of activities

If you get stuck, don't forget Table 10.2!

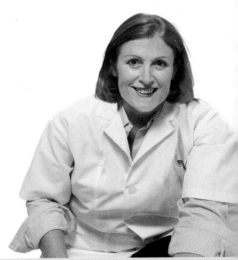

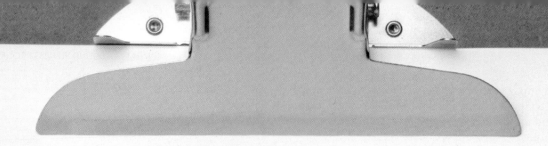

GAME PLAN
Tips for Increasing Your Physical Activity

There are 1,440 minutes in every day. Spend just 30 of those minutes in physical activity, and you'll be taking an important step toward improving your health. Here are some tips adapted from the Centers for Disease Control and Prevention and the United States Department of Health and Human Services for working activity into your daily life:[6,7]

❑ Walk as often and as much as possible: park your car farther away from your dorm, lecture hall, or shops; walk to school or work; go for a brisk walk between classes; get on or off the bus one stop away from your destination.

❑ Take the stairs instead of the elevator.

❑ Exercise while watching television, for example by doing sit-ups, stretching, or using a treadmill or stationary bike.

❑ Put on a CD and dance!

❑ Get an exercise partner: join a friend for walks, hikes, cycling, skating, tennis, or a fitness class.

❑ Take up a group sport.

❑ Register for a class from the physical education department in an activity you've never tried before, maybe yoga, fencing, or bowling!

❑ Register for a dance class, such as jazz, tap, or ballroom.

❑ Join a health club, gym, or YMCA and use the swimming pool, weights, rock-climbing wall, and other facilities.

❑ Join an activity-based club such as a skating or hiking club.

If you have been inactive for a while, use a sensible approach by starting out slowly. Gradually build up the time you spend doing the activity by adding a few minutes every few days until you reach 30 minutes a day. As this 30-minute minimum becomes easier, gradually increase the length of time you spend in activity, the intensity of the activities you choose, or both.[6]

RECAP *To improve fitness, you must place an appropriate overload on your body. Follow the FIT principle: FIT stands for frequency, intensity, and time of activity. Frequency refers to the number of activity sessions per week. Intensity refers to how difficult the activity is to perform. Time refers to how long each activity session lasts. Warm-up exercises prepare the muscles for exertion by increasing blood flow and temperature. Low-intensity cool-down activities help prevent injury and may help reduce muscle soreness.*

What Fuels Our Activities?

adenosine triphosphate (ATP)
The common currency of energy for virtually all cells of the body.

In order to perform physical activity, or muscular work, we must be able to generate energy. The common currency of energy for virtually all cells in the body is a molecule called **adenosine triphosphate (ATP)**. As you might guess from its name, a molecule of ATP includes an organic compound called adenosine and three phosphate

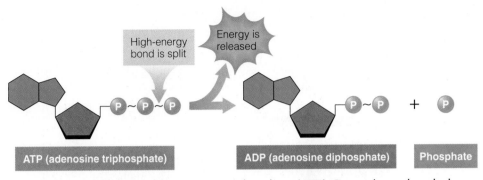

High-energy
bond is split

Energy is
released

P~P~P

ATP (adenosine triphosphate)

P~P   +   P

ADP (adenosine diphosphate)

Phosphate

FIGURE 10.5 Structure of adenosine triphosphate (ATP). Energy is produced when ATP is split into adenosine diphosphate (ADP) and inorganic phosphate (P).

groups (FIGURE 10.5). Scientists call ATP "the energy molecule" because whenever one of the phosphates is broken away from the rest of the molecule, energy is released.

Adenosine Triphosphate and Creatine Phosphate Stored in Our Muscles Fuel Brief Activities

The amount of ATP stored in a muscle cell is very limited; it can keep the muscle active for only about 1 to 3 seconds. When more energy is needed, our bodies break down a high-energy compound called **creatine phosphate (CP),** which is also stored in our muscles. As with ATP, when the phosphate bond in this molecule is broken, energy is released.

Muscle tissue contains about 4 to 6 times as much CP as ATP, but that is still not enough to fuel long-term activities. We tend to use CP the most during very intense, very short bouts of activity such as lifting, jumping, and sprinting (FIGURE 10.6). To fuel activities for longer periods of time, our bodies generate ATP from the breakdown of the energy nutrients, primarily carbohydrate and fat and to a lesser extent protein. As you will see, the type, intensity, and duration of the activities we perform determine the amount of ATP we need and therefore the type of energy we use.

The Breakdown of Carbohydrates Provides Energy for Brief and Long-Term Activity

During activities lasting longer than 30 seconds, we cannot generate enough ATP from the breakdown of CP alone to fully support our efforts. Thus, our bodies begin to break down carbohydrates, specifically glucose, in a process called **glycolysis.** We get this glucose from glycogen stored in our muscles and from the glucose present in our blood. As shown in FIGURE 10.7, for every glucose molecule that goes through glycolysis, two ATP molecules are produced. That's not much, but fortunately the process doesn't end there.

Glycolysis produces not only ATP but also **pyruvic acid.** In the presence of adequate oxygen, the body breaks down pyruvic acid into 36 to 38 molecules of ATP. That's enough ATP to keep us going for a while; in fact, our bodies use **aerobic** metabolism of glucose (that is, metabolism in the presence of oxygen) to fuel our muscles during activities lasting from 3 minutes to 4 hours.

During high-intensity exercise, the amount of oxygen we inhale is not sufficient to allow us to generate all of the ATP we need through aerobic metabolism. In this state, our bodies send some of the pyruvic acid produced during glycolysis into a metabolic pathway that does not require oxygen. In this pathway, the pyruvic acid is converted to **lactic acid** (see the blue portion of Figure 10.7). As you might guess, this reaction is described as **anaerobic,** because it occurs in the absence of oxygen. For years it was assumed that lactic acid was a useless, even potentially toxic by-product of high-intensity exercise. We now know that lactic acid is important in glucose breakdown and that it plays a critical role

creatine phosphate (CP) A high-energy compound that can be broken down for energy and used to regenerate ATP.

glycolysis The breakdown of glucose; yields two ATP molecules and two pyruvic acid molecules for each molecule of glucose.

pyruvic acid The primary end product of glycolysis.

aerobic Means "with oxygen." Term used to refer to metabolic reactions that occur only in the presence of oxygen.

lactic acid A compound that results when pyruvic acid is metabolized.

anaerobic Means "without oxygen." Term used to refer to metabolic reactions that occur in the absence of oxygen.

FIGURE 10.6 The relative contributions of ATP-CP, carbohydrate, and fat to activities of various durations and intensities.

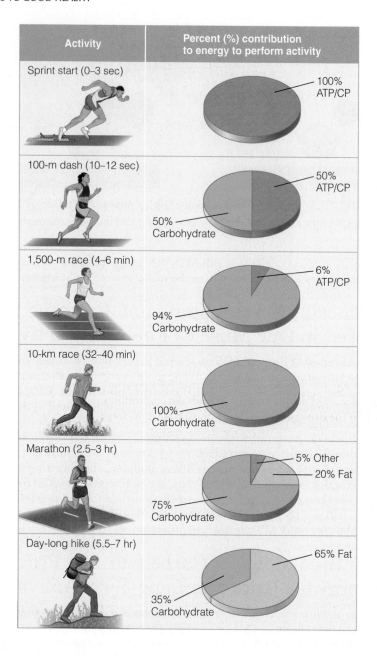

Activity	Percent (%) contribution to energy to perform activity
Sprint start (0–3 sec)	100% ATP/CP
100-m dash (10–12 sec)	50% ATP/CP 50% Carbohydrate
1,500-m race (4–6 min)	6% ATP/CP 94% Carbohydrate
10-km race (32–40 min)	100% Carbohydrate
Marathon (2.5–3 hr)	5% Other 20% Fat 75% Carbohydrate
Day-long hike (5.5–7 hr)	65% Fat 35% Carbohydrate

in supplying fuel for working muscles, the heart, and resting tissues (see Nutrition Myth or Fact?: Does Lactic Acid Cause Muscle Fatigue and Soreness? on page 315).

As you learned in Chapter 4, we can store only a limited amount of glycogen in our bodies. An average, well-nourished man who weighs about 154 lb (or 70 kg) can store about 200 g to 500 g of muscle glycogen, which is equal to 800 kcal to 2,000 kcal of energy. Athletes have larger glycogen stores than inactive people, but even they do not have enough stored glycogen to provide an unlimited glucose supply. Thus, in addition to glucose, we need a fuel source that is abundant and can support activities of lower intensity and longer duration. This fuel source is fat.

Aerobic Breakdown of Fats Supports Exercise of Low Intensity and Long Duration

When we refer to fat as a fuel source, we mean the triglyceride molecule, which is the primary storage form of fat in our cells. As you learned in Chapter 4, a triglyceride molecule is composed of a glycerol backbone attached to three fatty acid

NUTRITION MYTH OR FACT?

Does Lactic Acid Cause Muscle Fatigue and Soreness?

Theo and his teammates won their basketball game last night, but just barely. With two of the players sick, Theo got more court time than usual, and when he got back to the dorm, he could hardly get his legs to carry him up the stairs. This morning, Theo's muscles ache all over, and he wonders if a build-up of lactic acid is to blame.

Lactic acid is a by-product of glycolysis. For many years, it was believed that lactic acid caused both muscle fatigue and soreness. Does recent scientific evidence support this belief?

The exact causes of muscle fatigue are not known, and there appear to be many contributing factors. Recent evidence suggests that fatigue may be due not only to the accumulation of acids and other metabolic by-products but also to the depletion of creatine phosphate and changes in calcium in the cells that affect muscle contraction. In addition, depletion of muscle glycogen, liver glycogen, and blood glucose, as well as psychological factors, can all contribute to fatigue.[8] Thus, lactic acid contributes to fatigue but does not appear to cause fatigue independently.

So what factors cause muscle soreness? As with fatigue, there are probably many contributors. It is theorized that soreness usually results from microscopic tears in the muscle fibers as a result of strenuous exercise. This damage triggers an inflammatory reaction that causes an influx of fluid and various chemicals to the damaged area. These substances work to remove damaged tissue and initiate tissue repair; however, they may also stimulate pain.[8] However, it appears highly unlikely that lactic acid is an independent cause of muscle soreness.

Recent studies indicate that lactic acid is produced even under aerobic conditions! This means it is produced at rest as well as during low-, moderate-, and high-intensity exercise. The reasons for this constant production of lactic acid are still being studied. What we do know is that lactic acid is an important fuel for resting tissues and also for working cardiac and skeletal muscles. That's right—skeletal muscles not only *produce* lactic acid, but they also *use* it for energy, both directly and after it is converted to glucose and glycogen in the liver.[9,10] We also know that endurance training improves the ability of muscles to use lactic acid for energy. Thus, contrary to being a waste product of glucose metabolism, lactic acid is actually an important energy source for muscle cells during rest and exercise.

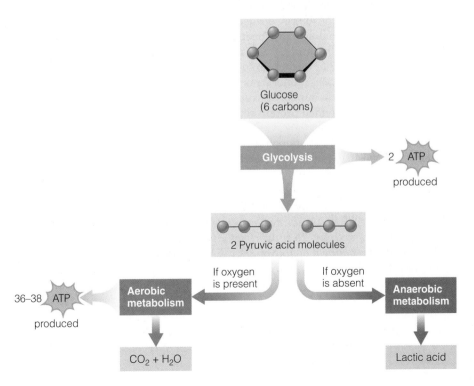

Glucose
(6 carbons)

Glycolysis → 2 ATP produced

2 Pyruvic acid molecules

If oxygen is present — Aerobic metabolism → 36–38 ATP produced

Aerobic metabolism → $CO_2 + H_2O$

If oxygen is absent — Anaerobic metabolism → Lactic acid

FIGURE 10.7 The breakdown of one molecule of glucose, or the process of glycolysis, yields two molecules of pyruvic acid and two ATP molecules. The further metabolism of pyruvic acid in the presence of insufficient oxygen (anaerobic process) results in the production of lactic acid. The metabolism of pyruvic acid in the presence of adequate oxygen (aerobic process) yields 36 to 38 molecules of ATP.

molecules (see Figure 4.1 on page 100). These fatty acid molecules provide much of the energy we need to support long-term activity.

There are two major advantages of using fat as a fuel. First, fat is a very abundant energy source, even in lean people. For example, a man who weighs 154 lb (or 70 kg) who has a body fat level of 10% has approximately 15 lb of body fat, which is equivalent to more than 50,000 kcal of energy! This is significantly more energy than can be provided by muscle glycogen (800 to 2,000 kcal). Second, fat provides 9 kcal of energy per gram, whereas carbohydrate provides only 4 kcal per gram, which means that fat supplies more than twice as much energy per gram as carbohydrate. The primary disadvantage of using fat as a fuel is that the breakdown process is relatively slow; thus, fat is used predominantly as a fuel source during activities of lower intensity and longer duration. Fat is also our primary energy source during rest, sitting, and standing in place.

What specific activities are primarily fueled by fat? Walking long distances uses fat stores, as do other low- to moderate-intensity forms of exercise. Fat is also an important fuel source during endurance events such as marathons (26.2 miles) and ultramarathons (49.9 miles). Endurance exercise training improves our ability to use fat for energy, which may be one reason that endurance athletes tend to have lower body fat levels than people who do not exercise.

Our bodies are continually using some combination of carbohydrate and fat for energy. At rest, we use very little carbohydrate, relying mostly on fat. During maximal exercise (at 100% effort), we are using mostly carbohydrate and very little fat. However, most activities we do each day involve some use of both fuels.

When it comes to eating properly to support regular physical activity or exercise training, the nutrient to focus on is carbohydrate. This is because most people store more than enough fat to support exercise, whereas our storage of carbohydrate is limited. It is especially important that we maintain adequate stores of glycogen for moderate to intense exercise. Dietary recommendations for fat, carbohydrate, and protein are reviewed later in this chapter.

Amino Acids Are Not Major Sources of Fuel During Exercise

Proteins, or more specifically amino acids, are not major energy sources during exercise. Depending on the intensity and duration of the activity, amino acids may contribute about 3% to 6% of the energy needed.[11]

Given this, why is it that so many people are concerned about their protein intake? As we discussed in Chapter 9, our muscles are not stimulated to grow when we eat extra protein, whether as food or supplements. Only appropriate physical training can achieve that. Most Americans, including sedentary Americans, eat more than enough protein to support tissue recovery for even the most highly competitive athletes! Recommended protein requirements for active people are identified shortly.

Recall that if we do not eat enough carbohydrate, our bodies will draw on our protein stores for energy. Thus, it is important to consume enough carbohydrate to support physical activity.

RECAP *Adenosine triphosphate, or ATP, is the common energy source for all cells of the body. ATP and creatine phosphate stored in our muscle cells can only fuel brief spurts of activity. To support activities that last longer, energy is produced from the breakdown of glucose. Fat is broken down slowly to support activities of low intensity and long duration. Amino acids help build and repair tissues after exercise but contribute only 3% to 6% of the energy needed during exercise. We generally consume more than enough protein in our diets to support regular exercise and do not need protein or amino acid supplements.*

What Kind of Diet Supports Physical Activity?

Lots of people wonder, "Will my nutrient needs change if I become more physically active?" The answer to this question depends on the type, intensity, and duration of the activity. It is not necessarily true that our requirement for every nutrient is greater if we are physically active.

If you enter your activity level in www.MyPyramid.gov, it will provide you with general nutritional guidelines to follow. In addition, Table 10.3 provides an overview of the nutrients that can be affected by regular, vigorous exercise training. Each of these nutrients is described in more detail in this section.[12]

TABLE 10.3 Suggested Intakes of Nutrients to Support Vigorous Exercise

Nutrient	Functions	Suggested Intake
Energy	Supports exercise, activities of daily living, and basic body functions	Depends upon body size and the type, intensity, and duration of activity For many female athletes: 1,800 to 3,500 kcal/day For many male athletes: 2,500 to 7,500 kcal/day
Carbohydrate	Provides energy, maintains adequate muscle glycogen and blood glucose; high-complex-carbohydrate foods provide vitamins, minerals, and fiber	At least 55% of total energy intake Depending upon sport and gender, should consume 6–10 grams of carbohydrate per kg body weight per day
Fat	Provides energy, fat-soluble vitamins, and essential fatty acids; supports production of hormones and transport of nutrients	15%–25% of total energy intake
Protein	Helps build and maintain muscle; provides building material for glucose; energy source during endurance exercise; aids recovery from exercise	12%–20% of total energy intake Endurance athletes: 1.4–1.6 grams per kg body weight Strength athletes: 1.0–1.7 grams per kg body weight
Water	Maintains temperature regulation (adequate cooling); maintains blood volume and blood pressure; supports all cell functions	Consume fluid before, during, and after exercise Consume enough to maintain body weight Consume at least 8 cups (or 64 fl. oz) of water daily to maintain regular health and activity Athletes may need up to 10 liters (or 170 fl. oz) every day; more is required if exercising in a hot environment
B vitamins	Critical for energy production from carbohydrate, fat, and protein	May need slightly more (1–2 times the RDA) for thiamin, riboflavin, and vitamin B_6
Calcium	Builds and maintains bone mass; assists with nervous system function, muscle contraction, hormone function, and transport of nutrients across cell membrane	Meet the current AI: 14–18 y: 1,300 mg/day 19–50 y: 1,000 mg/day 51 y and older: 1,200 mg/day
Iron	Primarily responsible for the transport of oxygen in blood to cells; assists with energy production	Consume at least the RDA: Males: 14–18 y: 11 mg/day 19 y and older: 8 mg/day Females: 14–18 y: 15 mg/day 19–50 y: 18 mg/day 51 y and older: 8 mg/day

Vigorous Exercise Increases Energy Needs

Highly active people generally have higher energy needs than moderately active or sedentary people. The amount of extra energy they need is determined by the type, intensity, and duration of their activity. In addition, the energy needs of men are generally higher than those of women, because men weigh more, have more muscle mass, and will expend more energy during activity than women. This is relative, of course: a large woman who trains 3 to 5 hours each day will need more energy than a wsmall man who trains 1 hour each day. The energy needs of athletes can range from only 1,500 to 1,800 kcal per day for a small female gymnast to more than 7,500 kcal per day for a male cyclist competing in the Tour de France cross-country cycling race!

FIGURE 10.8 shows a sample of meals that total 1,800 kcal per day and 4,000 kcal per day, with the carbohydrate content of these meals meeting more than 60% of total energy intake. As you can see, athletes who need more than 4,000 kcal per day need to consume very large quantities of food. However, the heavy demands of daily physical training, work, school, and family responsibilities often leave these athletes with little time to eat adequately. Thus, many athletes meet their energy demands by planning regular meals and snacks and **grazing** (eating small meals throughout the day) consistently. They may also take advantage of the energy-dense snack foods and meal replacements specifically designed for athletes participating in vigorous training. These steps help athletes to maintain their blood glucose and energy stores to maximize their performance.

For athletes, weight maintenance is generally recommended to maximize performance. If an athlete is losing body weight, then his or her energy intake is inadequate. Conversely, weight gain may indicate that energy intake is too high. If weight loss is warranted, food intake should be lowered no more than 200 to 500 kcal per day, and athletes should try to lose weight prior to the competitive season if at all possible. Weight gain may be necessary for some athletes and can usually be accomplished by consuming 500 to 700 kcal per day more than needed for weight maintenance.

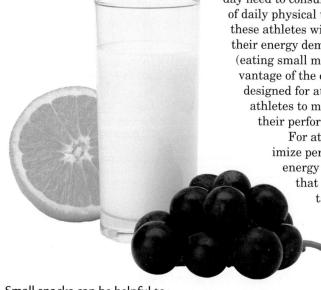

Small snacks can be helpful to meet daily energy demands.

Carbohydrate Needs Increase for Many Active People

Active people require adequate carbohydrate to maintain their glycogen stores and provide quick energy.

How Much of an Athlete's Diet Should Be Carbohydrates?

You may recall from Chapter 3 that the AMDR for carbohydrates is 45% to 65% of total energy intake. It is suggested that athletes consume at least 55% of their total energy intake as carbohydrates, which falls within this recommended range. Athletes who are participating in strength-type activities, sprinting, or other explosive-type events or are not training for more than 1 hour each day may find that consuming 50% of their total energy intake as carbohydrate is sufficient.

When Should Carbohydrates Be Consumed?

It is important for athletes not only to consume enough carbohydrate to maintain glycogen stores but also to time their intake optimally. Our bodies store glycogen very rapidly during the first 24 hours of recovery from exercise, with the highest storage rates occurring during the first few hours.[13] Athletes who must perform or participate in training bouts that are scheduled less than 8 hours apart should try to

grazing   Consistently eating small meals throughout the day; done by many athletes to meet their high-energy demands.

1,800 kcal/day	4,000 kcal/day
1½ cup Cheerios 4 oz skim milk 1 medium banana 8 fl. oz orange juice	3 cups Cheerios 8 fl. oz skim milk 1 medium banana 2 slices whole-wheat toast 1 tbsp. butter 16 fl. oz orange juice

Turkey sandwich with:
  2 slices whole-wheat bread
  3 oz turkey lunch meat
  1 oz Swiss cheese slice
  1 leaf iceberg lettuce
  2 slices tomato
  1 cup tomato soup
   (made with water)
	Two turkey sandwiches with:
	  2 slices whole-wheat bread
	  3 oz turkey lunch meat
	  1 oz Swiss cheese slice
	  1 leaf iceberg lettuce
	  2 slices tomato
	  2 cups tomato soup
	   (made with water)
	Two 8-oz containers of
	  low-fat fruit yogurt
	24 fl. oz of Gatorade

4 oz grilled skinless
  chicken breast
1½ cup mixed salad greens
1 tbsp. French salad dressing
1 cup steamed broccoli
1 cup cooked brown rice
8 fl. oz skim milk
	6 oz grilled skinless
	  chicken breast
	3 cups mixed salad greens
	3 tbsp. French salad dressing
	2 cups cooked
	  spaghetti noodles
	1 cup spaghetti sauce
	  with meat
	16 fl. oz skim milk

FIGURE 10.8 High-carbohydrate (approximately 60% of total energy) meals that contain approximately 1,800 kcal per day (on left) and 4,000 kcal per day (on right). Athletes must plan their meals carefully to meet energy demands, particularly those with very high energy needs.

consume enough carbohydrate in the few hours after training to allow for ample glycogen storage. However, with a longer recovery time (such as 12 hours or more), athletes can eat when they choose, and glycogen levels should be restored as long as the total carbohydrate eaten is sufficient. Failure to replenish glycogen stores after activity may result in suboptimal energy levels for the next workout or event.

What Food Sources of Carbohydrates Support Athletic Training?

What are good carbohydrate sources to support vigorous training? In general, fiber-rich, less-processed carbohydrate foods such as whole grains and cereals, fruits, vegetables, and juices are excellent sources that also supply vitamins, minerals and fiber. The guideline for intake of simple sugars is less than 10% of total energy intake, but some athletes who need very large energy intakes to support training may be able to consume more.

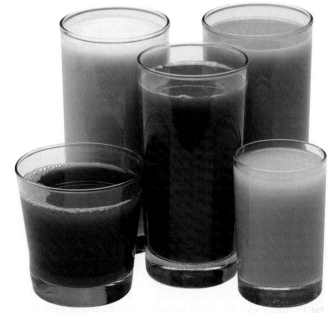

Fruit and vegetable juices can be a good source of carbohydrates.

TABLE 10.4 Carbohydrate and Total Energy in Various Foods and Sport Bars

Food	Amount	Carbohydrate (grams)	Energy from Carbohydrate (%)	Total Energy (kcal)
Sweetened applesauce	1 cup	50	97	207
Large apple Saltine crackers	1 each 8 each	50	82	248
Whole-wheat bread Jelly Skim milk	1-oz. slice 4 tsp 12 fl. oz	50	71	282
Spaghetti noodles (cooked) Tomato sauce	1 cup ¼ cup	50	75	268
Brown rice (cooked) Mixed vegetables Apple juice	1 cup ½ cup 12 fl. oz	100	88	450
Grape Nuts cereal Raisins Skim milk	½ cup ⅜ cup 8 fl. oz	100	84	473
Clif Bar (chocolate chip)	2.4 oz	45	72	250
Meta-Rx (fudge brownie)	3.53 oz	48	60	320
Power Bar (chocolate)	2.25 oz	42	75	225
PR Bar Ironman	2 oz	24	42	230

Source: Reprinted with permission from Manore, M. and J. Thompson. 2000. *Sport Nutrition for Health and Performance.* (Champaign, IL: Human Kinetics), 42, 49.

carbohydrate loading Also known as glycogen loading. A process that involves altering training and carbohydrate intake so that muscle glycogen storage is maximized.

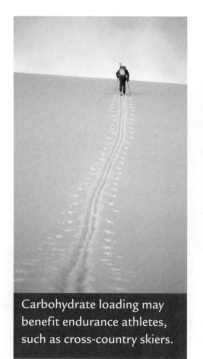

Carbohydrate loading may benefit endurance athletes, such as cross-country skiers.

Many snack bars have been designed to assist athletes with increasing carbohydrate intake. The carbohydrate and energy content of some of these products is identified in Table 10.4, along with several less-expensive foods high in carbohydrate.

When Does Carbohydrate Loading Make Sense?

Because of the importance of carbohydrates as an exercise fuel and our limited capacity to store them, discovering ways to maximize our storage of carbohydrates has been at the forefront of sports nutrition research for many years. The practice of **carbohydrate loading,** also called *glycogen loading,* involves altering both exercise duration and carbohydrate intake such that it maximizes the amount of muscle glycogen. Table 10.5 provides a schedule for carbohydrate loading for an endurance athlete. Athletes who may benefit from maximizing muscle glycogen stores are those competing in marathons, ultramarathons, long-distance swimming, cross-country skiing, and triathlons. Athletes who compete in baseball, American football, 10K runs, walking, hiking, weight lifting, and most swimming events will not gain any performance benefits from this practice, nor will people who regularly participate in moderately intense physical activities to maintain fitness.

Carbohydrate loading does not always improve performance and can be accompanied by many adverse side effects, including extreme gastrointestinal distress, particularly diarrhea. In addition, we store water along with the extra glycogen in our muscles, which leaves many athletes feeling heavy and sluggish. Athletes who want to try carbohydrate loading should experiment prior to competition to determine if it is beneficial for them.[14]

TABLE 10.5 Recommended Carbohydrate Loading Procedure for Endurance Athletes

Days Prior to Event	Exercise Duration (minutes)	Carbohydrate Content of Diet (grams per kg of body weight)
6	90	5
5	40	5
4	40	5
3	20	10
2	20	10
1	None (rest day)	10
Day of Race	Competition	Precompetition food and fluid

Source: Coleman, E. 2006. Carbohydrate and exercise. In Marie Dunford, ed. *Sports Nutrition.* 4th ed. Chicago, IL. The American Dietetic Association.

RECAP *The type, intensity, and duration of activities we participate in will determine our nutrient needs. Men generally need more energy than women because of their higher muscle mass and larger body weight. In general, athletes should consume at least 55% of their total energy as carbohydrate. Consuming carbohydrate sources within the first few hours of recovery can maximize carbohydrate storage rates. Carbohydrate loading involves altering physical training and the diet such that the storage of muscle glycogen is maximized in an attempt to enhance endurance performance.*

Moderate Fat Consumption Is Enough to Support Most Activities

Fat is an important energy source for both moderate physical activity and vigorous endurance training. When athletes reach a physically trained state, they are able to use more fat for energy; in other words, they become better "fat burners." This can also occur in people who are not athletes but who regularly participate in aerobic-type fitness activities. This effect occurs for a number of reasons, including an increase in enzymes involved in fat metabolism, improved ability of the muscles to store fat, and improved ability to extract fat from the blood for use during exercise.

Many people concerned with their weight and physical appearance eat less than 15% of their total energy intake as fat, but this is inadequate. Instead, a fat intake of 15% to 25% of total energy intake is generally recommended, with less than 10% of total energy intake as saturated fat. Recall that fat provides not only energy but also fat-soluble vitamins and essential fatty acids that are critical to maintaining general health. People who have chronic disease risk factors such as high blood lipids, high blood pressure, or unhealthful blood glucose levels should work with their physician to adjust their intake of fat and carbohydrate according to their health risks.

Active People Need More Protein, but Many Already Eat Enough

The protein intakes suggested for active people range from 0.8 to 1.7 g/kg body weight. At the lower end of this range are people who exercise 4 to 5 times a week for 30 minutes or less. At the upper end are athletes who train 5 to 7 times a week for more than an hour a day. Studies do not support the contention that consuming more than 2 g of protein per kilogram of body weight improves protein synthesis, muscle strength, or performance.[15]

Most inactive people and many athletes in the United States consume more than enough protein to support their needs.[16] However, some athletes do not consume enough protein, including those with very low energy intakes, vegetarians or vegans who do not consume high-protein food sources, and young athletes who are growing and are not aware of their higher protein needs.

In 1995, Dr. Barry Sears published *The Zone: A Dietary Road Map,* a book that claims numerous benefits of a high-protein, low-carbohydrate diet for athletes.[17] This and other low-carbohydrate, high-protein diets have become quite popular, especially among people who want to lose weight. Unlike many of these diets, the Zone Diet was developed and marketed specifically for competitive athletes. It recommends that athletes eat a 40-30-30 diet, or one composed of 40% carbohydrate, 30% fat, and 30% protein. Dr. Sears claims that high-carbohydrate diets impair athletic performance because of unhealthful effects of insulin. These claims have not been supported by research, and in fact, many of Dr. Sears's claims are not consistent with human physiology. The primary problem with the Zone Diet for athletes is that it is too low in both energy and carbohydrate to support training and performance.

As described in Chapter 5, high-quality protein sources include lean meats, poultry, fish, eggs, low-fat dairy products, legumes, and soy products. By following their personalized MyPyramid, people of all fitness levels can consume more than enough protein without the use of supplements or specially formulated foods.

> RECAP *Athletes and physically active people use more fat for energy. A dietary fat intake of 15% to 25% is generally recommended, with less than 10% of total energy intake as saturated fat. Protein needs can be somewhat higher for athletes, but most people in the United States already consume more than twice their daily needs. Although low-carbohydrate, high-protein diets have been marketed to athletes, they are generally too low in carbohydrate and total energy to support training and competition.*

Regular Exercise Increases Our Need for Fluids

A detailed discussion of fluids is provided in Chapter 8. In this chapter, we will briefly review the role of water during exercise.

Cooling Mechanisms

When we exercise, our bodies generate heat. In fact, heat production can increase 15 to 20 times during heavy exercise! The primary way in which we dissipate this heat is through sweating, which is also called **evaporative cooling.** When body temperature rises, more blood (which contains water) flows to the skin. Heat is carried in this way from the core to the surface of the body. By sweating, the water (and body heat) leaves the body and the air around us picks up (or evaporates) this water from the skin, cooling the body.

Dehydration and Heat-Related Illnesses

Exercising or performing manual labor in extreme heat and humidity is very dangerous for two reasons: the extreme heat dramatically raises body temperature, and the high humidity prohibits evaporative cooling. During periods of high humidity, the environmental air is so saturated with water that it is unable to pull the water from the surface of the skin. In addition, during intense activity in the heat, our muscles and skin are constantly competing for blood flow. When there is no longer enough blood flow to simultaneously provide adequate blood to our muscles and to our skin, muscle blood flow takes priority over the skin, which prevents us from cooling ourselves. Under these conditions, heat illnesses are likely to occur.

Dehydration significantly increases the risk for heat illnesses. FIGURE 10.9 identifies specific symptoms of dehydration during heavy exercise.

Heat illnesses include heat syncope, heat cramps, heat exhaustion, and heatstroke:

● **Heat syncope** is dizziness that occurs when people stand for too long in the heat, and the blood pools in their lower extremities. It can also occur

evaporative cooling   Another term for sweating, which is the primary way in which we dissipate heat.

heat syncope   Dizziness that occurs when people stand for too long in the heat or when they stop suddenly after a race or stand suddenly from a lying position; results from blood pooling in the lower extremities.

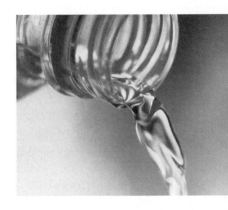
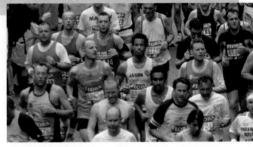

Symptoms of Dehydration during Heavy Exercise:
- Decreased exercise performance
- Increased level in perceived exertion
- Dark yellow or brown urine color
- Increased heart rate at a given exercise intensity
- Decreased appetite
- Decreased ability to concentrate
- Decreased urine output
- Fatigue and weakness
- Headache and dizziness

FIGURE 10.9 Symptoms of dehydration during heavy exercise.

when people stop suddenly after a race or stand suddenly from a lying position.

- **Heat cramps** are muscle spasms that can occur during exercise or several hours after strenuous exercise or manual labor. They are most commonly felt in the legs, arms, or abdomen after a person cools down. They occur during times when sweat losses and fluid intakes are high, urine volume is low, and sodium intake is inadequate to replace losses.

- **Heat exhaustion** and **heatstroke** occur on a continuum, with unchecked heat exhaustion leading to heatstroke. Early signs of heat exhaustion include excessive sweating, cold and clammy skin, rapid but weak pulse, weakness, nausea, dizziness, headache, and difficulty concentrating. As this condition progresses, consciousness becomes impaired. Signs that a person is progressing to heatstroke are hot, dry skin, rapid and strong pulse, vomiting, diarrhea, a body temperature greater than or equal to 104°F, hallucinations, and coma. Prompt medical care is essential to save the person's life.

Guidelines for Proper Fluid Replacement

If we rely only on our feelings of thirst, we will not consume enough fluid to replace the amount lost during exercise. Instead, fluid replacement recommendations are based on maintaining body weight. Athletes who are training and competing in hot environments should weigh themselves on the same scale before and after the training session or event and should regain the weight lost during the event over the subsequent 24-hour period. They should avoid losing more than 2% to 3% of body weight during exercise. Performance can be impaired with fluid losses as small as 1% of body weight (e.g., as little as 1.5 lb for a 150-lb person).

Table 10.6 provides guidelines for proper fluid replacement. For activities lasting less than 1 hour, plain water is generally adequate to replace fluid losses. However, for training and competition lasting longer than 1 hour in any weather, sports beverages containing carbohydrate and electrolytes are recommended. These beverages are also recommended for people who will not drink enough water because they don't like the taste. If drinking these beverages will promote adequate hydration, they are appropriate to use. For more specific information about sports beverages, refer to Chapter 8.

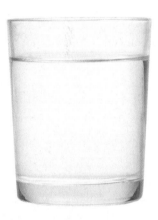

Water is essential for maintaining fluid balance and preventing dehydration.

heat cramps Muscle spasms that occur several hours after strenuous exercise; most often occur when sweat losses and fluid intakes are high, urine volume is low, and sodium intake is inadequate.

heat exhaustion A heat illness that is characterized by excessive sweating, weakness, nausea, dizziness, headache, and difficulty concentrating. Unchecked heat exhaustion can lead to heatstroke.

heat stroke A potentially fatal heat illness that is characterized by hot, dry skin, rapid heart rate, vomiting, diarrhea, body temperature greater than or equal to 104°F, hallucinations, and coma.

TABLE 10.6   Guidelines for Fluid Replacement

Activity Level	Environment	Fluid Requirements (liters per day)
Sedentary	Cool	2–3
Active	Cool	3–6
Sedentary	Warm	3–5
Active	Warm	5–10

Before Exercise or Competition:

- Drink adequate fluids during 24 hours before event; should be able to maintain body weight
- Slowly drink about 0.17 to 0.24 fl. oz per kg body weight of water or a sports drink at least 4 hours prior to exercise or event to allow time for excretion of excess fluid prior to event
- Slowly drink another 0.10 to 0.17 fl. oz per kg body weight about 2 hours before the event
- Consuming beverages with sodium and/or small amounts of salted snacks at a meal will help stimulate thirst and retain fluids consumed

During Exercise or Competition:

- Drink early and regularly throughout event to sufficiently replace all water lost through sweating
- Amount and rate of fluid replacement depends on individual sweating rate, exercise duration, weather conditions, and opportunities to drink
- Fluids should be cooler than the environmental temperature and flavored to enhance taste and promote fluid replacement

During Exercise or Competition That Lasts More Than 1 Hour:

- Fluid replacement beverage should contain 5%–10% carbohydrate to maintain blood glucose levels; sodium and other electrolytes should be included in the beverage in amounts of 0.5–0.7 grams of sodium per liter of water to replace the sodium lost by sweating

Following Exercise or Competition:

- Consume about 3 cups of fluid for each pound of body weight lost
- Fluids after exercise should contain water to restore hydration status, carbohydrates to replenish glycogen stores, and electrolytes (for example, sodium and potassium) to speed rehydration
- Consume enough fluid to permit regular urination and to ensure the urine color is very light or light yellow in color; drinking about 125%–150% of fluid loss is usually sufficient to ensure complete rehydration

In General:

- Products that contain fructose should be limited, as these may cause gastrointestinal distress
- Caffeine and alcohol should be avoided, as these products increase urine output and reduce fluid retention
- Carbonated beverages should be avoided, as they reduce the desire for fluid intake due to stomach fullness

Source: Adapted from R. Murray. 1997. Drink more! Advice from a world class expert. *ACSM's Health and Fitness Journal* 1:19–23; American College of Sports Medicine. 2007. Position Stand, Exercise and fluid replacement. *Med. Sci. Sports Exerc.* 39(2):377–390; and Casa, D. J., L. E. Armstrong, S. K. Hillman, S. J. Montain, R. V. Reiff, B. S. E. Rich, W. O. Roberts, and J. A. Stone. 2000. National Athletic Trainers' Association position statement: Fluid replacement for athletes. *J. Athletic Training* 35: 212–224.

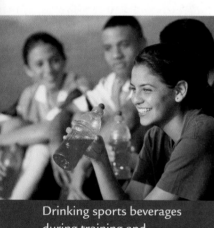

Drinking sports beverages during training and competition lasting more than 1 hour replaces fluid, carbohydrates, and electrolytes.

Inadequate Intakes of Some Vitamins and Minerals Can Diminish Health and Performance

If you're training vigorously for athletic events, your requirements for certain vitamins and minerals may be altered. These include the B-complex vitamins, calcium, and iron.

B Vitamins

The B-complex vitamins are directly involved in energy metabolism. There is reliable evidence that the requirements of active people for thiamin, riboflavin, and vitamin B_6 may be slightly higher than the current RDA.[14] However, these increased needs are easily met by consuming adequate energy and plentiful fiber-rich carbohydrates. Vegan athletes may be at risk for inadequate intake of vitamin B_{12}; food sources enriched with this nutrient include most soy and cereal products.

Calcium

Calcium supports proper muscle contraction and ensures bone health. Calcium intakes are inadequate for many men and women in the United States. Although vigorous training does not appear to increase the body's need for calcium, we do need to consume enough calcium to support bone health. If we do not, stress fractures and severe loss of bone density can result. For athletes who do not consume dairy products or calcium-fortified foods, supplementation may be needed to meet recommendations.

Iron

Iron is a part of the hemoglobin molecule and is critical for the transport of oxygen in the blood to the cells and working muscles. Iron also is involved in energy production. Research has shown that active individuals lose more iron in the sweat, feces, and urine than sedentary people and that endurance runners lose iron when their red blood cells break down in their feet because of the impact of running.[18] Thus, many athletes are at higher risk of iron deficiency. Depending on its severity, poor iron status can impair athletic performance and our ability to maintain regular physical activity.

Females of reproductive age lose iron because of menstrual blood losses and tend to eat less iron in their diet. Thus, physically active young women are at particularly high risk of suffering from iron deficiency.[19,20] Because of this, it is suggested that dietary iron intakes and blood tests of iron stores be routinely done for active females.[14] Some female athletes, such as those who are also vegans, may not be able to meet their iron needs through their diet, and supplementation may be necessary. Iron supplementation should be done with a physician's approval and supervision.

Sports anemia is a transient decrease in iron stores that occurs at the start of an exercise program for some people and is also seen in athletes who increase their training intensity. Exercise training increases the amount of water in our blood (called *plasma volume*); however, the amount of hemoglobin does not increase until later into the training period. Thus, early in training, the iron *content* in the blood appears to be low, but in fact only the *ratio* of iron is depressed because of the increased plasma volume. Sports anemia, because it is not true iron-deficiency anemia, does not affect performance.

> RECAP *Regular exercise increases our fluid needs. Adequate fluid cools the body core and prevents dehydration and heat illnesses, including heat syncope, heat cramps, heat exhaustion, and heatstroke. Active people may need more thiamin, riboflavin, and vitamin B_6 than inactive people. Exercise itself does not increase calcium needs, but many active people do not consume enough calcium. Iron deficiency is a concern for some female athletes and vegetarian athletes.*

NUTRI-CASE THEO

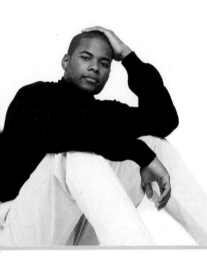

"Ever since I learned about carbs in my nutrition class, I've been watching my carb intake. Lately, I've been getting close to 500 grams of carbs a day. But now I'm beginning to wonder, am I getting enough protein? I'm starting to feel really wiped out, especially after games. We've won four out of the last five games, and I'm giving it everything I've got, but today I was really dragging myself through practice. I'm eating about 150 grams of protein a day, but I think I'm going to try one of those protein powders they sell at my gym. I guess I just feel like, when I'm competing, I need some added insurance."

Theo's weight averages about 170 lb (77 kg) during practice season. Given what you've learned about the role of nutrition in vigorous physical activity, what do you think might be causing Theo to feel "wiped out"? Should Theo try the protein supplement? What other strategies might be helpful for him to consider? (Hint: If you get stuck, check out Table 10.3.)

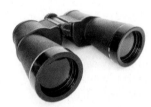

HEALTHWATCH
Are Ergogenic Aids Necessary for Active People?

Many competitive athletes, body builders, and even some recreationally active people continually search for that "something extra" that will enhance their performance, strength, and body composition. Though they might not know it, they're looking for **ergogenic aids,** the technical term for substances used to improve exercise and athletic performance.

Nutritional products such as sports bars and beverages can be classified as ergogenic aids, as these products can help athletes maintain their nutrition and hydration before, during, and after training and performance. Other ergogenic aids include vitamin, mineral, and amino acid supplements and anabolic steroids and other pharmaceuticals. Many of these supplements and pharmaceuticals are expensive and ineffective, and some are actually dangerous. Ergogenic aids, classified as supplements, do not require FDA approval prior to marketing and are not tested for safety, quality, purity, or effectiveness by the FDA.

For the average consumer, it is virtually impossible to track the latest research findings for ergogenic aids. In fact, many have not been adequately studied, and unsubstantiated false claims surrounding them are rampant. So how can you become a more educated consumer?

Be on the lookout for the common deceptive practices used to sell ergogenic aids and nutritional supplements.[21,22] These practices are identified in the accompanying Highlight. For example, in many cases, research done on a product is misrepresented or is conducted by an inexperienced or biased investigator. Some companies claim that research is being conducted but state that the findings cannot be shared with the public. This is a warning sign, as there is no need to hide research findings. The use of a celebrity spokesperson is also very common, as celebrity testimonials help to sell products. However, celebrities often do not actually use the product they are being paid to endorse. Finally, it is critical to realize that a patent on a product does not guarantee the effectiveness or safety of that product. Recall from Chapter 1 that

ergogenic aids Substances used to improve exercise and athletic performance.

HIGHLIGHT

Nine Deceptive Practices Used to Market Ergogenic Aids

1. *General misrepresentation of research:*
   - Published research is taken out of context, or findings are applied in an unproven manner.
   - Claims that the product is university-tested may be true, but the investigator may be inexperienced, or the manufacturer may control all aspects of the study.
   - Research may not have been done, but the company falsely claims it has been conducted.

2. *Company claims that research is currently being done:* Although many companies claim they are doing properly controlled research, when asked to provide specific information about this research, many are unable to do so.

3. *Company claims that research is not available for public review:* Consumers have a right to obtain proof about performance claims, and there is no rationale to support hiding research findings.

4. *Testimonials:* Celebrities who endorse a product may only be doing so for the money. Testimonials can be bought, exaggerated, and even faked. If the product does work for one celebrity, its perceived effectiveness may be due to the placebo effect. The **placebo effect** means that even though a product has been proved to have no physiological benefits, a person believes so strongly in the product that his or her performance improves. It is estimated that there is a 40% chance that any substance will enhance mental or physical performance through the placebo effect.

5. *Patents:* These are granted to indicate distinguishable differences among products. Patents do not indicate effectiveness or safety of a product and can be given without any research being done on a product.

6. *Inappropriately referenced research:*
   - References may include poorly designed and inadequately controlled studies.
   - The company may refer to research that was published in another country and is not accessible in the United States or may base claims on unsubstantiated rumors or unconfirmed reports.
   - The company may cite outdated research that has not been validated or fail to quote studies that do not support its claims.

7. *Media approaches:* Advertising modes include infomercials and mass-media marketing videos. Although the Federal Trade Commission (FTC) regulates false claims in advertising, products are generally investigated only if they pose significant danger to the public.

8. *Mail-order fitness evaluations:* Used to attract consumers to their products. Most of these evaluations are not specific enough to be useful to the consumer, and their accuracy is highly questionable.

9. *Anabolic measurements:* Some companies perform in-house tests of hair and blood to give consumers information on protein balance. Often these tests are used inappropriately and only to sell the ergogenic products. The test results may be inaccurate or may indicate nutritional deficiencies that can be remedied with proper nutrition.

Adapted from Lightsey, D. M., and J. R. Attaway. 1992. Nine deceptive tactics used in marketing purported ergogenic aids. *Natl. Strength Cond. Assoc. J.* 14:26–31.

---

patents are granted solely to distinguish differences among products; indeed, they can be granted on a product that has never been scientifically tested for effectiveness or safety.

New ergogenic aids are available virtually every month. It is therefore not possible to discuss every available product in this chapter. However, a brief review of a number of currently popular ergogenic aids is provided.

Anabolic Products Are Promoted as Muscle and Strength Enhancers

Many ergogenic aids are said to be **anabolic,** meaning that they build muscle and increase strength. Most anabolic substances promise to increase testosterone, which is the hormone associated with male sex characteristics that increases muscle size

placebo effect Improved performance based on the belief that a product is beneficial although the product has been proved to have no physiologic benefits.

anabolic Refers to a substance that builds muscle and increases strength.

and strength. Although some anabolic substances are effective, they are generally associated with harmful side effects.

Anabolic Steroids

In 2007–2008, an Olympic track star, a trio of record-breaking baseball players, and a cyclist were just a few of the many athletes whose reputations were forever tarnished by federal allegations that they owed their triumphs—at least in part—to their illegal use of anabolic steroids. As we discussed in Chapter 9, steroids are testosterone-based drugs that are known to be effective in increasing muscle size, strength, power, and speed. However, they cause serious and irreversible side effects, including stunted growth, infertility, liver dysfunction, high blood pressure, increased aggressiveness, feminization in men, and masculinization in women. In fact, one of the most damaging testimonies linking a female cyclist to steroids was that of an endocrinologist who, during a medical examination, observed facial and chest hair that she concluded had grown as a result of the cyclist's use of steroids.[23] These products are illegal in the United States, and their use is banned by all major collegiate and professional sports organizations, in addition to both the U.S. and the International Olympic Committees.

Androstenedione and Dehydroepiandrosterone

Androstenedione ("andro") and dehydroepiandrosterone (DHEA) are precursors of testosterone. Manufacturers of these products claim that taking them will increase muscle mass strength, but no studies support these claims. Because of concerns related to the harmful steroid-like effects of precursors, the FDA in 2004 required the removal of androstenedione from dietary supplements. Studies have also found that androstenedione increases the risk of heart disease in men aged 35 to 65 years.[24]

Gamma-Hydroxybutyric Acid

Gamma-hydroxybutyric acid, or GHB, was once promoted as an alternative to anabolic steroids for building muscle. The production and sale of GHB were never approved in the United States; however, it was illegally produced and sold on the black market. For many users, GHB caused only dizziness, tremors, or vomiting, but others experienced severe side effects, including seizures. Many people were hospitalized and some died.

After GHB was banned, a similar product (gamma-butyrolactone, or GBL) was marketed in its place. This product was also found to be dangerous and was removed from the market by the FDA. Recently, another replacement product called BD, or 1,4-butanediol, was also banned by the FDA because it has caused at least 71 deaths, with 40 more under investigation. BD is an industrial solvent and is listed on ingredient labels as tetramethylene glycol, butylene glycol, or sucol-B. Side effects include wild, aggressive behavior, nausea, incontinence, and sudden loss of consciousness.

Creatine

Creatine is a supplement that has become wildly popular with strength and power athletes. Creatine, or creatine phosphate, is found in meat and fish and stored in our muscles. As described earlier in this chapter, we use creatine phosphate (or CP) to regenerate ATP. By taking creatine supplements, it is theorized that more CP is available to replenish ATP, which will prolong a person's ability to train and perform in short-term, explosive activities such as weight lifting and sprinting. Between 1994 and 2008, more than 700 research articles related to creatine and exercise in humans were published. Creatine does not seem to enhance performance in aerobic-type events but has been shown to enhance sprint performance in swimming, running, and cycling.[15,25–27] In addition, some studies have shown that creatine increases the amount of work performed, and the amount of strength gained, during resistance exercise.[27–29]

In January 2001, the *New York Times* reported that the French government claimed that creatine use could lead to cancer.[30] The news spread quickly across

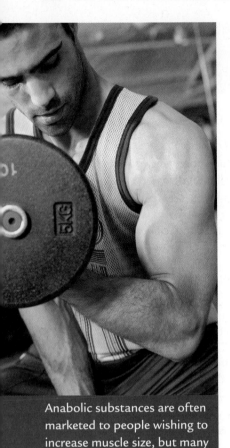

Anabolic substances are often marketed to people wishing to increase muscle size, but many cause harmful side effects.

national and international news organizations and over the Internet. These claims were found to be false, as there are absolutely no studies in humans that suggest an increased risk of cancer with creatine use. In fact, numerous studies show an anti-cancer effect.[31,32] Although side effects such as dehydration, muscle cramps, and gastrointestinal disturbances have been reported with creatine use, we have very little information on how long-term use of creatine affects health. A recent study found that the incidence of muscle cramps, injuries, or other side effects for athletes who had never used creatine was similar to that in those using creatine up to 4 years.[33]

Some Products Are Said to Optimize Fuel Use during Exercise

Certain ergogenic aids are said to increase energy levels and improve athletic performance by optimizing our use of fat, carbohydrate, and protein. The products reviewed here include caffeine, ephedrine, carnitine, chromium, and ribose.

Caffeine

Caffeine is a stimulant that makes us feel more alert and energetic, decreasing feelings of fatigue during exercise. In addition, caffeine has been shown to increase the use of fat as a fuel during endurance exercise, which spares muscle glycogen and improves performance.[34,35] Caffeine is a controlled or restricted drug in the athletic world, and athletes can be banned from Olympic competition if urine levels are too high. However, the amount of caffeine that is banned is quite high, equivalent to about 5 to 10 cups of standard coffee, and most athletes would need to consume caffeine in pill form to reach this level. Side effects of caffeine use include increased blood pressure, increased heart rate, dizziness, insomnia, headache, and gastrointestinal distress.

Ephedrine

Ephedrine, also known as ephedra, Chinese ephedra, or *ma huang,* is a strong stimulant marketed as a weight-loss supplement and energy enhancer. In reality, many products sold as Chinese ephedra (or herbal ephedra) contain ephedrine from the laboratory and other stimulants such as caffeine. The use of ephedra does not appear to enhance athletic performance, but supplements containing both caffeine and ephedra have been shown to prolong the amount of exercise that can be done until exhaustion is reached.[36] Ephedra is known to reduce body weight and body fat in sedentary women, but its impact on weight loss and body fat levels in athletes is unknown. Side effects of ephedra use include headaches, nausea, nervousness, anxiety, irregular heart rate, and high blood pressure, and at least 17 deaths have been attributed to its use.[37] As discussed in Chapter 9, it is currently illegal to sell ephedra-containing supplements in the United States.

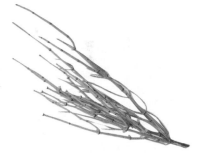

Ephedrine is made from the herb *Ephedra sinica* (Chinese ephedra).

Carnitine

Carnitine is a compound made from amino acids that is found in the membrane of mitochondria. As you learned in Chapter 2, mitochondria are tiny energy-generators inside our cells. Carnitine helps shuttle fatty acids into the mitochondria so they can be used for energy. It has been theorized that exercise depletes our cells of carnitine and that supplementation should increase the amount of carnitine in our mitochondrial membranes and improve our use of fat as fuel. Thus, carnitine is marketed not only as a performance-enhancing substance but also as a "fat burner." Research studies of carnitine supplementation do not support these claims, as neither the transport of fatty acids nor their oxidation appears to be enhanced with supplementation.[38,39] Use of carnitine supplements has not been associated with improved performance nor with detrimental side effects.

Chromium

Chromium is a trace mineral that enhances the action of insulin. It is found in whole-grain foods, cheese, nuts, mushrooms, and asparagus. It is theorized that

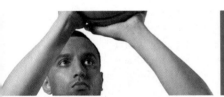

Where I'm at now...

Now that you've read this chapter, do you feel that increased physical activity is an important goal for you?

Yes or **No**

If **Yes**, jot down here a specific, measurable goal that is personalized to you and that you are confident you can begin to meet starting today:

many people are chromium deficient, that supplementation will enhance nutrient uptake into muscle cells, and that this increased uptake will promote muscle growth and strength. Like carnitine, chromium is marketed as a "fat burner," as it is speculated that its effect on insulin stimulates the brain to decrease food intake.[37] Chromium supplements are available as chromium picolinate and chromium nicotinate. Early studies of chromium supplementation showed promise, but more recent, better-designed studies do not support any benefit of chromium supplementation on muscle mass, muscle strength, body fat, or exercise performance.[40]

Ribose

Ribose is a five-carbon sugar that is critical to the production of ATP. Ribose supplementation is claimed to improve athletic performance by increasing work output and by promoting a faster recovery time from vigorous training. Although ribose has been shown to improve exercise tolerance in patients with heart disease,[41] several studies have reported that ribose supplementation has no impact on athletic performance.[42–44]

From this review of ergogenic aids, you can see that most of these products are not effective in enhancing athletic performance or in optimizing muscle strength or body composition. It is important to be a savvy consumer when examining these products to avoid wasting your money or putting your health at risk by using them.

> RECAP *Ergogenic aids are substances used to improve exercise and athletic performance. Many are ineffective, and some are dangerous. Anabolic steroids and GHB have been banned in the United States because of serious health consequences. Neither androstenedione nor DHEA has been shown to increase muscle mass or strength, and androstenedione has been linked to heart disease. Creatine supplements can enhance sprint performance and strength gained in resistance exercise. Caffeine increases the use of fat during exercise. Ephedrine is a stimulant that has been banned from the United States due to its potentially fatal side effects. Neither carnitine nor chromium supplements burn fat or improve athletic performance. Ribose supplementation is claimed to enhance work output and recovery from training, but no studies support these claims.*

REVIEW QUESTIONS

Circle the correct choice.

1. For achieving and maintaining physical fitness, the intensity range during exercise typically recommended is:
   a. 25% to 50% of your estimated maximal heart rate.
   b. 35% to 75% of your estimated maximal heart rate.
   c. 64% to 90% of your estimated maximal heart rate.
   d. 75% to 95% of your estimated maximal heart rate.

2. The amount of ATP stored in a muscle cell can keep a muscle active for about:
   a. 1 to 3 seconds.
   b. 10 to 30 seconds.
   c. 1 to 3 minutes.
   d. 1 to 3 hours.

3. To support a long afternoon of gardening, the body predominantly uses which nutrient for energy?
   a. carbohydrate
   b. fat
   c. amino acids
   d. lactic acid

4. Creatine:
   a. seems to enhance performance in aerobic-type events.
   b. appears to increase an individual's risk for bladder cancer.
   c. seems to increase strength gained in resistance exercise.
   d. is stored in the liver.

5. Athletes participating in an intense athletic competition lasting more than 1 hour should drink:
   a. beverages containing caffeine.
   b. beverages containing carbohydrates and electrolytes.
   c. plain, room-temperature water.
   d. nothing.

6. True or False? A sound fitness program overloads the body.

7. True or False? A dietary fat intake of 10% to 15% is generally recommended for active people.

8. True or False? Carbohydrate loading involves altering duration and intensity of exercise and intake of carbohydrate such that the storage of fat is minimized.

9. True or False? Sports anemia is a chronic decrease in iron stores that occurs in some athletes who have been training intensely for several months to years.

10. True or False? FIT stands for frequency, intensity, and time.

WEB LINKS

www.americanheart.org
American Heart Association

The Healthy Lifestyle section of this site has sections on health tools, exercise and fitness, healthy diet, managing your lifestyle, and more.

www.acsm.org
American College of Sports Medicine

Look under Health and Fitness Information for guidelines on healthy aerobic activity, calculating your exercise heart rate range, and the ACSM's Fit Society Page newsletter.

www.webmd.com
WebMD Health

Visit this site to learn about a variety of lifestyle topics, including fitness and exercise.

www.hhs.gov
U.S. Department of Health and Human Services

Review this site for multiple statistics on health, exercise, and weight, as well as information on supplements, wellness, and more.

http://win.niddk.nih.gov/publications/physical.htm
Physical Activity and Weight Control

Find out more about healthy fitness programs.

http://dietary-supplements.info.nih.gov
NIH Office of Dietary Supplements

Look on this National Institutes of Health site to learn more about the health effects of specific nutritional supplements.

http://fnic.nal.usda.gov
Food and Nutrition Information Center

Visit this site for links to detailed information about ergogenic aids and sports nutrition.

http://nutrition.arizona.edu/new
Nutrition Exercise Wellness

Check this University of Arizona site for information for athletes on nutrition, fluid intake, and ergogenic aids.

TEST YOURSELF ANSWERS

1. **True.** Up to 55% of Americans do not do enough physical activity, and another 26% report doing no physical activity at all, not even on the job.

2. **False.** Walking, vigorous housework, heavy gardening, and other forms of moderate physical activity do yield significant health benefits if you engage in these activities for approximately 30 minutes a day most days of the week.

3. **False.** Our muscles are not stimulated to grow when we eat extra protein, whether as food or supplements. Weight-bearing exercise appropriately stresses the body and produces increased muscle mass and strength.

4. **True.** Most ergogenic aids are ineffective, or do not produce the results that are advertised. Some, such as anabolic steroids and ephedra, are banned because of their serious side effects.

5. **False.** Carbohydrate loading may help improve performance for endurance events such as marathons and triathlons, but does not improve performance in nonendurance types of athletic events such as a 1,500-meter run.

REFERENCES

1. U.S. Department of Health and Human Services. 1996. *Physical Activity and Health: A Report of the Surgeon General.* Atlanta, GA: U.S. Department of Health and Human Services, Centers for Disease Control and Prevention, National Centers for Chronic Disease Prevention and Health Promotion.
2. Caspersen, C. J., K. E. Powell, and G. M. Christensen. 1985. Physical activity, exercise, and physical fitness: Definitions and distinctions for heath-related research. *Public Health Rep.* 100:126–131.
3. Heyward, V. H. 1998. *Advanced Fitness Assessment and Exercise Prescription.* 3rd ed. Champaign, IL: Human Kinetics Publishers.
4. Centers for Disease Control and Prevention (CDC). 2003. Prevalence of physical activity, including lifestyle activities among adults—United States, 2000–2001. *MMWR* 52(32):764–769.
5. U.S. Department of Health and Human Services. 2000. *Healthy People 2010* (conference edition, in two volumes). Washington, DC: U.S. Department of Health and Human Services.

6. Centers for Disease Control and Prevention. 2005. Physical Activity for Everyone: Making Physical Activity Part of Your Life: Tips for Being More Active. Available at http://www.cdc.gov/nccdphp/dnpa/physical/life/tips.htm.

7. United States Department of Health and Human Services. 2005. Get Active: Goals. Available at http://www.smallstep.gov/step_3/step_3_goals.html.

8. Brooks, G. A., T. D. Fahey, T. P. White, K. M. Baldwin. 2000. *Exercise Physiology. Human Bioenergetics and Its Applications.* Mountain View, CA: Mayfield Publishing Company.

9. Brooks, G. A. 2000. Intra- and extra-cellular lactate shuttles. *Med. Sci. Sports Exerc.* 32:790–799.

10. Gladden, L. B. 2000. Muscle as a consumer of lactate. *Med. Sci. Sports Exerc.* 32:764–771.

11. Tarnopolsky, M. 2000. Protein and amino acid needs for training and bulking up. In: Burke, L., and V. Deakin, eds. *Clinical Sports Nutrition.* Sydney, Australia: McGraw-Hill.

12. American College of Sports Medicine, American Dietetic Association, and Dietitians of Canada. 2000. Nutrition and athletic performance. Joint position statement. *Med. Sci. Sports Exerc.* 32:2130–2145.

13. Burke, L. 2000. Nutrition for recovery after competition and training. In: Burke, L., and V. Deakin, eds. *Clinical Sports Nutrition.* 2nd ed. Sydney, Australia: McGraw-Hill, pp. 396–427.

14. Manore, M., and J. Thompson. 2000. *Sports Nutrition for Health and Performance.* Champaign, IL: Human Kinetics Publishers.

15. Tarnopolsky, M. A., and D. P. MacLennan. 2000. Creatine monohydrate supplementation enhances high-intensity exercise performance in males and females. *Int. J. Sport Nutr. Exerc. Metab.* 10:452–463.

16. Manore, M. M., S. I. Barr, and G. E. Butterfield. 2000. Nutrition and athletic performance. Joint Position Statement of the American College of Sports Medicine, American Dietetic Association, and Dietitians of Canada. *Med. Sci. Sports Exerc.* 32(12):2130–2145.

17. Sears, B. 1995. *The Zone. A Dietary Road Map.* New York: HarperCollins.

18. Weaver, C. M., and S. Rajaram. 1992. Exercise and iron status. *J. Nutr.* 122:782–787.

19. Haymes, E. M. 1998. Trace minerals and exercise. In: Wolinsky, I., ed. *Nutrition and Exercise and Sport.* Boca Raton, FL: CRC Press, pp. 1997–2218.

20. Haymes, E. M., and P. M. Clarkson. 1998. Minerals and trace minerals. In: Berning J. R., and S. N. Steen, eds. *Nutrition and Sport and Exercise.* Gaithersburg, MD: Aspen Publishers, pp. 77–107.

21. Lightsey, D. M., and J. R. Attaway. 1992. Deceptive tactics used in marketing purported ergogenic aids. *Natl. Strength Cond. Assoc. J.* 14:26–31.

22. Federal Trade Commission (FTC). 2001. FTC Fact for Consumers. "Miracle" Health Claims: Add a Dose of Skepticism. Available at www.ftc.gov/bcp/conline/pubs/health/frdheal.pdf.

23. Schmidt, M. S. Sports briefing/doping: Cyclist linked to steroids. *The New York Times,* March 26, 2008.

24. Broeder, C. E., J. Quindry, K. Brittingham, et al. 2000. The Andro Project: Physiological and hormonal influences of androstenedione supplementation in men 35 to 65 years old participating in a high-intensity resistance training program. *Arch. Intern. Med.* 160:3093–3104.

25. Balsom, P. D., K. Söderlund, B. Sjödin, and B. Ekblom. 1995. Skeletal muscle metabolism during short duration high-intensity exercise: Influence of creatine supplementation. *Acta Physiol. Scand.* 1154:303–310.

26. Grindstaff, P. D., R. Kreider, R. Bishop, M. Wilson, L. Wood, C. Alexander, and A. Almada. 1997. Effects of creatine supplementation on repetitive sprint performance and body composition in competitive swimmers. *Int. J. Sport Nutr.* 7:330–346.

27. Kreider, R. B., M. Ferreira, M. Wilson, et al. 1998. Effects of creatine supplementation on body composition, strength, and sprint performance. *Med. Sci. Sports Exerc.* 30:73–82.

28. Almada, A., R. Kreider, M. Ferreira, et al. 1997. Effects of calcium β-HMB supplementation with or without creatine during training on strength and sprint capacity. *FASEB J.* 11:A374.

29. Volek, J. S., N. D. Duncan, S. A. Mazzetti, et al. 1999. Performance and muscle fiber adaptations to creatine supplementation and heavy resistance training. *Med. Sci. Sports Exerc.* 31:1147–1156.

30. Reuters. 2001. Creatine use could lead to cancer, French government reports. *The New York Times,* January 25.

31. Jeong, K. S., S. J. Park, C. S. Lee, et al. 2000. Effects of cyclocreatine in rat hepatocarcinogenesis model. *Anticancer Res.* 20(3A):1627–1633.

32. Ara, G., L. M. Gravelin, R. Kaddurah-Daouk, and B. A. Teicher. 1998. Antitumor activity of creatine analogs produced by alterations in pancreatic hormones and glucose metabolism. *In Vivo* 12:223–231.

33. Schilling, B. K., M. H. Stone, A. Utter, J. T. Kearney, M. Johnson, R. Coglianese, L. Smith, H. S. O'Bryant, A. C. Fry, M. Starks, R. Keith, and M. E. Stone. 2001. Creatine supplementation and health variables: A retrospective study. *Med. Sci. Sports Exerc.* 33:183–188.

34. Anderson, M. E., C. R. Bruce, S. F. Fraser, N. K. Stepto, R. Klein, W. G. Hopkins, and J. A. Hawley. 2000. Improved 2000-meter rowing performance in competitive oarswomen after caffeine ingestion. *Int. J. Sport Nutr. Exerc. Metab.* 10:464–475.

35. Spriet, L. L., and R. A. Howlett. 2000. Caffeine. In: Maughan, R. J., ed. *Nutrition in Sport.* Oxford: Blackwell Science, pp. 379–392.

36. Bucci, L. 2000. Selected herbals and human exercise performance. *Am. J. Clin. Nutr.* 72:624S–636S.

37. Williams, M. H. 1998. *The Ergogenics Edge.* Champaign, IL: Human Kinetics Publishers.

38. Hawley, J. A. 2002. Effect of increased fat availability on metabolism and exercise capacity. *Med. Sci. Sports Exerc.* 34(9):1485–1491.

39. Heinonen, O. J. 1996. Carnitine and physical exercise. *Sports Med.* 22:109–132.

40. Vincent, J. B. 2003. The potential value and toxicity of chromium picolinate as a nutritional supplement, weight loss agent and muscle development agent. *Sports Med.* 33(3):213–230.

41. Pliml, W., T. von Arnim, A. Stablein, H. Hofmann, H. G. Zimmer, and E. Erdmann. 1992. Effects of ribose on exercise-induced ischaemia in stable coronary artery disease. *Lancet* 340(8818):507–510.

42. Earnest, C. P., G. M. Morss, F. Wyatt, A. N. Jordan, S. Colson, T. S. Church, Y. Fitzgerald, L. Autrey, R. Jurca, and A. Lucia. 2004. Effects of a commercial herbal-based formula on exercise performance in cyclists. *Med. Sci. Sports Exerc.* 36(3):504–509.

43. Hellsten, Y., L. Skadhauge, and J. Bangsbo. 2004. Effect of ribose supplementation on resynthesis of adenine nucleotides after intense intermittent training in humans. *Am. J. Physiol. Regul. Integr. Comp. Physiol.* 286:R182–R188.

44. Kreider, R. B., C. Melton, M. Greenwood, C. Rasmussen, J. Lundberg, C. Earnest, and A. Almada. 2003. Effects of oral D-ribose supplementation on anaerobic capacity and selected metabolic markers in healthy males. *Int. J. Sport Nutr. Exerc. Metab.* 13(1):76–86.

11 Nutrition Throughout the Life Cycle

TEST YOURSELF

Are these statements true or false? Circle your guess.

1 Despite popular belief, very few pregnant women actually experience morning sickness, food cravings, or food aversions. **TRUE or FALSE**

2 Most infants begin to require solid foods by about 3 months (12 weeks) of age. **TRUE or FALSE**

3 After their first birthday, children should be given nonfat dairy products to reduce their risk for obesity. **TRUE or FALSE**

4 It is now believed that diet has virtually no role in the development of adolescent acne. **TRUE or FALSE**

5 More than 1 in 10 American households with children and 1 in 20 with seniors experience food insecurity. **TRUE or FALSE**

Test Yourself answers can be found at the end of the chapter.

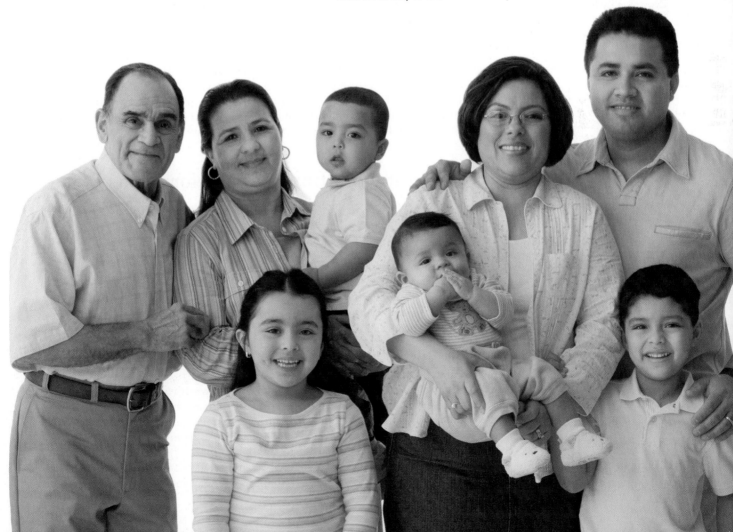

ON SUNDAY AFTERNOONS, the Sophat family gathers for dinner at the Long Beach apartment of their 88-year-old matriarch, Leng. Only 5 feet tall, Leng is as thin as a rail, as are her 70-year-old daughter and 67-year-old son. But when her granddaughters, who are cooking the family meal, send everyone to the table, a change becomes evident. Almost all of Leng's grandchildren and their spouses are overweight, as are most of her great-grandchildren. Even her "darling" 2-year-old great-great-granddaughter, Jewel, is chubby. Leng worries about everyone's weight. Back home in Cambodia, overweight was rare and a sign of health, but here in America, it seems to bring illness. One of her grandsons had a heart attack last year. During her pregnancy with Jewel, Leng's great-granddaughter developed gestational diabetes, and several other family members have been diagnosed with type 2 diabetes. Leng's family isn't alone in their weight problems: more than 17% of American children and adolescents (age 6 to 19 years) are overweight, along with more than 66% of American adults.[1] And type 2 diabetes, which afflicts about 10% of Asian Americans, occurs in about 6% of all Americans.[2]

Why have rates of obesity and its associated chronic diseases skyrocketed in the past 10 years, and what can be done to promote weight management across the lifespan? How do our nutrient needs change as we grow and age, and what other nutrition-related concerns develop in each life stage? This chapter will help you answer these questions.

Starting Out Right: Healthful Nutrition in Pregnancy

At no stage of life is nutrition more crucial than during fetal development and infancy. From conception through the end of the first year of life, adequate nutrition is essential for tissue formation, neurological development, and bone growth, modeling, and remodeling. Our ability to reach peak physical and intellectual potential as adults is in part determined by the nutrition we receive during fetal development and the first year of life.

Why Is Nutrition Important Before Conception?

conception (also called *fertilization*) The uniting of an ovum (egg) and sperm to create a fertilized egg.

teratogen Any substance that can cause a birth defect.

Several factors make nutrition important even before **conception**—the point at which a woman's ovum (egg) is fertilized with a man's sperm. First, some deficiency-related problems develop extremely early in the pregnancy, typically before the mother even realizes she is pregnant. An adequate and varied preconception diet reduces the risk of such problems, providing "insurance" during those first few weeks of life. For example, inadequate levels of folate in the first 28 days after conception may cause the spinal cord tissues to fail to close, resulting in problems ranging from paralysis to absence of brain tissue. For this reason, all women capable of becoming pregnant are encouraged to consume 400 µg of folic acid from fortified foods such as cereals or supplements daily, in addition to natural sources of folate from a varied, healthful diet.

Second, adopting a healthful diet and lifestyle prior to conception requires women to avoid alcohol, illegal drugs, and other known **teratogens** (substances that cause birth defects). Women should also consult their healthcare providers about their consumption of caffeine, prescription medications, herbs, and supplements. Smoking increases the risk for a low-birth-weight baby and infant mortality, so women should quit smoking prior to getting pregnant.[3]

Third, a healthful diet and regular physical activity can help women achieve and maintain an optimal body weight prior to pregnancy. Women with a healthy prepreg-

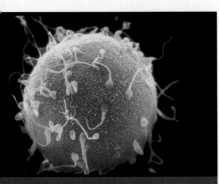

During conception, a single sperm will succeed in fertilizing the woman's egg.

nancy weight have the best chance of an uncomplicated pregnancy and delivery, with low risk of negative outcomes such as prolonged labor and cesarean section.[4] Women who are underweight or overweight prior to conception are at greater risk for pregnancy-related complications.

Finally, maintaining a balanced and nourishing diet before conception reduces a woman's risk of developing a nutrition-related disorder during her pregnancy. These disorders, which we discuss later in the chapter, include a form of diabetes and a disorder in which the mother's blood pressure becomes dangerously high. Although some problems, such as genetic defects, are beyond the woman's control, maintaining a healthful lifestyle and eating a nourishing diet prior to conception are two things a woman can do to help her fetus develop into a healthy baby.

The man's nutrition prior to pregnancy is important as well, because malnutrition contributes to abnormalities in sperm.[5] Both sperm number and motility (ability to move) are reduced by alcohol consumption, as well as the use of certain prescription and illegal drugs. Finally, infections accompanied by a high fever can destroy sperm; so, to the extent that adequate nutrition keeps the immune system strong, it also promotes a man's fertility.

Why Is Nutrition Important During Pregnancy?

A balanced, nourishing diet throughout pregnancy provides the nutrients needed to support fetal growth and development without depriving the mother of nutrients she needs to maintain her own health. It also minimizes the risks of excessive weight gain.

In clinical practice, the calculation of weeks in a pregnancy begins with the date of the first day of a woman's last menstrual period. A full-term pregnancy lasts 38 to 42 weeks and is divided into three **trimesters,** with each trimester lasting about 13 to 14 weeks.

During the First Trimester, the Embryo Is Extremely Vulnerable

The first trimester (approximately weeks 1 to 13) begins when the ovum and sperm unite to form a single, fertilized cell. Over the next few weeks, layers of cells develop into the distinct tissues of the developing **embryo.**

By about week 8, the embryo's tissues and organs have differentiated dramatically. A primitive skeleton and muscles have begun to develop. A primitive heart has begun to beat, and distinct digestive organs (stomach, liver, etc.) are forming. During the next few weeks, the embryo continues to grow and change dramatically into a recognizable human **fetus.**

Given such remarkable development, it isn't surprising that the embryo is most vulnerable to teratogens and malnutrition during the first trimester (FIGURE 11.1). Not only alcohol and illegal drugs but also prescription and over-the-counter medications, megadoses of supplements such as vitamin A, certain herbs, viruses, cigarette smoking, and radiation can interfere with embryonic development and cause birth defects.[5] In addition, deficiencies of nutrients such as folate can result in serious birth defects. In some cases, the damage is so severe that the pregnancy is naturally terminated in a **spontaneous abortion** (*miscarriage*). Not surprisingly, miscarriages occur most often in the first trimester.

It is also during the first trimester that the **placenta** forms, the organ that provides nutrients to the fetus and removes wastes. The placenta is connected to the fetus via the **umbilical cord,** an extension of fetal blood vessels emerging from the fetus's navel (see the top photo in Figure 11.1).

The Second and Third Trimesters Are Characterized by Remarkable Growth

During the second trimester (approximately weeks 14 to 27 of pregnancy), the fetus grows to approximately 10 inches and gains about 2 lb. Bones become harder and organ systems continue to develop and mature.

trimester Any one of three stages of pregnancy, each lasting 13 to 14 weeks.

embryo Human growth and developmental stage lasting from the third week to the end of the eighth week after fertilization.

fetus Human growth and developmental stage lasting from the beginning of the ninth week after conception to birth.

spontaneous abortion (also called *miscarriage*) Natural termination of a pregnancy and expulsion of fetus and pregnancy tissues because of a genetic, developmental, or physiological abnormality that is so severe that the pregnancy cannot be maintained.

placenta A pregnancy-specific organ formed from both maternal and embryonic tissues. It is responsible for oxygen, nutrient, and waste exchange between mother and fetus.

umbilical cord The cord containing arteries and veins that connects the baby (from the navel) to the mother via the placenta.

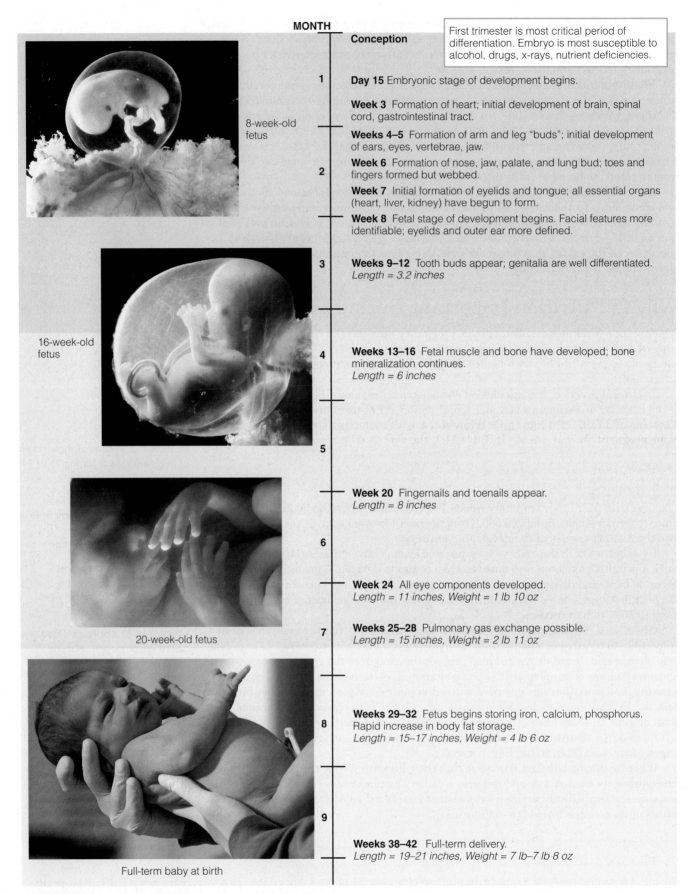

MONTH

Conception

First trimester is most critical period of differentiation. Embryo is most susceptible to alcohol, drugs, x-rays, nutrient deficiencies.

8-week-old fetus

1 — **Day 15** Embryonic stage of development begins.

Week 3 Formation of heart; initial development of brain, spinal cord, gastrointestinal tract.

Weeks 4–5 Formation of arm and leg "buds"; initial development of ears, eyes, vertebrae, jaw.

2 — **Week 6** Formation of nose, jaw, palate, and lung bud; toes and fingers formed but webbed.

Week 7 Initial formation of eyelids and tongue; all essential organs (heart, liver, kidney) have begun to form.

Week 8 Fetal stage of development begins. Facial features more identifiable; eyelids and outer ear more defined.

3 — **Weeks 9–12** Tooth buds appear; genitalia are well differentiated. *Length = 3.2 inches*

16-week-old fetus

4 — **Weeks 13–16** Fetal muscle and bone have developed; bone mineralization continues. *Length = 6 inches*

5 —

Week 20 Fingernails and toenails appear. *Length = 8 inches*

6 —

Week 24 All eye components developed. *Length = 11 inches, Weight = 1 lb 10 oz*

7 — **Weeks 25–28** Pulmonary gas exchange possible. *Length = 15 inches, Weight = 2 lb 11 oz*

20-week-old fetus

8 — **Weeks 29–32** Fetus begins storing iron, calcium, phosphorus. Rapid increase in body fat storage. *Length = 15–17 inches, Weight = 4 lb 6 oz*

9 —

Weeks 38–42 Full-term delivery. *Length = 19–21 inches, Weight = 7 lb–7 lb 8 oz*

Full-term baby at birth

FIGURE 11.1 A timeline of embryonic and fetal development.

During the third trimester (approximately weeks 28 to birth), the fetus gains nearly half its body length and three-quarters of its body weight! At the time of birth, an average baby will be approximately 18 to 22 inches long and about 7.5 lb. Brain growth (which continues to be rapid for the first 2 years of life) is also quite remarkable.

Impact of Nutrition on Newborn Maturity and Birth Weight

Generally, a birth weight of at least 5.5 lb is considered a marker of a successful pregnancy. An undernourished mother is likely to give birth to a **low-birth-weight** infant.[6] Any infant weighing less than 5.5 lb at birth is considered to be of low birth weight and is at increased risk of infection, learning disabilities, impaired physical development, and death in the first year of life. Although nutrition is not the only factor contributing to maturity and birth weight, its role cannot be overstated.

> RECAP *A full-term pregnancy lasts from 38 to 42 weeks and is traditionally divided into trimesters lasting 13 to 14 weeks. During the first trimester, cells differentiate and divide rapidly to form the various tissues of the human body. The fetus is especially susceptible to nutrient deficiencies, toxicities, and teratogens during this time. The second and third trimesters are characterized by profound growth and maturation. An adequate, nourishing diet increases the chance that a baby will be born after 37 weeks and weighing at least 5.5 lb.*

How Much Weight Should a Pregnant Woman Gain?

Recommendations for weight gain vary according to a woman's weight *before* she became pregnant. As you can see in Table 11.1, the average recommended weight gain for women of normal prepregnancy weight is 25 to 35 lb; underweight women should gain a little more than this amount, and overweight and obese women should gain somewhat less.[6] Adolescents, who may not have completed their own growth, are advised to gain at the upper end of these ranges, as they are at high risk for delivering low-birth-weight and premature infants. Small women, 5'2" or shorter, should aim for a total weight gain at the lower end of these ranges. Women who are pregnant with twins are advised to gain 35 to 45 lb.

Women who gain too little weight during their pregnancy increase their risk of having a preterm or low-birth-weight baby. They also risk dangerously depleting their own nutrient reserves. Gaining *too much* weight during pregnancy increases the risk that the fetus will be large, and large babies have an increased risk of trauma during vaginal delivery and of cesarean birth. Also, a high birth weight has been linked to increased risk of adolescent obesity.[7] In addition, the more weight gained during pregnancy, the more difficult it is for the mother to return to her prepregnancy weight and the more likely it is that her weight gain will be permanent.

In addition to the amount of weight, the *pattern* of weight gain is important. During the first trimester, a woman of normal weight should gain no more than a

TABLE 11.1 Recommended Weight Gain for Women During Pregnancy

Prepregnancy Weight Status	Body Mass Index (kg/m^2)	Recommended Weight Gain (lb)
Normal	18.5–25.0	25–35
Underweight	< 18.5	28–40
Overweight	25.1–29.9	15–25
Obese	≥ 30.0	No more than 15

low birth weight A weight of less than 5.5 lb at birth.

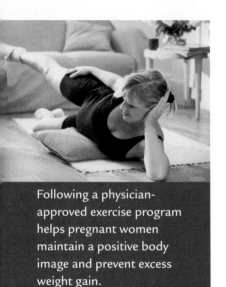

Following a physician-approved exercise program helps pregnant women maintain a positive body image and prevent excess weight gain.

total of 3 to 5 lb. During the second and third trimesters, an average of about 1 lb a week is considered healthful.

In a society obsessed with thinness, it is easy for pregnant women to worry about weight gain. Focusing on the quality of food consumed, rather than the quantity, can help women feel more in control. In addition, following a physician-approved exercise program helps women maintain a positive body image and prevent excessive weight gain. Women should never diet during pregnancy, even if they begin the pregnancy overweight, as this can lead to nutrient deficiencies for both the mother and fetus. Instead, women concerned about their weight should consult their physician or a registered dietitian experienced in working with prenatal populations.

A pregnant woman may also feel less anxious about her weight gain if she understands how that weight is distributed. Of the total weight gained in pregnancy, 10 to 12 lb are accounted for by the fetus itself, the amniotic fluid, and the placenta (FIGURE 11.2). Another 3 to 8 lb represents a natural increase in the volume of the mother's blood and extracellular fluid. A woman can expect to be about 10 to 12 lb lighter immediately after the birth and, within about 2 weeks, another 5 to 8 lb lighter because of fluid loss.

After the first 2 weeks, losing the remainder of pregnancy weight depends on more energy being expended than is taken in. Appropriate physical activity can help women lose those extra pounds. Also, because production of breast milk requires significant energy, breastfeeding helps many new mothers lose the remaining weight.

What Are a Pregnant Woman's Nutrient Needs?

The requirements for nearly all nutrients increase during pregnancy to accommodate the growth and development of the fetus without depriving the mother of the nutrients she needs to maintain her own health. The DRI tables on the last pages of this textbook identify the DRIs for pregnant women in three age groups.

Macronutrient Needs of Pregnant Women

Given what you've just learned about pregnancy weight gain, you've probably figured out that energy requirements increase only modestly during pregnancy. In fact,

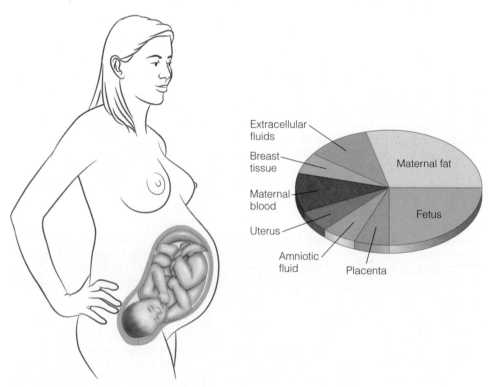

FIGURE 11.2 The weight gained during pregnancy is distributed between the mother's own tissues and the pregnancy-specific tissues.

during the first trimester, a woman should consume approximately the same number of calories daily as during her nonpregnant days. Instead of eating more, she should attempt to maximize the nutrient density of what she eats. For example, drinking low-fat milk or calcium-fortified soy milk is preferable to drinking soft drinks. Low-fat milk and fortified soy milk provide valuable protein, vitamins, and minerals to feed the fetus's rapidly dividing cells, whereas soft drinks provide nutritionally empty calories.

During the last two trimesters of pregnancy, energy needs increase by about 350 to 450 kcal/day. For a woman normally consuming 2,000 kcal/day, an extra 400 kcal represents only a 20% increase in energy intake, a goal that can be met more easily than many pregnant women realize. For example, one cup of low-fat yogurt and two pieces of whole-wheat toast spread with a tablespoon of peanut butter is about 400 kcal. At the same time, some vitamin and mineral needs increase by 50% or more, so again, the key for getting adequate micronutrients while not consuming too many extra calories is choosing nutrient-dense foods.

During pregnancy, protein needs increase to about 1.1 g per day per kilogram body weight over the entire 9-month period. This is an increase of about 25 g of protein per day. Remember that yogurt and toast with peanut butter we just mentioned? This light meal provides the additional 25 g of protein most women need. As an example of total daily protein needs, a pregnant woman weighing approximately 142 lb should consume about 71 g of protein per day.

Pregnant women should aim for a carbohydrate intake of at least 175 g per day.[8] Glucose is the primary metabolic fuel of the developing fetus; thus, pregnant women need to consume healthful sources of carbohydrate throughout the day. All pregnant women should be counseled on the potential hazards of very-low-carbohydrate diets.

The guideline for the percentage of daily calories that comes from fat does not change during pregnancy. Pregnant women should be aware that, because new tissues and cells are being built, adequate consumption of dietary fat is even more important than in the nonpregnant state. In addition, during the third trimester, the fetus stores most of its own body fat, which is a critical source of fuel in the newborn period. Without adequate fat stores, newborns cannot effectively regulate their body temperature.

An omega-3 polyunsaturated fatty acid known as *docosahexaenoic acid (DHA)* has been found to be uniquely critical for both neurologic and eye development. Because the fetal brain grows dramatically during the third trimester, DHA is especially important in the mother's diet at this time. Good sources of DHA are oily fish such as anchovies, mackerel, salmon, and sardines. It is also found in lesser amounts in tuna, chicken, and eggs (some eggs are DHA-enhanced by feeding hens a DHA-rich diet).

Pregnant women who eat fish should be aware of the potential for mercury contamination, as even a limited intake of mercury during pregnancy can impair a fetus's developing nervous system. Large fish such as swordfish, shark, tile fish, and king mackerel have high levels of mercury and should be avoided. The National Healthy Mothers, Healthy Babies Coalition recommends that women who are pregnant or breastfeeding should eat at least 12 oz of most other types of fish, such as salmon, mackerel, sardines, and tuna, per week, as long as it is adequately cooked.[9]

Micronutrient Needs of Pregnant Women

The need for certain micronutrients increases during pregnancy. Refer to Table 11.2 for an overview of these changes. The key micronutrients are discussed in this section.

Folate As noted earlier, adequate folate is critical during the first 28 days after conception, when it is required for the formation and closure of the **neural tube**—an embryonic structure that eventually becomes the brain and spinal cord. Folate deficiency is associated with neural tube defects such as **spina bifida** (FIGURE 11.3) and **anencephaly,** a fatal defect in which there is partial absence of brain tissue.[10] To reduce the risk of a neural tube defect, all women capable of becoming pregnant are encouraged to consume 400 µg of folic acid per day from supplements, fortified foods, or both in addition to a variety of foods naturally high in folates. Adequate folate

neural tube Embryonic tissue that forms a tube, which eventually becomes the brain and spinal cord.

spina bifida Embryonic neural tube defect that occurs when the spinal vertebrae fail to completely enclose the spinal cord, allowing it to protrude.

anencephaly A fatal neural tube defect in which there is partial absence of brain tissue most likely caused by failure of the neural tube to close.

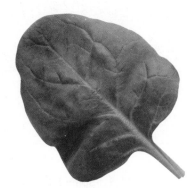

Spinach is a good source of folate.

TABLE 11.2 Changes in Nutrient Recommendations with Pregnancy for Adult Women

Micronutrient	Prepregnancy	Pregnancy	% Increase
Folate	400 µg/day	600 µg/day	50
Vitamin B$_{12}$	2.4 µg/day	2.6 µg/day	8
Vitamin C	75 mg/day	85 mg/day	13
Vitamin A	700 µg/day	770 µg/day	10
Vitamin D	5 µg/day	5 µg/day	0
Calcium	1,000 mg/day	1,000 mg/day	0
Iron	18 mg/day	27 mg/day	50
Zinc	8 mg/day	11 mg/day	38
Sodium	1,500 mg/day	1,500 mg/day	0
Iodine	150 µg/day	220 µg/day	47

intake does not guarantee normal neural tube development, as the precise cause of neural tube defects is unknown, and, in some cases, there is a genetic component.

Of course, folate remains very important even after the neural tube has closed. Folate deficiency can result in macrocytic anemia (a condition in which blood cells do not mature properly) and has been associated with low birth weight, preterm delivery, and failure of the fetus to grow properly. The RDA for folate for pregnant women is 600 µg/day, a full 50% increase over the RDA for a nonpregnant female.[10]

Vitamin B$_{12}$ Vitamin B$_{12}$ (cobalamin) is vital during pregnancy because it regenerates the active form of folate. The RDA for vitamin B$_{12}$ for pregnant women is shown in Table 11.2. It can easily be obtained from animal food sources; however, deficiencies have been observed in vegan women. Fortified foods or supplementation provide these women with the necessary B$_{12}$.

Vitamin C Vitamin C is necessary for the synthesis of collagen, a component of connective tissue (including skin, blood vessels, and tendons) and part of the organic matrix of bones. As shown in Table 11.2, the RDA for vitamin C during pregnancy is increased by a little more than 10% over the RDA for nonpregnant women. Women

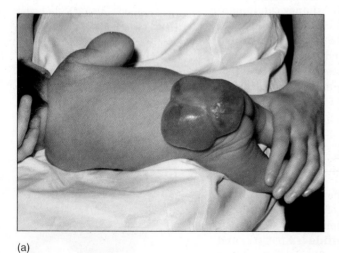

(a)

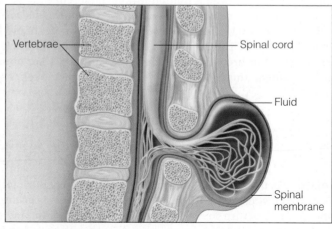

Vertebrae

Spinal cord

Fluid

Spinal membrane

(b)

FIGURE 11.3 Spina bifida, a common neural tube defect. (a) An external view of an infant with spina bifida. (b) An internal view of the protruding spinal cord tissue and fluid-filled sac.

who smoke during pregnancy should consume even higher levels, because smoking lowers both serum and amniotic fluid levels of vitamin C.

Vitamin A As shown in Table 11.2, vitamin A needs increase during pregnancy, and deficiency has been linked to low birth weight and preterm delivery. However, consumption of excessive vitamin A, particularly during the first trimester, increases the risk for birth of an infant with cleft lip or palate, heart defects, and abnormalities of the central nervous system.[11] A well-balanced diet supplies sufficient vitamin A, so supplementation even at low levels is not recommended. Note that beta-carotene (which is converted to vitamin A in the body) has not been associated with birth defects.

Vitamin D Despite the role of vitamin D in calcium absorption, the AI for this nutrient does not increase during pregnancy. However, pregnant women with darkly pigmented skin and/or limited sun exposure who do not regularly drink milk will benefit from vitamin D supplementation. Most prenatal vitamin supplements contain 10 µg/day (400 IU) of vitamin D, which is considered safe and acceptable.[12]

Calcium Growth of the fetal skeleton requires as much as 30 g of calcium, most during the last trimester. However, the AI for calcium does not change during pregnancy; it remains at 1,300 mg/day for pregnant adolescents and 1,000 mg/day for adult pregnant women for two reasons. First, pregnant women absorb calcium from the diet more efficiently than nonpregnant women. Second, the extra demand for calcium has not been found to cause permanent demineralization of the mother's bones or to increase fracture risk.[12]

Iron Iron is important in the formation of red blood cells, which transport oxygen throughout the body. During pregnancy, the demand for red blood cells increases to accommodate the needs of the expanded maternal blood volume, growing uterus, placenta, and the fetus itself.[11] Thus, more iron is needed (see Table 11.2). Fetal demand for iron increases even further during the last trimester, when the fetus stores iron in the liver for use during the first few months of life. This iron storage is protective because breast milk is low in iron.

Severely inadequate iron intake certainly has the potential to harm the fetus, resulting in an increased rate of low birth weight, preterm birth, stillbirth, and death of the newborn in the first weeks after birth. However, in most cases, the fetus builds adequate stores by "robbing" maternal iron, prompting iron-deficiency anemia in the mother. During pregnancy, maternal iron deficiency causes pallor and exhaustion, but at birth it endangers her life: anemic women are more likely to die during or shortly after childbirth because they are less able to tolerate blood loss and fight infection. To ensure adequate iron during pregnancy, an iron supplement (as part of, or distinct from, a total prenatal supplement) is routinely prescribed during the last two trimesters.

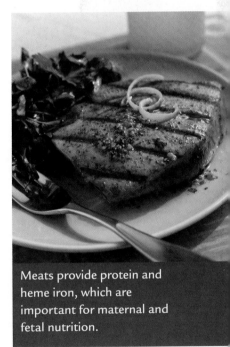

Meats provide protein and heme iron, which are important for maternal and fetal nutrition.

Zinc Because zinc has critical roles in DNA and protein synthesis, it is imperative that adequate zinc status be maintained during pregnancy to facilitate proper growth and development of both maternal and fetal tissues. The RDA for zinc for adult pregnant women is 11 mg per day and increases to 12 mg per day for pregnant adolescents (see Table 11.2).[11]

Sodium and Iodine The AI for sodium does not change during pregnancy.[13] Although too much sodium is associated with fluid retention and bloating, as well as high blood pressure, increased body fluids are a normal and necessary part of pregnancy, and some sodium is necessary to maintain fluid balance.

As shown in Table 11.2, iodine needs increase significantly during pregnancy, but the RDA is easy to achieve by using a modest amount of iodized salt during cooking.

Do Pregnant Women Need Supplements?

Prenatal multivitamin and mineral supplements are not strictly necessary during pregnancy, but most healthcare providers recommend them. Meeting all the nutrient needs would otherwise take careful and somewhat complex dietary planning.

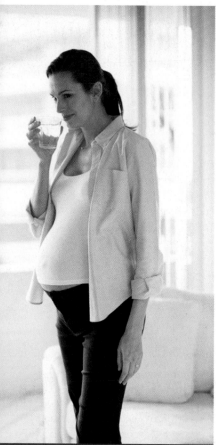

It is important that pregnant women drink about 10 cups of fluid a day.

Prenatal supplements are especially good insurance for vegans, adolescents, and others whose diet might be low in one or more micronutrients. It is important that pregnant women understand, however, that supplements are to be taken *in addition to,* not as a substitute for, a nutrient-rich diet.

Fluid Needs of Pregnant Women

Fluid plays many vital roles during pregnancy. It allows for the necessary increase in the mother's blood volume, acts as a lubricant, aids in regulating body temperature, and is necessary for many metabolic reactions. Fluid that the mother consumes also helps maintain the **amniotic fluid** that surrounds, cushions, and protects the fetus in the uterus. The AI for fluid intake includes approximately 2.3 L (10 cups) of fluid as beverages, including drinking water.[13]

> RECAP *During the last two trimesters of pregnancy, energy needs increase by about 350 to 450 kcal/day. Pregnant women should consume enough energy from nutrient-dense foods to support an appropriate weight gain, typically 25 to 35 lb. Protein, carbohydrates, and fats provide the building blocks for fetal growth. Folate deficiency has been associated with neural tube defects. Most healthcare providers recommend prenatal supplements as well as an iron supplement for pregnant women to ensure that sufficient micronutrients are consumed. More fluid is needed during pregnancy to provide for increased maternal blood volume and amniotic fluid.*

Nutrition-Related Concerns for Pregnant Women

Pregnancy-related conditions involving a particular nutrient, such as neural tube defects and iron-deficiency anemia, have already been discussed. The following sections describe some of the most common discomforts and disorders of pregnant women that are related to their general nutrition.

Morning Sickness

More than half of all pregnant women experience **morning sickness,** or *nausea and vomiting of pregnancy (NVP).* The symptoms vary from occasional mild queasiness to constant nausea with bouts of vomiting. In truth, "morning sickness" is not an appropriate name because about 80% of pregnant women report that their symptoms last all day. Except in severe cases, the mother and fetus do not suffer lasting harm. However, some women experience such frequent vomiting that they require hospitalization.

Morning sickness is thought to be prompted at least in part by the effect of pregnancy-related hormones on the brain stem and gastrointestinal (GI) tract. Some researchers speculate that emotional factors may contribute.

There is no cure for morning sickness. However, some women find it helpful to snack lightly throughout the day rather than consuming three larger meals. Greasy and high-fat foods should be avoided, as should strong cooking odors. Some women find that cold or room-temperature foods are less likely to cause nausea. Alternative therapies such as meditation, biofeedback, and acupressure wrist bands may also help.

Food Cravings

It seems as if nothing is more stereotypical about pregnancy than the image of a frazzled husband getting up in the middle of the night to run to the convenience store to get his pregnant wife some pickles and ice cream. This image, although humorous, is far from reality. Although some women have specific cravings, most crave a type of food (such as "something sweet" or "something salty") rather than a particular food.

Most cravings are, of course, for edible substances. But a surprising number of pregnant women crave nonfoods like laundry starch, chalk, and clay. This craving, called **pica,** is the subject of the accompanying Highlight box.

amniotic fluid The watery fluid contained within the innermost membrane of the sac containing the fetus. It cushions and protects the growing fetus.

morning sickness Varying degrees of nausea and vomiting associated with pregnancy, most commonly in the first trimester.

pica An abnormal craving to eat something not fit for food, such as clay, paint, and so forth.

HIGHLIGHT

The Danger of Nonfood Cravings

A few weeks after her nurse told her she was pregnant, Darlene started feeling "funny." She'd experience bouts of nausea lasting several hours every day, and her appetite seemed to disappear. At the grocery store, she'd wander through the aisles with an empty cart, confused about what foods she should be choosing for her growing baby, and unable to find anything that appealed to her. Eventually, she'd return home with a few things: frozen prepared macaroni and cheese, cereal bars, orange and grape soda—and a large bag of ice. She took cupfuls of ice from the soda machine at the assembly plant where she worked and ate it throughout the day. Each weekend, she went through more than a boxful of popsicles to "settle her stomach." Even her favorite strawberry ice cream no longer appealed to her.

At Darlene's next check-up, her nurse became concerned because she had lost weight. "I want to eat the stuff like in those pictures you gave me," Darlene confessed, "but I don't like it very much." She was too embarrassed to admit to anyone, even the nurse, that the only thing she really wanted to eat was ice.

Some people contend that a pregnant woman with unusual food cravings is intuitively seeking needed nutrients. Arguing against this theory is the phenomenon of *pica*—the craving and consumption of nonfood material, which often occurs during pregnancy. A woman with pica may crave ice, clay, dirt, chalk, coffee grounds, baking soda, laundry starch, and many other substances. The cause of these nonfood cravings is not known; however, people with developmental disabilities are at increased risk.[14] Underlying biochemical disorders such as decreased activity of neurotransmitters in the brain, lower socioeconomic status, and family stress have also been implicated, as have cultural factors. For example, in the United States, pica is more common among pregnant African American women than women from other racial or ethnic groups.[15] The practice of eating clay has been traced to central Africa, and researchers theorize that people taken from central Africa and sent as slaves to the United States brought the practice with them. In addition, nutrient deficiencies have been associated with pica, although it is not at all clear that nutrient deficiencies cause it. In fact, inhibition of nutrient absorption caused by the ingestion of clay and other substances may produce nutrient deficiency.[15]

No matter the cause, pica is dangerous. Consuming ice can lead to inadequate weight gain if, as with Darlene, the ice substitutes for food. Ingestion of clay, starch, and other substances can not only inhibit absorption of nutrients but also cause constipation, intestinal blockage, and even excessive weight gain. Ingestion of certain substances, such as dish-washing liquid in one case, can lead to such severe vomiting and diarrhea that the individual experiences electrolyte disturbances that lead to seizures or death.[14]

Some pregnant women with pica find food items they can substitute for the craved nonfood; for instance, peanut butter for clay or nonfat powdered milk for starch. If a woman experiences pica, she should talk with her healthcare provider immediately to identify strategies to avoid consuming dangerous substances and to consume healthful foods that will support optimal growth and development of her fetus.

Gestational Diabetes

Gestational diabetes, which occurs in approximately 7% of all U.S. pregnancies, is defined as any degree of glucose intolerance that begins or is first diagnosed during pregnancy. It is usually a temporary condition in which a pregnant woman is unable to produce sufficient insulin or becomes insulin resistant, resulting in elevated levels of blood glucose.

Fortunately, gestational diabetes has no ill effects on either the mother or the fetus if blood glucose levels are strictly controlled through diet, physical activity, and/or medication. If uncontrolled, gestational diabetes can result in a type of high blood pressure discussed in the next section. It can also result in a baby that is too large as a result of receiving too much glucose across the placenta during fetal life. Infants who are overly large are at risk for early birth and trauma during vaginal birth and may need to be delivered by cesarean section.

gestational diabetes Insufficient insulin production or insulin resistance that results in consistently high blood glucose levels, specifically during pregnancy; condition typically resolves after birth occurs.

NUTRI-CASE JUDY

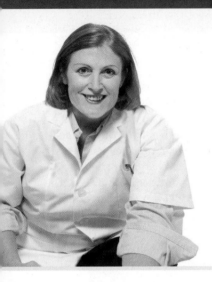

"Back when I was pregnant with Hannah, the doctor told me I had gestational diabetes but I shouldn't worry about it. He said I didn't need any medication, and I don't remember changing my diet. In fact, I just kept eating whatever I wanted, and by the time Hannah was born, I had gained almost 60 pounds. I never did lose all that extra weight, and of course my blood sugar never got back to normal. If I'd known then what I know now, I might have done things differently."

Review what you learned about diabetes in Chapter 3. What information would have been important for Judy to learn while she was pregnant? What are some things Judy could do now to improve her blood glucose levels?

Hypertension

In the United States, approximately 7% to 8% of pregnant women develop some form of hypertension, or high blood pressure, yet it accounts for almost 15% of pregnancy-related deaths. If left untreated, hypertension during pregnancy can lead to seizures and kidney failure that is life-threatening for both the mother and fetus.

No one knows exactly what causes hypertension during pregnancy, but deficiencies in dietary protein, vitamin C, vitamin E, calcium, and magnesium seem to increase the risk. Pregnant adolescents and women who are pregnant for the first time are at higher risk, as are African American and low-income women. High levels of blood triglycerides (associated with high-sugar diets) have also been correlated with increased risk.

Management focuses mainly on blood pressure control. Typical treatment includes bed rest and medical oversight. In nearly all women without a prior history of hypertension, blood pressure returns to normal within about a day after childbirth.

Adolescent Pregnancy

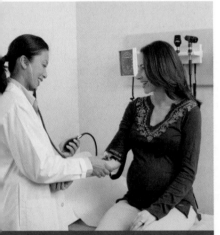

Pregnant women have their blood pressure measured to test for hypertension.

Although the rate of adolescent pregnancies in the United States has declined by almost 25% since 1995, approximately 750,000 U.S. teenagers gave birth in 2002.[16] Adolescents who become pregnant face greater nutritional challenges than adult women for several reasons:

- An adolescent's body is still changing and growing: peak bone mass has not yet been reached, and full stature may not have been attained. This demand for tissue growth keeps nutrient needs during adolescence very high.

- Many adolescents have not established healthful nutritional patterns and many are underweight; thus, the added burden of pregnancy on an adolescent body can create a nutrient demand that can be very difficult to meet.

- Pregnant adolescents are less likely than older women to receive early and regular prenatal care.

- Pregnant adolescents are more likely to smoke and less likely to understand the medical consequences of prenatal smoking, alcohol consumption, and drug abuse.

These factors make adolescent mothers more likely than older mothers to have preterm births, low-birth-weight babies, and other complications, including iron deficiency anemia. In addition, the rate of infant mortality is higher among infants born to adolescent mothers.

Vegetarianism

With the possible exception of iron and zinc, vegetarian women who consume dairy products and eggs (lacto-ovo-vegetarians) have no nutritional concerns beyond those encountered by every pregnant woman. In contrast, women who are vegan need to be more vigilant than usual about their intake of nutrients that are derived primarily or wholly from animal products. These include vitamin D (unless regularly exposed to sunlight throughout the pregnancy), vitamin B_6, vitamin B_{12}, calcium, iron, and zinc. Supplements and/or fortified foods containing these nutrients are usually necessary.

> RECAP *About half of all pregnant women experience morning sickness during pregnancy. Pica is a craving for nonfood items experienced by some pregnant women. Gestational diabetes and hypertension are nutrition-related disorders that can seriously affect maternal and fetal health. As adolescents' bodies are still growing and developing, their nutrient needs during pregnancy become so high that adequate nourishment for the mother and baby becomes difficult. Women who follow a vegan diet usually need to consume multivitamin and mineral supplements during pregnancy.*

Consumption of Caffeine

Caffeine is a naturally occurring stimulant found in several foods, including coffee, tea, soft drinks, and chocolate. Caffeine readily crosses the placenta and thus quickly reaches the fetus, but at what dose and to what extent it causes fetal harm is still a subject of controversy and study. Current thinking holds that women who consume less than about 200 mg of caffeine per day (the equivalent of one to two 8-ounce cups of coffee) are not harming the fetus. Evidence suggests that consuming higher daily doses of caffeine (the higher the dose, the more compelling the evidence) may slightly increase the risk of miscarriage, preterm delivery, and low birth weight. It is sensible, then, for pregnant women to limit daily caffeine intake to no more than the equivalent of 2 cups of coffee.[17]

Consumption of Alcohol

As discussed in Chapter 8, alcohol is a known teratogen that readily crosses the placenta and accumulates in the fetal bloodstream. The immature fetal liver cannot readily metabolize alcohol, and its presence in fetal blood and tissues is associated with a variety of birth defects, including fetal alcohol syndrome, the subject of a *Healthwatch* in Chapter 8. According to the March of Dimes, approximately 40,000 babies are born in the United States each year with some type of alcohol-induced damage.[18]

Heavy drinking during the first trimester typically results in fetal malformations such as heart defects and facial abnormalities. Because many women do not even realize they are pregnant until several weeks after conception, public health officials recommend not only that pregnant women abstain from all alcoholic beverages, but also that women who are trying to become pregnant or suspect they may be pregnant abstain.

Smoking

Despite the well-known consequences of cigarette smoking and the growing social stigma associated with smoking during pregnancy, between 18% and 19% of pregnant U.S. women smoke.[19] Adolescents are more likely to smoke during pregnancy compared to older mothers, and the rate of smoking among pregnant teens continues to increase.

Several components and metabolites of tobacco are toxic to the fetus, including lead, cadmium, cyanide, nicotine, carbon monoxide, and polycyclic aromatic hydrocarbons. Fetal nourishment, growth, and development may be impaired by reduced oxygen levels in fetal blood and reduced placental blood flow.

Maternal smoking greatly increases the risk of miscarriage, stillbirth, placental abnormalities, poor fetal growth, preterm delivery, and low birth weight. The effects of maternal smoking continue after birth: sudden infant death syndrome and respiratory illnesses occur with greater frequency in the children of smokers than the children of nonsmokers.

Illegal Drugs

Although the specific effects of every illegal drug are not fully known, pregnant women should assume any use of illegal drugs will be harmful to the development and growth of their babies. Most drugs pass through the placenta into the fetal blood; as with alcohol, the fetal liver is too immature to efficiently break down these substances, so the drugs tend to accumulate in fetal blood and tissue. Many illegal drugs decrease oxygen delivery to the fetus and/or impair placental blood flow, thereby reducing the transfer of nutrients from the mother to the developing fetus.

All women are strongly advised to stop taking drugs *before* becoming pregnant. If a woman using illegal drugs discovers she is pregnant, she should seek immediate medical care and request assistance to stop her drug use as soon as possible. There is no safe level of use for illegal drugs during pregnancy; they are harmful to the mother and the developing fetus and result in serious long-term health deficits in the child.

Food Safety

A few specific foods may be unsafe for women who are pregnant. These include unpasteurized milk; raw or partially cooked eggs; raw or undercooked meat, fish, or poultry; unpasteurized juices; and raw sprouts.[20] Certain soft cheeses such as Brie, feta, Camembert, Roquefort, and Mexican-style cheeses, also called *queso blanco* or *queso fresco,* should be avoided unless they are labeled as made with pasteurized milk.

As discussed earlier, fish is an excellent source of the omega-3 essential fatty acid DHA and, in appropriate amounts, is a healthful addition to a balanced prenatal diet. However, certain types of fish should be avoided because of their high mercury content.[9] All fish should be thoroughly cooked to kill any disease-causing bacteria or parasites. Pregnant women should avoid sushi and other raw fish as well as raw oysters and clams.

Exercise

Exercise can help keep a woman physically fit during pregnancy. In addition, exercise is a great mood booster, helping women feel more in control of their changing bodies and reducing postpartum depression. Expending additional energy through exercise will also allow intake of compensatory energy when a ravenous appetite kicks in. Moreover, regular moderate exercise will reduce the risk of gestational diabetes, help keep blood pressure down, and confer all the cardiovascular benefits that it does for nonpregnant individuals.[21,22] Regular exercise can also shorten the duration of active labor. Finally, a woman who keeps fit during pregnancy will have an easier time resuming a fitness routine and losing weight after pregnancy.

If a woman was not active prior to pregnancy, she should begin an exercise program slowly and progress gradually under the guidance of her healthcare provider. If a woman was physically active before pregnancy, she can continue to be physically active during pregnancy, within comfort and reason. Low- or no-impact exercises such as brisk walking, hiking, swimming, and water aerobics are excellent choices. Women who have been avid runners before pregnancy can often continue to run, as long as they feel comfortable. However, they should probably limit the distance and intensity of their runs as the pregnancy progresses.

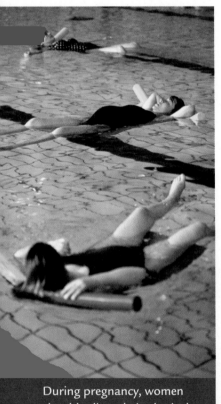

During pregnancy, women should adjust their physical activity to comfortable low-impact exercises.

RECAP *Caffeine intake should not exceed 2 cups of coffee per day throughout pregnancy. Alcohol and illegal drugs are teratogens and should not be consumed in any amount during pregnancy. Cigarette smoking impairs fetal growth and development; pregnant women should not smoke nor expose themselves to secondhand smoke. Safe food-handling practices are especially important during pregnancy. Exercise (provided the mother has no contraindications) can enhance the health of a pregnant woman.*

Nutrition in Infancy

In the first year of life, infants generally grow about 10 inches and triple their weight—a growth rate more rapid than will ever occur again. At the same time, their limited physical activity means that the majority of their energy expenditure is to support growth.

What Are the Benefits of Breastfeeding?

Throughout most of human history, infants have thrived on only one food: breast milk. Breastfeeding is universally recognized as the ideal method of infant feeding because of the nutritional quality and health benefits of breast milk.[23] However, the technique does require patience and practice. La Leche League International is an advocacy group for breastfeeding: its publications, Web site (www.lalecheleague.org), and local meetings are all valuable resources for breastfeeding mothers and their families. Many hospitals and HMOs also offer breastfeeding classes.

Nutritional Quality of Breast Milk

In the first few days after birth, the breast milk is called **colostrum.** This yellowish fluid is rich in protein, vitamins A and E, and antibodies that help protect the newborn from infection. It also contains a factor that promotes the growth of helpful intestinal bacteria and has a laxative effect that helps the newborn to expel the sticky first stool.

Within 2 to 4 days, colostrum is replaced by mature breast milk. The amount and types of proteins in breast milk are ideally suited to the human infant: they are easily digested in the infant's immature GI tract, reducing the risk of gastric distress; they prevent the growth of harmful bacteria; and they include antibodies that help prevent infection while the infant's immune system is still immature.

The primary carbohydrate in breast milk is lactose, a disaccharide composed of glucose and galactose. The galactose component is important in nervous system development. Lactose provides energy and promotes the growth of beneficial bacteria. It also aids in the absorption of calcium. Breast milk has more lactose than cow's milk.

As with protein, the amount and types of fat in breast milk are ideally suited to the human infant. The fats in breast milk, especially omega-3 DHA and omega-6 arachidonic acid (ARA), have been shown to be essential for the growth and development of the infant's nervous system and the retina of the eyes. Many people are surprised to learn that the fat content of breast milk is higher than that of whole cow's milk. The energy provided by these fats, however, supports the rapid rate of growth during the first year of life.

The fat content of breast milk changes according to the age of the infant, providing a ratio of fatty acids unique to the growing infant's needs. The fat content also changes during the course of every feeding: The milk that is initially released is watery and is thought to satisfy the infant's initial thirst. As the feeding progresses, the milk acquires more fat until the very last 5% or so of the milk produced is similar to cream. This milk is thought to satiate the infant. Breast milk is also relatively high in cholesterol, which supports the rapid growth and development of the brain and nervous system.

In terms of micronutrients, breast milk is a good source of readily absorbed calcium and magnesium. It is low in iron, but the iron it does contain is easily absorbed (recall that the fetus stores iron in preparation for the first few months of life). Most experts agree that breast milk can meet the iron needs of full-term healthy infants for the first 6 months, after which iron-rich foods are needed.

Because its nutrient composition changes as the baby grows, breast milk alone is entirely sufficient to sustain an infant for the first 6 months of life. Throughout the next 6 months of infancy, as solid foods are gradually introduced, breast milk remains the baby's primary source of superior-quality nutrition. The American Academy of Pediatrics (AAP) encourages exclusive breastfeeding (no food or other source of nourishment) for the first 6 months of life, continuing breastfeeding for at least

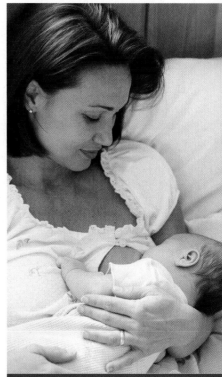

Breastfeeding has benefits for the mother and infant.

colostrum The first fluid made and secreted by the breasts from late in pregnancy to about a week after birth. It is rich in immune factors and protein.

the first year of life and, if acceptable within the family unit, into the second year of life or longer.[23]

Immunologic Benefits for Breast-fed Infants

Immune factors from the mother, including antibodies and immune cells, are passed directly from the mother to the newborn through breast milk. These factors provide important disease protection for the infant while its immune system is still immature. It has been shown that breast-fed infants have a lower incidence of bacterial infections. Breast-fed infants also demonstrate an enhanced immune response to polio, tetanus, and diphtheria immunizations.[24] In the United States, infant mortality rates are reduced by 21% in breast-fed infants.[23]

In addition, breast milk is nonallergenic, and breastfeeding is associated with a reduced risk of allergies during childhood and adulthood. Breastfed babies also die less frequently from **sudden infant death syndrome (SIDS)** and have a decreased chance of developing diabetes, overweight and obesity, hypercholesterolemia, and chronic digestive disorders.[23]

Physiologic Benefits for the Mother

Breastfeeding causes uterine contractions that quicken the return of the uterus to prepregnancy size and reduce bleeding. Many women also find that breastfeeding helps them lose the weight they gained during pregnancy, particularly if they breastfeed for more than 6 months.

Breastfeeding also suppresses **ovulation,** lengthening the time between pregnancies and giving a mother's body the chance to recover before she conceives again. Ovulation may not cease completely, however, so it is still possible to become pregnant while breastfeeding. The benefits of breastfeeding are summarized in Table 11.3.

Effects of Drugs and Other Substances on Breast Milk

Many substances make their way into breast milk. Among them are illegal and prescription drugs, over-the-counter drugs, and even substances from foods the mother eats. All illegal drugs should be assumed to pass into breast milk and should be avoided by breastfeeding mothers. Prescription drugs vary in the degree to which they pass into breast milk. Breastfeeding mothers should inform their physicians that they are breastfeeding. In some cases, the physician may advise that a woman switch to formula feeding while she is taking a certain medication.

Caffeine and alcohol rapidly enter breast milk. Caffeine can make the baby agitated and fussy, whereas alcohol can make the baby sleepy, depress the central nervous system, and, over time, slow motor development, in addition to inhibiting the mother's milk supply. Nicotine also passes into breast milk; therefore, it is best for the woman to quit smoking. A recent study showed that women who smoke while breastfeeding often stop nursing their babies sooner than nonsmokers.[25] Smoking while breastfeeding also interferes with infant sleep patterns.[26]

Food components that pass into the breast milk may not seem harmful; however, some substances that the mother eats, such as chemicals found in garlic, onions, peppers, broccoli, and cabbage, are distasteful enough to the infant to prevent proper feeding. Some high-risk babies have allergic reactions to foods the mother ate, such as wheat, cow's milk, eggs, strawberries, or citrus, and suffer GI upset, diaper rash, or another reaction.

Although environmental contaminants can enter the breast milk, the benefits of breastfeeding almost always outweigh potential risks. Fresh fruits and vegetables should be thoroughly washed and peeled to minimize exposure to pesticides and fertilizer residues. Maternal exposure to solvents, paints, gasoline fumes, furniture strippers, and similar products should also be limited.

sudden infant death syndrome (SIDS) The sudden death of a previously healthy infant; the most common cause of death in infants more than 1 month of age.

ovulation The release of an ovum (egg) from a woman's ovary.

TABLE 11.3   Benefits of Breastfeeding

Benefits to Infant	Benefits to Mother	Benefits to Family/Society
Provides superior level and balance of nutrients for infant growth, health, and development. Decreases incidence and severity of a wide range of infectious diseases, including diarrhea, bacterial meningitis, and respiratory infections. Is associated with decreased risk for both type 1 and type 2 diabetes. Has possible protective effect against sudden infant death syndrome (SIDS), several chronic digestive diseases, leukemia, lymphoma, Hodgkin's disease, asthma, and allergies. Is associated with reduced risk for childhood and adulthood overweight and obesity. Associated with enhanced cognitive development.	Increases level of oxytocin, resulting in less postpartum bleeding and more rapid return of uterus to prepregnant state. Delays resumption of menstrual periods, causing reduced menstrual blood loss over the months after the birth and preserving maternal iron. Delays resumption of ovulation and thereby increases spacing between pregnancies Promotes an earlier return to prepregnancy weight. Improves bone remineralization in months after birth. Reduces the woman's risk of ovarian cancer and premenopausal breast cancer.	Reduces healthcare costs and employee absenteeism for care attributable to infant/child illness. Decreases family food expenditures: cost of purchasing extra food for lactating mother is less than half the cost of purchasing infant formula. Decreases environmental burden for production and transport of formula, bottles, artificial nipples, etc. Reduces caregiver time away from infant/siblings to prepare infant food: breast milk requires no preparation and is always the perfect temperature.

Source: The benefits identified in this table are derived from American Academy of Pediatrics, Section on Breastfeeding. February 2005. Policy Statement: Breastfeeding and the use of human milk. *Ped* 115(2):496–506. In addition to these benefits, the La Leche League and other breastfeeding advocacy organizations identify emotional and psychologic benefits of skin-to-skin suckling.

The human immunodeficiency virus, HIV, which causes AIDS, can be transmitted from mother to baby through breast milk. Thus, HIV-positive women in the United States and Canada are encouraged to feed their infants formula.[27] Women with tuberculosis should not breastfeed until they have completed at least 2 weeks of antituberculin therapy. Women with cancer should avoid breastfeeding while on chemotherapy.

What Are a Breastfeeding Woman's Nutrient Needs?

You might be surprised to learn that breastfeeding requires even more energy and nutrients than pregnancy! This is because breast milk has to supply an adequate amount of all of the nutrients an infant needs to grow and develop. The current DRIs during breastfeeding, also called *lactation,* are listed in the tables on the final pages of this textbook.

Nutrient Recommendations for Breastfeeding Women

It is estimated that milk production requires about 700 to 800 kcal/day. It is generally recommended that breastfeeding women aged 19 years and above consume 330 kcal/day above their prepregnancy energy needs during the first 6 months of breastfeeding and 400 additional kcal/day during the second 6 months.[8] This additional energy is sufficient to support adequate milk production. At the same time, the remaining energy deficit helps women gradually lose any excess fat and body weight gained during pregnancy. It is critical that breastfeeding women avoid severe energy restriction, as this practice can result in decreased milk production.

Of the macronutrients, carbohydrate and protein needs are increased. An additional 15 to 25 g of protein/day and 80 g of carbohydrate/day above prepregnancy requirements are recommended.

For the micronutrients, the needs of several vitamins and minerals increase over the requirements of pregnancy. These include vitamins A, C, E, riboflavin, vitamin B_{12}, biotin, and choline, and the minerals copper, chromium, manganese, iodine, selenium, and zinc. Requirements for iron decrease significantly to a mere 9 mg/day. This is because iron is not a significant component of breast milk and, in addition, breastfeeding usually suppresses menstruation for at least a few months, reducing iron losses. The recommended intake for calcium for a lactating woman is the same as for all women between the ages of 19 and 50 years, that is, 1,000 mg/day. Because of their own continuing growth, however, teen mothers who are breastfeeding should continue to consume 1,300 mg/day.

Do Breastfeeding Women Need Supplements?

If a breastfeeding woman appropriately increases her energy intake and does so with nutrient-dense foods, her nutrient needs can usually be met without supplements. However, there is nothing wrong with taking a basic multivitamin for insurance, as long as it is not considered a substitute for proper nutrition. Breastfeeding women should consume omega-3 fatty acids either in fish or supplements to support the infant's developing nervous system, and women who don't consume dairy products should monitor their calcium and vitamin D intakes carefully. Women following a vegan diet should consume a vitamin B_{12} supplement or include B_{12} fortified foods in their diet.

Fluid Recommendations for Breastfeeding Women

Because extra fluid is expended with every feeding, lactating women need to consume about an extra quart (about 1L) of fluid per day. The AI for fluid recommends about 13 cups of beverages to facilitate milk production and prevent dehydration.[13]

What Is the Nutritional Quality of Infant Formula?

Women with certain infectious diseases are advised not to breastfeed, as are women using certain prescription medications and women who abuse drugs.[23] If breastfeeding is not feasible, several types of commercial formulas provide nutritious alternatives. Most formulas are based on cow's milk that is modified to make it more appropriate for human infants. Soy-based formulas are a viable alternative for infants who are lactose intolerant (although this is rare in infants) or cannot tolerate the proteins in cow's milk–based formulas. Soy formulas may also satisfy the requirements of families who are strict vegans. However, soy-based formulas are not without controversy. Because soy contains isoflavones, or plant forms of estrogens, there is some concern over the effects these compounds have on growing infants. In addition, soy is a common allergen.

Cow's milk should not be introduced to infants until after 1 year of age. Cow's milk is too high in protein, the protein is difficult to digest, and the poor digestibility may contribute to gastrointestinal bleeding. In addition, cow's milk has too much sodium, too little iron, and a poor balance of other vitamins and minerals. Goat's milk, soy milk, and rice milk are also inappropriate for infants.

When feeding an infant formula, parents and caretakers need to pay close attention to their infants' cues for hunger and fullness. Although most parents instinctively recognize when their baby needs to eat, it is often harder for them to know when to stop. Some infants turn their head away from the nipple or tightly close their lips; others simply nod off or fall asleep. Older infants may actually push away the bottle or initiate play-like behaviors.

Once the baby's teeth start coming in, he or she should not be allowed to fall asleep while sucking on the bottle. This practice allows the formula to pool around the teeth and, without the normal release of saliva that occurs when the baby is awake, can lead to a form of severe dental decay known as *baby bottle syndrome* (FIGURE 11.4).

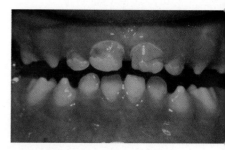

FIGURE 11.4 Allowing an infant or toddler to fall asleep with a bottle containing any carbohydrate-rich fluid such as breast milk, formula, cow's milk, or juice can result in the tooth decay of baby bottle syndrome.

What Are an Infant's Nutrient Needs?

Three characteristics of infants combine to make their nutritional needs unique. These are (1) their high energy needs as compared to their body weight; (2) their immature digestive tracts and kidneys; and (3) their small size. The DRIs for infants are based on the nutrient values of breast milk and are listed in the tables on the final pages of this textbook.

Macronutrient Needs of Infants

Infants are not small versions of adults; they are growing rapidly compared to the typically stable adult phase of life. Infants need to consume about 40 to 50 kcal/pound of body weight per day, with newborns at the higher end of the range and those aged 6 to 12 months at the lower end.

About 40% to 50% of an infant's caloric intake should come from fat during the first year of life. Fat intakes below this level can be harmful before the age of 2 years. Omega-6 and omega-3 fatty acids are essential for the rapid brain growth, retinal maturation, and nervous system development that happens in the first 1 to 2 years of life.

Although carbohydrate and protein are also essential for infant growth and development, no more than 20% of an infant's daily energy requirement should come from protein. Immature infant kidneys are not able to process and excrete the excess nitrogen from higher-protein diets.

Micronutrient Needs of Infants

Breast milk and commercial formulas provide most of the vitamins and minerals infants need. However, there are several micronutrients that may warrant supplementation.

All infants are routinely given an injection of vitamin K shortly after birth. This provides vitamin K until the infant's intestine can develop its own healthful bacteria, which then provide the needed vitamin K.

Breast milk is low in vitamin D, and deficiencies of this nutrient have been detected in breast-fed infants with dark skin and in those with limited sunlight exposure. Breast-fed infants are often prescribed a supplement containing vitamin D until they are about 6 months of age.[23]

Breastfed infants also require additional iron beginning no later than 6 months of age because the infant's iron stores become depleted and breast milk is a poor source of iron. Iron is extremely important for cognitive development and prevention of iron-deficiency anemia. Infant rice cereal fortified with iron, an excellent choice as a first food, can serve as an additional iron source, as can pureed meats.

Depending on the fluoride content of the household water supply, breast-fed infants over the age of 6 months may need a fluoride supplement. Most brands of bottled water have low levels of fluoride, and many home water treatment systems remove fluoride. On the other hand, fluoride toxicity may be a risk for infants simultaneously exposed to fluoridated toothpaste and rinses, fluoridated water, and fluoride supplements.

There are special conditions in which additional supplements may be needed for breast-fed infants. For example, if a woman is a vegan, her breast milk may be low in vitamin B_{12}, and a supplement of this vitamin should be given to the baby.

For formula-fed infants, the need for supplementation depends on the formula composition and other factors. Many formulas are already fortified with iron, for example; thus, no additional iron supplement is necessary. If the baby is getting adequate vitamin D through either the ingestion of at least 2 cups of vitamin D–fortified formula or via regular brief sun exposure, then an extra supplement may not be necessary.

Fluid Recommendations for Infants

Fluid is critical for everyone, but for infants the balance is more delicate for two reasons. First, because infants are so small, they proportionally lose more water through evaporation than adults. Second, their kidneys are immature and unable to concentrate urine. Hence, they are at increased risk of dehydration. An infant needs about 2 fl oz of fluid per pound of body weight, and either breast milk or formula is almost always adequate in providing this amount. Experts recently confirmed that "infants exclusively fed human milk do not require supplemental water."[13] The practice common among some low-income families of diluting infant formula with extra water is extremely dangerous. Overhydration can cause nutrient imbalances such as hyponatremia (low blood sodium) as well as inadequate weight gain and failure to thrive.

> RECAP *Breast milk provides superior nutrition and heightened immunity for infants. Mothers who breastfeed experience the benefit of increased postpregnancy weight loss and suppressed ovulation. If breastfeeding is not feasible, several types of commercial formulas provide nutritious alternatives. Vitamin D supplements may be recommended for exclusively breast-fed infants; iron and fluoride supplements may be prescribed for infants older than 6 months of age.*

When Do Infants Begin to Need Solid Foods?

Before 4 to 6 months of age, most infants are not physically or developmentally able to consume solid food. The suckling response, present at birth, depends on a particular movement of the tongue that draws liquid out of a breast or bottle. When very young infants are spoon-fed solid food, this tongue movement, known as the extrusion reflex, causes most of the food to be pushed back out of the mouth. This reflex action must begin to subside before solid foods can be successfully introduced, typically after 4 to 6 months of age.

In addition, to minimize the risk of choking or gagging, the infant must have gained muscular control of the head and neck. The infant must also be able to sit up (with or without support).

An infant is also not ready for solid foods until the digestive system has matured. Infants are able to digest and absorb lactose from the time of their birth; however, they lack adequate levels of the enzyme amylase, for the digestion of starch, until the age of 3 to 4 months. If an infant is fed solid foods too soon, starches remain undigested, contributing to diarrhea and bloating, and proteins can be absorbed intact and undigested, setting the stage for allergies. In addition, the kidneys must have matured so that they are better able to process electrolytes and nitrogen waste products as well as properly concentrate urine.

When deciding which foods to introduce first, parents must consider their infant's nutrient needs and the risk of an allergic reaction. At about 6 months of age, infant iron stores become depleted; thus, the first food introduced is typically iron-fortified infant rice cereal. Rice is a good first grain, because it rarely triggers an allergic response and is easy to digest. Infant rice cereal can be mixed with breast milk or formula to the desired consistency. Most babies start with only 1 to 2 teaspoons of cereal a day and gradually work up to portions of about ¼ cup. Cereal and other solid foods should always be fed to the infant from a spoon, not placed into a bottle.

The extrusion reflex will push solid food out of an infant's mouth.

Parents should not introduce another new food for at least 4 to 5 days in order to carefully watch for signs of a food allergy or intolerance, including a rash, unexplained diarrhea, runny nose, or wheezing. If all goes well with the rice cereal, another single-grain cereal (other than wheat, which is highly allergenic) can be introduced, or the family may choose to introduce a different single-item food such as a strained vegetable or meat. Some nutritionists recommend meat, because it is a good source of iron and zinc, while others encourage the introduction of vitamin C–rich vegetables. It is wise to introduce strained vegetables before fruits because once a child becomes accustomed to the sweetness of bananas, peaches, and other fruits, the relative blandness of most vegetables may be less appealing. To allow time to monitor for allergic reactions, parents should wait 4 to 5 days between the introduction of each new food.

Gradually, a variety of foods should be introduced to the infant by the end of the first year. Throughout the first year, solid foods should only be a supplement to, not a substitute for, breast milk or iron-fortified formula. Infants still need the nutrient density and energy that breast milk and formula provide.

What *Not* to Feed an Infant

The following foods should never be offered to an infant:

- *Foods that could cause choking.* Foods such as grapes, chunks of hot dogs, nuts, popcorn, raw carrots, raisins, and hard candies cannot be chewed adequately by infants and can cause choking.

- *Corn syrup and honey.* These may contain spores of the bacterium *Clostridium botulinum*. These spores can produce a toxin that can be fatal. Children older than 1 year can safely consume these substances because their digestive tracts are mature enough to kill any *C. botulinum* spores.

- *Goat's milk.* Goat's milk is notoriously low in many nutrients that infants need, such as folate, vitamin C, vitamin D, and iron.

- *Cow's milk.* For infants under 1 year, cow's milk is too concentrated in minerals and protein and contains too few carbohydrates to meet infant energy needs. Children can begin to consume whole cow's milk after the first birthday.

- *Large quantities of fruit juices.* Fruit juices are poorly absorbed in the infant digestive tract, causing diarrhea if consumed in excess. It is considered safe for infants older than 6 months to consume 4 to 8 oz of pure fruit juice (no sweeteners added) per day, with no more than 2 to 4 oz given at a time; however, plain water will also effectively quench an infant's thirst. Diluting fruit juice with water is another option.

- *Too much salt and sugar.* Infant foods should not be seasoned with salt or other seasonings. Naturally occurring sugars such as those found in fruits can provide needed energy. Cookies, cakes, and other excessively sweet, processed foods should be avoided.

- *Too much breast milk or formula.* As nutritious as breast milk and/or formula are, once infants reach the age of 6 months, solid foods should be introduced gradually. Six months of age is a critical time, as it is when a baby's iron stores begin to be depleted. Overreliance on breast milk or formula, to the exclusion or displacement of iron-rich foods, can result in a condition known as *milk anemia*.

RECAP *In the absence of breastfeeding, commercial formulas provide adequate nutrition for infants. Solid foods can gradually be introduced into an infant's diet at 4 to 6 months of age beginning with rice cereal, then moving to single-item vegetables or meats. Parents should avoid foods that represent a choking hazard, foods containing honey or corn syrup, cow's and goat's milk, and foods and beverages high in sugar.*

Nutrition-Related Concerns for Infants

Nutrition is one of the biggest concerns of new parents. Infants cannot speak, and their cries are sometimes indecipherable. Feeding time can be very frustrating for parents, especially if the child is not eating, not growing appropriately, or has problems such as diarrhea, vomiting, or persistent skin rashes. Following are some nutrition-related concerns for infants.

Allergies

As noted earlier, breastfeeding minimizes the risk of allergy development, as does delaying introduction of solid foods until 6 months of age. One of the most common allergies in infants is to the proteins in cow's milk–based formulas. Egg whites, peanuts and other nuts, wheat, soy, and citrus are other common allergens.

As stated, every food should be introduced in isolation, so that any allergic reaction can be identified and the particular food avoided. If there is a strong family history of food allergies, parents should be particularly watchful when introducing new foods to their infant; labels should be closely examined for offending ingredients.

Colic

Perhaps nothing is more frustrating to new parents than the relentless crying spells of some infants, typically referred to as **colic.** In this condition, infants who appear happy, healthy, and well nourished suddenly begin to cry or even shriek and continue for hours no matter what their caregiver does to console them. The spells tend to occur at the same time of day, typically late in the afternoon or early in the evening, and often occur daily for a period of several weeks. Overstimulation of the nervous system, feeding too rapidly, swallowing of air, and intestinal gas pain are considered possible culprits, but the precise cause is unknown. For breast-fed infants, colic spells are sometimes reduced when the mother switches to a bland diet. For formula-fed infants, a change in type of formula sometimes helps.

Gastroesophageal Reflux

Particularly common in preterm infants, gastroesophageal reflux occurs in about 3% of newborns. Typically, as the gastrointestinal tract matures within the first 12 months of life, this condition resolves. Caretakers should avoid overfeeding the infant, keep the infant upright after each feeding, and watch for choking or gagging. Some infants improve when fed whey-enriched formulas.

Iron-Deficiency Anemia

As stated earlier, full-term infants are born with sufficient iron stores to last for approximately the first 6 months of life. In older infants and toddlers, however, iron is the mineral most likely to be deficient. Iron-deficiency anemia causes pallor, lethargy, and impaired growth. Iron-fortified formula and rice cereal are good sources of this mineral. Overconsumption of cow's milk remains a common cause of anemia among U.S. infants and children.

Dehydration

Whether the cause is diarrhea, vomiting, prolonged fever, or inadequate fluid intake, dehydration is extremely dangerous to infants and if left untreated can quickly result in death. Treatment includes providing fluids, a task that is difficult if vomiting is occurring. In some cases, the physician may recommend that a pediatric electrolyte solution, readily available at most grocery and drug stores, be administered on a temporary basis. In more severe cases, hospitalization and administration of intravenous fluids may be necessary.

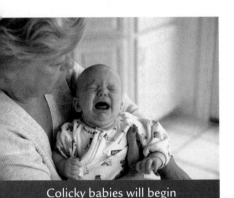

Colicky babies will begin crying for no apparent reason even if they otherwise appear well nourished and happy.

colic Unconsolable infant crying of unknown origin that lasts for hours at a time.

RECAP *Risk for food allergies can be reduced by breastfeeding and delaying the introduction of solid foods until the infant is at least 6 months of age. Infants with colic or gastroesophageal reflux present special challenges, but both conditions generally improve over time. Iron-deficiency anemia is easily prevented through the use of iron-fortified cereals. Dehydration is extremely dangerous to infants, and prompt, balanced fluid replacement is essential.*

Nutrition for Toddlers

The rapid growth rate of infancy begins to slow during toddlerhood—the period from 12 to 36 months of age. During the second and third years of life, a toddler will grow a total of about 5.5 to 7.5 inches and gain an average of 9 to 11 lb. Toddlers expend more energy to fuel increasing levels of activity as they explore their ever-expanding world and develop new skills. They progress from taking a few wobbly steps to running, jumping, and climbing with confidence, and they begin to dress, feed, and toilet themselves. Thus, their diet should provide an appropriate quantity and quality of nutrients to fuel their growth and activity. Table 11.4 identifies nutrient recommendations for toddlers, children, and adolescents.

What Are a Toddler's Nutrient Needs?

A toddler's energy needs per day vary according to age, body weight, and level of activity. However, a healthy toddler generally requires about 1,000 kcal per day. Healthy toddlers of appropriate body weight need more fat than adults, up to 40% of total calories, and should not be given low-fat or skim milk or other dairy products

TABLE 11.4 Nutrient Recommendations for Children and Adolescents

Nutrient	Toddlers (1 to 2 years)	Children (3 to 8 years)	Children (9 to 13 years)	Adolescents (14 to 18 years)
Carbohydrate	130 g/day	130 g/day	130 g/day	130 g/day
Fat	No DRI	No DRI	No DRI	No DRI
Protein	1.10 grams/kg body weight per day	0.95 grams/kg body weight per day	0.95 grams/kg body weight per day	0.85 grams/kg body weight per day
Vitamin A	300 µg/day	400 µg/day	600 µg/day	Boys = 900 µg/day Girls = 700 µg/day
Vitamin C	15 mg/day	25 mg/day	45 mg/day	Boys = 75 mg/day Girls = 65 mg/day
Vitamin E	6 mg/day	7 mg/day	11 mg/day	15 mg/day
Calcium	500 mg/day	800 mg/day	1,300 mg/day	1,300 mg/day
Iron	7 mg/day	10 mg/day	8 mg/day	Boys = 11 mg/day Girls = 15 mg/day
Zinc	3 mg/day	5 mg/day	8 mg/day	Boys = 11 mg/day Girls = 9 mg/day
Fluid	1.3 liters/day	1.7 liters/day	Boys = 2.4 liters/day Girls = 2.1 liters/day	Boys = 3.3 liters/day Girls = 2.3 liters/day

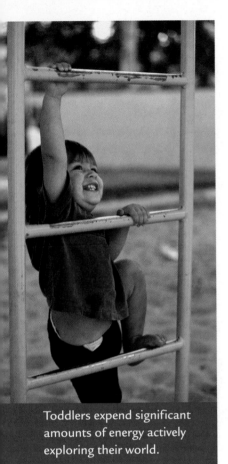

Toddlers expend significant amounts of energy actively exploring their world.

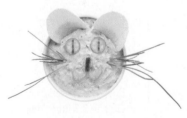

Most toddlers are delighted by food prepared in a "fun" way.

until at least age 2. Toddlers' protein and carbohydrate needs increase modestly; most of the carbohydrates eaten should be complex, and refined carbohydrates should be kept to a minimum. As toddlers grow, their micronutrient needs increase. Of particular concern are adequate intakes of the micronutrients associated with fruits and vegetables, such as vitamins A, C, and E, as well as the minerals calcium, iron, and zinc. See Table 11.4 for nutrient recommendations.

Toddlers sometimes become so busy playing that they ignore or fail to recognize the thirst sensation, so caregivers need to make sure an active toddler is drinking adequately. The recommended total fluid intake for toddlers includes about 4 cups of beverages.[13] Suggested beverages include plain water, milk and soy milk, and diluted fruit juices. Given their typically erratic eating habits, toddlers can develop nutrient deficiencies. That's why many pediatricians recommend a multivitamin and mineral supplement formulated especially for toddlers. As always, if a supplement is given, the recommended dose should not be exceeded. A supplement should not contain more than 100% of the daily value of any nutrient per dose.

> RECAP *Growth during toddlerhood is slower than during infancy; however, toddlers are highly active and need to consume enough energy to fuel growth and activity. Total energy, fat, and protein requirements are higher for toddlers than for infants. Many toddlers will not eat vegetables, so micronutrients of concern include vitamins A, C, and E. Until age 2, healthy toddlers of appropriate weight should drink whole milk rather than reduced-fat (2% or lower) milk to meet calcium requirements and sustain adequate fat intake.*

Encouraging Nutritious Food Choices with Toddlers

Parents and pediatricians have long recognized that toddlers tend to be choosy about what they eat. Some avoid entire foods groups, such as all meats or vegetables. Others will abruptly refuse all but one or two favorite foods (such as peanut butter on crackers) for several days or longer. Still others eat in extremely small amounts, seemingly satisfied by a single slice of apple or two bites of toast. These behaviors frustrate and worry many parents, but in fact, studies have consistently shown that, as long as healthful food is abundant and choices are varied, toddlers have an innate ability to match their intake with their needs. It is the whole nutrition profile over time that matters most, and the toddler will most likely make up for one day's deficiency later on in the week. Parents who offer only foods of high nutritional quality can feel confident that their children are getting the nutrition they need even if their choices seem odd or erratic on any particular day. Food should never be "forced" on a child; doing so sets the stage for eating and control issues later in life.[28]

To encourage nutritious food choices in toddlers, it's important to recognize that their stomachs are still very small and they cannot consume all of the calories they need in three meals. They need small meals, interspersed with nutritious snacks, and should eat every 2 to 3 hours. Toddlers should not be forced to sit still until they finish every bite. A successful snack-time technique used by many experienced parents is to create a snack tray filled with small portions of nutritious food choices, such as one-third of a banana, two pieces of cheese, and three whole-grain pretzels, and leave it within reach of the child's play area. The child can then "graze" on these healthful foods while he or she plays. A snack tray plus a spill-proof cup of milk or water is particularly useful on car trips.

Firm, raw foods such as nuts, carrots, grapes, raisins, and cherry tomatoes are difficult for a toddler to chew, as are cooked, cut-up hotdogs. Such foods pose a choking hazard. Foods should be soft and sliced into strips or wedges that are easy for children to grasp. As the child develops more teeth and becomes more coordinated, the food repertoire can become more varied.

Foods prepared for toddlers should also be fun. Parents can use cookie-cutters to turn a peanut-butter sandwich into a pumpkin face or arrange cooked peas or carrot slices to look like a smiling face on top of mashed potatoes. Juice and low-fat yogurt can be frozen into "popsicles" or blended into "milkshakes."

Even at mealtime, portion sizes should be small. One tablespoon of a food for each year of age constitutes a serving throughout the preschool years (FIGURE 11.5). Realistic portion sizes can give toddlers a sense of accomplishment when they "eat it all up" and lessen parents' fears that their child is not eating enough.

Introduce new foods gradually. Most toddlers are leery of new foods, spicy foods, hot (temperature) foods, mixed foods such as casseroles, and foods with strange textures. A helpful rule is to require the child to eat at least one bite of a new food: if the child does not want the rest, nothing negative should be said and the child should be praised just for the willingness to try. Parents should reintroduce the food a few weeks later because, over time, toddlers will often accept foods they once rejected.

Providing limited healthful alternatives early on will also help toddlers to make nutritious food choices. For example, parents might say, "It's snack time! Would you like apples and cheese or bananas and yogurt?" Toddlers can also help select from a limited range of nutritious foods at the grocery store.

Nutrition-Related Concerns for Toddlers

Just as toddlers have their own specific nutrient needs, they also have toddler-specific nutrition concerns. Some continue from infancy, whereas others are new.

Continued Allergy Watch

As during infancy, new foods should be presented one at a time, and the toddler should be monitored for allergic reactions for 4 to 5 days before introducing additional new foods. To prevent the development of food allergies, even foods that are established in the diet should be rotated rather than served every day.

Vegetarian Families

For toddlers, a lacto-ovo vegetarian diet in which dairy foods and eggs are included can be as wholesome as a diet including meats and fish. However, because meat is an excellent source of zinc and heme iron, the most bioavailable form of iron, families who do not serve meat must be careful to include enough zinc and iron from other sources in their child's diet.

In contrast, a vegan diet, in which no foods of animal origin are consumed, poses several potential nutritional risks for toddlers. For this reason, the practice of feeding children a vegan diet is highly controversial. See the Nutrition Myth or Fact? box for more information about this issue.

RECAP *Toddlers require small, frequent, nutritious meals and snacks, and food should be cut in small pieces so it is easy to handle, chew, and swallow. Because toddlers are becoming more independent and can self-feed, parents need to be alert for choking and should watch for allergies and monitor weight gain. Role modeling by parents and access to ample healthful foods can help toddlers make nutritious choices for snacks and meals. Feeding vegan diets to toddlers is controversial because it poses potential deficiencies for several nutrients.*

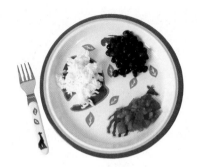

FIGURE 11.5 Portion sizes for preschoolers are much smaller than for older children. Use the following guideline: 1 tablespoon of the food for each year of age equals 1 serving. For example, the meal shown here—2 tablespoons of rice, 2 tablespoons of black beans, and 2 tablespoons of chopped tomatoes—is appropriate for a 2-year-old toddler.

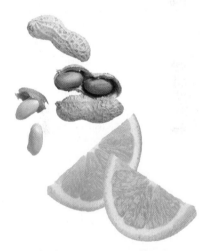

Foods that may cause allergies, such as peanuts and citrus fruits, should be introduced to toddlers one at a time.

Nutrition Throughout Childhood

Children experience an average growth of 2 to 4 inches per year throughout childhood. Distinct developmental markers such as increased language fluency, physical coordination and dexterity, and decision-making skills are characteristic of the childhood years. Between the ages of 3 and 13, children begin to make some of their own food choices. The impact of these decisions on children's health can be profound, so age-appropriate nutrition education is critical.

NUTRITION MYTH OR FACT?

Are Vegan Diets Inappropriate for Young Children?

The practice of feeding a vegan diet to young children is a subject of heated controversy. Many proponents of veganism feel that consumption of any type of animal product is immoral, that feeding animal products to children fosters a lifetime of obesity and chronic disease, and that consumption of animal products wastes natural resources and contributes to environmental damage. In contrast, opponents emphasize that feeding a vegan diet to young children deprives them of a healthful level of essential nutrients that can only be obtained if the child consumes animal products. Some people even suggest that veganism for young children is, in essence, a form of child abuse.

As with many controversies, there are valid concerns on both sides. For example, there have been documented cases of children failing to thrive, and even dying, on extreme vegan diets.[29] Cases have been cited of vitamin B_{12}, calcium, zinc, and vitamin D deficiencies in vegan children. These nutrients are found primarily or almost exclusively in animal products, and deficiencies can have serious and lifelong consequences. For example, not all of the neurologic impairments caused by vitamin B_{12} deficiency can be reversed by timely B_{12} supplement intervention. In addition, inadequate zinc, calcium, and vitamin D can result in impaired bone growth and strength and failure to reach peak bone mass.

However, close inspection of the cases of nutrition-related illness in children that cite veganism as the culprit reveals that lack of education, fanaticism, and/or extremism is usually at the root of the problem. Informed parents following responsible vegan diets are rarely involved. On the other hand, such cases do point out that veganism is not a lifestyle one can safely undertake without thorough education regarding the necessity of supplementation of those nutrients not available in plant products. For example, it is very difficult for a young child to maintain iron status without including sources of heme iron, which are totally absent in a vegan diet. Parents also need to understand that typical vegan diets are high in fiber and low in fat, and that this combination can be dangerous for very young children. Moreover, certain staples of the vegan diet, such as wheat, soy, and nuts, commonly provoke allergic reactions in children; when this happens, finding a plant-based substitute that contains adequate nutrients can be challenging.

On the other hand, both the American Dietetic Association and the American Academy of Pediatrics have stated that a vegan diet can promote normal growth and development—*provided* that adequate supplements and/or fortified foods are consumed to account for the nutrients that are normally found in animal products. However, most health-care organizations stop short of outright endorsement of a vegan diet for young children. Instead, many advocate a more moderate approach during the early childhood years. Reasons for this level of caution include acknowledgment of several factors:

- Some vegan parents are not adequately educated on the planning of meals, the balancing of foods, and the inclusion of supplements to ensure adequate levels of all nutrients.
- Most young children are picky eaters and are hesitant to eat certain food groups, particularly vegetables, a staple in the vegan diet.
- The high fiber content of vegan diets may not be appropriate for very young children.
- Young children have small stomachs, and they are not able to consume enough plant-based foods to ensure adequate intakes of all nutrients and energy.

Because of these concerns, most nutrition experts advise parents to take a more moderate dietary approach, one that emphasizes plant foods but also includes some animal-based foods, such as fish, dairy, and/or eggs. Once children reach school age, the low fat, abundant fiber, antioxidants, and many micronutrients in a carefully planned vegan diet will promote their health as they progress into adulthood.

What Are a Child's Nutrient Needs?

By age 3, children exposed to a wide variety of foods typically have developed a varied diet. Nevertheless, children cannot be expected to consume all of the nutrients they need in three meals. Thus, nutrient-dense snacks continue to be important. Table 11.4 identifies the nutrient needs of children age 3 to 8 and 9 to 13.

Macronutrient Recommendations for Children

Fat remains a key macronutrient in childhood, and children's fat intakes should be around 25% to 35% of total energy.[8] A diet lower in fat is not recommended for healthy children of school age, as they are still growing, developing, and maturing.

Total need for protein increases, but the need for carbohydrate remains the same as for toddlers. Fiber-rich carbohydrates are important and simple sugars should come from fruits and fruit juices, with refined-carbohydrate items such as cakes, cookies, and candies saved for occasional indulgences. Too much fiber, however, can be detrimental because it can make a child feel full and interfere with food intake and nutrient absorption.

Micronutrient Recommendations for Children

Children who fail to consume the recommended 5 or more servings of fruits and vegetables each day may become deficient in vitamins A, C, and E. Minerals of concern continue to be calcium, iron, and zinc, which come primarily from animal-based foods (see Table 11.4). Notice that calcium needs increase dramatically in children age 9 to 13 to allow for increased bone growth and density.

If there is any doubt that a child's nutrient needs are not being met for any reason (for instance, breakfasts are skipped, lunches are traded, parents lack money for nourishing food, etc.), a vitamin/mineral supplement that provides no more than 100% of the daily value for the micronutrients may help to correct any existing deficit.

Fluid Recommendations for Children

Fluid recommendations for children are shown in Table 11.4. The exact amount of fluid a child needs varies according to level of physical activity and weather conditions. Under most circumstances, water remains the beverage of choice; sports beverages, fruit drinks, and sodas provide excess calories that can, over time, contribute to inappropriate weight gain.

RECAP *Children experience an average growth of 2 to 4 inches per year. They need a lower percentage of fat calories than toddlers but slightly more than adults (25% to 35% of energy). Micronutrient needs increase because of growth and maturation. Children can become easily dehydrated, especially during vigorous activity in warm weather.*

Encouraging Nutritious Food Choices with Children

Most children can understand that some foods will "help them grow up healthy and strong" and that other foods will not. Because children want to grow as quickly as possible, parents can capitalize on this natural desire and, using age-appropriate language, encourage foods high in fiber-rich carbohydrates, protein, and micronutrients.

However, peer pressure can be extremely difficult for both parents and their children to deal with during this life stage. If a popular child is eating chips and drinking sugared soft drinks, it may be hard for a child to eat her tuna-on-whole-wheat sandwich, apple, and milk without embarrassment.

Continuing education is helpful. Parents can go online with their child to the MyPyramid.gov site and print out a personalized pyramid and the MyPyramid for Kids poster (FIGURE 11.6). The MyPyramid for Kids poster provides age-appropriate nutrition information in a colorful cartoon symbol that tells children to "Eat Right. Exercise. Have Fun." Also available with the poster are an interactive game, coloring page, worksheet, tips for families, and lesson plans for teachers.

Parents can also continue to involve children in food choices.[28] For instance, children can have their own weekly shopping list on which they can write nutritious

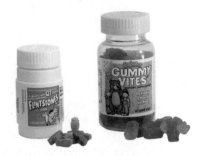

Children's multivitamins often appear in shapes or bright colors.

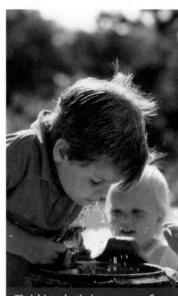

Fluid intake is important for children, who may become so involved in their play that they ignore the sensation of thirst.

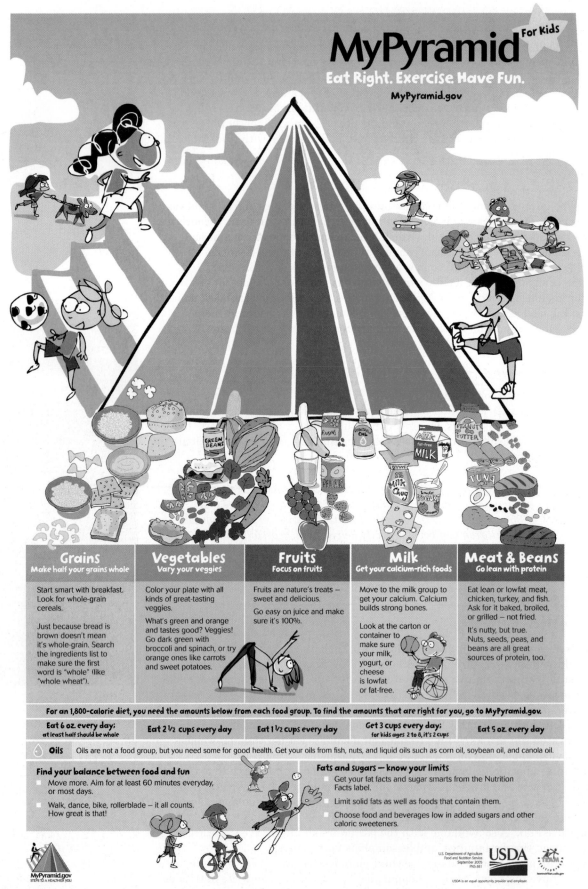

FIGURE 11.6 MyPyramid for Kids. This symbol modifies the MyPyramid graphic for the nutrition needs of children aged 6 to 11, and teaches them to "Eat Right. Exercise. Have Fun."

favorites like strawberries or whole-wheat pretzels that they'd like their parents to buy. If children have input into what is going into their bodies, they may be more likely to take an active role in their health.

What Is the Effect of School Attendance on Nutrition?

School attendance can affect a child's nutrition in several ways. First, in the hectic time between waking and getting out the door, many children minimize or skip breakfast completely. Students who don't eat breakfast are more likely to do poorly on schoolwork, have decreased attention spans, and have more behavioral problems than their peers who do eat breakfast.[30-31] Public schools are required to offer low-cost school breakfasts that are free of charge to low-income families. Taking advantage of these breakfasts can help children avoid hunger in the classroom. We discuss the benefits of eating breakfast in more detail in the Nutrition Myth or Fact? box later in this chapter (page 366).

Another consequence of attending school is that, with no one monitoring what they eat, children do not always consume adequate amounts of food. They may spend their lunch time conversing or playing with friends rather than eating. If a school lunch is purchased, they might not like the foods being served, or their peers might influence them to skip certain foods with comments such as, "This broccoli is yucky!" Even homemade lunches that contain nutritious foods may be left uneaten or traded for less nutritious fare.

Are school lunches nutritious? On the surface, the answer to this question is "yes." All school lunches must meet certain nutrition requirements set forth by federal guidelines, including the Healthy Meals for Healthy Americans Act.[32] However, the actual proportion of nutrients a student *gets* depends on what the student actually *eats*. School lunch programs do not have to meet the federal guidelines every day and for each individual meal, but only over the course of a full week's meals. Thus, the school lunches that students actually eat tend to be high in fat and low in nutrients because students choose foods they like, such as pizza, hamburgers, hot dogs, or French fries, instead of veggie lasagna, lentil soup, a baked potato, or carrots. In addition, some schools actually have fast-food restaurants selling their food in competition with the school lunch program! The School Nutrition Association promotes "nutrition integrity" for all schools, including the provision of healthful foods and beverages, nutrition education, physical activity, and a healthful school environment.[33] Locally developed school-based nutrition education programs and implementation of recent USDA-mandated wellness policies, supported by parental involvement, can help improve students' food choices and activity patterns, thus enhancing lifelong health.[32]

Despite recent federal and state legislation, along with new industry-sponsored initiatives to limit the sales of snack foods, some schools still provide vending machines filled with foods and beverages that are high in energy, sugar, and fat. Eating too many of these foods, either in place of or in addition to lunch, can lead to overweight and potential nutrient deficiencies. Nutrition standards have recently been developed to encourage schools to sell only those foods and beverages that promote a healthful diet.[34]

Nutrition-Related Concerns for Children

Two significant nutrition-related concerns for children are food insecurity and overweight. These are discussed in the following sections.

Childhood Food Insecurity

Although most children in the United States grow up with an abundant and healthful supply of food, a small but persistent percentage of children are faced with food insecurity and hunger. *Food insecurity* occurs when a family is not able to ensure a predictable supply of safe and nutritious food or is unable to acquire food in a

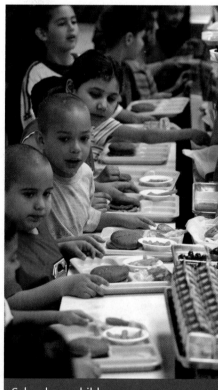

School-age children may receive a standard school lunch, but many young people choose to eat less healthful foods when given the opportunity.

socially acceptable manner; in other words, the parents might have to steal food, forage for food in trash receptacles, or beg for food.[35] Approximately 12% of U.S. households with children can be classified as food insecure.[35] More than 80% of these households limit the variety of foods offered to their children, more than 50% are not always able to afford foods for balanced meals, and 25% indicate their children don't get enough to eat because of lack of money.

The effects of food insecurity can be very harmful to young children. Impaired nutrient status can blunt children's immune responses, making them more susceptible to common childhood illnesses. Poorly nourished preschoolers often fail to achieve their full growth potential, falling off their normal growth curve. Iron-deficiency anemia can develop, and deficiencies of vitamin D and/or calcium can keep children from attaining optimal bone density.

Options for families facing food insecurity include government programs such as WIC (Women, Infants, and Children), the USDA Child and Adult Care Food Program (CACFP), and school breakfast and lunch programs. Private and church-based food pantries and kitchens can provide a narrow range of foods for a limited period of time but cannot be relied on to meet the nutritional needs of young children and their families over an extended period of time.

Obesity Watch: Encouraging an Active Lifestyle

As with adults, the problem of overweight and obesity in children is now approaching epidemic proportions in the United States.[1] Nationwide, about 19% of U.S. school-aged children 6 to 11 years of age are overweight, as are 17% of 12 to 19 year olds.[1] These children are at higher risk of several health problems: overweight can exacerbate asthma, contribute to the development of type 2 diabetes, cause sleep apnea, impair the child's mobility, and lead to intense teasing, low self-esteem, and social isolation.

In the past decade, the skyrocketing rate of childhood obesity has become a concern of nutritionists, physicians, educators, and policy makers. Experts agree that the main culprits are similar to those involved in adult obesity: eating too much and moving around too little. Thus, they recommend a two-pronged approach: establishing healthful eating practices that work for the whole family, as well as increasing physical activity (see Chapter 10).

Because of the high nutrient needs of children, restrictive diets are not advised. Rather, parents should strive to consistently provide nutritious food choices. Families should also sit down together to a shared family meal each evening. The television should be off throughout dinner to encourage slow eating and true enjoyment of the food.

To encourage activity throughout the day, parents should limit their own and their children's television watching to no more than 2 hours per day. Time spent watching television not only reduces time available for physical activity but can increase energy intake: children often snack excessively on high-calorie, low-nutrient snack foods while they watch television. Moreover, an abundance of television commercials during children's programs advertise less healthful foods, such as sweetened breakfast cereals made with refined grains, high-sugar yogurt products, candies, pastries, and high-fat snacks. Even parents who limit television watching should sit with their children during several commercials and explain to them, in age-appropriate language, that these foods are made to look appealing to kids and are not healthful choices.

Parents should encourage children to replace television watching, computer games, and other sedentary activities with physical activity, especially shared activities such as ball games, hikes, and so forth. Newly developed electronic game systems encourage indoor physical activity through virtual tennis, bowling, dancing, and other sport simulations. When parents and children are active together, healthful activity patterns are established early. Over time, overweight children who are encouraged to be active can "catch up" to their weight as they grow taller without restricting their intake of healthful foods. Increased activity also helps young children acquire motor skills and muscle strength and develop self-esteem as they feel themselves becoming faster, stronger, and more skilled.

The Institute of Medicine recommends that children participate in daily physical activity and exercise for at least an hour each day.[8] Children should be exposed to a

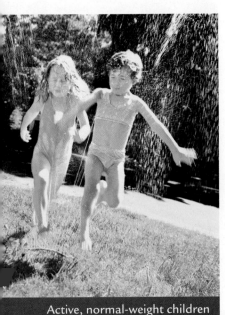

Active, normal-weight children are less likely to become overweight adults.

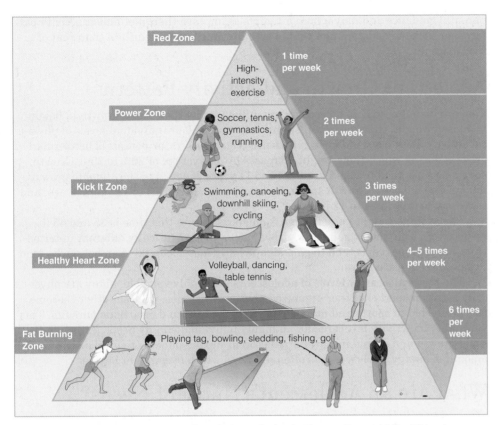

Red Zone
High-intensity exercise
1 time per week

Power Zone
Soccer, tennis, gymnastics, running
2 times per week

Kick It Zone
Swimming, canoeing, downhill skiing, cycling
3 times per week

Healthy Heart Zone
Volleyball, dancing, table tennis
4–5 times per week

6 times per week

Fat Burning Zone
Playing tag, bowling, sledding, fishing, golf

FIGURE 11.7 The American Dietetic Association's Fitness Pyramid for Kids gives guidelines for the duration, intensity, and frequency of various types of activities that are appropriate for children aged 2 to 11 years.
(*Source:* Reprinted from *Journal of the American Dietetic Association,* V. 104, Position of the American Dietetic Association: Dietary Guidance for Healthy Children Ages 2 to 11 years, pp. 660–667. © 2004, with permission from Elsevier.)

variety of activities so that they move different muscles, play at various intensities, avoid boredom, and find out what they like and don't like to do. The American Dietetic Association has designed a Fitness Pyramid for Kids to help guide children toward a physically active lifestyle (FIGURE 11.7).

RECAP *Peer pressure has a strong influence on children's nutritional choices. Educating children and involving them in food purchasing and preparation can help them make more healthful choices. School breakfasts and lunches must meet federal nutrition guidelines, but the foods that children actually choose to eat can be high in fat, sugar, and energy and low in nutrients. Food insecurity is a significant nutritional concern for U.S. children. Rates of childhood overweight and obesity are rising, and all children should be encouraged to be active at least 1 hour every day.*

Nutrition for Adolescents

The adolescent years begin with the onset of **puberty,** the period in life in which secondary sexual characteristics develop and there is the capacity for reproducing. Adolescence is characterized by increasing independence and autonomy, when the adolescent establishes a personal sense of identity and works toward greater self-reliance. All teens deal with their emerging sexuality, and many experiment with behaviors, such as smoking and drinking, that lie outside their traditional cultural or social boundaries. During this developmental phase, they may be unresponsive to

puberty The period in life in which secondary sexual characteristics develop and people are biologically capable of reproducing.

parental guidance and may ignore attempts to improve their diet and/or activity patterns, or they may adopt a diet that is actually much more healthful than that of their parents.

Adolescent Growth and Activity Patterns

The nutritional needs of adolescents are influenced by their rapid growth in height, increased weight, changes in body composition, and their individual levels of physical activity. Both boys and girls experience *growth spurts,* or periods of accelerated growth, during which their height increases by an average of 20% to 25%. Growth spurts for girls tend to begin around 10 to 11 years of age, and they tend to grow a total of 2 to 8 inches. Growth spurts for boys begin around 12 to 13 years of age, and they tend to grow by 4 to 12 inches.[36]

The average weight gained by girls and boys during this time is 35 and 45 lb, respectively. The weight gained by girls and boys is dramatically different in terms of its composition. Girls tend to gain significantly more body fat than boys, who tend to gain more muscle mass.

The physical activity levels of adolescents are highly variable. Many are physically active in sports or other organized physical activities, whereas others become less interested in sports and more interested in intellectual or artistic pursuits. This variability in activity levels results in highly individual energy needs. Although the rapid growth and sexual maturation that occur during puberty require a significant amount of energy, adolescence is often a time in which overweight begins.

What Are an Adolescent's Nutrient Needs?

The nutrient needs of adolescents are influenced by rapid growth, weight gain, and sexual maturation, in addition to the demands of physical activity.

Energy and Macronutrient Recommendations for Adolescents

Adequate energy intake is necessary to maintain adolescents' health, support their dramatic growth and maturation, and fuel their physical activity. Because of these competing demands, the energy needs of adolescents can be quite high. Dieting to lose weight should only be undertaken under the guidance of a physician or registered dietitian, and fad diets should be strictly avoided.

Because adolescents are at risk for the same chronic diseases as adults, they are advised to consume 25% to 35% of total energy from fat and to consume no more than 10% of total energy from saturated fat. Adolescents should consume about 45%

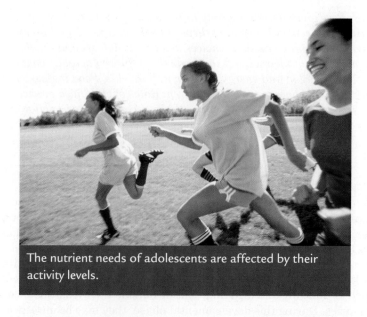

The nutrient needs of adolescents are affected by their activity levels.

to 65% of their total energy as carbohydrate, and most carbohydrate should come from fiber-rich sources. The RDA for protein for adolescents is similar to that of adults, at 0.85 g of protein per kilogram of body weight per day. This amount is assumed to be sufficient to support health and to cover the additional needs of growth and development during the adolescent stage.

Micronutrient Recommendations for Adolescents

Micronutrients of particular concern for adolescents include calcium, iron, and vitamin A. Adequate calcium intake is critical to achieve peak bone density. The AI for calcium remains high throughout adolescence and can be difficult to consume for teens who do not drink milk or calcium-fortified beverages.

As shown in Table 11.4, the iron needs of adolescents are relatively high to replace the blood lost during menstruation in girls and to support the growth of muscle mass in boys. If energy intake is adequate and adolescents consume animal products each day, they should be able to meet the RDA for iron. However, some young people adopt a vegetarian lifestyle during this life stage, or they consume foods that have limited nutrient density. Both of these situations can prevent adolescents from meeting the RDA for iron.

Vitamin A is critical to support the rapid growth and development that occurs during adolescence. Consuming at least 5 servings of fruits and vegetables each day can help teens meet their RDA (see Table 11.4).

If an adolescent is unable or unwilling to eat adequate amounts of nutrient-dense foods, then a multivitamin and mineral supplement that provides no more than 100% of the Daily Value for the micronutrients could be beneficial as a safety net. As with younger children and adults, a supplement should not be considered a substitute for a balanced, healthful diet.

Fluid Recommendations for Adolescents

The AI for total fluid for adolescent boys includes about 11 cups as beverages, including drinking water. The AI for girls includes about 8 cups as beverages. Boys are generally more active than girls and have more lean tissue, so they require a higher fluid intake. Highly active adolescents who are exercising in the heat may have higher fluid needs than the AI and should drink often to avoid dehydration.

> RECAP *Adolescents experience rapid increases in height, weight, and lean body mass and fat mass, so energy needs can be very high. Percentages of fat, carbohydrate, and protein intake should be similar to that of adults. Because many adolescents fail to eat a variety of nutrient-dense foods, intakes of some nutrients may be deficient. Calcium is needed to optimize bone growth and to achieve peak bone density, and iron needs are increased due to increased muscle mass in boys and to menstruation in girls.*

Encouraging Nutritious Food Choices with Adolescents

Adolescents make most of their own food choices, and many are also buying and preparing a significant amount of the foods they consume. Although parents can still be effective role models, adolescents are generally strongly influenced by their peers, mass media, and their own developing sense of what foods compose a healthful and adequate diet.

Of frequent concern in the adolescent diet is a lack of vegetables, fruits, dairy, and whole grains. Many teens eat on the run from fast-food restaurants, convenience stores, and vending machines, where these healthful foods may not be available. In addition, many teens skip meals. For instance, adolescent girls often skip breakfast because they believe it might make them fat and are concerned about gaining weight. Other teens skip breakfast because they're rushing to get to school.[37] Whatever the reason, many nutrition experts believe that adolescents who skip

NUTRITION MYTH OR FACT?

Is Breakfast the Most Important Meal of the Day?

What did you eat for breakfast this morning? Whole-grain cereal with low-fat milk? A strawberry Pop-Tart? Or nothing? What does it matter, anyway? Sure, you've heard the saying that breakfast is the most important meal of the day, but that's just a myth—isn't it? As long as you eat a nutritious meal at lunch and dinner, why should skipping breakfast matter?

Over the past two decades, literally dozens of published studies have pointed to the importance of a healthful breakfast. Most of these studies cite two key health benefits: First, breakfast supports our physical and mental functioning. Second, it helps us maintain a healthful weight. Let's examine the evidence for each of these claims.

The word *breakfast* was initially used as a verb meaning "to break the fast"; that is, to end the hours of fasting that naturally occur during a night of sleep. When we fast, our bodies break down stored nutrients to provide energy to fuel the resting body. First, cells break down glycogen stores in the muscle tissues and liver, using the "freed" glucose for energy. These stores last about 12 hours. But people who skip breakfast fast much longer than that: if they finish dinner around 7:00 p.m. and don't eat again until noon the next day, they're going without fuel for 17 hours! Long before this point, essentially all stored glycogen is used up, and the body turns to fatty acids and amino acids as fuel sources.

If you're like most people, when your blood glucose is low, you experience not only hunger, but also weakness, shakiness, irritability, and poor concentration. So it's not surprising that children and teens who skip breakfast don't function as well—either physically or academically—as their breakfast-eating peers.[30-31] The Food Research & Action Center (FRAC) cites more than 20 studies supporting the following conclusions:[38]

- Missing breakfast and experiencing hunger impair children's ability to learn. These children exhibit slower memory recall, score lower on cognitive tests, have more behavioral and emotional problems, and are more likely to have to repeat a grade than children who arrive at school in a well-nourished state.

- Eating breakfast at school helps children perform better on demanding mental tasks, and improves attention and memory. Children who eat a complete breakfast make fewer mistakes and work faster in math and vocabulary.

- Breakfast improves students' behavior, including improving their reaction to frustration, reducing disciplinary office referrals, decreasing tardiness, and increasing school attendance rates.

But what about the claim that eating breakfast helps us maintain a healthful weight? Although it seems counterintuitive, the evidence that eating breakfast helps prevent weight gain is striking. For instance, a 2005 study found that girls who ate breakfast were more likely to have a lower BMI than girls who skipped breakfast.[39] A 2006 study of adolescents with one or two obese parents found that those teens who ate breakfast every day were more likely to have BMIs within a healthy range than those who tended to skip breakfast.[40] Additionally, a 2008 study of more than 2,000 adolescents reported that the more often adolescents ate breakfast, the lower their BMI. Why eating breakfast is linked to lower BMI is unclear, but researchers noted that both boys and girls who consistently ate breakfast also had an overall diet higher in fiber. They speculated that consumption of fiber-rich foods such as cereals at breakfast may improve blood glucose and insulin levels, making adolescents feel satisfied and less likely to eat more later in the day.[41]

Skeptics say the studies' conclusions suggest an *association* between eating breakfast and health benefits, but not a *cause*. They say, for example, that the same parents who insist their kids eat a healthful breakfast are likely to be those who also make sure their kids get adequate sleep, help with their kids' homework, and monitor their TV watching. Others speculate that kids who avoid breakfast may, in general, be slow starters, and may be poorly adapted to academic work or physical activity in the morning as well.

What do you think? Is breakfast the most important meal of the day? And what—if anything—will you be having for breakfast tomorrow?

breakfast are hurting both their performance in school and their health. Is breakfast the most important meal of the day? Check out the Nutrition Myth or Fact? box above to find the answer.

Parents and school food-service programs can capitalize on adolescents' preferences for pizza, burgers, spaghetti, and sandwiches by providing more healthful versions of these foods, as well as appealing vegetable-based sides. In addition, keeping on hand raw fruits and vegetables that are already cleaned and sliced may encourage adolescents to consume more of these foods as between-meal snacks. Teens should also be encouraged to consume adequate milk and other calcium-enriched beverages.

Nutrition-Related Concerns for Adolescents

Nutrition-related concerns for adolescents continue to include bone density and overweight. Additional concerns include disordered eating, acne, and the use of alcohol and tobacco products.

Bone-Density Watch

Early adolescence, 13 to 15 years of age, is a crucial time for ensuring adequate dietary calcium in order to maximize bone mineral density over the next several years.[12] Achieving and maintaining optimal bone density during adolescence and into young adulthood is critical for reducing the risk of osteoporosis.

Meeting the adolescent DRI for calcium (1,300 mg/day) requires a daily consumption of at least 4 servings (4 cups) of milk or other dairy foods, calcium-fortified foods and beverages, or supplements. It is extremely challenging to meet the adolescent DRI for calcium from plant-based foods alone. Yet, by age 18, average fluid milk consumption has fallen below 1 cup per day while soda intake has doubled.[42] While not the only factor, milk consumption during adolescence is strongly linked to higher bone mineral content and lower risk of adult bone fractures.[43]

Obesity Watch: Balancing Food and Physical Activity

Although expected and healthful, weight gain during adolescence can become excessive if increased energy intake is not balanced with adequate physical activity. Only 36% of U.S. high school students report completing at least 60 minutes of physical activity on most or all days of the week, clear evidence that activity is often inadequate during adolescence.[44] By offering daily physical education in school and by providing more opportunities and encouragement for adolescents to participate in regular physical activity outside of school, the prevalence of overweight and obesity among adolescents can be reduced.

Disordered Eating and Eating Disorders

An initially healthful concern about body image and weight can turn into a dangerous obsession during this emotionally challenging life stage. Clinical eating disorders frequently begin during adolescence and can occur in boys as well as girls. Parents, teachers, and friends should be aware of the warning signs, which include rapid and excessive weight loss, a preoccupation with weight and body image, going to the bathroom regularly after meals, and signs of frequent vomiting or laxative use. Refer to Chapter 9 for a discussion of eating disorders.

Adolescent Acne and Diet

The hormonal changes that occur during puberty are largely responsible for the acne flare-ups that plague many adolescents. Emotional stress, genetic factors, and personal hygiene are most likely secondary contributors. But what about foods? For decades, chocolate, fried foods, fatty foods, and other foods have been wrongfully linked to acne; it is now believed that diet has virtually no role in its development.[45] On the other hand, a healthful diet, rich in fruits, vegetables, whole grains, and lean meats, can provide vitamin A, vitamin C, zinc, and other nutrients to optimize skin health and maintain an effective immune system.

Prescription medications, including a vitamin A derivative called Accutane, effectively control severe forms of acne. Neither Accutane nor any other prescription vitamin A derivative should be used by women who are pregnant or who may become pregnant. Accutane is a known teratogen, causing severe fetal malformations. Women of childbearing age who want to treat their acne with vitamin A–derivative prescription drugs must register in a risk management program developed by the

FDA called iPLEDGE. This program requires patients and their physicians to agree to assume specific responsibilities to ensure that patients do not become pregnant while taking the drug. In addition to its known role in birth defects, Accutane has been associated with depression, psychosis, suicidal thoughts or actions, aggressive or violent behavior, and serious brain problems.[46] For these reasons, the drug should be considered only for teens who have severe, disfiguring acne, and anyone using it should be monitored closely for signs of depression, irritability, and other emotional changes.

Use of Alcohol and Tobacco

Many adolescents experiment with alcohol and tobacco. The risks of alcohol consumption among teens and adults were discussed extensively in Chapter 8. Cigarette smoking diminishes appetite, interferes with nutrient metabolism, reduces physical fitness, damages the lungs, increases the incidence of respiratory illness, and promotes addiction to nicotine. Most people who begin smoking during adolescence continue to smoke throughout adulthood, increasing their risks for lung cancer, heart disease, osteoporosis, and emphysema.

Cigarette smoking may interfere with nutrient metabolism.

RECAP *The food choices of adolescents are influenced by peer pressure, personal preferences, and their own developing sense of what foods are healthful. Adolescents are at risk for skipping meals and selecting fast-food meals and low-nutrient snack foods. Milk is commonly replaced with soft drinks. Obesity can occur during adolescence because of increased appetite and food intake and decreased physical activity. Disordered eating behaviors, consumption of alcohol, and cigarette smoking are additional risks in this age group.*

Nutrition for Older Adults

The U.S. population is getting older each year. In 2003, almost 36 million people aged 65 and older lived in the United States, representing about 12% of the population.[47] It is estimated that by the year 2030, the elderly will account for about 20% of Americans, or more than 71 million adults (FIGURE 11.8).

In 2004, the average U.S. **life expectancy,** which is the average number of years that a person may be expected to live, reached 77.8 years.[48] Whereas some researchers have argued that the growing rate of obesity and its medical consequences will drive down U.S. life expectancy over the next several decades, others refute this claim, saying that future advances in healthcare will balance this factor.

Life span is the age to which the longest-living member of the species has lived. Madame Jeanne Calment, born in 1875, survived to the age of 122 and is generally acknowledged as having lived longer than anyone else in the world. Researchers have made great progress toward understanding the aging of humans, but much remains unknown. Scientists can't even agree when the aging process begins: some believe it starts at birth, others argue it begins after peak reproductive age.[49] While the debate continues, however, gerontologists agree that humans can positively impact the aging process through personal choices, such as eating a nourishing diet, participating in regular physical activity, and avoiding smoking and substance abuse.

Physiologic Changes That Accompany Aging

Aging is natural and inevitable; however, the changes that typically accompany aging are at least partly within your control. For instance, decreased muscle strength is partly due to low physical activity levels. Older adults who regularly participate in strengthening exercises and aerobic-type activities experience less muscle atrophy and weakness.

For most of us, eating is a social and pleasurable process; the sights, sounds, odors, and textures associated with food are integral to the stimulation and continuation of appetite. With age comes the decline of taste, odor, and tactile and visual

life expectancy   The expected number of years remaining in one's life; typically stated from the time of birth: children born in the United States in 2003 could expect to live, on average, 77.6 years.

life span   The highest age reached by any member of a species; currently, the human life span is 122 years.

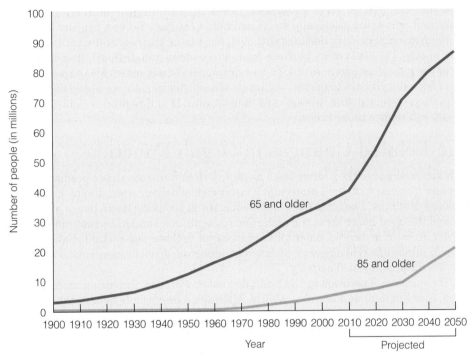

FIGURE 11.8 Growth in the population of older adults in the United States. Data for age 65 and older and age 85 and older are provided. Data for 2010–2050 are projections. Notice that between 2010 and 2050, researchers anticipate a sharp increase in the population of Americans age 65 and older.

perception: the more each of these functions becomes impaired, the greater the potential impact on the person's food intake. For example, loss of visual acuity may result in difficulty reading food labels, including nutrient information and "pull dates" for perishable foods. Driving skills decline, limiting the ability of some older Americans to get to markets that sell healthful, affordable foods. Older adults may no longer be able to read their favorite recipes or distinguish the small markings on temperature knobs on ovens and stoves. Their diet may thus consist of a few foods that are easy to prepare, such as cereal with milk and sandwiches with cold cuts, and may lack the variety necessary to prevent nutrient deficiencies.

With increasing age, salivary production declines. Thus, teeth are more susceptible to decay, chewing and swallowing become more difficult, and the risk for choking increases. Achlorhydria, a severe reduction in gastric acid production, limits the absorption of minerals such as calcium, iron, and zinc and food sources of folic acid and vitamin B_{12}. Lack of intrinsic factor reduces the absorption of vitamin B_{12}, whether from food or supplements. Older adults may also experience a delay in gastric emptying, resulting in a prolonged sense of fullness and a reduced appetite. Because only about 30% of older adults retain an "adequate" level of lactase activity, many restrict their milk intake and fail to consume adequate calcium.

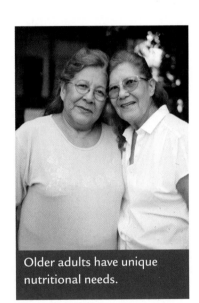

Older adults have unique nutritional needs.

Age-Related Changes in Body Composition

With aging, muscle mass declines. It has been estimated that women and men lose 20% to 25% of their lean body mass, respectively, as they age from 35 to 70 years.[49] Decreased production of certain hormones and chronic diseases contribute to this loss of muscle, as do poor diet and an inactive lifestyle. Along with adequate dietary intake, regular physical activity, including strength or resistance training, can help older adults maintain or enhance their muscle mass and strength.

Body fat increases from young adulthood through middle age, peaking at approximately 55 to 65 years of age. It remains somewhat stable through about age 70 and then tends to decline. With aging, body fat shifts from subcutaneous stores, just

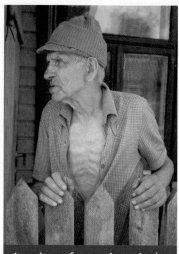

A variety of gastrointestinal and other physiologic changes can lead to weight loss in older adults.

below the skin, to internal or visceral fat stores. Maintaining an appropriate energy intake and remaining physically active can help keep body fat to a healthy level.

Bone mineral density declines with age, increasing the risk of fracture. Among older women, the onset of menopause leads to a sudden and dramatic loss of bone due to the lack of estrogen. Although less dramatic, elderly males also experience loss of bone due in part to decreasing levels of testosterone. A nourishing diet with adequate protein, calcium, phosphorus, and vitamin D and regular weight-bearing activity can reduce these losses.

Age-Related Changes in Organ Function

With increasing age, the kidney loses its ability to concentrate waste products, leading to an increase in urine output and greater risk of dehydration. Bladder control also often declines. The aged liver is less efficient at breaking down drugs and alcohol, and the aged heart lacks the endurance to sustain a sudden increase in physical activity. In most instances, older adults can adapt to these age-related changes through minor lifestyle adjustments such as reducing alcohol consumption and gradually increasing physical activity.

The number of neurons in the brain decreases with age, impairing memory, reflexes, coordination, and learning ability. Although many people believe that dementia is an inevitable part of the aging process, this is not true: diet, physical activity, intellectual stimulation, social contact, and other factors can help preserve the health of the brain as well as the body.

Factors That Accelerate the Aging Process

It is never too late to change our personal habits. Many older adults can enhance their remaining years by paying close attention to their diet, activity, and personal health practices.

The Genetics of Aging

There is no doubt that genes exert tremendous influence on the aging process. Siblings of centenarians, those who live to be 100 years old or greater, are four times more likely to live into their nineties than others.[49] The brother of Madame Calment, previously introduced as the world's oldest human, himself survived to the age of 97. A number of studies currently under way suggest that our genetic makeup does influence our cellular aging and life span.

The Biochemistry of Aging

As cells age, they undergo many changes in structure and function.[49] Some cells, such as skeletal and cardiac muscle, atrophy or decrease in size, whereas others, including fat cells, enlarge. Many gerontologists have linked the aging process to a progressive accumulation of free radicals, known to damage DNA and various cell proteins. Others cite a progressive failure in DNA repair. Still others point to abnormal attachment of glucose to proteins in our tissues. Cell membrane function certainly declines with age, allowing waste products to accumulate within the cell and preventing normal uptake of nutrients and oxygen.

Lifestyle and Environmental Influences on Aging

The way we live greatly influences the way we age. While **chronologic age** is immovable, **biologic age** is in large part due to our personal choices. Accelerated or unsuccessful aging is marked by premature loss of function, high rates of disability, and multiple disease complications. It is now possible to estimate how long you are likely to live by answering a series of scored questions related to smoking habits, sun exposure, family history, weight status, alcohol consumption, food choices, and other factors. Are you curious about your longevity? Check out the quiz at http://preventdisease.com/healthtools/articles/health_age.html to find out!

chronologic age Age as defined by calendar years, from date of birth.

biologic age Physiologic age as determined by health and functional status; often estimated by scored questionnaires.

> RECAP *The physiological changes that occur with aging include sensory declines, loss of muscle mass and lean tissue, increased fat mass, decreased bone density, and impaired ability to absorb and metabolize various nutrients. Body organs lose functional capacity and are less tolerant of stressors. Many of these changes influence the nutritional needs of older adults and their ability to consume a healthful diet.*

What Are an Older Adult's Nutrient Needs?

The requirements for many nutrients are the same for older adults as for young and middle-aged adults. A few nutrient requirements increase, and a few are actually lower. Table 11.5 identifies nutrient recommendations important to older adults.

Energy and Macronutrient Recommendations for Older Adults

The energy needs of older adults are lower than those of younger adults. This decrease is primarily due to a loss of muscle mass and lean tissue, which results in a lower basal metabolic rate, and a less physically active lifestyle, which lowers total energy requirements. Some of this decrease in energy expenditure is an inevitable response to aging, but some of the decrease can be delayed or minimized by staying physically active. Because energy needs are lower, older adults need to pay particularly close attention to consuming a diet high in nutrient-dense foods but not too high in energy in order to avoid weight gain. Refer to the Highlight at the end of this chapter to learn more about the theory of caloric restriction, which proposes that energy-restricted diets may significantly prolong our life span.

The DRIs for total fat, protein, and carbohydrate for older adults are the same for adults of all ages. After age 50, however, fiber needs decrease slightly: 30 g of fiber per day for men and 21 g per day for women is assumed sufficient to reduce the risks for constipation and diverticular disease, maintain healthful blood levels of glucose and lipids, and to provide good sources of nutrient-dense, low-energy foods.

Micronutrient Recommendations for Older Adults

The vitamin and mineral recommendations that change for older adults are identified in Table 11.5. Although zinc recommendations are the same for all adults, zinc is a critical nutrient for optimizing immune function and wound healing in older adults. Intakes of both zinc and iron can be inadequate in older adults if they may eat less red meat, poultry, and fish. These foods are relatively expensive and older adults on a limited income may not be able to afford to eat them regularly. Also, some older adults find it difficult to chew meats properly.

Vitamin A requirements are also the same for adults of all ages; however, older adults should be careful not to consume more than the RDA, as absorption of vitamin A is actually greater in older adults. Thus, this group is at greater risk for vitamin A toxicity, which can cause liver damage, neurological problems, and increased risk of bone fracture. However, consuming foods high in beta-carotene or other carotenoids is safe and does not lead to vitamin A toxicity.

Older adults need to pay close attention to consuming adequate amounts of the B-complex vitamins, particularly vitamin B_{12}, vitamin B_6, and folate. Inadequate intakes of these vitamins increases blood levels of homocysteine, an amino acid that some researchers have linked to increased risk of heart disease and dementia. Older adults need larger amounts of vitamin B_6 in their diets and, as discussed in Chapter 6, they should get most of their vitamin B_{12} from supplements or fortified foods.

Fluid Recommendations for Older Adults

The AI for fluid is the same for older and younger adults. Many elderly do not perceive thirst as effectively as do younger adults and can develop dehydration. Some older adults will intentionally limit their beverage intake because they have urinary

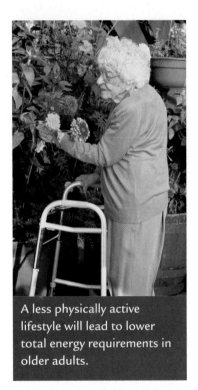

A less physically active lifestyle will lead to lower total energy requirements in older adults.

TABLE 11.5   Nutrient Recommendations of Importance with Increased Age

Key Nutrient Recommendations	Rationale
Vitamin D *Increased need* for vitamin D from 5 μg/day for young adults to 10 μg/day for adults 51 to 70 years and to 15 μg/day for adults over age 70 years.	Decreased bone density Decreased ability to synthesize vitamin D in our skin Decreased absorption of dietary calcium
Calcium *Increased need* for calcium from 1,000 mg/day for young adults to 1,200 mg/day for adults 51 years of age and older.	Decreased bone density Decreased absorption of dietary calcium
B Vitamins *Increased need* for vitamin B_6 and need for vitamin B_{12} *as a supplement or from fortified foods*	Lower levels of stomach acid Decreased absorption of food B_{12} from gastrointestinal tract Increased need to reduce homocysteine levels and to optimize immune function
Fiber *Decreased need* for fiber from 38 grams/day for young men to 30 grams/day for men 51 years and older. Decreases for women are from 25 grams/day for young women to 21 grams/day for women 51 years and older.	Decreased energy intake
Iron *Decreased need* for iron from 18 mg/day for young women to 8 mg/day for women 51 years and older. No change in iron recommendations for men 51 years and older.	Cessation of menstruation in women; some loss of muscle and lean tissue in both men and women, although the loss of muscle mass in men is not enough to change iron guidelines. Intake of heme iron from meats/fish/poultry may be limited because of their expense and the difficulty of chewing certain cuts of meat.
Zinc No change in recommendations; however, special attention to adequacy may be important for older adults.	Optimizes immune function Enhances wound healing Intake from meats and poultry may be limited because of their expense and the difficulty of chewing certain cuts of meat
Vitamins C and E No change in recommendations; however, special attention to adequacy may be important for older adults.	Counteract the increased oxidative stress of chronic diseases and the aging process
Vitamin A No change in recommendations; however, older adults are at higher risk for vitamin A toxicity.	Inappropriately high use of vitamin A supplements may increase risk of bone fractures, liver damage, and neurologic problems.

T U F T S

Food Guide Pyramid for Older Adults

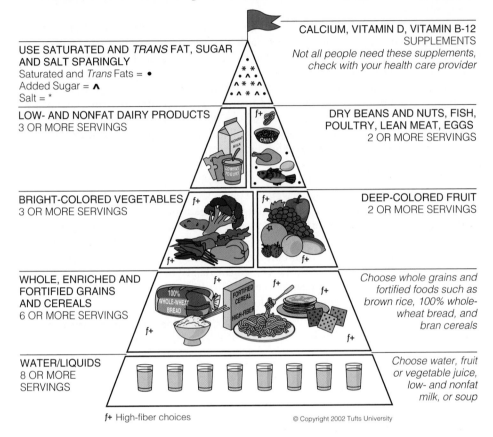

CALCIUM, VITAMIN D, VITAMIN B-12
SUPPLEMENTS
*Not all people need these supplements,
check with your health care provider*

USE SATURATED AND *TRANS* FAT, SUGAR
AND SALT SPARINGLY
Saturated and *Trans* Fats = ●
Added Sugar = ∧
Salt = *

LOW- AND NONFAT DAIRY PRODUCTS
3 OR MORE SERVINGS

DRY BEANS AND NUTS, FISH,
POULTRY, LEAN MEAT, EGGS
2 OR MORE SERVINGS

BRIGHT-COLORED VEGETABLES
3 OR MORE SERVINGS

DEEP-COLORED FRUIT
2 OR MORE SERVINGS

WHOLE, ENRICHED AND
FORTIFIED GRAINS
AND CEREALS
6 OR MORE SERVINGS

*Choose whole grains and
fortified foods such as
brown rice, 100% whole-
wheat bread, and
bran cereals*

WATER/LIQUIDS
8 OR MORE
SERVINGS

*Choose water, fruit
or vegetable juice,
low- and nonfat
milk, or soup*

f+ High-fiber choices   © Copyright 2002 Tufts University

FIGURE 11.9 Tufts Modified Food Guide Pyramid for Mature (70+) Adults. This pyramid follows the design of the previous USDA Food Guide Pyramid and emphasizes fluid and food choices appropriate for older adults.
(*Source:* Tufts Food Guide for Older Adults. © 2002 Tufts University)

incontinence or do not want to be awakened for nighttime urination. This practice can endanger their health, so it is important for these individuals to seek treatment for the incontinence and continue to drink plenty of fluids. Notice that the foundation of the Tufts Modified Food Pyramid for older adults shown in FIGURE 11.9 is fluids. At least eight 1-cup (8-oz) servings of water or other fluid is recommended.

RECAP *Older adults have lower energy needs due to their loss of lean tissue and lower physical activity levels. Fat, protein, and carbohydrate recommendations are the same as for younger adults, but fiber needs decrease slightly. Micronutrients of concern for older adults include calcium, vitamin D, zinc, vitamin B_{12}, vitamin B_6, and folate. Older adults are at increased risk for dehydration, so ample fluid intake should be encouraged.*

Nutrition-Related Concerns for Older Adults

Older adults have a number of unique medical, social, and nutritional concerns that are closely interrelated.

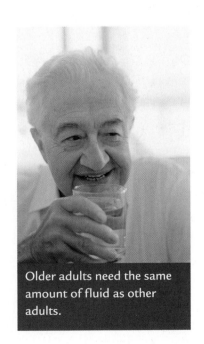

Older adults need the same amount of fluid as other adults.

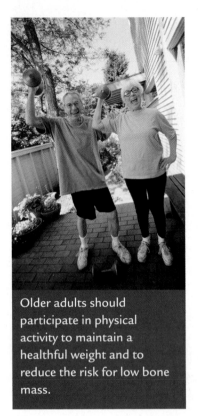

Older adults should participate in physical activity to maintain a healthful weight and to reduce the risk for low bone mass.

Overweight and Underweight: A Delicate Balancing Act

Not surprisingly, overweight and obesity are of concern to older adults. Although adults 75 years and older are less likely to be overweight or obese compared to other age groups, it is estimated that over 30% of U.S. elderly are currently obese and that the incidence will increase to as high as 37% of all older adults by the year 2010.[50] The elderly population as a whole has a high risk for heart disease, hypertension, type 2 diabetes, and cancer, and these diseases are more prevalent in people who are overweight or obese.

Although some healthcare providers question the value of attempting treatment at the age of 70 or 75 years of age, even moderate weight loss in obese elderly can improve physical functioning. The interventions are the same as for younger adults: use of dietary modifications to achieve an energy deficit while retaining adequate nutrient intakes, gradual and medically appropriate initiation of physical activity, and culturally appropriate behavior modification. There is little information on the effectiveness and safety of weight-loss drugs in the elderly; thus this option is rarely selected.[51] Obese elderly are typically at high risk for surgical complications and are usually not viewed as appropriate candidates for weight-loss surgery such as gastric bypass.

Underweight may actually be more risky for older adults than overweight, as mortality rates are higher in underweight elderly. According to the Nutrition Screening Initiative, many older adults lose weight as a result of illness, medication, loss of ability to perform self-care, tooth loss or mouth pain, alcoholism, smoking, or economic hardship.[52] In addition, depression and reduced social contact, which can develop after the death of family members and friends, or when adult children move out of the area, can cause older adults to lose the desire to prepare nourishing meals for themselves. Impaired vision can make it difficult to read labels and recipes, and a reduced sense of taste can contribute to loss of appetite. Dementia can cause older adults to forget to eat, to eat only an extremely limited diet, or to store foods inappropriately (e.g., meats or milk in a cabinet rather than in the refrigerator). Any of these several factors can result in underweight and frailty, significantly increasing the person's risk of serious illness, injuries such as fractures, and death.

Osteoporosis

As discussed in Chapter 7, osteoporosis is a complex disease that develops over an extended period of time. Bone density and structure are impaired, and fractures of the hip, wrist, and spine are common. It is estimated that 50% of females and 25% of males over the age of 50 will have an osteoporosis-related bone fracture within their lifetime.[53] Close to 25% of elderly hip fracture patients will die of complications related to the fracture within 1 year.[53]

Age-Related Eye Disorders

Cataracts, a cloudiness of the lens of the eye that impairs vision, develop in almost 70% of adults in their eighties. *Macular degeneration,* deterioration of the retina of the eye that causes a loss or distortion of vision, is the most common cause of blindness in U.S. elderly. Sunlight exposure and smoking are factors that increase the risk of each condition.

Recent research suggests, but does not definitively prove, that dietary choices may slow the progress of these degenerative eye diseases. For example, studies suggest that vitamins C and E, zinc, and two phytochemicals, lutein and zeaxanthin, may provide protection against these diseases. Although the research is not yet conclusive, older adults can benefit by including foods rich in these nutrients, primarily richly colored fruits and vegetables, nuts, and whole grains.

Dementia

Dementia is a progressive deterioration of cognitive function. Although the incidence increases in older adults, it is by no means a normal or inevitable part of aging.

Lifelong dietary choices may influence an individual's risk for dementia. Some, but not all, research suggests that long-term intake of antioxidants such as vitamin

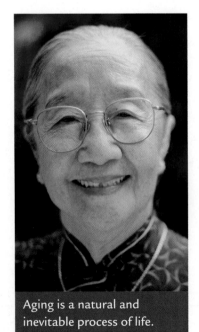

Aging is a natural and inevitable process of life.

E and phytochemicals may lower the risk.[54] Recent studies also suggest that adequate intakes of vitamins B_{12} and D can improve cognitive function in older adults.[55–56] Other research suggests a protective role for specific types of food including fish and fruits and vegetables.[57–58] While not conclusive, these studies emphasize the critical importance to older adults of consuming a balanced, healthful diet and, as needed, nutrient supplementation.

Interactions Between Medications, Supplements, and Nutrition Status

The average number of filled prescriptions for older Americans in the year 2000 was 30 per year.[47] Although the elderly account for less than 15% of the U.S. population, they experience almost 40% of adverse drug effects, in part because of **polypharmacy,** the use of three or more drugs at the same time. These drugs can interact with one another in a way that is harmful to the consumer.

Drugs can also interact adversely with nutrients. Some medications affect appetite, either increasing or decreasing food intake, and others alter nutrient digestion and absorption. Several drugs negatively impact the activation or metabolism of nutrients such as vitamin D, folate, and vitamin B_6, while others increase the kidney's excretion of nutrients.

Conversely, nutrient intake can also affect the action of certain drugs. For example, excessive vitamin K can block the action of anticoagulant drugs. Table 11.6 summarizes a few of the more common drug–nutrient interactions that may place older adults at risk.

In addition to the interactions between drugs and individual nutrients, certain foods and beverages are known to alter drug metabolism. Both ibuprofen (e.g., Motrin) and acetaminophen (Tylenol) are commonly prescribed for muscle, joint, and headache pain, but taking these drugs with alcoholic beverages increases the risk for liver damage and bleeding, so alcohol should not be consumed with them. Certain foods such as grapefruit juice, spinach, and aged cheese are known to react negatively with certain drugs; thus, pharmacists and/or dietitians should provide pertinent nutritional guidance to consumers.

TABLE 11.6   Examples of Common Drug–Nutrient Interactions

Category of Drug	Common Nutrient/Food Interactions
Antacids	May decrease the absorption of iron, calcium, folate, vitamin B_{12}
Antibiotics	May reduce the absorption of calcium, fat-soluble vitamins; reduce the production of vitamin K by gut bacteria
Anticonvulsants	Interfere with activation of vitamin D
Anticoagulants ("blood thinners")	Oppose the clotting activity of vitamin K
Antidepressants	May cause weight gain as a result of increased appetite
Antiretroviral Agents (treatment of HIV/AIDS)	Reduce the absorption of most nutrients
Aspirin	Lowers blood folate levels; increases loss of iron due to GI bleeding
Diuretics	Some types may increase urinary loss of potassium, sodium, calcium, magnesium; others cause retention of potassium and other electrolytes
Laxatives	Increase fecal excretion of dietary fat, fat-soluble vitamins, calcium, and other minerals

polypharmacy   Concurrent use of three or more medications.

Supplement usage continues to grow among all segments of the U.S. population, including the elderly. There is intriguing but contradictory research linking supplement use with decreased risk of age-related conditions such as cataracts, age-related macular degeneration, and dementia. Should older adults use supplements and, if so, what types? Do the potential risks outweigh potential benefits?

The Institute of Medicine, in establishing the DRI for vitamin B_{12}, specifically stated that adults over the age of 50 years should obtain most of their B_{12} "by consuming foods fortified with B_{12} or a B_{12}-containing supplement."[10] The Tufts Modified Food Guide Pyramid for older adults recommends calcium and vitamin D supplements as well (Figure 11.9). Older adults who eat fewer than two full meals per day or have limited food choices due to dental problems also should be encouraged to use a multivitamin/mineral supplement. Those under medical care for osteoporosis, gastrointestinal diseases, anemia, and other chronic diseases also benefit from specific nutrient supplements when used at prescribed levels of intake. In contrast, unsupervised use of high-potency supplements of vitamins A, C, D, and E pose real risks, as does inappropriate use of iron supplements. Healthcare providers should evaluate all nutrient supplements and related products (herbs and other remedies) used by their older clients and discuss their relative risks and benefits.

NUTRI-CASE GUSTAVO

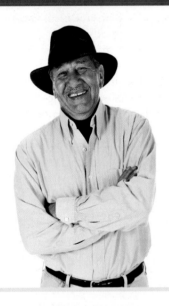

" I don't believe in taking vitamins. If you eat good food, you get everything you need, and it's the way nature intended it. My daughter kept nagging at my wife and me to start taking B vitamins. She said when people get to be our age they have problems with their nerves and their blood pressure if they don't. I didn't fall for it, but my wife did, and then her doctor told her she needed calcium pills and vitamin D, too. The kitchen counter is starting to look like a medicine chest! You know what I think? I think this whole vitamin thing is just a hoax to get you to empty your wallet."

Would you support Gustavo's decision to avoid taking a B-complex vitamin supplement? Given what you have learned in previous Nutri-Cases about Gustavo's wife, would you support or oppose her taking a vitamin B, calcium, or vitamin D supplement? Explain your choices.

What Social Programs Provide Food to Older Adults in Need?

Approximately 6% of households with older adults experience food insecurity at some point during any given year.[35] The most common cause of food insecurity and hunger among older adults is lack of income and poverty.[35] Older adults in poverty may live in areas with few or no supermarkets, may not be able to afford transportation to buy healthful food, and may fear leaving their home to shop for groceries. Low-income elderly households may lack working refrigerators and/or stoves, limiting the types of foods that can be bought, stored, and prepared.

The federal government has developed an extensive network of food and nutrition services for older Americans. Many of these services are coordinated with

HIGHLIGHT

Can We Live Longer by Eating a Low-Energy Diet?

How old do you want to live to be—80 years, 100 years, 120 years? If you were to discover that you could live to be 125 years of age by eating a little more than half of your current energy intake and still be healthy as you age, would you do it? Believe it or not, some people are already doing this in response to studies suggesting that low-energy diets can significantly increase the life span of animals.

Existing research shows that feeding certain small species of animals a low-energy diet, a practice referred to as *caloric restriction,* can significantly extend the life span of these animals; most of this research has been done in rats, mice, fish, flies, and yeast cells.[59-60] Until recently, we did not know if this same effect would be seen in larger animals, including humans. But a 2007 summary of ongoing studies of caloric restriction suggests that the practice can improve various metabolic, hormonal, and functional measures of health, which may then possibly translate into an extended lifespan in humans as well.[61]

How can caloric restriction prolong life span? It is speculated that the reduction in metabolic rate that occurs with restricting energy intake results in a much lower production of free radicals, which in turn significantly reduces oxidative damage and can prolong life. Caloric restriction also causes marked improvements in insulin sensitivity and results in hormonal changes that result in a lower incidence of chronic diseases such as heart disease and diabetes. In fact, caloric restriction in small animals has been shown to alter gene expression, which can reduce the effects of aging and prevent diseases such as cancer.[61] Some of the effects of prolonged caloric restriction in rodents include:[62]

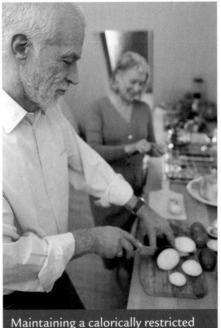

Maintaining a calorically restricted diet that is also highly nutritious requires significant planning and preparing of meals.

- Decreased insulin levels and improved insulin sensitivity
- Decreased body temperature
- Decreased energy expenditure
- Decreased oxidative stress
- Decreased fat mass and lean body mass
- Increased levels of voluntary physical activity

It is important to emphasize that species that live longer due to caloric restriction are fed exceptionally nutritious diets. The macro- and micronutrients of each meal are precisely balanced to achieve the optimum health benefit for the lower energy consumed. Unhealthful energy-restriction situations such as starvation, wasting caused by diseases such as cancer, prolonged fasting, and eating disorders such as anorexia nervosa do not result in prolonged life. In fact, these situations are associated with increased risks for illness and premature death.[63]

Okay, so caloric restriction can extend the lives of some animals, but how can we be confident that the same effect would occur in humans? For now, scientists are measuring *markers* of the aging process, such as hormones or metabolites, in short-term research projects. Long-term studies that could fully answer this question will likely never be conducted because of ethical and logistical concerns. Finding enough people to participate in such a study over their entire lifetime would be extremely difficult. Most people find it challenging to follow a caloric-restricted diet for just a few months; compliance to this type of diet over 80 years or more could be almost impossible. Institutional committees that review research studies are hesitant to approve caloric-restriction research in humans not only because of this logistical problem but also because of the considerable potential for malnutrition in study participants.

You may be wondering how much less energy you would have to consume to meet the caloric-restriction levels studied in animals. Most studies have found a significant extension of life span when animals are fed 30% to 40% less energy than control animals. If you are a woman who normally eats about 2,000 kcal/day, this level of reduction would result in an energy intake of about 1,200 to 1,400 kcal/day. Although this amount of energy reduction does not seem excessive, it is very difficult to achieve this reduction every day over a lifetime! You must also keep in mind that this diet must be of *extraordinarily high nutritional quality,* which presents a huge number of challenges, including meticulous planning of meals, preparation of most, if not all, of your own foods, limited options for eating meals outside of the

(continued)

Can We Live Longer by Eating a Low-Energy Diet? *(continued)*

home, and the challenge of working the demands of your special diet around the eating behaviors of family members and friends.

Anyone considering caloric restriction should know that some research in humans indicates that being underweight can actually *increase* the risk for premature mortality, or death.[64] It is well-known that people who are heavy smokers, chronic alcoholics, and people with cancer or other wasting diseases are underweight and die prematurely. However, even when researchers control for these factors, people with a body mass index of less than 18.5 have a significantly higher rate of premature death. Because this research is observational in nature, and researchers have not fed individuals an energy-restricted diet over a lifetime to determine

its impact, it is still unclear why underweight people may have a shortened life span. There is also no evidence to suggest that humans eating a calorie-restricted diet will die prematurely, assuming their diet is adequate in nutrients.

Considering the potential benefits and risks of caloric restriction, do you think it is worth following this type of diet? Are you willing to make the sacrifices and lifestyle changes required, even though no one knows for sure whether or not this practice could prolong your life? If we do find that caloric restriction increases longevity, should it be recommended for all people? This debate will continue as more research is conducted, possibly for generations to come.

---

state and local governments as well as nonprofit or community organizations. They include the following:

- *Food Stamp Program:* This USDA program is designed to meet the basic nutritional needs of eligible households or individuals. Participants are provided with a monthly allotment, typically in the form of a prepaid debit card or food coupons. There are very few restrictions on the foods that can be purchased under this plan.

- *Child and Adult Care Program:* This program provides healthful meals and snacks to older and functionally impaired adults in qualified adult day-care settings.

- *Commodity Supplemental Food Program:* Unlike food stamps, this program is not intended to provide a complete array of foods. Instead, specific commodity foods are distributed, including cereals, peanut butter, dry beans, rice or pasta, and canned juice, fruits, vegetables, meat, poultry, and tuna. On occasion, other surplus foods are distributed.

- *Seniors' Farmers Market Nutrition Program:* This program is sponsored by the U.S. Department of Agriculture and provides coupons to low-income seniors so they can buy eligible foods at farmers' markets, roadside stands, and community-supported agricultural programs. Seniors benefit from the nutritional advantages of fresh produce and are often able to increase the variety of foods within their meals.

- *Nutrition Services Incentive Program:* The Department of Health and Human Services, through the Administration on Aging, provides cash and USDA commodity foods to individual state agencies for meals for senior citizens. There is no income criteria; any person 60 years or above (plus their spouse, even if younger) can take part in this program. Meals, designed to provide one-third of the RDA for key nutrients, are served at senior centers located in community complexes, public housing units, religious centers, schools, or similar locations. Some centers provide "bag dinners" for evening meals and

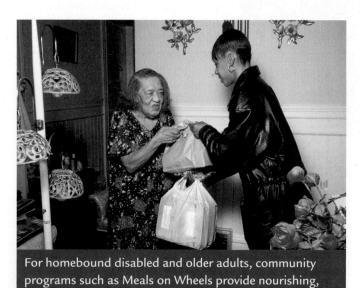

For homebound disabled and older adults, community programs such as Meals on Wheels provide nourishing, balanced meals, as well as vital social contact.

others send home meals on Fridays for use over the weekend. This program also provides nutrition and health education and usually offers transportation to and from the meal site. For qualified elders, meals can be delivered to their homes through the Meals on Wheels program.

- *The Emergency Food Assistance Program:* The USDA purchases commodity foods and distributes them to state agencies for use by local food banks, food pantries, and soup kitchens. Each state or agency establishes eligibility criteria, if any.

Participation in nutrition programs for the elderly improves the dietary quality and nutrient intakes of older adults.[65] Unfortunately, many of these programs have long waiting lists and are unable to meet the current demands of their communities. With the ever-increasing number of elderly, legislators must continue to commit adequate funding for these essential services.

RECAP *Both overweight and underweight can contribute to poor health in older adults. Osteoporosis is increasingly common in both men and women in this age group, as are fracture-related deaths. Risk for cataracts and macular degeneration, two eye disorders common in older adults, may be affected by intake of antioxidants and phytochemicals. Nutrient intake or status may also influence the development of dementia. An older adult's nutrition can influence the effectiveness of certain medications, and some drugs affect nutrient status. Appropriate use of supplements can enhance the health of older adults; however, unsupervised use of high-potency supplements can carry significant risk. A number of social services are available to older adults who are unable to secure a healthful diet.*

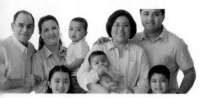

REVIEW QUESTIONS

Circle the correct choice.

1. Folate deficiency in the first weeks after conception has been linked with which of the following problems in the newborn?

  a. high blood pressure

  b. neural tube defects

  c. abnormally high birth weight

  d. poor bone mineralization

2. Which of the following nutrients should be added to the diet of breast-fed infants when they are around 6 months of age?

  a. fiber

  b. fat

  c. iron

  d. vitamin C

3. The AI for calcium for adolescents is

  a. less than that for young children.

  b. less than that for adults.

  c. less than that for pregnant adults.

  d. greater than that for children, adults, and pregnant adults.

4. Which of the following nutrients is needed in increased amounts in older adulthood?

  a. fiber

  b. vitamin D

  c. carbohydrate

  d. vitamin A

5. Why are older adults often at risk for inappropriate weight loss?

  a. certain drugs interfere with normal appetite

  b. depression and social isolation decrease food intake

  c. many elderly have limited incomes and have no transportation to shop for healthful foods

  d. all of the above

6. True or False? Major developmental errors and birth defects are most likely to occur in the third trimester of pregnancy.

7. True or False? For infants, honey is a safer choice of sweetener than white sugar.

8. True or False? Toddlers are too young to be influenced by their parents' examples.

9. True or False? The rate of obesity among adolescents has increased in the past decade.

10. True or False? Sensory deficits such as impaired vision can contribute to nutrient deficiencies.

WEB LINKS

http://aappolicy.aappublications.org
American Academy of Pediatrics

Visit this Web site for information on infants' and children's health. Clinical information as well as guidelines for parents and caregivers can be found. Searches can be performed for topics such as "neural tube defects" or "infant formulas." Benefits, challenges, and outright contraindications to breastfeeding are discussed in the AAP policy statement on breastfeeding.

www.health.gov/dietaryguidelines/dga2005/
Dietary Guidelines for Americans, 2005

This Web site provides the most recent revision of the *Dietary Guidelines for Americans;* it also provides links to other government sites. Materials, including food plans, are available.

www.fns.usda.gov
Food and Nutrition Service, U.S. Department of Agriculture

This Web site provides information on federal programs for low-income children and elderly, such as the Child and Adult Care Food Program and Congregate Meals.

www.nal.usda.gov/fnic
Food and Nutrition Information Center

Click on "Topics A–Z" and then "Child Nutrition and Health." This page provides a list of topics for infant nutrition, as well as a listing of child nutrition programs, links, and resources.

www.emedicine.com/ped
eMedicine: Pediatrics

This Web site provides references for numerous infant health and nutrition issues. Search for "Toxicity, Iron" to learn about iron poisoning and its signs in children and infants.

www.marchofdimes.com
March of Dimes

Click on "Pregnancy & Newborn" to find links on nutrition during pregnancy, breastfeeding, and baby care.

www.diabetes.org
American Diabetes Association

Search for "gestational diabetes" to find information about diabetes that develops during pregnancy. The Web site also provides recipes, advice, and resources for those with diabetes.

www.llli.org
La Leche League

This Web site provides information about breastfeeding, including multiple articles on the health effects of breastfeeding for mother and infant, as well as tips for successful breastfeeding.

www.obgyn.net
OBGYN.net

Visit this Web site to learn about pregnancy health and nutrition, breastfeeding, and infant nutrition.

www.nofas.org
National Organization on Fetal Alcohol Syndrome

This Web site provides news and information relating to fetal alcohol syndrome.

www.iom.edu
Institute of Medicine

Click on "Food & Nutrition" to learn more about the Institute of Medicine's projects and reports concerning nutrition for different life stages.

http://teamnutrition.usda.gov/kids-pyramid.html
MyPyramid for Kids

This site contains the MyPyramid symbol designed specifically for children aged 6 to 11, as well as lesson plans, tips, worksheets, and an interactive game.

www.aarp.org
AARP

A national advocacy group for the elderly; adults 50 years and above can join this organization of 35 million older Americans. The Web site has links to articles focusing on all aspects of health, finances, housing, and legal issues that are of importance to the elderly.

www.aoa.gov
Administration on Aging

Follow legislative updates on this Web site, including information related to Congregate Meal and Meals on Wheels programs.

www.aafp.org/PreBuilt/NSI_DETERMINE.pdf
American Academy of Family Physicians' Determine Your Nutritional Health

This Web page provides a checklist for determining whether an older adult you know is at nutritional risk. It also explains the warning signs of poor nutritional health.

www.cdc.gov
The Centers for Disease Control and Prevention

Select "Life Stages & Populations" for accurate information on health issues across the life cycle.

www.eatright.org
The American Dietetic Association

This Web site offers information on nutrition for people of all ages.

www.healthandage.com
Health and Age

This Web site features comprehensive information about nutrition and exercise for older adults.

http://nihseniorhealth.gov
NIH Senior Health

This Web site, written in large print, offers up-to-date information on popular health topics for older Americans.

www.livingto100.com
The Living to 100 Healthspan Calculator

By answering a series of scored questions related to smoking habits, sun exposure, family history, weight status, alcohol consumption, food choices, and other factors, you can find out how long you are likely to live!

TEST YOURSELF ANSWERS

1. **False.** More than half of all pregnant women experience morning sickness, and food cravings or aversions are also common.

2. **False.** Most infants do not have a physiologic need for solid food until about 6 months of age.

3. **False.** As a percent of total calories, young toddlers have a higher need for fat than do older children or adults, so nonfat dairy foods are not appropriate choices.

4. **True.** Hormonal changes, emotional stress, genetic factors, and personal hygiene are the most likely contributors to adolescent acne.

5. **True.** About 12% of American households with children and 6% of households with elderly are unable to acquire adequate, nutritious food throughout the year.

REFERENCES

1. Centers for Disease Control and Prevention. 2007. National Center for Health Statistics. Fast Stats. Overweight. Available at www.cdc.gov/nchs/fastats/overwt.htm.
2. National Diabetes Information Clearinghouse (NDIC). National Diabetes Statistics. National Institutes of Health Publication No. 06–3892. 2005. Available at http://diabetes.niddk.nih.gov/dm/pubs/statistics/index.htm.
3. Matthews, T. J., and M. F. MacDorman. 2007. Infant mortality statistics from the 2004 period linked birth/infant death data set. *National Vital Statistics Reports* 55(15):1–32. Hyattsville, MD: National Center for Health Statistics.
4. Robinson, H. E., C. M. O'Connell, K. S. Joseph, and N. L. McLeod. 2005. Maternal outcomes in pregnancies complicated by obesity. *Obstet. Gynecol.* 106:1357–1364.
5. Olds, S. B., M. L. London, P. W. Ladewig, and M. R. Davidson. 2003. *Maternal-Newborn Nursing and Women's Health Care.* 7th ed. Upper Saddle River, NJ: Prentice Hall Health.

6. March of Dimes. 2008. Weight Gain. Available at www.marchofdimes.com/printableArticles/159_153.asp.

7. Gillman, M. W., S. Rifas-Shiman, C. S. Berkey, A. E. Field, and G. A. Colditz. 2003. Maternal gestational diabetes, birth weight, and adolescent obesity. *Pediatrics* 111(3):e221–226.

8. Institute of Medicine, Food and Nutrition Board. 2002. *Dietary Reference Intakes for Energy, Carbohydrate, Fiber, Fat, Fatty Acids, Cholesterol, Protein, and Amino Acids.* Washington, DC: National Academies Press.

9. National Healthy Mothers, Healthy Babies Coalition. October 4, 2007. Seafood Recommendations During Pregnancy. Available at www.brainybabieshealthykids.org/seafood-recommendations-for-pregnancy/.

10. Institute of Medicine, Food and Nutrition Board. 1998. *Dietary Reference Intakes for Thiamin, Riboflavin, Niacin, Vitamin B₆, Folate, Vitamin B₁₂, Pantothenic Acid, Biotin, and Choline.* Washington, DC: National Academies Press.

11. Institute of Medicine, Food and Nutrition Board. 2001. *Dietary Reference Intakes for Vitamin A, Vitamin K, Arsenic, Boron, Chromium, Copper, Iodine, Iron, Manganese, Molybdenum, Nickel, Silicon, Vanadium, and Zinc.* Washington, DC: The National Academy of Sciences.

12. Institute of Medicine, Food and Nutrition Board. 1997. *Dietary Reference Intakes for Calcium, Phosphorus, Magnesium, Vitamin D, and Fluoride.* Washington, DC: National Academies Press.

13. Institute of Medicine, Food and Nutrition Board. 2004. *Dietary Reference Intakes for Water, Potassium, Sodium, Chloride, and Sulfate.* Washington, DC: National Academies Press.

14. National Institute for Occupational Safety and Health. 2005. *Pica.* Available at www.cdc.gov/niosh/wdd-issue6.html.

15. Ellis, C. R., and C. J. Schnoes. 2006. *Eating disorder: Pica.* Available at www.emedicine.com/ped/topic1798.htm.

16. Ventura, S. J., J. C. Abma, W. D. Mosher, and S. K. Henshaw. 2006. Recent trends in teenage pregnancy in the United States, 1990–2002. Health E-stats. Hyattsville, MD: National Center for Health Statistics.

17. March of Dimes. 2005a. Caffeine in Pregnancy. Available at www.modimes.com/printableArticles/14332_1148.asp.

18. March of Dimes. 2005b. Drinking Alcohol During Pregnancy. Available at www.modimes.com/printableArticles/14332_1170.asp.

19. U.S. Department of Health and Human Services. Centers for Disease Control and Prevention. 2005. Pregnancy Nutrition Surveillance System (PNSS): 2005 Pregnancy Nutrition Surveillance. Summary of Health Indicators. Available at www.cdc.gov/pednss/pnss_tables/index.htm.

20. U.S. Department of Health and Human Services and U.S. Department of Agriculture. 2005. *Dietary Guidelines for Americans 2005.* 6th ed. Washington, DC: U.S. Government Printing Office. Available at www.healthierus.gov/dietaryguidelines.

21. American College of Obstetricians and Gynecologists. 2002. Exercise during pregnancy and the postpartum period. ACOG Committee Opinion 267. *Obstet. Gynecol.* 99:171–173.

22. Pivarnik, J. M., H. O. Chambliss, J. F. Clapp, S. A. Dugan, M. C. Hatch, C. A. Lovelady, M. F. Mottola, and M. A. Williams. 2006. Impact of physical activity during pregnancy and postpartum on chronic disease risk. *Med. Sci. Sports. Exerc.* 38:989–1006.

23. American Academy of Pediatrics, Section on Breastfeeding. 2005. Policy statement: Breastfeeding and the use of human milk. *Pediatrics* 115(2):496–506.

24. The National Women's Health Information Center. 2005. Benefits of Breastfeeding. Available at www.4woman.gov/breastfeeding/print-bf.cfm?page=227.

25. Liu, J., K. D. Rosenberg, and A. P. Sandoval. 2006. Breastfeeding duration and perinatal cigarette smoking in a population-based cohort. *Am. J. Public Health* 96:309–314.

26. Mennella, J. A., L. M. Yourshaw, and L. K. Morgan. 2007. Breastfeeding and smoking: short-term effects on infant feeding and sleep. *Pediatrics* 120:497–502.

27. Jackson, D. J., M. Chopra, C. Witten, and M. J. Sengwana. 2003. HIV and infant feeding: Issues in developed and developing countries. *J. Obst. Gynecol. Neonatal Nurs.* 32(1):117–127.

28. Satter, E. 2005. *Your Child's Weight: Helping Without Harming, Birth Through Adolescence.* Madison, WI: Kelcy Press.

29. Stern, R. 2007. Diet from hell. *Phoenix New Times,* May 10, 2007. Available at www.phoenixnewtimes.com/2007-05-10/news/diet-from-hell/.

30. Rampersaud, G. C., M. A. Pereira, B. L. Girard, J. Adams, and J. D. Metzl. 2005. Breakfast habits, nutritional status, body weight, and academic performance in children and adolescents. *J Am Diet Assoc* 105:743–760.

31. Mahoney, C. R., H. A. Taylor, R. B. Kanarek, and P. Samuel. 2005. Effect of breakfast composition on cognitive processes in elementary school children. *Physiology & Behavior* 85:635–645.

32. Pilant, V. B. 2006. Position of the American Dietetic Association: Local support for nutrition integrity in schools. *J. Am. Diet Assoc.* 106:122–133.

33. School Nutrition Association. Nutrition Integrity in School Food & Nutrition Programs. Available at www.schoolnutrition.org/Index.aspx?id=1107. (Accessed April 2008.)

34. Stallings, V. A., and A. L. Yaktine. Eds. 2007. *Nutrition Standards for Foods in Schools: Leading the Way Toward Healthier Youth.* Washington, DC: National Academies Press.

35. Nord, M., M. Andrews, and S. Carlson. 2004. Household food security in the United States, 2003. *ERS Research Brief.* Food Assistance and Nutrition Research Report No. (FANRR42). Washington, DC: Economic Research Service.

36. Polan, E. U., and D. R. Taylor. 2003. *Journey Across the Lifespan.* 2nd ed. Philadelphia: F. A. Davis.

37. Cohen, B., S. Evers, S. Manske, K. Bercovitz, and H. G. Edward. 2003. Smoking and physical activity and breakfast consumption among secondary school students in a southwestern Ontario community. *Can. J. Public Health* 94:41–44.

38. Food Research & Action Center. Breakfast for Learning: Child Nutrition Fact Sheet. Available at www.frac.org. (Accessed April 2008.)

39. Barton, B. A., A. L. Elderidge, D. Thompson, S. G. Affenito, R. H. Striegel-Moore, D. L. Franko, A. M. Albertson, and S. J. Crockett. 2005. The relationship of breakfast and cereal consumption to nutrient intake and body mass index: the National Heart, Lung, and Blood Institute Growth and Health Study. *J. Am. Heart Assoc* 105(9):1383–1389.

40. Fiore, H., S. Travis, A. Whalen, P. Auinger, and S. Ryan. 2006. Potentially protective factors associated with healthful body mass index in adolescents with obese and nonobese parents: A secondary data analysis of the Third National Health and Nutrition Examination Survey, 1988–1994. *J. Am. Diet Assoc* 106:55–64.

41. Bakalar, N. 2008. Skipping cereal and eggs, and packing on pounds. *The New York Times,* March 25, 2008. Available at www.nytimes.com/2008/03/25/health/nutrition/25brea.html.

42. Rampersaud, G. C., L. B. Bailey, and G. P. A. Kauwell. 2003. National survey beverage consumption data for children and adolescents indicate the need to encourage a shift toward more nutritive beverages. *J. Am. Diet. Assoc.* 103:97–100.

43. Kalkwarf, H. J., J. C. Khoury, and B. P. Lanphear. 2003. Milk intake during childhood and adolescence, adult bone density, and osteoporotic fractures in US women. *Am. J. Clin. Nutr.* 77:257–265.

44. Centers for Disease Control and Prevention. 2006. Youth risk behavior surveillance, United States, 2005. *Morbidity & Mortality Weekly Report* 55(SS-5):1–108.

45. Magin, P., D. Pond, W. Smith, and A. Watson. 2005. A systematic review of the evidence for "myths and misconceptions" in acne management: Diet, face-washing, and sunlight. *Family Practice* 22:62–70.

46. U.S. Food and Drug Administration. 2005. *Alert for Healthcare Professionals: Isotretinoin (Accutane).* Rockville, MD: U.S. Food and Drug Administration.

47. Federal Interagency Forum on Aging-Related Statistics. 2004. *Older Americans 2004: Key Indicators of Well-Being.* Washington DC: U.S. Government Printing Office.

48. Minino, A. M., M. P. Heron, S. L. Murphy, and K. D. Kochanek. 2007. Deaths: Final Data for 2004. *National Vital Statistics Reports* 55:1–120.

49. National Institute on Aging, National Institutes of Health. 2002. *Aging under the Microscope: A Biological Quest.* NIH Publ. No. 02-2756. Bethesda, MD: National Institutes of Health.

50. Ogden, C. L., M. D. Carroll, L. R. Curtin, M. A. McDowell, C. J. Tabak, and K. M. Flegal. 2006. Prevalence of overweight and obesity in the United States, 1999–2004. *J. Am. Med. Assoc.* 295:1549–1555.

51. Jensen, G. L., and M. Berg. Obesity in middle and older age. 2004. In: Bales, C. W., and C. S. Ritchie. Eds. *Handbook of Clinical Nutrition and Aging.* Totowa, NJ: Humana Press, pp. 517–530.

52. Nutrition Screening Initiative. 2005. *Determine Your Nutritional Health.* Available at www.aafp.org/x16087.xml.

53. National Osteoporosis Foundation. 2008. Fast Facts. Available at www.nof.org/osteoporosis/diseasefacts.htm.

54. Van Dyk, K. 2007. The impact of nutrition on cognition in the elderly. *Neurochem. Res.* 32:893–904.

55. Clarke, R., J. Birks, E. Nexo, P.M. Ueland, J. Schneede, J. Scott, A. Molloy, and J.G. Evans. 2007. Low vitamin B-12 status and risk of cognitive decline in older adults. *Am. J. Clin. Nutr.* 86:1384.

56. Przybelski, R. J., and N. C. Binkley. 2007. Is vitamin D important for preserving cognition? A positive correlation of serum 25-hydroxyvitamin D concentration with cognitive function. *Arch. Biochem. Biophysics* 460:202–205.

57. Nurk, E., C. A. Drevon, H. Refsum, K. Solvoll, S. E. Vollset, O. Nygard, H. A. Nygaard, K. Engedal, G. S. Tell, and A. D. Smith. 2007. Cognitive performance among the elderly and dietary fish intake: The Hordaland Health Study. *Am. J. Clin. Nutr.* 86:1470–1478.

58. Kang, J. H., A. Ascherio, and F. Grodstein. 2005. Fruit and vegetable consumption and cognitive decline in aging women. *Ann. Neurol.* 57:713–720.

59. Dhahbi, J. M., H.-J. Kim, P. L. Mote, R. J. Beaver, and S. R. Spindler. 2004. Temporal linkage between the phenotypic and genomic responses to caloric restriction. *Proce. Natl. Acad. Sci. USA* 101(15):5524–5529.

60. Wang, C., R. Weindruch, J. R. Fernández, C. S. Coffey, P. Patel, and D. B. Allison. 2004. Caloric restriction and body weight independently affect longevity in Wistar rats. *Int. J. Obesity* 28(3):357–362.

61. Fontana, L., and S. Klein. 2007. Aging, adiposity, and calorie restriction. *J. Am. Med. Assoc.* 297:986–994.

62. Heilbronn, L. K., and E. Ravussin. 2003. Calorie restriction and aging: Review of the literature and implications for studies in humans. *Am. J. Clin. Nutr.* 78(3):361–369.

63. Kostoff, R. N. 2001. Energy restriction. *Am. J. Clin. Nutr.* 74(4):556–557.

64. Calle, E. E., M. J. Thun, J. M. Petrilli, C. Rodriguez, and C. W. Heath, Jr. 1999. Body-mass index and mortality in a prospective cohort of U.S. adults. *N. Engl. J. Med.* 341:1097–1105.

65. Ponza, M., J. C. Ohls, and B. A. Millen. 1996. *Serving Elders at Risk: The Older Americans Act Nutriton Programs— National Evaluation of the Elderly Nutrition Programs, 1993–1995.* Washington, DC: Mathematica Policy Research, Inc.

12 Nutrition Issues: The Safety and Security of the World's Food Supply

TEST YOURSELF

Are these statements true or false? Circle your guess.

1 Freezing destroys any microorganisms that might be lurking in your food. **TRUE** or **FALSE**

2 Mold is the most common cause of food poisoning. **TRUE** or **FALSE**

3 Research has not proven that organic foods are consistently more nutritious than nonorganic foods. **TRUE** or **FALSE**

4 More than 10% of Americans are unable to obtain enough food to meet their physical needs every day. **TRUE** or **FALSE**

5 The most common nutrient deficiency in the world is protein deficiency. **TRUE** or **FALSE**

Test Yourself answers can be found at the end of the chapter.

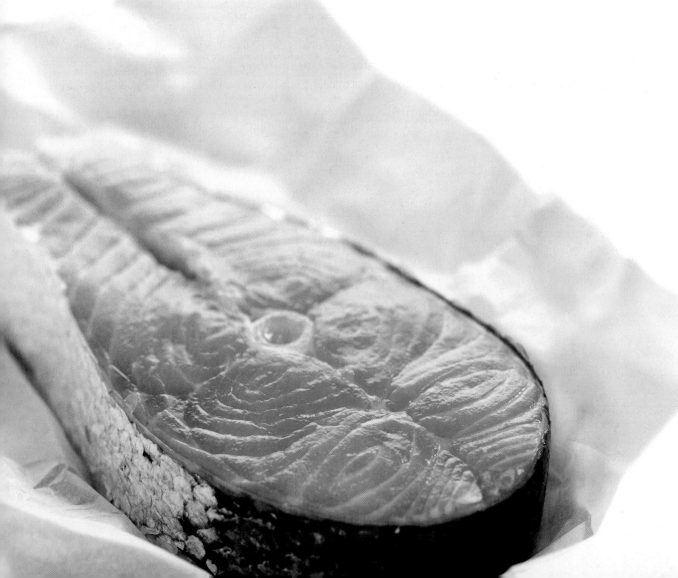

THE FALL OF 2006 was not a good season for produce. In September, more than 200 people became ill and 3 died after consuming raw spinach contaminated with a type of bacteria called *E. coli*. This was quickly followed by an outbreak of salmonellosis, another food-borne bacterial illness, in more than 150 people who consumed fresh tomatoes. In November, *E. coli* struck again, this time contaminating shredded iceberg lettuce consumed in Taco Bell restaurants in New York, New Jersey, and Pennsylvania and causing illness in more than 400 people.[1] The outbreaks prompted a national debate on food safety, with many experts calling for greater oversight by the United States Food and Drug Administration (FDA), the agency charged with protecting American produce. But fresh fruits and vegetables are not the only source of contamination in our food supply. For example, *E. coli* is a common resident of raw meats: in 1993, it caused more than 500 cases of severe illness and 3 deaths in people who consumed undercooked hamburgers in a restaurant chain in Washington State. *Salmonella* bacteria are routinely found in raw poultry and eggs, and in early 2007 showed up in two national brands of peanut butter. Mercury, a toxic metal, can collect in the tissues of fish swimming in polluted waters, and bacteria and pollutants can even contaminate drinking water.

How do disease-causing organisms enter our food and water supplies, and how can we protect ourselves from them? What makes foods spoil, and what techniques help keep foods fresh longer? Are pesticides and food additives helpful or harmful, and are organic foods safer or more nutritious? Is there anything we can do to increase everyone's access to safe, adequate, and wholesome foods, not only throughout the United States but also in other nations? We explore these and other questions in this chapter.

What Causes Food-Borne Illness?

Food-borne illness is a term used to encompass any symptom or illness that arises from ingesting food or water that contains harmful microscopic organisms (called *microorganisms*) or their products. You probably refer to food-borne illness as *food poisoning*. Some researchers also consider *food allergy*, a topic we discussed in Chapter 2, a type of food-borne illness.

According to the Centers for Disease Control and Prevention (CDC), approximately 76 million Americans report experiencing food-borne illness each year. Of these, more than 300,000 are hospitalized, and 5,000 die.[2] The people most at risk of serious illness from food-borne illness include:

- developing fetuses, infants, and young children, whose immune systems are still immature;
- the very old and the frail elderly, whose immune systems may be compromised;
- people with chronic illnesses such as diabetes;
- people with acquired immunodeficiency syndrome (AIDS); and
- people who are receiving immune-system suppressing drugs, such as transplant recipients and cancer patients.

Microorganisms or their toxic by-products cause most cases of food-borne illness. However, as we will discuss later in the chapter, chemical pollutants and residues in foods can also cause illness and death.

food-borne illness An illness transmitted through food or water either by an infectious agent, a poisonous substance, or a protein that causes an immune reaction.

Several Types of Microorganisms Contaminate Foods

Two types of food-borne illness are common: *food infections* result from the consumption of food containing living microorganisms, whereas *food intoxications* result from consuming food in which microorganisms have secreted poisonous substances called *toxins*.[3] The microorganisms that most commonly cause food infections are bacteria and viruses; however, helminths, molds, and prions also contaminate foods.

According to the CDC, the majority of food infections are caused by **bacteria** (Table 12.1).[2] Of the several species involved, *Campylobacter jejuni* is one of the most common culprits, causing more than 2 million cases each year in the United States (FIGURE 12.1). Most cases result from eating foods or drinking milk or water contaminated with animal feces. The bacteria cause fever, pain, and bloody and frequent diarrhea.[3]

Salmonella is also a leading bacterial culprit in food infections. Raw and undercooked eggs, poultry, meat, and seafood are commonly infected. Salmonellosis is the disease caused by eating food contaminated with this bacterium. Its symptoms include diarrhea, nausea, and vomiting. Cells of some strains of *Salmonella* can

bacteria Microorganisms that lack a true nucleus and have a chemical called peptidoglycan in their cell walls.

TABLE 12.1 Common Bacterial Causes of Food-Borne Illness

Bacteria	Incubation Period	Duration	Symptoms	Foods Most Commonly Affected	Usual Source of Contamination	Steps for Prevention
Campylobacter jejuni	1–7 days	7–10 days	Fever; headache and muscle pain followed by diarrhea (sometimes bloody); nausea; abdominal cramps	Raw and undercooked meat, poultry, or shellfish Raw eggs Cake icing Untreated water Unpasteurized milk	Intestinal tracts of animals and birds Raw milk Untreated water and sewage sludge	Only drink pasteurized milk Cook foods properly Avoid cross contamination
Salmonella (over 2,300 types)	12–24 hours	4–7 days	Diarrhea, abdominal pain, chills, fever, vomiting, dehydration	Raw or undercooked eggs Undercooked poultry and meat Raw milk and dairy products Seafood Fruits and vegetables	Intestinal tract and feces of poultry *Salmonella enteritidis* in raw eggs	Cook thoroughly Avoid cross contamination Use sanitary practices
Escherichia coli (O157:H7 and other strains that can cause human illness)	2–4 days	5–10 days	Diarrhea (may be bloody), abdominal cramps, nausea, can lead to kidney and blood complications	Contaminated water Raw milk Raw or rare ground beef, sausages Unpasteurized apple juice or cider Uncooked fruits and vegetables	Intestinal tracts of cattle Raw milk Unchlorinated water	Thoroughly cook meat Avoid cross contamination

TABLE 12.1 Common Bacterial Causes of Food-Borne Illness (*continued*)

Bacteria	Incubation Period	Duration	Symptoms	Foods Most Commonly Affected	Usual Source of Contamination	Steps for Prevention
Clostridium botulinum	12–36 hours	1–8 days	Nausea, vomiting, diarrhea, fatigue, headache, dry mouth, double vision, muscle paralysis (droopy eyelids), difficulty speaking and swallowing, difficulty breathing	Improperly canned or vacuum-packed food Meats Sausage Fish Garlic in oil Honey	Widely distributed in nature Soil, water, on plants, and in intestinal tracts of animals and fish Grows only in little or no oxygen	Properly can foods following recommended procedures Cook foods properly Children under 16 months should not consume raw honey
Staphylococcus	1–6 hours	2–3 days	Severe nausea and vomiting, abdominal cramps, diarrhea	Custard- or cream-filled baked goods and cream sauces Ham and poultry Dressings and gravies Eggs Mayonnaise-based salads and sandwiches	Human skin Infected cuts Pimples Noses and throats	Refrigerate foods Use sanitary practices
Shigella (over 30 types)	12–50 hours	2 days–2 weeks	Bloody and mucus-containing diarrhea, fever, abdominal cramps, chills, vomiting	Contaminated water Salads Milk and dairy products	Human intestinal tract Rarely found in other animals	Use sanitary practices
Listeria monocytogenes	2 days–3 weeks	None reported	Fever, muscle aches, nausea, diarrhea; headache, stiff neck, or convulsions can occur if infection spreads to nervous system; infections during pregnancy can lead to miscarriage or stillbirth, premature delivery, or infection of newborn	Uncooked meats and vegetables Soft cheeses Lunch meats and hot dogs Unpasteurized milk	Intestinal tract and feces of animals Soil and manure used as fertilizer Raw milk	Thoroughly cook all meats Wash raw vegetables before eating Keep uncooked meats separate from vegetables and cooked foods Avoid unpasteurized milk or foods made from unpasteurized milk

Source: Iowa State University Extension. 2000. Food Safety and Quality Project 2000, Safe Food: It's Your Job Too! Available at www.extension.iastate.edu/foodsafety/Lesson/L1.html. (Accessed July 2003.); U.S. Food and Drug Administration (FDA). 2008. How Can I Prevent Foodborne Illness? Available at www.cfsan.fda.gov/~dms/qa-fdb1.html. (Accessed April 2008.); Centers for Disease Control and Prevention (CDC), Division of Bacterial and Mycotic Diseases. 2005. Disease Information, Foodborne Illness. Available at www.cdc.gov/ncidod/dbmd/diseaseinfo/foodborneinfections_g.htm.

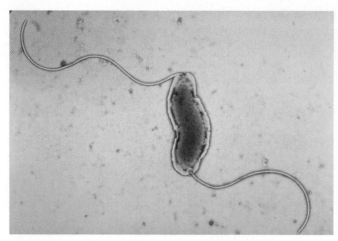

FIGURE 12.1 The bacteria called *Campylobacter jejuni* causes more than 2 million cases of food infection each year in the United States.

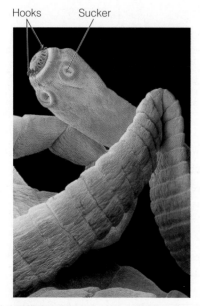

Hooks   Sucker

FIGURE 12.2 Tapeworms have hooks and suckers that help them to attach to human tissues and have long, worm-like bodies.

viruses A group of infectious agents that are much smaller than bacteria, lack independent metabolism, and are incapable of growth or reproduction outside of living cells.

helminth Multicellular microscopic worm.

giardiasis A diarrheal illness caused by the intestinal parasite *Giardia intestinalis* (or *Giardia lamblia*).

perforate the intestines and enter the bloodstream to be carried to other tissues and organs.

Although bacteria are the primary cause of food infections, some food-borne **viruses** also cause disease. In terms of sheer numbers, the rotaviruses are among the most serious: in the United States, they cause about 50,000 cases of severe diarrhea in children each year, and worldwide they are responsible for about 1 million childhood deaths annually. The hepatitis A and E viruses can contaminate foods during harvesting, production, or preparation if work areas are unclean or workers have poor personal hygiene. Infection can result in symptoms ranging from mild gastrointestinal distress to liver damage. The Norwalk virus can contaminate water supplies and foods in contact with the contaminated water, causing diarrhea, nausea, and vomiting.

Helminths are commonly called worms and include tapeworms, flukes, and roundworms (**FIGURE 12.2**). These microorganisms release their eggs into the environment, such as in vegetation or water. Animals, most commonly cattle, pigs, or fish, then consume the contaminated matter. The eggs hatch inside their host, and larvae develop in the host's tissue. The larvae can survive in the flesh long after the host is killed for food. Thoroughly cooking beef, pork, or fish destroys the larvae. In contrast, if you eat contaminated meat or fish either raw or under-cooked, you consume living larvae, which then mature into adult worms in your small intestine. Some worms cause mild symptoms such as nausea and diarrhea, but others can grow large enough to cause intestinal obstruction. Some spread beyond the gastrointestinal tract to damage other organs, such as the liver, bladder, or lungs. Some helminths can cause death.

A parasite known as *Giardia intestinalis* (or *Giardia lamblia*) causes a diarrheal illness called **giardiasis.** *Giardia* lives in the intestines of infected animals and humans, and it is passed into the environment from their stools. It is one of the most common causes of waterborne disease in humans in the United States. You can consume *Giardia* by putting something in your mouth that has come into contact with the stool of an infected person or animal, by swallowing contaminated water (in lakes, streams, rivers, swimming pools, hot tubs, or fountains), or by eating contaminated uncooked food. Symptoms, which include diarrhea, stomach cramps, and upset stomach, usually begin within 1 to 2 weeks of being infected and generally last 2 to 6 weeks.

Mold is a thread-like type of **fungi.** Growth of mold on foods is common but rarely causes food-borne illness. This is due in part to the fact that very few species of fungi cause serious disease in people with healthy immune systems, and those that do cause disease in humans are not typically food-borne.[3] In addition, unlike bacterial growth, which is invisible, mold typically grows on the surface of a food, making it look so unappealing that we quickly discard it (**FIGURE 12.3**).

A food-borne illness that has had front-page exposure in recent years is mad cow disease, or *bovine spongiform encephalopathy (BSE)*. This neurological disorder is caused by a **prion,** a proteinaceous infectious particle. Prions are normal proteins of animal tissues that can misfold and become infectious. When they do, they can transform other normal proteins into abnormally shaped prions until they eventually cause illness.[4] Cattle contract BSE from eating feed contaminated with tissue and blood from other infected animals. Prions are not destroyed with cooking, and thus BSE can be passed to humans who consume cooked, contaminated meat or tissue. For more information on mad cow disease, check out the Highlight in Chapter 5 on page 149, Mad Cow Disease: What's the Beef?

Some Bacteria and Fungi Release Toxins

The microorganisms just discussed cause illness by directly infecting and destroying body cells. In contrast, some bacteria and fungi cause illness indirectly, by secreting chemicals called **toxins** into foods. We consume the toxins when we consume the food. For example, one of the most common and deadly toxins is produced by the bacteria *Clostridium botulinum*. The botulism toxin blocks nerve transmission to muscle cells, causing paralysis, including of the muscles required for breathing. Common sources of contamination are split or pierced bulging cans, foods improperly canned at home, and raw honey.

Some fungi produce poisonous chemicals called *mycotoxins*. (The prefix *myco-* means "fungus.") These toxins are typically found in grains, peanuts, and other crops stored in moist environments. Long-term consumption of mycotoxins can cause organ damage or cancer.

A highly visible fungus that causes food intoxication is the poisonous mushroom. Most mushrooms are not toxic, but a few, such as the "death cap" mushroom (*Amanita phalloides*), can be fatal. Some poisonous mushrooms are quite colorful (FIGURE 12.4), a fact that helps to explain why the victims of mushroom poisoning are often children.[3]

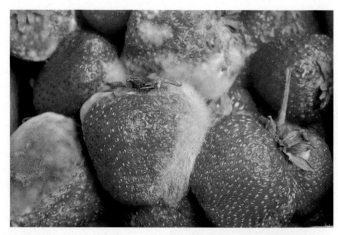

FIGURE 12.3 Molds rarely cause human illness, in part because they look so unappealing that we throw the food away.

Toxins Develop Naturally in Potatoes Exposed to Light

Prolonged exposure to light causes potatoes to turn green. Potatoes that have turned green contain the toxin solanine, which is a substance that forms during the greening process. The green color is actually due to the formation of the pigment chlorophyll, which is harmless. Although the production of solanine occurs simultaneously with the greening process, these are two separate, unrelated processes.[5] There is the potential for toxicity if the solanine content increases to very high levels.

Solanine formation occurs near the potato's skin, so the green areas can be cut away to remove any toxins. A good guide is to taste a small piece of the potato after the green areas have been removed. If the potato tastes bitter, then throw it away. If in doubt, or if serving the potato to someone with allergies, you should also discard the potato. You can avoid the greening of potatoes by storing them for only short periods in a dark cupboard or brown paper bag in a cool area. Wash the potato to expose any green areas, and cut away and discard any green areas. Cooked potatoes cannot turn green or produce solanine, but cooking green potatoes does not remove chlorophyll or solanine that may have formed prior to cooking.

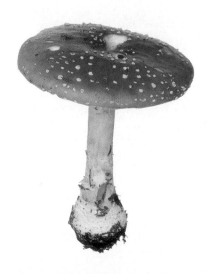

FIGURE 12.4 Some mushrooms, such as this fly agaric, contain toxins that can cause illness or even death.

Our Bodies Respond to Food-Borne Microorganisms and Toxins with Acute Illness

Many food-borne microorganisms are killed in the mouth by antimicrobial enzymes in saliva or in the stomach by hydrochloric acid. Microorganisms that survive these chemical assaults may get a chance to reproduce in the body to cause symptoms within several hours or days (see Table 12.1). As the population of microorganisms multiplies, the person begins to experience vomiting or diarrhea, mechanisms the body uses to try to get rid of the offenders. Simultaneously, the white blood cells of the immune system are activated, and a generalized inflammatory response will cause the person to experience nausea, fatigue, fever, and muscle cramps. In contrast, toxins in foods will usually trigger vomiting and/or diarrhea within several minutes to a few hours as the gastrointestinal tract attempts to expel the substance. The person's state of health, the precise microorganism or toxin involved, and the amount of contaminated food ingested all determine the severity and duration of the symptoms.

Treatment usually involves keeping the person hydrated and comfortable, because most food-borne illness tends to be self-limiting. In severe illnesses such as botulism, the patient's intestinal tract will be repeatedly flushed to remove the microorganism, and antibodies will be injected to neutralize its deadly toxin.

fungi Plantlike spore-forming organisms that can grow either as single cells or multicellular colonies.

prion A protein that misfolds and becomes infectious; prions are not living cellular organisms or viruses.

toxin Any harmful substance; in microbiology, a chemical produced by a microorganism that harms tissues or causes harmful immune responses.

Certain Environmental Conditions Help Microorganisms Multiply in Foods

Given the correct conditions, microorganisms can thrive in many types of food. Four factors affect the survival and reproduction of food microorganisms:

- *Temperature.* Many microorganisms capable of causing human illness thrive at warm temperatures, from about 40°F to 135°F (4°C to 57°C). You can think of this range of temperatures as the **danger zone**. (Note that the upper limit has recently been decreased from its previous value of 140°F.[6]) These microorganisms can be destroyed by thoroughly heating or cooking foods, and their reproduction can be slowed by refrigeration and freezing. We identify safe cooking and food-storage temperatures later in this chapter.

- *Humidity.* Many microorganisms require a high level of moisture, and thus foods such as boxed dried pasta do not make suitable microbial homes, though cooked pasta left at room temperature would prove hospitable.

- *Acidity.* Most microorganisms have a preferred range of acidity, or pH, in which they thrive. For instance, *Clostridium botulinum* thrives in alkaline environments. It cannot grow or produce its toxin in acidic environments, so the risk of botulism is decreased in citrus fruits, pickles, and tomato-based foods. In contrast, alkaline foods such as fish and low-acid vegetables are a magnet for *C. botulinum*.

- *Oxygen content.* Many microorganisms require oxygen to function; thus, food-preservation techniques that remove oxygen, such as industrial canning and bottling, keep foods safe for consumption. Because *C. botulinum* thrives in an oxygen-free environment, the canning process heats foods to an extremely high temperature to destroy this organism.

In addition, microorganisms need an entryway into a food. Just as our skin protects our bodies from microbial invasion, the peels, rinds, and shells of many foods seal off access to the nutrients within. Eggshells are a good example of a natural food barrier. Once such a barrier is removed, however, the food loses its primary defense against contamination.

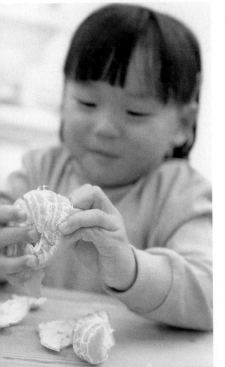

Peels protect foods against microorganisms.

> RECAP *Food infections result from the consumption of food containing living microorganisms, such as bacteria, viruses, and helminths. Food intoxications result from consuming food in which microorganisms have secreted toxins. In order to reproduce in foods, microorganisms require a precise range of temperature, humidity, acidity, and oxygen content, as well as access to the food.*

How Can You Prevent Food-Borne Illness?

The United States Department of Agriculture's FightBAC! logo identifies four basic rules for food safety, each of which is explored in detail shortly (FIGURE 12.5):

1. Wash your hands and kitchen surfaces often.
2. Separate foods to prevent **cross contamination**—that is, the spread of microorganisms from one food to another. This commonly occurs when raw foods such as chicken and vegetables are cut using the same knife or stored on the same plate.
3. Chill foods to prevent microorganisms from growing.
4. Cook foods to their proper temperatures.

Wash Hands and Surfaces Often

The first rule for "Fighting BAC" is to wash your hands and kitchen surfaces often. This is one of the easiest and most effective ways to prevent food-borne illness.

danger zone Range of temperature (about 40°F to 135°F [4°C to 57°C]) at which many microorganisms capable of causing human disease thrive.

cross contamination Contamination of one food by another via the unintended transfer of microorganisms through physical contact.

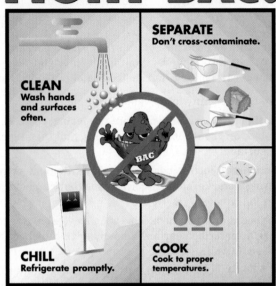

FIGHT BAC!

CLEAN
Wash hands and surfaces often.

SEPARATE
Don't cross-contaminate.

CHILL
Refrigerate promptly.

COOK
Cook to proper temperatures.

Keep Food Safe From Bacteria™

FIGURE 12.5 The Fight BAC! logo is the food safety logo of the United States Department of Agriculture.

Wash your hands before you begin to prepare food, and after working with each food before progressing to the next one. Scrub for at least 20 seconds with a mild soap under warm running water. Hot water is too harsh: it causes the surface layer of the skin to break down, increasing the risk that microorganisms will be able to penetrate your skin. Make sure to wash the areas underneath your fingernails and between your fingers. Rinse your hands thoroughly, rubbing them together, and then dry on a clean towel or use paper towels.

It's a good idea to remove any rings or bracelets before you begin working with food, because jewelry can harbor bacteria. Also keep your sleeves rolled up.

A clean work area and tools are also essential in reducing cross contamination. Wash utensils, containers, and cutting boards in the dishwasher or with hot soapy water before and after contact with food. If a cutting board, plate, countertop, or other surface has held raw meat, poultry, or seafood, sanitize it with a solution of 1 teaspoon of chlorine bleach to 1 quart of water, or use a commercial kitchen cleaning agent.[7] It's also important to wash utensils, faucets, cabinet knobs, or other areas you have touched with hot soapy water. Rinse, then air dry or dry with fresh paper towels.

Dishtowels, cloths, and aprons should be washed in hot water and detergent often. It's a good idea to wash sponges in the dishwasher each time you run it and to replace them regularly. If you don't have a dishwasher, put sponges in boiling water for 3 minutes to sterilize them on a routine basis. Paper towels should be disposed of immediately.

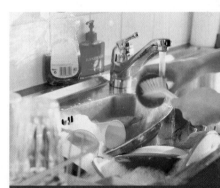

Washing dishes, utensils, and cutting boards with hot, soapy water reduces the chances for food contamination.

Separate Foods to Avoid Cross Contamination

The second step in keeping food safe from bacteria is to separate foods to prevent cross contamination. This commonly occurs when the bacteria in juices from raw meats, poultry, or fish contact ready-to-eat foods, such as bread or salad greens. It also occurs when unwashed raw foods are cut on the same cutting board or served together in the same dish. So how do you prevent cross contamination?

First, wash your hands! Then, before cutting or otherwise preparing fruits or vegetables, rinse them under running water and, if firm, either rub or scrub with a vegetable brush. For leafy greens, discard outer leaves and rinse inner leaves well. Always wash produce before peeling or slicing, even if the peel is to be entirely discarded. If you slice with a clean knife into an unwashed orange, for example, the knife can transport bacteria from the peel surface into the fruit. Removing the peel at that point would be ineffective.

Raw meat, poultry, and seafood harbor an array of microorganisms and can easily contaminate other foods through direct contact or through the juices they leave behind. To prepare raw meat, poultry, and seafood safely, follow these tips:[7]

- As always, before touching any food, wash your hands!
- Do not wash meat, poultry, or seafood before preparing. Instead, remove and discard wrapping, place on clean cutting board, slice, and then place on grill, pan, or other cooking surface.
- Use a smooth, nonporous cutting board made of hard maple or smooth plastic.[7] Make sure it is free of cracks, cuts, and scratches that can hold juices and harbor bacteria.
- Wash the cutting board or other surface as soon as you have removed the raw food, then sanitize as described earlier. Remember that dishcloths and sponges need to be sanitized as well.
- Never place any foods on a countertop, cutting board, or plate that has held raw meat, seafood, or poultry unless it has first been sanitized.
- Consider keeping a separate cutting board for use only when slicing ready-to-eat foods such as bread, cheese, and fresh fruit.
- Don't forget to wash your hands after preparing foods.

When preparing meat, poultry, or fish with a marinade, make sure you reserve some of the marinade in a clean container before adding raw ingredients, if you will need some noncontaminated marinade to use later in the cooking process. Always marinate raw foods in the refrigerator.

Keep Foods Cold

The third rule for keeping food safe from bacteria is to promptly refrigerate or freeze it. Remember the danger zone: microorganisms that cause food-borne illness can reproduce in temperatures above 40°F. So to keep them from multiplying in your food, keep it cold. Refrigeration (storage between 32°F and 40°F) and freezing (storage below 32°F) do not kill all microorganisms, but they diminish their ability to reproduce themselves in quantities large enough to cause illness. Also, many naturally occurring enzymes that cause food spoilage are deactivated at cold temperatures.

Shopping for Perishable Foods

When shopping for food, purchase refrigerated and frozen foods last. Many grocery stores are actually designed so that these foods are in the last aisles. Put packaged meat, poultry, or fish into a plastic bag before placing it in your shopping cart.[8] This prevents drippings from the food from coming into contact with other foods in your cart.

When choosing perishable foods, check the "sell by" or "best used by" date on the label. The "sell by" date indicates the last day a product can be sold and still maintain its quality during normal home storage and consumption. The "best used by" date tells you how long a product will maintain optimum quality before eating.[9] If the date stamped has passed, don't purchase the item, and notify the store manager. These foods should be promptly removed from the shelves.

Do not purchase foods with punctured or otherwise damaged packaging. Dented or bulging cans are especially dangerous, as they could harbor potentially deadly bacteria. Report any damaged packaging to the store manager.

Watch for unsanitary practices and conditions inside the store. For example, the unsafe displaying of food products, such as cooked shrimp on the same bed of ice as raw seafood, is illegal, as is slicing cold cuts with the same knife used to trim raw meat. Report such unsanitary practices or conditions to your local health authorities.[8]

After you purchase perishable foods, get them home and into the refrigerator or freezer within 1 hour. If your trip home will be longer than an hour, bring along a cooler to transport them in.

Refrigerating Foods at Home

As soon as you get home from shopping, put meat, poultry, and seafood in the back of the refrigerator away from the door so that they stay cold and on the lowest shelf so that their juices do not drip onto any other foods. If you are not going to use raw meat, poultry, or seafood within 48 hours of purchase, store it in the freezer.[9]

Eggs, cheeses, milk, and any other perishable foods should also be kept refrigerated. Avoid overstocking your refrigerator or freezer, because air needs to circulate around food to cool it quickly and continuously.

After a meal, refrigerate leftovers promptly—even if still hot—to discourage microbial growth. The standard rule for storing leftovers is *2 hours / 2 inches / 4 days:*

- Food should be refrigerated *within 2 hours* of serving. If the temperature is 90°F or higher, such as at a picnic, then foods should be refrigerated within 1 hour.[10]

- Because a larger quantity of food takes longer to cool and will allow more microorganisms to thrive, food should be stored at a depth of no greater than *2 inches*. The interior of deeper containers of foods can remain warm long after the surface of the food has cooled.

- Leftovers should only be refrigerated for *up to 4 days*. If you don't plan on using the food within 4 days, freeze it. A guide for storing foods in your refrigerator is provided in FIGURE 12.6.

Freezing and Thawing Foods

The temperature in your freezer should not get any warmer than 32°F (0°C). Use a thermometer and check it periodically. If your electricity goes out, avoid opening the freezer until the power is restored. When the power does come back on, check the

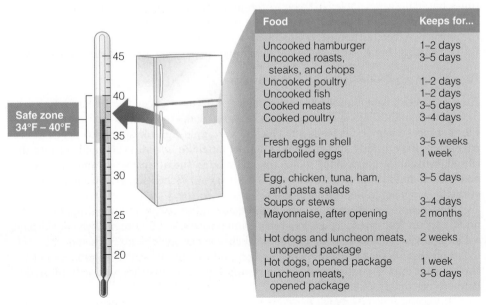

Food	Keeps for...
Uncooked hamburger	1–2 days
Uncooked roasts, steaks, and chops	3–5 days
Uncooked poultry	1–2 days
Uncooked fish	1–2 days
Cooked meats	3–5 days
Cooked poultry	3–4 days
Fresh eggs in shell	3–5 weeks
Hardboiled eggs	1 week
Egg, chicken, tuna, ham, and pasta salads	3–5 days
Soups or stews	3–4 days
Mayonnaise, after opening	2 months
Hot dogs and luncheon meats, unopened package	2 weeks
Hot dogs, opened package	1 week
Luncheon meats, opened package	3–5 days

Safe zone 34°F – 40°F

FIGURE 12.6 While it's important to keep a well-stocked refrigerator, it's also important to know how long foods will keep.
(From U.S. Department of Agriculture, Food Safety and Inspection Service. November 2005. Fact Sheets. Safe Food Handling. Refrigeration and Food Safety. Available at www.fsis.usda.gov/Fact_Sheets/Refrigeration_&_Food_Safety/index.asp.)

TABLE 12.2   A Guide to Thawing Poultry

Method Needed	Size of Poultry	Approximate Length of Time
Refrigerator	1–3 pounds, small chickens, pieces	1 day
	3–6 pounds, large chickens, ducks, small turkeys	2 days
	6–12 pounds, large turkeys	3 days
	12–16 pounds, whole turkey	3–4 days
	16–20 pounds, whole turkey	4–5 days
Microwave (read instructions)	1–3 pounds, small chickens, pieces	8–15 minutes* (standing time 10 minutes)
	3–6 pounds, large chickens, ducks, small turkeys	15–30 minutes* (standing time 20 minutes)

Source: R. W. Lacey, *Hard to Swallow: A Brief History of Food.* 1994. Cambridge: Cambridge University Press, pp. 85–187; U.S. Department of Agriculture, Food Safety and Inspection Service. 2000. Turkey Basics: Safe Thawing. Available at www.fsis.usda.gov/Fact_Sheets/Poultry_Preparation_Fact_Sheets/index.asp. *Approximate, read microwave's instructions.

Note: Turkeys purchased stuffed and frozen with the USDA or state mark of inspection on the packaging are safe because they have been processed under controlled conditions. These turkeys *should not* be thawed before cooking. Follow package directions for handling.

temperature on the top shelf. If it is warmer than 40°F (about 5°C), inspect your freezer's contents and discard any items that are not firmly frozen.

When freezing items, be aware that smaller packages will freeze more quickly. So rather than attempting to freeze an entire casserole or a whole batch of home-made spaghetti sauce, divide the food into multiple small portions (no more than 2 inches deep) in freezer-safe containers, then freeze.

Sufficient thawing will ensure adequate cooking throughout, which is essential to preventing food-borne illness. Thaw poultry on the bottom shelf of the refrigerator, in a large bowl to catch its juices. Table 12.2 shows recommended poultry thawing times based on weight. Never thaw frozen meat, poultry, or seafood on a kitchen counter or in a basin of warm water. Room temperatures allow growth of bacteria on the surface of food, although the inside may still be frozen.[9] A microwave is also useful for thawing, but be sure to follow your microwave's instructions carefully.

Dealing with Molds in Refrigerated Foods

Have you ever taken cheese out of the refrigerator and noticed that it had a fuzzy blue growth on it? This is mold, a type of fungus. Some molds like cool temperatures. For instance, when acidic foods such as leftover applesauce or spaghetti sauce are refrigerated, they readily support the growth of mold. So how did the mold get into the closed, refrigerated jar? Mold spores are common in the atmosphere, and they randomly land on food in open containers at your home. If the temperature and acidity of the food is hospitable, they will grow.

Most people throw away moldy foods because they are so unappealing, but as we noted earlier, food-borne illnesses aren't commonly caused by fungi. If the surface of a small portion of a solid food such as hard cheese becomes moldy, it is generally safe to cut off that section down to about an inch and eat the unspoiled portion. If soft cheese, sour cream, yogurt, tomato sauce, applesauce, or another soft or fluid product becomes moldy, discard it.

Cook Foods Thoroughly

Thoroughly cooking food is a sure way to kill the intestinal worms discussed earlier and many other microorganisms. The appropriate internal temperatures for doneness of meat, poultry, seafood, and eggs vary, as shown in FIGURE 12.7.

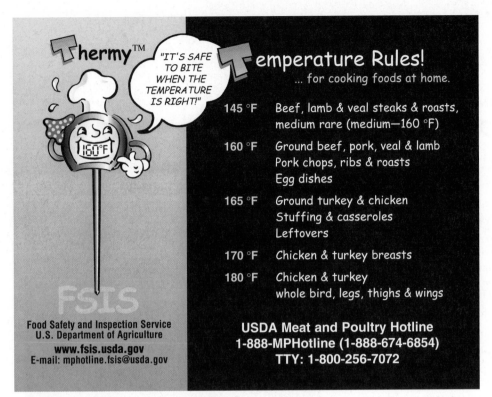

FIGURE 12.7 The United States Department of Agriculture's "Thermy" provides temperature rules for safely cooking foods at home.

Tips for Cooking Meat, Poultry, Fish, and Eggs

The color of cooked meat can be deceiving. Grilled meat and poultry often brown very quickly on the outside but may not be thoroughly cooked on the inside. The only way to be sure meat is thoroughly cooked is to test it with a food thermometer. Test your food in several places to be sure it has cooked evenly, and remember to wash the thermometer after each use. If you don't have a thermometer available, do not eat hamburger that is still pink inside.[10] See the Game Plan: Food Safety Tips for Your Next Barbecue on the following page for more tips about grilling and barbequing.

Microwave cooking is convenient, but you need to be sure your food is thoroughly and evenly cooked and that there are no cold spots in the food where bacteria can thrive. For best results, cover food, stir often, and rotate for even cooking.[10] If you are microwaving meat or poultry, use a thermometer to check internal temperatures in several spots, because temperatures vary more in microwave cooking than in conventional ovens.[9]

Raw and semiraw (such as marinated or partly cooked) fish delicacies, including sushi, sashimi, and so forth, may be tempting, but their safety cannot be guaranteed. Always cook fish thoroughly. When done, fish should be opaque and flake easily with a fork. If you're wondering how sushi restaurants can guarantee the safety of their food, the short answer is, they can't. All fish to be used for sushi must be flash frozen at –31°F (–35°C) or below for 15 hours or be regularly frozen to –4°F (–20°C) or below for 7 days.[11] Although this effectively kills any parasites that might be in the fish, it does not kill bacteria or viruses. Thus, eating raw seafood remains risky, and the FDA advises that people with compromised immunity, children, pregnant women, and the elderly avoid it.[8]

You may have memories of licking the cake batter off a spoon when you were a kid, but such practices are no longer considered safe. That's because most cake batter contains raw eggs, and an estimated one-third of chicken eggs in the United States is contaminated with *Salmonella*. The USDA recommends that you cook eggs until the yolk and whites are firm. Scrambled eggs should not be runny. If you are

GAME PLAN
Food Safety Tips for Your Next Barbecue

It's the end of the term and you and your friends are planning a lakeside barbecue to celebrate! Here are some tips from the Center for Food Safety and Applied Nutrition at the U.S. Food and Drug Administration for preventing food-borne illness at any outdoor gathering.

❑ **Wash your hands, utensils, and food preparation surfaces.** Even in outdoor settings, food safety begins with hand washing. Bring along a water jug, some soap, and paper towels, or a box of moist disposable towelettes. Keep all utensils and platters clean when preparing foods.

❑ **Keep foods cold during transport.** Use coolers with ice or frozen gel packs to keep food at or below 40°F. It's easier to maintain a cold temperature in small coolers. Consider packing three: put beverages in one cooler; washed fruits and vegetables and containers of potato salad, etc., in another; and wrapped, frozen meat, poultry, and seafood in another. Keep coolers in the air-conditioned passenger compartment of your car rather than in a hot trunk.

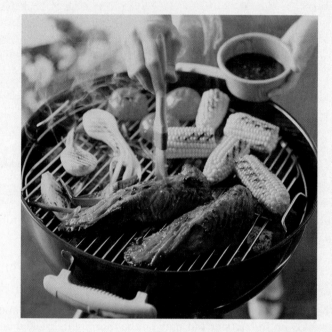

❑ **Grill foods thoroughly.** Use a food thermometer to be sure the food has reached an adequate internal temperature before serving. For example:

- ● Steaks should reach 145°F for medium rare, 160°F for medium, and 170°F for well done.
- ● Ground beef should reach 160°F.
- ● Poultry breasts should reach 170°F.
- ● Fish should reach 145°F or until flesh is opaque and separates easily with a fork.

❑ **Avoid cross contamination.** When bringing food from the grill to the table, never use the same platter or utensils that previously held raw meat or seafood!

❑ **Keep hot foods hot.** Keep grilled food hot until it is served by moving it to the side of the grill, just away from the coals, so that it stays at or above 135°F. If grilled food isn't going to be eaten right away, wrap it well and place it in an insulated container.

❑ **Keep cold foods cold.** Cold foods like chicken salad should be kept in a bowl of ice during your barbecue. Drain off water as the ice melts and replace the ice frequently. Don't let any perishable food sit out longer than 2 hours. In temperatures above 90°F, don't let food sit out for more than 1 hour.

Source: U.S. Food and Drug Administration, Center for Food Safety and Applied Nutrition. 2007. Food Facts. Eating Outdoors. Handling Food Safely.

using eggs in a casserole or custard, make sure that the internal temperature reaches at least 160°F.

Protect Yourself from Toxins in Foods

Killing microorganisms with heat is an important step in keeping food safe, but it won't protect you against their toxins. That's because many toxins are unaffected by heat and are capable of causing severe illness even when the microorganisms that produced them have been destroyed. For example, let's say you prepare a casserole for a team picnic. Too bad you forget to wash your hands before serving it to your teammates, because you contaminate the casserole with the bacteria *Staphylococcus aureus*, which is commonly found on moist skin folds.[3] You and your friends go off and play soccer, leaving the food in the sun, and a few hours later, you take the rest of the casserole home. At supper, you heat the leftovers thoroughly, thinking as you do so that this will kill any bacteria that might have multiplied while it was left out. That night you experience nausea, severe vomiting, and abdominal pain. What happened? While your food was left out, the bacteria from your hands multiplied in the casserole and produced a toxin (FIGURE 12.8). When you reheated the food, you killed

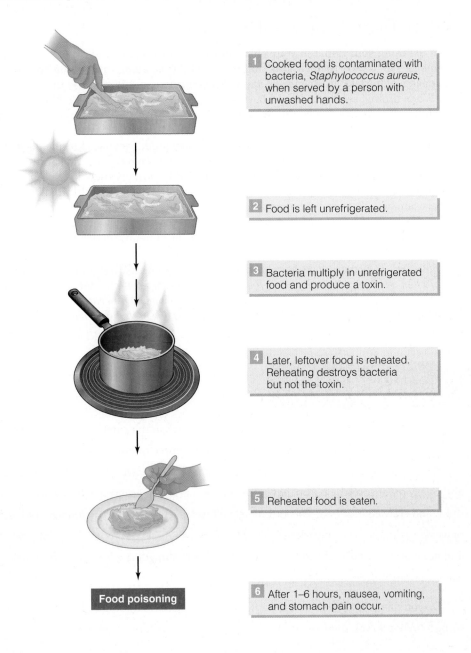

FIGURE 12.8 Food intoxication can occur long after the microorganism itself has been destroyed.

1 Cooked food is contaminated with bacteria, *Staphylococcus aureus*, when served by a person with unwashed hands.

2 Food is left unrefrigerated.

3 Bacteria multiply in unrefrigerated food and produce a toxin.

4 Later, leftover food is reheated. Reheating destroys bacteria but not the toxin.

5 Reheated food is eaten.

Food poisoning

6 After 1–6 hours, nausea, vomiting, and stomach pain occur.

the microorganisms, but their toxin was unaffected by the heat. When you then ate the food, the toxin made you sick. Fortunately, in the case of *S. aureus*, symptoms typically resolve on their own in healthy people in about 24 hours.

When Eating Out

When choosing a place to eat out, avoid restaurants that don't look clean. Grimy tabletops and dirty restrooms indicate indifference to hygiene. On the other hand, cleanliness of areas used by the public doesn't guarantee that the kitchen is clean. That is why health inspections are important. Public health inspectors randomly visit and inspect the food preparation areas of all businesses that serve food, whether eaten in or taken out. You can usually find the results of these inspections by contacting your local health department or by checking the inspection results posted in the restaurant.

Another way to protect yourself when dining out is by ordering foods to be cooked thoroughly. If you order a hamburger and it arrives pink in the middle, or scrambled eggs and they arrive runny, send the food back to be cooked thoroughly.

When Traveling to Other Countries

When planning your trip, tell your physician your travel plans and ask about vaccinations needed or any medications that you should take along in case you get sick. Also pack a waterless antibacterial hand cleanser and use it frequently during your trip. When dining, select foods and beverages carefully. All raw food has the potential for contamination. See the Highlight in Chapter 2 (page 62) on avoiding traveler's diarrhea.

Tap water is seldom a safe option, even if chlorinated, because chlorine doesn't kill all organisms that can cause disease. In regions where hygiene and sanitation are suspect, only consume canned, bottled, or boiled beverages such as tea. Ask for drinks without ice, because freezing contaminated water does not kill all microorganisms. You can find more information about how to ensure food and water safety when traveling by visiting the CDC's Web site, www.cdc.gov/travel/contentSafeFoodWater.aspx, or by contacting your local health department.

> RECAP *To prevent food-borne illness, follow these tips: Wash your hands and kitchen surfaces often. Separate foods to prevent cross contamination. Store foods in the refrigerator or freezer. Cook foods to their proper temperatures. When traveling, avoid raw foods and choose beverages that are boiled, bottled, or canned, without ice.*

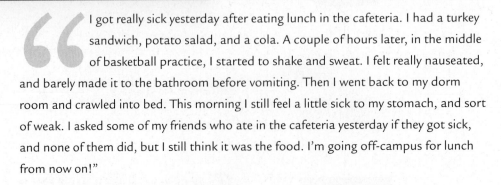

NUTRI-CASE THEO

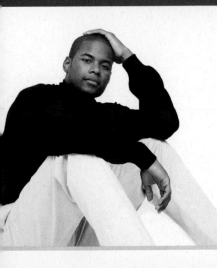

"I got really sick yesterday after eating lunch in the cafeteria. I had a turkey sandwich, potato salad, and a cola. A couple of hours later, in the middle of basketball practice, I started to shake and sweat. I felt really nauseated, and barely made it to the bathroom before vomiting. Then I went back to my dorm room and crawled into bed. This morning I still feel a little sick to my stomach, and sort of weak. I asked some of my friends who ate in the cafeteria yesterday if they got sick, and none of them did, but I still think it was the food. I'm going off-campus for lunch from now on!"

Do you think that Theo's illness was food-borne? If so, what food(s) do you most suspect? What do you think of his plan to go off-campus for lunch from now on?

How Is Food Spoilage Prevented?

Both enzymes naturally found in foods and microorganisms that colonize foods cause them to spoil over time.

Spoilage makes food unsafe to eat: because decomposition of foods is accomplished in part by microorganisms, if you eat a food that has spoiled, you risk developing a food-borne illness. Fortunately, spoilage usually degrades the appearance, texture, and smell of food so much that we throw it away uneaten. Would you eat fish with a strong odor or a tomato that has turned to "mush"?

Modern science and technology have given us a wide array of techniques to produce, preserve, and transport food. But these advances have not eliminated the threat of food spoilage, which can occur at any point on the journey from farm to table. Any food that has been harvested and that people aren't ready to eat must be preserved in some way, or before long it will spoil. Here, we look at some techniques that people have used for centuries to preserve food, as well as more modern techniques used in the food industry.

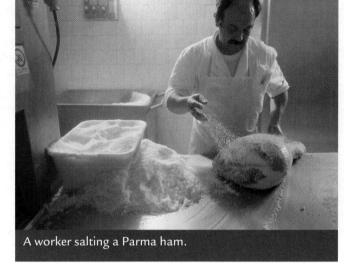

A worker salting a Parma ham.

Natural Methods of Preserving Foods Have Been Used for Thousands of Years

The most ancient methods of preserving foods employ naturally derived substances such as salt, sugars, and smoke or techniques such as drying and cooling.

Salting, Sugaring, Drying, and Smoking

Salting, sugaring, drying, and smoking preserve food by drawing the water out of the plant or animal cells. By dehydrating the food, these methods make it inhospitable to microorganisms, and dramatically slow the action of enzymes that would otherwise degrade the food:

- Salt is often used for curing meats and fish. A good example is the Parma ham from Italy, which is cured with sea salt.[12]
- Sugar is used to preserve foods such as fruits. Before families had electric refrigerators and freezers, they used sugaring to preserve summer's fruit harvest for winter consumption in the form of jellies and jams.
- Drying is used for fruits, herbs, and spices, and the modern technique of *freeze-drying* is used to preserve coffee, tea, and powdered milk.
- Smoking has been used for centuries for preservation of meats, poultry, and fish. If food was not drying well, it would be hung near the campfire or chimney so the smoke of the fire would permeate the food, further drying it. The type of wood used to smoke foods contributes to the food's flavor. Unfortunately, smoking does not guarantee that a food is safe to eat. Contamination in smoked fish, for example, is common. *Listeria monocytogenes* is a common bacterial culprit (see Table 12.1).

Cooling

As the temperature of a food is lowered, the functioning of any bacteria in the food is slowed, and it becomes less able to multiply or produce toxins. So what did people use to cool and store foods before they had electric refrigerators?

For thousands of years, people have stored foods in underground cellars, caves, running streams, and even "cold pantries"—north-facing rooms of the house that

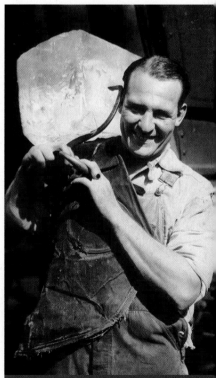

Before the modern refrigerator, an "iceman" would deliver ice to homes and businesses.

were kept dark and unheated and often were stocked with ice. The forerunner of our refrigerator, the miniature icehouse, was developed in the early 1800s, and in cities and towns, the local "iceman" would make rounds delivering ice to homes.

Many Food Producers Use Heat to Preserve Foods

Three synthetic food preservation techniques use heat:

- *Canning.* The French inventor Nicolas Appert developed the canning process in the late 1700s. It involves washing and blanching the food, placing it in cans, siphoning out air, sealing the cans, and then heating them to a very high temperature. Canned food has an average shelf life of at least 2 years from the date of purchase; however, the U.S. Army has found canned foods in "excellent states of preservation" after 46 years.

- *Pasteurization.* In 1864, the French microbiologist Louis Pasteur developed the pasteurization technique to destroy microorganisms that spoiled wine. **Pasteurization** exposes a beverage or other food to heat high enough to destroy microorganisms but for a length of time short enough so that the taste and quality of the food is not affected. For example, in *flash pasteurization*, milk or other liquids are heated to 162°F (72°C) for 15 seconds.

- *Aseptic packaging.* You probably know **aseptic packaging** best as "juice boxes" (FIGURE 12.9). Food and beverages are first heated, then cooled, then placed in the sterile container. The process uses less energy than traditional canning, and the cartons use less material than any comparable container. By eliminating the need for refrigeration or preservatives, aseptic packaging also reduces subsequent energy use.[13]

New Techniques Expand Food Choices but Raise Concerns About Safety

In the past several decades, manufacturers have developed many new food-preservation techniques, such as the addition of preservative chemicals and irradiation of foods. In addition, genetic modification can produce foods with a longer shelf life. Although these techniques have expanded our food choices, technologic manipulation of food also raises food-safety concerns among many people.

Addition of Preservatives

Most processed foods contain **food preservatives,** substances added to foods to prevent or slow spoilage. All preservatives must be listed in the ingredients, but you must know a wide array of chemical names to recognize them. Some of the most commonly used are:

- *Vitamins C and E.* These antioxidant micronutrients help protect foods from oxidation.

- *Sulfites.* A small segment of the population is sensitive to **sulfites,** preservatives used in many beers and wines and some other processed foods. These people can experience asthma, headaches, or other symptoms after eating food containing the offending preservatives.

- *Nitrites.* Commonly used to preserve processed meats, **nitrites** are of concern to many food safety experts, because they can be easily converted to *nitrosamines* during the cooking process. Nitrosamines have been found to be carcinogenic in animals, so the U.S. Food and Drug Administration (FDA) has required all foods with nitrites to contain additional antioxidants to decrease the formation of nitrosamines.

Table 12.3 on page 404 lists some other common preservatives and the types of foods you might expect to find them in.

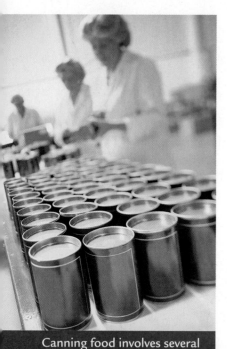

Canning food involves several steps to ensure all microorganisms in the food are killed.

pasteurization A form of sterilization using high temperatures for short periods of time.

aseptic packaging Sterile packaging that does not require refrigeration or preservatives while seal is maintained.

food preservatives Chemicals that help prevent microbial spoilage and enzymatic deterioration.

sulfites A mold inhibitor that is very effective in controlling growth in grapes and wine.

nitrites Chemicals used in meat curing to develop and stabilize the pink color associated with cured meat, also functions as an antibacterial agent.

irradiation A sterilization process in which food is exposed to gamma rays or high-energy electron beams to kill microorganisms. Irradiation does not impart any radiation to the food being treated.

genetic modification/genetically modified organisms (GMOs) Terms used to signify that the organism has been created through manipulation of the genetic material.

Irradiation

Irradiation is a process that exposes foods to gamma rays from radioactive metals. Energy from the rays penetrates food and its packaging, killing microorganisms in the food or leaving them incapable of reproducing. The process leaves no residue and does not cause foods to become radioactive!

In the United States, many foods are approved for preservation using irradiation; among them are spices, grains, fruits, pork products, beef, and poultry. A few nutrients, including vitamins A, E, K, and thiamin, are lost with irradiation, but these losses are also incurred in conventional processing and preparation.

Although irradiated food has been shown to be safe, the FDA requires that all irradiated foods be labeled with a "radura" symbol and a caution against irradiating the food again (FIGURE 12.10). Irradiated foods can be contaminated during handling, so consumers still need to be diligent in their storage and preparation of these foods.

Genetic Modification

In **genetic modification**, the DNA of an organism is altered to bring about specific changes in its seeds or offspring, for instance making tomatoes plumper, juicier, and more pest-resistant, or using selective breeding to produce beef cattle that are resistant to heat and humidity and produce high-quality meat. The relative benefits and harm of genetic modification have been debated worldwide and are the subject of the accompanying Highlight: Genetically Modified Organisms: A Blessing or a Curse?

> RECAP *Salting, sugaring, drying, and smoking are techniques that draw water out of foods, making them inhospitable to microorganisms. Storage in icehouses and other cold areas has been used for centuries to preserve food. Canning, pasteurization, and aseptic packaging use high heat to destroy microorganisms. Preservatives such as vitamins C and E, sulfites, and nitrites are often added to keep foods fresher longer. Irradiation involves the use of energy to destroy the microorganisms in foods. The DNA of plants and animals can be genetically modified to enhance certain qualities of foods, such as the ability of a plant to resist pests.*

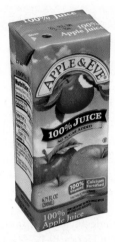

FIGURE 12.9 Aseptic packaging allows foods to be stored unrefrigerated for several months without spoilage.

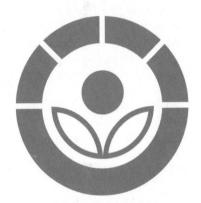

FIGURE 12.10 Radura—the international symbol of irradiated food—is required by the Food and Drug Administration to be displayed on all irradiated food sold in the United States.

What Are Food Additives, and Are They Safe?

Have you ever picked up a loaf of bread and started reading its ingredients? You'd expect to see flour, yeast, water, and some sugar, but what are all those other items? They are collectively called *food additives*, and they are in almost every processed food. **Food additives** are not foods in themselves but rather natural or synthetic chemicals added to foods to enhance them in some way. For instance, "yellow #6" colors a processed cheese spread, and calcium increases the nutrient value of orange juice. The preservatives we discussed earlier are also food additives: without them, that loaf of bread would go stale within a day or two. More than 3,000 different food additives are currently used in the United States. Table 12.3 identifies only a few of the most common.

Food Additives Include Flavorings, Colorings, Nutrients, and Other Agents

Roughly half of all food additives are **flavoring agents,** which are used to replace the natural flavors lost during food processing.[14] In contrast, *flavor enhancers* have little or no flavor of their own but accentuate the natural flavor of foods. One of the most common flavor enhancers used is MSG (monosodium glutamate). In some people, MSG causes symptoms such as headaches, difficulty breathing, and heart palpitations.

food additive A substance or mixture of substances intentionally put into food to enhance its appearance, safety, palatability, and quality.

flavoring agents Obtained from either natural or synthetic sources; they allow manufacturers to maintain a consistent flavor from batch to batch.

HIGHLIGHT

Genetically Modified Organisms: A Blessing or a Curse?

Current advances in biotechnology have opened the door to one of the most controversial topics in food science, **genetically modified organisms (GMOs).** GMOs are organisms that are created through a type of genetic engineering called *recombinant DNA technology*, in which DNA from two organisms of different species are combined to create a new type of organism. The process, which is shown in Figure 12.11, usually begins when scientists isolate a segment of DNA coding for a desirable protein—for example, a protein that confers a helpful trait such as ability to tolerate salty soil. Scientists extract and copy that DNA segment, then insert it into cells of organisms lacking that trait. As the cells multiply, they produce new organisms that express the desired trait.

In 1994, the Flavr Savr tomato became the first commercially sold GMO. The process for developing this tomato involved manipulating the gene that codes for an enzyme that causes ripening in the tomato. As a result, the enzyme was not synthesized, and ripening slowed dramatically—making the tomato appear "fresh" longer and enabling it to maintain a longer shelf life.[15]

Since 1994, hundreds of plants and animals have been genetically modified and incorporated into our food supply. For example, in 2000, approximately 54% of all soybeans and 25% of all the corn grown in the United States were GMOs.[16] Genetic engineering of animals has led to the development of cattle, sheep, pigs, and poultry that grow more quickly, with a higher disease resistance and lower fat levels. Genetically modified salmon are significantly larger than their wild relatives and are more resistant to disease.

Proponents of genetic modification suggest that genetically engineered plants and animals could solve several food production problems encountered worldwide by improving nutrient content, increasing yield, decreasing the need for pesticides, and allowing plants to grow in inhospitable soils. They also argue that genetic engineering is simply an extension of traditional plant and animal breeding methods. In

traditional plant breeding, farmers save seeds from the best plants, or pair one plant with another of a similar species—as with tangelos, which are a combination of grapefruit and tangerines. In animals, innovation occurs via selective breeding. For example, Brahman cattle (which have poor meat but are highly resistant to both heat and humidity) are bred with English shorthorn cattle (which have excellent meat but do not resist heat and humidity) to produce Santa Gertrudis cattle (which have good meat and are resistant to heat and humidity).

Opponents of genetic engineering argue that traditional methods are safer and more natural than genetic engineering. Their concerns regarding GMOs include environmental hazards, human health risks, and economic concerns. A particular concern is unintended transfer of genes to nontarget species, which occurs, for example, when pollen from a GMO crop is carried on the wind or by bees or birds to other, non-GMO crops. If a plant that had been engineered for herbicide tolerance were to disperse genes to weeds, the result could be a "super weed"—a plant tolerant to herbicides, thereby requiring that newer and stronger chemicals be produced.

An increased risk of allergens is another legitimate concern. Introducing a gene from one plant into another may create a new allergen, or cause susceptible people to experience an allergic reaction to a previously safe food because it now contains genetic material from an allergenic food.[16] In the United States, legislation passed in 1992 requires all new GMOs to be tested and labeled for allergy sensitivity if the DNA introduced is from any food containing a common allergen. However, processed foods that contain GMOs are exempt from this labeling requirement. Many U.S. consumer groups are pressuring the government to require labeling for all foods containing GMOs.

As you can see, despite many benefits of GMOs, there are also many risks to their development and use. Nutrition scientists estimate that it will take several generations before the full impact of genetically modified organisms is known.

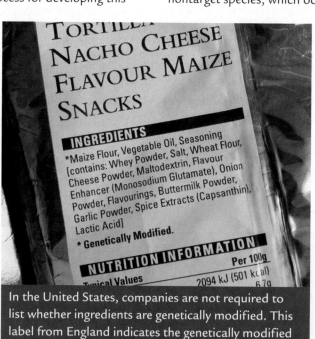

In the United States, companies are not required to list whether ingredients are genetically modified. This label from England indicates the genetically modified content of the food.

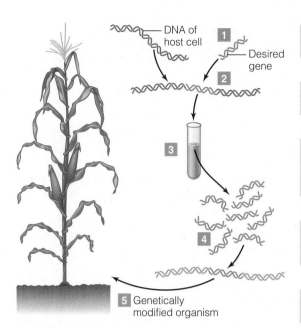

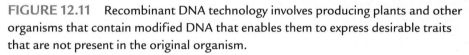

DNA of host cell

1

Desired gene

2

3

4

5 Genetically modified organism

1 Gene that expresses desired trait is extracted from cell.

2 Gene is combined with DNA of host cell that lacks this gene.

3 Host cell containing recombinant DNA is cultured, resulting in many copies of the gene.

4 Gene is extracted and inserted into DNA of cells of an organism that lacks this gene.

5 Cells produce organism that expresses the desired trait.

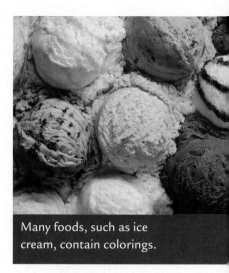

Many foods, such as ice cream, contain colorings.

FIGURE 12.11 Recombinant DNA technology involves producing plants and other organisms that contain modified DNA that enables them to express desirable traits that are not present in the original organism.

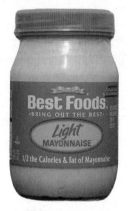

Mayonnaise contains emulsifiers to prevent separation of fats.

Common food colorings include beet juice, which gives a red color, beta-carotene, which gives a yellow color, and caramel, which adds brown color. The coloring tartrazine (FD&C yellow #5) causes an allergic reaction in some people, and its use must be indicated on the product packaging.

Vitamins and minerals are added to foods as preservatives or as nutrients. Vitamin E is usually added to fat-based products to keep them from going rancid, and vitamin C is used as an antioxidant in many foods. Iodine is added to table salt to help decrease the incidence of goiter, a condition that causes the thyroid gland to enlarge. Vitamin D is added to milk, and calcium is added to soy milk, rice milk, and some juices to help prevent osteoporosis.

Texturizers such as calcium chloride are added to foods to improve their texture. For instance, they are added to canned tomatoes and potatoes so they don't fall apart. **Stabilizers** also give foods "body" and help them maintain a desired texture or color. **Thickening agents** absorb water and keep the complex mixtures of oils, water, acids, and solids in processed foods balanced.[17] **Emulsifiers** help to keep fats evenly dispersed within foods.

Moisture content is a critical component of food. **Humectants** such as glycerin and sorbitol keep foods like marshmallows, chewing gum, and shredded coconut moist and stretchy. **Desiccants** prevent moisture absorption from the air; for example, they are used to prevent table salt from forming clumps.

Are Food Additives Safe?

Federal legislation was passed in 1958 to regulate food additives. The Delaney Clause, also enacted in 1958, states that "No additive may be permitted in any amount if tests show that it produces cancer when fed to man or animals or by other appropriate tests." Before a new food additive can be used in food, the producer of the additive must demonstrate its safety to the FDA by submitting data on its reasonable safety. The FDA makes a determination of the additive's safety based on these data.

During this same year, the U.S. Congress recognized that many substances added to foods would not require this type of formal review by the FDA prior to marketing and use, as their safety had already been established through long-term use or because their safety had been recognized by qualified experts through scientific

texturizer A chemical used to improve the texture of various foods.

stabilizer A chemical that helps maintain smooth texture and uniform color and flavor in some foods.

thickening agents Natural or chemically modified carbohydrates that absorb some of the water present in food, making the food thicker.

emulsifiers Chemicals that improve texture and smoothness in foods; stabilize oil–water mixtures.

humectants Chemicals that help retain moisture in foods, keeping them soft and pliable.

desiccants Chemicals that prevent foods from absorbing moisture from the air.

TABLE 12.3 Examples of Common Food Additives

Food Additive	Foods Found In
Coloring Agents	
Beet extract	Beverages, candies, ice cream
Beta carotene	Beverages, sauces, soups, baked goods, candies, macaroni and cheese mixes
Caramel	Beverages, sauces, soups, baked goods
Tartrazine	Beverages, cakes and cookies, ice cream
Preservatives	
Alpha-tocopherol (vitamin E)	Vegetable oils
Ascorbic acid (vitamin C)	Breakfast cereals, cured meats, fruit drinks
BHA	Breakfast cereals, chewing gum, oils, potato chips
BHT	Breakfast cereals, chewing gum, oils, potato chips
Calcium proprionate/Sodium proprionate	Bread, cakes, pies, rolls
EDTA	Beverages, canned shellfish, margarine, mayonnaise, processed fruits and vegetables, sandwich spreads
Propyl gallate	Mayonnaise, chewing gum, chicken soup base, vegetable oils, meat products, potato products, fruits, ice cream
Sodium benzoate	Carbonated beverages, fruit juice, pickles, preserves
Sodium chloride (salt)	Most processed foods
Sodium nitrate/sodium nitrite	Bacon, corned beef, luncheon meats, smoked fish
Sorbic acid/potassium sorbate	Cakes, cheese, dried fruits, jellies, syrups, wine
Sulfites (sodium bisulfite, sulfur dioxide)	Dried fruits, processed potatoes, wine
Texturizers, Emulsifiers, and Stabilizers	
Calcium chloride	Canned fruits and vegetables
Carageenan/pectin	Ice cream, chocolate milk, soy milk, frostings, jams, jellies, cheese, salad dressings, sour cream, puddings, syrups
Cellulose gum/guar gum/gum arabic/locust gum/xanthan gum	Soups and sauces, gravies, sour cream, ricotta cheese, ice cream, syrups
Gelatin	Desserts, canned meats
Lecithin	Mayonnaise, ice cream
Humectants	
Glycerin	Chewing gum, marshmallows, shredded coconut
Propylene glycol	Chewing gum, gummy candies

studies. These substances are exempt from the more stringent testing criteria for new food additives and are referred to as substances that are **Generally Recognized as Safe (GRAS).** The GRAS list identifies substances that have either been tested and determined by the FDA to be safe and approved for use in the food industry, or are deemed safe as a result of consensus among experts qualified by scientific training and experience.

In 1985, the FDA established the Adverse Reaction Monitoring System (ARMS). Under this system, the FDA investigates complaints from consumers, physicians, or food companies about food additives.

Generally Recognized as Safe (GRAS) list Established by Congress to identify substances used in foods that are generally recognized as safe based on a history of long-term use or on the consensus of qualified research experts.

RECAP *Food additives are chemicals intentionally added to foods to enhance their color, flavor, texture, nutrient density, moisture level, or shelf life. Although there is continuing controversy over food additives in the United States, the FDA regulates additives used in our food supply and considers safe those it approves.*

Do Residues Harm Our Food Supply?

Food **residues** are chemicals that remain in the foods we eat despite cleaning and processing. Three residues currently of global concern are persistent organic pollutants, pesticides, and growth hormones.

Persistent Organic Pollutants Can Pass into the Food Chain

Many different chemicals are released into the atmosphere as a result of industry, agriculture, automobile emissions, and improper waste disposal. These chemicals, collectively referred to as **persistent organic pollutants (POPs),** eventually enter the food supply through the soil or water. If a pollutant gets into the soil, a plant can absorb the chemical into its structure and can pass it on as part of the food chain. Animals can also absorb the pollutant into their tissues or can consume it when feeding on plants growing in the polluted soil. Fat-soluble pollutants are especially problematic, as they tend to accumulate in the animal's body tissues and are then absorbed by humans when the animal is used as a food source (**FIGURE 12.12**).

POP residues have been found in virtually all categories of foods, including baked goods, fruit, vegetables, meat, poultry, fish, and dairy products. It is believed that all living organisms on Earth carry a measurable level of POPs in their tissues.[18]

residues Chemicals that remain in the foods we eat despite cleaning and processing.

persistent organic pollutants (POPs) Chemicals released into the environment as a result of industry, agriculture, or improper waste disposal; automobile emissions also are considered POPs.

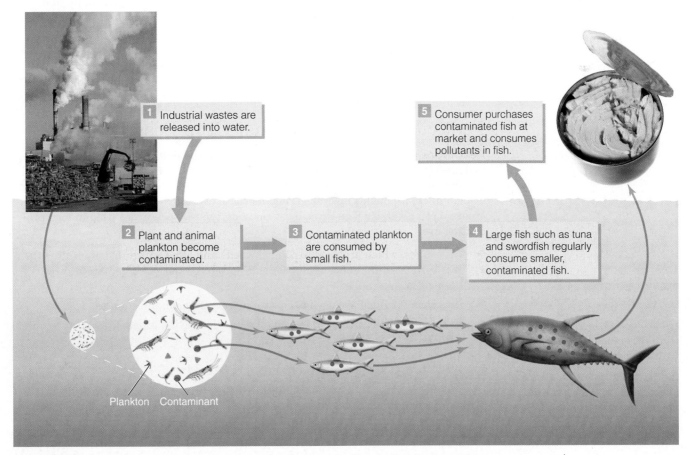

1 Industrial wastes are released into water.

5 Consumer purchases contaminated fish at market and consumes pollutants in fish.

2 Plant and animal plankton become contaminated.

3 Contaminated plankton are consumed by small fish.

4 Large fish such as tuna and swordfish regularly consume smaller, contaminated fish.

Plankton Contaminant

FIGURE 12.12 Bioaccumulation of persistent organic pollutants in the food supply.

Mercury and Lead Are Nerve Toxins Found in the Environment

Mercury, a naturally occurring element, is found in soil, rocks, and water. It is also released into the air by pulp and paper processing and the burning of garbage and fossil fuels. As mercury falls from the air, it finds its way to streams, rivers, lakes, and the ocean, where it accumulates. Fish absorb mercury as they feed on aquatic organisms. This mercury is passed on to us when we consume the fish. As mercury accumulates in the body, it has a toxic effect on the nervous system.

Large predatory fish, such as swordfish, shark, King mackerel, and tilefish tend to contain the highest levels of mercury.[19] Because mercury is especially toxic to the developing nervous system of fetuses and growing children, pregnant and breast-feeding women and young children are advised to avoid eating these types of fish. Canned tuna, salmon, cod, pollock, sole, shrimp, mussels, and scallops do not contain high levels of mercury and are safe to consume; however, the FDA recommends that pregnant women and young children eat no more than two servings (12 oz) per week of any type of fish.[19] To learn more about the risks of mercury in seafood, visit the FDA's food safety Web site at http://vm.cfsan.fda.gov/list.html or call the FDA's 24-hour information line at 1(888) SAFEFOOD.

Lead can also be found naturally in the soil, water, and air. It also occurs as industrial waste from leaded gasoline, lead-based paints, and lead-soldered cans, now outlawed but decomposing in landfills. Some ceramic mugs and other dishes are fired with lead-based glaze. Thus, residues can build up in foods. Excessive lead exposure can cause learning and behavioral impediments in children and cardiovascular and kidney disease in adults.

Industrial Pollutants Also Create Residues

Polychlorinated biphenyls (PCBs) and dioxins are two industrial pollutants that have been found in food worldwide. Dioxins from discarded transformers and PCBs, which are by-products of waste incineration, enter the soil and can persist in the environment for years, easily accumulating in fatty tissues. PCBs and dioxins along with other POPs have been linked to cancer, learning disorders, impaired immune function, and infertility.[18]

Pesticides Protect Against Crop Losses

Pesticides are a family of chemicals used in both the field and farm storage areas to decrease destruction and crop losses caused by weeds, animals, insects, and fungus. Pesticides also help to reduce the potential spread of disease by decreasing the level of microorganisms on crops. They increase overall crop yield and allow for greater crop diversity. The three most common types of pesticides used in food production are:

- *Herbicides,* which are used to control weeds and other unwanted plant growth. It is estimated that 65% of all pesticides produced in the United States are herbicides.
- *Insecticides,* which are used to control insects that can infest crops.
- *Fungicides,* which are used to control plant-destroying fungal growth.

Pesticides Can Be Natural or Synthetic

Despite the negative connotations associated with pesticides, many pesticides used today are naturally derived and/or have a low impact on the environment. Gardeners and farmers are starting to use **biopesticides,** which are species-specific and work

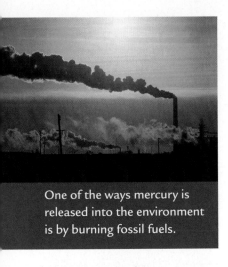

One of the ways mercury is released into the environment is by burning fossil fuels.

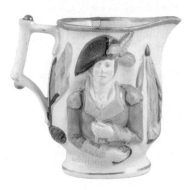

Antique porcelain is often coated with lead-based glaze.

pesticides Chemicals used either in the field or in storage to decrease destruction by predators or disease.

biopesticides Primarily insecticides, these chemicals use natural methods to reduce damage to crops.

to suppress a pest's population, not eliminate it. For example, pheromones are a biopesticide that disrupts insect mating by attracting males into traps. Biopesticides also do not leave residues on crops—most degrade rapidly and are easily washed away with water. In addition, many common products such as salt, boric acid, dried blood, or diatomaceous earth (soil made up of a type of algae called *diatoms*) are used as pesticides.

Pesticides can also be synthetically derived. Many are made from petroleum-based products. Examples include fungicides commonly used to prevent contamination of potatoes and apples.

Pesticides Are Potential Toxins

The liver is responsible for detoxifying the chemicals that enter our bodies. But if the liver is immature, as in a fetus, infant, or child, or is stressed by disease or other toxins, such as excessive alcohol, then it cannot effectively remove pesticide residues. When pesticide residues are not effectively removed, they can damage body tissues. Some are fat-soluble and can be deposited in adipose tissues. Others target nerves and endocrine cells. Thus, although originally intended for other organisms, pesticides do have the potential to cause problems in humans. It is therefore essential to wash all produce carefully.

Government Regulations Control the Use of Pesticides

The Environmental Protection Agency (EPA) is the government agency responsible for regulating the labeling, sale, distribution, use, and disposal of all pesticides in the United States. The EPA also sets a tolerance level, which is the maximum residue level of a pesticide permitted in or on food or feed grown in the United States or imported into the United States from other countries.[20]

Before a pesticide can be accepted by the EPA for use, it must be determined that it performs its intended function with minimal impact to the environment. Once the EPA has certified a pesticide, states can set their own regulations for its use. Canadian regulation of pesticides closely resembles American laws, with provinces and territories given free range to limit pesticide use.

NUTRI-CASE GUSTAVO

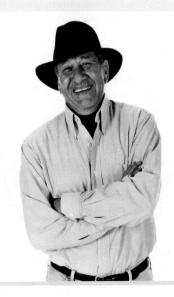

"   All of a sudden, a feisty bunch of newcomers to town are complaining about vineyards around here using too many pesticides. They're worried that somehow the pesticides we use are going to hurt them, but that's not possible because winemaking destroys all those bad chemicals before you drink it. I've been working with pesticides for 50 years, and they haven't hurt me!"

What do you think of Gustavo's claim that pesticides are not harmful? Before you answer, think not only about their effect on the grapes used to make wine but also about other potential forms of contamination.

Growth Hormones Are Injected into Cows that Produce Meat and Milk

Introduced in the U.S. food supply in 1994, **recombinant bovine growth hormone (rBGH)** is a genetically engineered growth hormone. It is used in beef herds to induce animals to grow more muscle tissue and less fat. It is also injected into dairy cows to increase milk output. Currently, there are no labeling requirements for products containing rBGH.

Although the FDA has allowed the use of rBGH in the United States, both Canada and the European Union have banned its use because of studies showing that there is an increased risk of illness in dairy cows administered rBGH.[21] These cows have an increased tendency to develop lameness, infertility, and mastitis (udder swelling), the latter of which requires medical treatment with antibiotics. The antibiotics then enter the cows' milk, possibly fostering the development of antibiotic-resistant strains of bacteria in humans, although this is also a topic of considerable controversy.

Advocates of rBGH say that its use allows farmers to use less feed for the same yield, reducing resource use by each ranch or farm. Thus, it is unlikely that there will be agreement regarding the use of rBGH in the near future.

> RECAP *Persistent organic pollutants (POPs) of concern include mercury, lead, polychlorinated biphenyls (PCBs), and dioxins. Pesticides are used to prevent or reduce food crop losses but are potential toxins; therefore, it is essential to wash all produce carefully. Recombinant bovine growth hormone (rBGH) is injected into meat and dairy cows to increase meat production and milk output. Concerns about rBGH include possible effects on human and bovine health.*

Are Organic Foods More Healthful?

The term *organic* is commonly used to describe foods that are grown without the use of synthetic pesticides. A recent national survey indicated that approximately 27% of U.S. consumers use organic foods on a daily or weekly basis.[22]

To Be Labeled Organic, Foods Must Meet Federal Standards

The National Organic Program (NOP) of the USDA came into law in October 2002. Its Organic Standards established uniform definitions for all organic products. Any label or product claiming to be organic must comply with the following definitions:

- *100% Organic:* Products containing only organically produced ingredients, excluding water and salt.
- *Organic:* Products containing 95% organically produced ingredients by weight, excluding water and salt, with the remaining ingredients consisting of those products not commercially available in organic form.
- *Made with organic ingredients:* A product containing more than 70% organic ingredients.

Processed products containing less than 70% organically produced ingredients cannot use the term *organic* in the principal display panel, but ingredients that are organically produced can be specified on the ingredients statement on the information panel.

Products that are "100% organic" and "organic" may display the USDA seal (FIGURE 12.13) or mark of certifying agents. Any product that is labeled as organic must identify each organically produced item in the ingredient statement of the label. The name and address of the certifying agency must also be on the label.

recombinant bovine growth hormone (rBGH) A genetically engineered hormone injected into dairy cows to enhance their milk output.

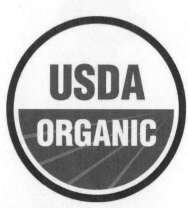

FIGURE 12.13 The USDA organic seal identifies foods that are at least 95% organic.

The USDA Regulates Organic Farming

The USDA regulates organic farming standards, and farms must be certified as organic by a government-approved certifier who inspects the farm and verifies that the farmer is following all USDA organic standards. Companies that handle or process organic food before it arrives at your local supermarket or restaurant must also be certified.[23] Organic farming methods are strict and require farmers to find natural alternatives to many common problems such as weeds and insects. Contrary to common belief, organic farmers can use pesticides as a final option for pest control when all other methods have failed or are known to be ineffective, but they are restricted to a limited number that have been approved for use based on their origin, environmental impact, and potential to persist as residues.[24]

Organic meat, poultry, eggs, and dairy products come from animals fed only organic feed, and if the animals become ill, they are removed from the others until well again. None of these animals are given growth hormones to increase their size or ability to produce milk. Irradiation is also prohibited.[24]

Studies Comparing Organic and Conventionally Grown Foods Are Limited

Recent studies at the University of California, Davis, and other institutions indicate that some organically grown foods are higher in vitamins E and C and in certain antioxidant phytochemicals than their non-organic counterparts.[25–27] Although these studies appear promising, they do not prove that organic foods are more nutritious than non-organic foods. To date, there are very few studies that have assessed the nutritional content of organically grown foods and compared them to the same foods grown non-organically. Thus, no consensus can be reached as to whether organic foods are more healthful than traditionally grown foods.

RECAP *The USDA regulates organic farming standards and inspects and certifies farms that follow all USDA Organic Standards. The USDA organic seal identifies foods that are at least 95% organic. Although a few recent studies indicate that some organic foods have higher levels of some nutrients and phytochemicals than nonorganic foods, there is insufficient evidence to support the claim that organic foods are more nutritious than nonorganic foods.*

Malnutrition Is a Concern Shared Throughout the World

Our ability to feed ourselves is influenced by many factors, some of which are beyond our personal control. These include environmental forces, such as a drought that leads to widespread crop failure resulting in famine; political forces, such as a war that causes people to flee their homes and gather in refugee camps; economic forces, such as a job loss that makes it difficult for a family to afford nourishing food; and marketing forces, such as advertising that entices children to consume nutrient-poor foods. These nutrition concerns are shared throughout the world and are met in different ways in different countries.

Food Security Is Elusive in the United States and Throughout the World

Food security means daily access to food with enough energy and nutrient quality to support a healthy, active life. The food is available because the people grow it themselves or because they have enough money to buy it from a vendor accessible to

food security A situation in which a person has daily access to a supply of safe foods with enough energy and sufficiently rich nutrient quality to promote a healthy, active life.

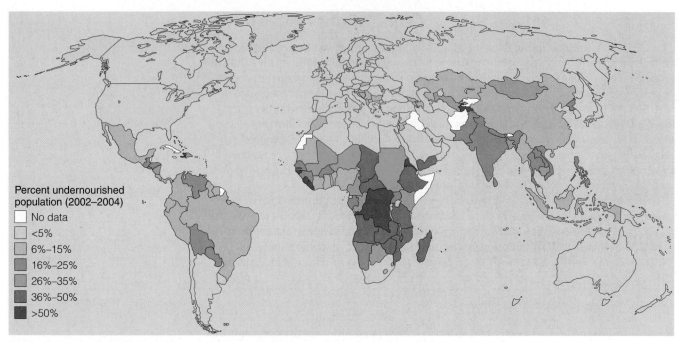

Percent undernourished
population (2002–2004)

- No data
- <5%
- 6%–15%
- 16%–25%
- 26%–35%
- 36%–50%
- >50%

FIGURE 12.14 Undernutrition is most prevalent in parts of sub-Saharan Africa and Southeast Asia.
(Source: © Food and Agriculture Organization of the United Nations. 2004. Undernourished Population [2002–2004]. Available at www.fao.org/es/ess/faostat/foodsecurity/FS%20Map/map14.htm. Reprinted by permission.)

them. Food security is enjoyed by 89% of the U.S. population; most individuals in developed nations enjoy food security.[28]

Food insecurity is an inability to obtain enough energy and nutrients to meet physical needs every day. Almost 4% of American households experience *very low food security*, meaning that they lack even basic foods to meet their energy needs and face the uneasiness and pain that accompany hunger pangs.[28] In the United States, food insecurity and hunger typically occur because of poverty; that is, adequate food is available in the neighborhood or area, but the individual or family does not have enough money to buy it or does not own enough land on which to grow it. Families consisting of a single mother with children are most at risk: in 2005, 30.8% of these families experienced food insecurity.[28] Other at-risk groups in the United States are the homeless, the unemployed, migrant laborers, and other unskilled workers in minimum-wage jobs.

Food insecurity is much more severe worldwide than it is in the United States, Canada, Australia, or Europe (FIGURE 12.14). The Food and Agriculture Organization (FAO) of the United Nations estimates that one in five people in the developing world is chronically hungry.[29]

The Three Types of Malnutrition Are Undernutrition, Nutrient Deficiency, and Overnutrition

Poor health can result from any of three main types of malnutrition:

- **Undernutrition** is an inadequate intake of energy. In some parts of the world, it is *endemic* (common throughout a region for many years) because of wars, floods, droughts, or farming practices that make widespread crop failure common. Undernourished adults and children appear **wasted,** with a low body weight for their height. Children who do not eat enough food to support their growth are often shorter than would be expected for their age, a condition known as **stunting.** In circumstances of extreme hunger, children can be both stunted and wasted.

food insecurity Situation in which one or more factors limit an individual's access to a safe and adequate nutrient-rich food supply.

undernutrition Malnutrition defined by an absolute lack of adequate energy leading to underweight.

wasting Very low weight for height.

stunting Low height for age.

- **Nutrient deficiency** is a state in which an insufficient amount of one or more essential nutrients is consumed. Although nutrient deficiency sometimes occurs as a result of consuming too little energy, it usually results from consuming a diet that has ample calories but is not varied.

- **Overnutrition** refers to a type of malnutrition in which energy intake is in excess of energy use so that body fat is stored and the person becomes overweight or obese. In Chapter 9 we discussed the problem of overweight and obesity in the developed world, but overnutrition is also becoming more common in developing nations.

Several Factors Contribute to Malnutrition

Malnutrition exists in every country of the world and has four main causes:

- *Famine.* A **famine** is a widespread food shortage that causes starvation and death. It most often occurs in nations that depend mainly on subsistence-level farming for food. Famines are often prompted by war that disrupts food production or distribution. Natural phenomena such as flood, drought, or pest infestations that destroy the major energy crop in a geographic area can also produce famine. Devastating as they are, famines are not the major cause of malnutrition.

- *Chronic food shortages.* The most persistent cause of undernutrition, chronic food shortages are usually due to inadequate production, distribution, and/or storage of food in a particular locality. Production may be inadequate because of poor soil, erosion, inadequate rainfall, or nutrient depletion of the soil from poor agricultural practices such as lack of crop rotation. Chronic food shortages occur seasonally in many countries as food from the previous harvest runs out before the next harvest. Chronic food shortage can also occur among women and girls when distribution of a limited food supply goes preferentially to men and boys, or among people of a certain religious group or ethnicity not favored by local authorities.

- *Poor-quality diet.* A high-quality diet requires a safe supply of grains, legumes, fruits, and vegetables. Quality can be augmented with small amounts of eggs, fish, poultry, meat, and dairy products. However, the usual diet in impoverished regions of the world often consists of starchy staples that are low in essential amino acids, fatty acids, vitamins, and minerals. These foods are the least expensive to buy and to store. Exclusive consumption of starchy staples provides adequate calories to prevent starvation but results in nutrient deficiency.

- *Overconsumption.* Overconsumption of a poor-quality diet, such as starchy staples or high-sugar, high-fat processed foods, can lead to nutrient deficiency and increase a population's risk for chronic disease.

Malnutrition and Infection Create a Vicious Cycle

Undernutrition and nutrient deficiency make populations more vulnerable to fatal infections among children. In impoverished nations, pneumonia and infectious diarrhea are the leading causes of death among children under 5 years of age.[30] Malnutrition reduces a child's general health, energy stores, and immune resistance, increasing the likelihood that the child will not survive infection. On the other hand, infections exacerbate malnutrition by decreasing appetite, causing vomiting and diarrhea, and generally weakening the immune system. A vicious cycle of malnutrition, infection, worsening malnutrition, and increased vulnerability to infection develops.

Other costs of malnutrition and infection include high infant-mortality rates, death of women during childbirth, preterm births, mental retardation, poor childhood growth, poor school performance, low work capacity in young adults, and short life expectancy. For example, in 2003, life expectancy of a newborn varied from a high of nearly 85 years in Japan to a low of 36 years in Sierra Leone, a country where malnutrition is endemic.[30]

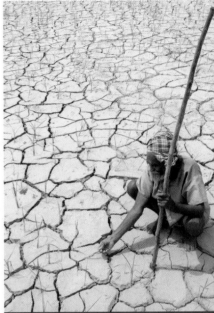

An Indian farmer inspects what is left of his crop during a drought.

nutrient deficiency Malnutrition defined by a poor-quality diet that may or may not be adequate in energy. One or more nutrient-deficiency diseases may occur.

overnutrition Malnutrition defined by an absolute excess of energy leading to overweight. Diet may be high-quality or poor-quality.

famine A widespread and severe food shortage that causes starvation and death in a large portion of a population in a region.

What Can Be Done to Relieve Malnutrition?

To combat malnutrition and achieve global food security, long-term solutions are critical. We discuss some of the most effective here.

Global Solutions

Among the most important long-term solutions for improving the survival and health of children worldwide are programs that encourage breastfeeding. This is because breast milk provides optimal nutrition for the newborn and contains antibodies that protect against infections, including infectious diarrhea. In contrast, feeding infants with formula increases the infant's risk of diarrhea if the powder is mixed with unsanitary water. The World Health Organization (WHO) sponsors programs to encourage breastfeeding throughout the developing world.

Campaigns to increase immunization of children are also helping to reduce the rate of infectious disease in children worldwide. At the same time, supplying local health agencies with oral rehydration therapy, a simple solution of fluids and electrolytes that can be administered to children with diarrhea, is helping to reduce deaths from dehydration.

Many international organizations help improve the nutrient status of the poor by enabling them to produce their own foods. For example, both USAID and the Peace Corps have agricultural education programs, the World Bank provides loans to fund small business ventures, and many non-profit and non-governmental organizations support community and family farms.

Another method for increasing local food production is **sustainable agriculture.** The goal of the sustainable agriculture movement is to develop local, site-specific farming methods that improve soil conservation, crop yields, and food security in a sustainable manner, minimizing the adverse environmental impact. For example, soil erosion can be controlled by terracing sloped land for the cultivation of crops (FIGURE 12.15), by tillage that minimizes disturbance to the topsoil, and by the use of herbicides to remove weeds rather than hoeing. Another practice associated with sustainable agriculture is the use of genetically modified plants that can be cultivated on marginally fertile land.

sustainable agriculture
Techniques of food production that preserve the environment indefinitely.

Local Solutions

In the United States, several government programs help low-income citizens acquire food over extended periods of time. Among these are the Food Stamp Program, which helps low-income individuals of all ages; the Special Supplemental Nutrition Program for Women, Infants and Children (WIC), which helps pregnant women and children to age 5; the National School Lunch and National School Breakfast Programs, which help low-income schoolchildren; and the Summer Food Service Program, which helps low-income children in the summer. The U.S. Department of Agriculture also sponsors programs to distribute emergency foods and surplus commodity foods to qualifying families. Foods may be distributed through charitable organizations or local or county agencies.

Get Involved!

Several times each year, college students from hundreds of campuses all over the United States gather to fight hunger. Members of the National Student Campaign Against Hunger and Homelessness, they hold Hunger Clean-Ups, staff relief agencies, solicit donations of food and money, and promote community activism. Their organization is just one of dozens in which you can get in-

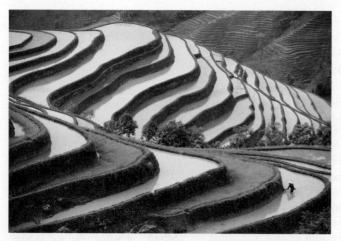

FIGURE 12.15 Terracing sloped land to avoid soil erosion is one practice of sustainable agriculture.

volved. For more information, see the Web links at the end of this chapter. In addition, the What About You box on the following page challenges you to find out how your actions affect global food security.

> RECAP *Food security is daily access to a supply of adequate, safe, and nutritious food. The three types of malnutrition are undernutrition, nutrient deficiency, and overnutrition. Globally, factors that contribute to malnutrition include famine, chronic food shortages, a poor-quality diet, and overconsumption. Malnutrition makes populations more susceptible to infection and childhood death. Strategies for relieving malnutrition include international, national, and private efforts.*

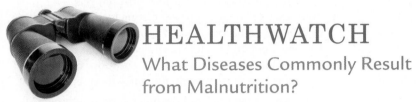

HEALTHWATCH
What Diseases Commonly Result from Malnutrition?

Malnutrition can cause a wide variety of disorders. Of these, only a few of the most common are discussed here.

Marasmus Results from Too Low an Intake of Energy

Marasmus is a disease of children that results from grossly inadequate food intake (FIGURE 12.16). Essentially, children with marasmus slowly starve to death. Marasmus commonly occurs when chronic food shortages due to poverty or other factors restrict children's diets to watery cereal drinks. Children with marasmus have minimal fat stores and severe muscle wasting. They are anemic. If marasmus continues over time, they become stunted and suffer impaired brain development and learning. Their weakened immune systems make them vulnerable to death from infectious disease. Other causes of death include dehydration or heart failure from a weakened heart muscle.

Kwashiorkor Results from Inadequate Consumption of Protein

Kwashiorkor is a disease of toddlers who have recently been weaned because a sibling is born and monopolizes breastfeeding (FIGURE 12.17 on page 415). The disease is known throughout the world by different names, but the name used throughout much of Africa, *kwashiorkor*, comes from the Ga language of Ghana and refers to the clinical syndrome, including the characteristic reddish hair, that develops when a child is suddenly deprived of protein-rich breast milk.[31] Typically, the breast milk is replaced with a watery cereal-based porridge with inadequate amounts of poor-quality protein and marginal amounts of total energy. In addition to protein deprivation, infection is thought to contribute to the onset of the disease.

The lack of dietary protein in children with kwashiorkor causes edema because the low level of protein in the blood is inadequate to keep fluids from seeping into the tissue spaces. This edema, along with a little subcutaneous fat, can make a child with kwashiorkor appear adequately nourished. The child's belly may also be swollen because of intestinal parasites. Lack of protein pigments causes the hair to turn reddish, and the skin also loses pigmentation. The child experiences severe wasting of muscle tissue, becomes inactive and apathetic, has little appetite, and easily succumbs to infection. If infection is controlled and adequate protein can be given in time, the child can recover. However, children with kwashiorkor often die from infection.

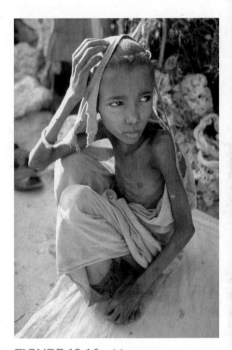

FIGURE 12.16 Marasmus results from grossly inadequate intake of energy and other nutrients.

marasmus   A form of malnutrition seen in children and resulting from grossly inadequate intakes of protein, carbohydrates, fats, and micronutrients.

kwashiorkor   A form of malnutrition that is typically seen in toddlers who are weaned because of the birth of a subsequent child. Denied breast milk, they are fed a cereal diet that provides adequate energy but inadequate protein.

WHAT ABOUT YOU?

Do Your Actions Contribute to Global Food Security?

Have you ever wondered whether or not your actions inadvertently contribute to the problem of world hunger? Or whether any efforts you make in your home or community can help feed people thousands of miles away? If so, you might want to reflect on your behaviors in each of three roles you play every day: consumer, student, and citizen of the world.

In your role as a consumer, ask yourself:

● What kinds of food products do I buy?
Your purchases influence the types of foods that are manufactured and sold. And buying less processed foods saves energy.

1. Choose fresh, locally grown, organic foods more often to support local sustainability.

2. Choose whole or less-processed versions of packaged foods (e.g., peanut butter made solely from ground peanuts or plain yogurt from a local dairy) rather than versions of foods made with high-fructose corn syrup, dyes, and other additives. This encourages increased production of the less-processed foods.

3. Limit purchases of nutrient-poor foods and beverages to discourage their profitability. Also limit high-calorie fast-food meals.

4. Consider how much packaging is used for a given food or fast-food meal and whether you will be able to recycle the package.

● How often do I eat vegetarian?
Vegetarian foods can be produced with less energy cost than animal-based foods, so every time you eat vegetarian, you save global energy.

1. Experiment with some recipes in a vegetarian cookbook. Try making at least one new vegetarian meal each week.

2. Introduce friends and family members to your new vegetarian dishes.

3. When eating out, choose restaurants that provide vegetarian menu choices. If the campus cafeteria or a favorite restaurant has no vegetarian choices, request that one or more be added to the menu.

● How much do I eat?
Eating just the calories you need to maintain a healthy weight provides more of the global harvest for others and will likely reduce your use of limited medical resources as well.

1. To raise your consciousness about the physical experience of hunger, consider fasting for 1 day. If health or other reasons prevent you from fasting safely, try keeping silent during each meal throughout 1 day so that you can more fully appreciate the food you're eating and reflect on those who do not enjoy food security.

2. For 1 week, keep track of how much food you throw away, and why. Do you put more food on your plate than you can eat? Do you allow foods stored in your refrigerator to spoil?

3. On a daily basis, check in with your body before and as you eat: are you really hungry, and if so, how much and what type of food does your body really need?

In your role as a student, ask yourself:

● How can I use what I have learned about nutrition to help feed my neighbors and the world?

1. Visit each of your local fast-food restaurants and ask for information about the nutritional value of their foods. Analyze the nutrition information, then summarize it in simple language. Offer to submit a series of articles about your findings to your school or local newspaper.

2. Research what local produce is available in each season. Write an article for your school newspaper listing what is in season each month of the year and include two healthy recipes using vegetables and fruits that are in season during the month your article will be published.

3. Create an entertaining skit or puppet show that encourages young children to eat healthful foods. Offer to entertain on the weekends at your local library, day-care center, or after-school community program.

4. Begin or join a food cooperative, community garden, or shared farming program. Donate a portion of your produce each week to a local food pantry.

● What careers could I consider to promote global food security?

1. If you are interested in teaching, you could become a member of the Peace Corps and teach nutrition in developing countries. If you want to teach in the United States, see the Feeding Minds Fighting Hunger Web site listed in this chapter's Web Links for information on teaching young people about global nutrition.

2. If you are interested in science, you could help develop higher-yielding crops, better irrigation methods, or projects to improve food or water safety.

3. If you plan a career in business, you could enter the food industry and help market healthful foods.

4. If you pursue a career in healthcare, you could join an international medical corps working among the poor.

In your role as a world citizen, ask yourself:

● **How can I improve the nutrition of people in my own community?**

1. You can volunteer at a local soup kitchen, homeless shelter, foodbank, or community garden.

2. Because obesity is likely to be a significant problem in your community, you can help increase opportunities for physical activity in your community. Start a walking group, or volunteer to coach children in your favorite sport.

● **How can I improve the nutrition of people in developing nations?**

1. Donate time or money to one of the international agencies that work to provide relief from famine or chronic hunger. Check out options for charitable contributions and volunteer efforts at www. charitynavigator.org.

2. Research the global effects of protectionist agricultural subsidies in the United States and Europe, then write letters to your school or community newspaper, your elected officials, and political action groups expressing your concerns.

3. Research the human rights records of international food companies whose products you buy. If you don't like what you find out, switch brands, and write to the company and tell them why you did.

4. Vote for elected officials who support policies that help impoverished Americans and promote agricultural equity around the world.

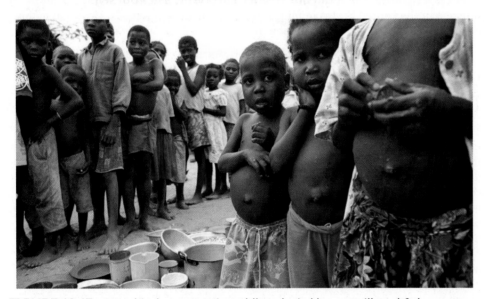

FIGURE 12.17 Kwashiorkor occurs in toddlers denied breast milk and fed a watery cereal that provides inadequate protein.

Vitamin A Deficiency Causes Night Blindness

Lack of sufficient vitamin A in the diet is a preventable cause of night blindness in children. (Night blindness is described in Chapter 6.) When the deficiency continues, permanent blindness results in as many as 500,000 children each year.[32] Because vitamin A is also critical for immune function, about half of these children die of infection within a year of becoming blind. In high-risk areas, pregnant women often become night-blind as well. Where vitamin A deficiency is widespread, the WHO

Where I'm

at now...

Now that you've read this chapter, jot down four simple things you can do to avoid food-borne illness:

1.

2.

3.

4.

Write down one action—if any—that you are willing to commit to taking to help relieve hunger in your neighborhood or across the world:

recommends breastfeeding and vitamin A supplementation for infants, fortification of commonly consumed foods, and the cultivation of vegetables and fruits rich in beta-carotene in home gardens.

Iron Deficiency Is the Most Common Nutrient Deficiency in the World

Iron deficiency is the world's most common nutrient deficiency. The WHO estimates that more than 30% of the world's population is anemic due to inadequate iron intake.[33] Malaria and worm infections also contribute to iron deficiency. Because iron deficiency affects so many people—increasing the risk of infection, premature birth, and low birth weight, rendering children less able to learn, impairing the ability of adults to work, and increasing the likelihood that women will die in childbirth—it is a global public health problem of unparalleled importance. The WHO advocates increasing iron intake by supplemental iron, promoting iron-rich diets through dietary diversification with incorporation of naturally iron-rich foods, and iron fortification of foods. It also advocates control of worm infections and malaria to aid in improving iron status in developing countries.

Iodine Deficiency Causes Preventable Brain Damage in Children

The most common cause of preventable mental impairment in children is low iodine intake during the mothers' pregnancy and the early childhood years. The WHO estimates that 13% of the world's population is affected by iodine deficiency disorders and another 30% is at risk.[34] Iodine is plentiful in saltwater fish, but iodine deficiency is a significant problem in 130 developing inland countries and was once a problem in the United States in midwestern and mountain regions. However, iodine deficiency has been largely eliminated in the United States and other countries that have adopted the use of iodized salt.

Obesity and Its Associated Diseases Are Increasing Throughout the World

Throughout the 20th century, advances in microbiology and public health efforts to improve access to safe water and vaccines led to a dramatic decline in mortality from infectious diseases in developed nations. As the incidence of infectious diseases dwindled, **noncommunicable diseases** such as heart disease, stroke, diabetes, and cancer became the leading causes of death. As we have discussed throughout this book, overweight and obesity are risk factors for most of these diseases. Once confined to a minority of the population worldwide, overweight and its associated diseases are now a global concern.

In our global economy, countries as diverse as India and Brazil are experiencing a shift in dietary pattern called the **nutrition transition.** That is, an increasing percentage of the population is food secure, there is a greater variety of foods from which to choose, and more high-fat, high-sugar processed foods are available. Greater access to motorized transportation and a decrease in occupational physical activity accompany the transition. Not surprisingly, transitioning countries have been experiencing an alarming increase in the prevalence of overweight and obesity and associated chronic diseases.[35] These countries are challenged to support economic prosperity without promoting overnutrition.

noncommunicable diseases Diseases that are not infectious but are largely determined by genetics and lifestyle. Chronic diseases are typically noncommunicable.

nutrition transition A shift in dietary pattern toward greater food security, greater variety of foods, and more foods with high energy density because of added fat and sugar. It is accompanied by access to motorized transportation, sedentary occupations, and economic growth.

RECAP *Marasmus is a disease of children that results from grossly inadequate intakes of all nutrients, whereas kwashiorkor is linked to inadequate protein intake. Vitamin A deficiency causes permanent blindness and increased vulnerability to infection. Iron deficiency increases the risk of infection, impaired development, and premature death, and iodine deficiency can cause mental impairment and other problems. As developing nations begin to prosper economically, they go through a nutrition transition and experience increased rates of obesity and its associated chronic diseases.*

REVIEW QUESTIONS

Circle the correct choice.

1. Monosodium glutamate (MSG) is

a. a thickening agent used in baby foods.

b. a flavor enhancer used in a variety of foods.

c. a mold inhibitor used on grapes and other foods.

d. an amino acid added as a nutrient to some foods.

2. Foods that are labeled *100% Organic:*

a. contain only organically produced ingredients, excluding water and salt.

b. may display the EPA's organic seal.

c. were produced without the use of pesticides.

d. contain no discernible level of toxic metals.

3. Of the following techniques for food preservation, which has the least effect on taste?

a. sugaring

b. smoking

c. salting

d. pasteurization

4. Which of the following childhood illnesses has been linked to inadequate intake of dietary protein?

a. cretinism

b. malaria

c. night blindness

d. kwashiorkor

5. The shift in dietary patterns seen in populations as poverty is relieved is called

a. the nutrition transition.

b. nutrient deficiency.

c. very low food security.

d. chronic food shortage.

6. True or False? You prepare a potato, egg, and red onion salad with mayonnaise at 10:00 AM for a 2:00 PM barbecue. It is safe to leave the salad at room temperature until the barbecue.

7. True or False? Children with night blindness have an increased risk for premature death.

8. True or False? In the United States, farms certified as organic are allowed to use pesticides under certain conditions.

9. True or False? Irradiation makes foods radioactive.

10. True or False? Chronic food shortage is a more significant cause of undernutrition than is famine.

WEB LINKS

www.foodsafety.gov
Foodsafety.gov

Use this Web site as a gateway to government food safety information; it contains news and safety alerts, an area to report illnesses and product complaints, information on food-borne pathogens, and much more.

www.fightbac.org
Partnership for Food Safety Education

Learn more about safe food handling, food-borne illness, and how to "Fight BAC!"

www.fsis.usda.gov
The USDA Food Safety and Inspection Service

A comprehensive Web site providing information on all aspects of food safety. Explore the site for information about food preparation, storage, handling, and other specific safety issues.

http://vm.cfsan.fda.gov/list.html
The FDA Center for Food Safety and Applied Nutrition

This Web site contains thorough information on topics such as national food safety programs, recent news, and food labeling. It also contains links to special program areas, such as regulation of mercury levels in fish, food colorings, and biotechnology.

www.epa.gov/pesticides
The U.S. Environmental Protection Agency: Pesticides

This Web site provides information about agricultural and home-use pesticides, pesticide health and safety issues, environmental effects, and government regulations.

www.ams.usda.gov
The USDA National Organic Program

Click on "National Organic Program" to find the site describing the NOP's standards and labeling program, consumer information, and publications.

www.ota.com
The Organic Trade Association

Visit this Web site to learn about consumer use of organic foods, sales of organic foods, and recent research into conventional versus organic farming and the effects of each on foods and the environment.

www.unicef.org
The United Nations Children's Fund

Visit this Web site to learn about international concerns affecting the world's children, including nutrient deficiencies and hunger.

www.who.int/nutrition/en
The World Health Organization: Nutrition

Visit this Web site to learn about global malnutrition, micronutrient deficiencies, nutrition transition, and other issues of world hunger.

www.feedingminds.org
Feeding Minds Fighting Hunger

Visit this international electronic classroom to explore the problems of hunger, malnutrition, and food insecurity.

www.studentsagainsthunger.org
National Student Campaign Against Hunger and Homelessness

Visit this site to learn what students like you are doing to fight hunger, and how you can get involved.

TEST YOURSELF ANSWERS

1. **False.** Freezing destroys some microorganisms but only inhibits the ability of other microorganisms to reproduce. When the food is thawed, these cold-tolerant microorganisms resume reproduction.

2. **False.** Bacteria cause the vast majority of cases of food-borne illness.

3. **True.** Although some studies have found higher levels of vitamins E and C and certain antioxidant phytochemicals in organic foods, there are not enough studies published on this topic to state with confidence that organic foods are consistently more nutritious than nonorganic foods.

4. **True.** Approximately 11% of Americans experience food insecurity.

5. **False.** Iron deficiency is the most common nutrient deficiency in the world, affecting more than 30% of the world's population.

REFERENCES

1. Food and Drug Administration (FDA). December 2006. Questions & Answers: Taco Bell E. Coli 0157:H7 Lettuce Outbreak. December 14, 2006. Available at www.cfsan.fda.gov/~dms/tacobqa.html#cause.
2. Centers for Disease Control and Prevention (CDC). October 2005. Division of Bacterial and Mycotic Diseases. Disease Listing. Foodborne Illness. Available at www.cdc.gov/ncidod/dbmd/diseaseinfo/foodborneinfections_ g.htm. (Accessed April 2008.)
3. Bauman, R. W. 2007. *Microbiology with Diseases by Taxonomy*. 2nd ed. San Francisco: Pearson Benjamin Cummings.
4. Food and Drug Administration (FDA). 2005a. Prions and Transmissible Spongiform Encephalopathies. Available at www.cfsan.fda.gov/~mow/prion.html.
5. Pavlista, A. D. 2001. Green Potatoes: The Problem and Solution. NebGuide. The University of Nebraska-Lincoln Cooperative Extension. Available at http://ianrpubs.unl.edu/horticulture/g1437.htm.
6. Food and Drug Administration (FDA). 2003. Supplement to the 2001 Food Code. Available at www.cfsan.fda.gov/~dms/fc01-sup.html.
7. Food and Drug Administration (FDA). 2000. The unwelcome dinner guest: Preventing foodborne illness, Jan.–Feb 1991. *FDA Consumer*. Available at www.cfsan.fda.gov/~dms/qa-prp6.html.
8. Food and Drug Administration (FDA). 2005b. Eating Defensively: Food Safety Advice for Persons with AIDS. Available at www.cfsan.fda.gov/~dms/aidseat.html.
9. Food Marketing Institute. 2003. *A Consumer Guide to Food Quality and Safe Handling: Meat, Poultry, Seafood, Eggs*. Washington, DC: Food Marketing Institute, pp. 1–5.
10. U.S. Department of Agriculture (USDA), News Release. 2003. For an Enjoyable Fourth, Consumers Should Practice Food Safety. Available at www.fsis.usda.gov/Frame/FrameRedirect.asp?main=http://www.fsis.usda.gov/OA/news/2003/july4.htm.
11. Food and Drug Administration (FDA). 2003. *Anisakis simplex* and related worms. *Foodborne Pathogenic Microorganisms and Natural Toxins Handbook*. Available at www.cfsan.fda.gov/~mow/chap25.html.
12. Shephard, S. 2000. *Pickled, Potted and Canned: The Story of Food Preserving*. London: Headline Publishing, pp. 17–85, 99–114, 155–167, 275–306.
13. Aseptic Packaging Council. 2005. The Award-Winning, Earth Smart Packaging for a Healthy Lifestyle. Available at www.aseptic.org/main.shtml.
14. Winter, R. 1994. *A Consumer's Dictionary of Food Additives*. New York: Three Rivers Press, pp. 1–32.

15. McHughen, A. 2000. *Pandora's Picnic Basket: The Potential and Hazards of Genetically Modified Foods*. Oxford: Oxford University Press, pp. 17–45.

16. Whitman, D. B. 2005. Genetically modified foods: Harmful or helpful? *Cambridge Scientific Abstracts, Hot Topics Series*. Available at www.csa.com/hottopics/gmfood/overview.php.

17. Center for Science in the Public Interest (CSPI). 2005. Food Safety. Chemical Cuisine. CSPI's Guide to Food Additives. Available at www.cspinet.org/reports/chemcuisine.htm.

18. Schafer, K. S., and S. E. Kegley. 2002. Persistent toxic chemicals in the US food supply. *J. Epidemiol Community Health* 56:813–817.

19. Food and Drug Administration (FDA). 2004. What you need to know about mercury in fish and shellfish. Available at www.cfsan.fda.gov/~dms/admehg3.html.

20. Environmental Protection Agency (EPA). 2003. About Pesticides. Available at www.epa.gov/pesticides/about/index.htm.

21. Health Canada. 1999. News Release. Health Canada Rejects Bovine Growth Hormone in Canada. Health Canada Online. Available at www.hc-sc.gc.ca/ahc-asc/media/nr-cp/1999/1999_03_e.html.

22. Organic Trade Association (OTA). 2004. *Organic Food & Beverage Trends 2004: Lifestyles, Language and Category Adoption*. Available at www.ota.com/organic/mt/consumer.html. (Accessed October 2005.)

23. Aiyana, J. 2002. What consumers should know about the new USDA organic labeling standard. *The Pulse of Oriental Medicine*. Available at www.pulsemed.org/usdaorganic.htm.

24. Heaton, S. 2003. *Organic Farming, Food Quality and Human Health: A Review of the Evidence*. Soil Association. Bristol: Briston House.

25. Asami, D. K., Y. J. Hong, D. M. Barrett, and A. E. Mitchell. 2003. Comparison of the total phenolic and ascorbic acid content of freeze-dried and air-dried marionberry, strawberry, and corn grown using conventional, organic, and sustainable agricultural practices. *J. Agric. Food Chem.* 51(5):1237–1241.

26. Carbonaro, M., M. Mattera, S. Nicoli, P. Bergamo, and M. Cappelloni. 2002. Modulation of antioxidant compounds in organic vs conventional fruit (peach, Prunus persica L., and pear, Pyrus communis L.). *J. Agric. Food Chem.* 50(19):5458–5462.

27. Grinder-Pedersen, L., S. E. Rasmussen, S. Bügel, L. O. Jørgensen, D. Vagn Gundersen, and B. Sandström. 2003. Effect of diets based on foods from conventional versus organic production on intake and excretion of flavonoids and markers of antioxidative defense in humans. *Agric. Food Chem.* 51 (19):5671–5676.

28. U.S. Department of Agriculture (USDA). (2006). Economic Research Service. Food security in the United States: Conditions and Trends. Available at www.ers.usda.gov/Briefing/FoodSecurity/trends.htm.

29. Food and Agriculture Organization (FAO). 2005. The spectrum of malnutrition. Available at www.fao.org/FOCUS/E/SOFI00/img/sofisum-e.pdf.

30. World Health Organization. 2003a. *The World Health Report: Shaping the Future*. Geneva: WHO.

31. Tropical Medicine Central Resource. Kwashiorkor (Protein-Calorie Malnutrition). Available at http://tmcr.usuhs.mil/tmcr/chapter16/Kwashiorkor.htm.

32. World Health Organization. 2003b. Micronutrient Deficiencies: Combating Vitamin A Deficiency. Available at www.who.int/nut/vad.htm.

33. World Health Organization. 2003c. Micronutrient Deficiencies: Battling Iron Deficiency Anaemia. Available at www.who.int/nut/ida.htm.

34. World Health Organization. 2003d. Micronutrient Deficiencies: Eliminating Iodine Deficiency Disorders. Available at www.who.int/nut/idd.htm.

35. Popkin, B. M., and P. Gordon-Larsen. 2004. The nutrition transition: Worldwide obesity dynamics and their determinants. *Int. J. Obesity* 28:S2–S9.

APPENDICES

APPENDIX A NUTRIENT VALUES OF FOODS

The following table of nutrient values is taken from the MyDietAnalysis diet analysis software that is available with this text.* The foods in the table are just a fraction of the foods provided in the software. When using the software, you can quickly find foods shown here by entering the MyDietAnalysis code in the search field. Values are obtained from the USDA Nutrient Database for Standard Reference, Release 19. A "0" indicates that nutrient value is determined to be zero; a blank space indicates that nutrient information is not available.

Ener = energy (kilocalories); *Prot* = protein; *Carb* = carbohydrate; *Fiber* = dietary fiber; *Fat* = total fat; *Mono* = monounsaturated fat; *Poly* = polyunsaturated fat; *Sat* = saturated fat; *Chol* = cholesterol; *Calc* = calcium; *Iron* = iron; *Mag* = magnesium; *Phos* = phosphorus; *Sodi* = sodium; *Zinc* = zinc; *Vit A* = vitamin A; *Vit C* = vitamin C; *Thia* = thiamin; *Ribo* = riboflavin; *Niac* = niacin; *Vit B$_6$* = vitamin B$_6$; *Vit B$_{12}$* = vitamin B$_{12}$; *Vit E* = vitamin E; *Fol* = folate; *Alc* = alcohol.

Index to Appendix A

*This food composition table has been prepared for Pearson Education, Inc., and is copyrighted by ESHA Research in Salem, Oregon—the developer of the MyDietAnalysis software program.

MDA Code	Food Name	Amt	Wt (g)	Ener (kcal)	Prot (g)	Carb (g)	Fiber (g)	Fat (g)	Mono (g)	Poly (g)
	BEVERAGES									
	Alcoholic									
22831	Beer	12 fl oz	360	157	1	13		0	0	0
34067	Beer, dark	12 fl oz	355.5	150	1	13		0	0	0
34053	Beer, light	12 fl oz	352.9	105	1	5	0	0	0	0
22606	Beer, nonalcoholic	12 fl oz	352.9	73	1	14	0	0	0	0
22849	Beer, pale ale	12 fl oz	360.2	179	2	17		0	0	0
22545	Daiquiri, frozen, from concentrate mix	1 ea	36	101	0	26	0	0	0	0
22514	Gin, 80 proof	1 fl oz	27.8	64	0	0	0	0	0	0
22544	Liqueur, coffee, 63 proof	1 fl oz	34.8	107	0	11	0	0	0	0
34085	Martini, prepared from recipe	1 fl oz	28.2	69	0	1	0	0	0	0
22593	Rum, 80 proof	1 fl oz	27.8	64	0	0	0	0	0	0
22515	Tequila, 80 proof	1 fl oz	27.8	64	0	0	0	0	0	0
22594	Vodka, 80 proof	1 fl oz	27.8	64	0	0	0	0	0	0
22670	Whiskey, 80 proof	1 fl oz	27.8	64	0	0	0	0	0	0
34084	Wine, cooking	1 tsp	4.9	2	0	0	0	0	0	0
22884	Wine, red, Cabernet Sauvignon	1 fl oz	29	24	0	1		0	0	0
22876	Wine, red, Pinot Noir	1 fl oz	29.4	24	0	1		0	0	0
22676	Wine, sake/saki, Japanese	1 fl oz	29.1	39	0	1	0	0	0	0
22861	Wine, white, Sauvignon Blanc	1 fl oz	29.3	24	0	1		0	0	0
	Coffee									
20012	Coffee, brewed w/tap water	1 cup	237	2	0	0	0	0	0	0
20686	Coffee, decaffeinated, brewed w/tap water	1 cup	236.8	0	0	0	0	0	0	0
20439	Coffee, espresso	1 cup	237	5	0	0	0	0	0	0.2
20972	Coffee, espresso, decaffeinated	1 cup	237	0	0	0	0	0	0	0.2
20091	Coffee, decaffeinated, instant	1 cup	179	4	0	1	0	0	0	0
20023	Coffee, instant, prep w/water	1 cup	238.4	5	0	1	0	0	0	0
20402	Coffee, instant, French vanilla cafe, fat & sugar free	1 ea	7	25	0	5	0	0		
	Dairy Mixed Drinks and Mixes									
44	Carob flavor, dry mix, prepared w/whole milk	1 cup	256	192	8	22	1	8	2	0.5
85	Chocolate milk, prepared w/syrup	1 cup	282	254	9	36	1	8	2.1	0.5
46	Hot cocoa, sugar free, w/aspartame, prepared w/water	1 cup	256	74	3	14	1	1	0.2	0
195	Hot cocoa, rich chocolate, w/o add sugar, dry pkt	1 ea	15	50	2	10	1	0		
172	Hot cocoa, rich chocolate, dry pkt	1 ea	28	112	1	21	1	4		
21	Hot cocoa, prep from recipe w/milk	1 cup	250	192	9	27	2	6	1.7	0.1
48	Hot cocoa, prep from dry mix w/water	1 cup	274.7	151	2	32	1	2	0.5	0
166	Hot cocoa, w/marshmallows, dry pkt	1 ea	28	112	1	21	1	4		
39	Drink, chocolate, prepared from dry mix w/whole milk	1 cup	266	226	9	32	1	9	2.2	0.5
34	Chocolate malted milk, prepared from powder w/whole milk	1 cup	265	225	9	30	1	9	2.2	0.6
29	Malted milk, natural, w/o add nutrients, prep from powder w/milk	1 cup	265	233	10	27	0	10	2.4	0.7
41	Drink, strawberry, prep from dry mix w/whole milk	1 cup	266	234	8	33	0	8	2.4	0.3
	Fruit and Vegetable Beverages and Juices									
71080	Apple juice, unsweetened	8.45 fl oz	262	123	0	31	0	0	0	0.1
3010	Apple juice, unsweetened, prepared from frozen concentrate	1 cup	239	112	0	28	0	0	0	0.1
3015	Apricot nectar, w/o add vitamin C, canned	1 cup	251	141	1	36	2	0	0.1	0
72092	Blackberry juice, canned	0.5 cup	120	46	0	9	0	1	0.1	0.4
20277	Capri Sun, fruit punch, pouch	1 ea	210	99	0	26	0	0	0	0
5226	Carrot juice, canned	1 cup	236	94	2	22	2	0	0	0.2
20042	Clam and tomato juice, canned	5.5 oz	166.1	80	1	18	1	0		
3042	Cranberry juice cocktail	1 cup	252.8	137	0	34	0	0	0	0.1

Sat (g)	Chol (mg)	Calc (mg)	Iron (mg)	Mag (mg)	Phos (mg)	Pota (mg)	Sodi (mg)	Zinc (mg)	Vit A (RAE)	Vit C (mg)	Thia (mg)	Ribo (mg)	Niac (mg)	Vit B6 (mg)	Vit B12 (µg)	Vit E (mg)	Fol (µg)	Alc (g)
0	0						9								0			14.3
0	0						34											17.06
0	0	11				59	11				0.04	0.04	1.41					14.12
0	0	19				54	10				0.04	0.07	1.41					1.78
0	0						9								0			14.7
0	0	3	0.13	1.1	7	34	123	0.1	0	3.2	0.01	0.01	0	0	0	0	0	0
0	0	0	0.01	0	1	1	0	0	0	0	0	0	0	0	0	0	0	9.29
0	0	0	0.02	1	2	10	3	0	0	0	0	0	0.05	0	0	0	0	9.05
0	0	0	0.01	0.6	1	5	1	0	0	0	0	0	0.01	0	0	0	0	9.56
0	0	0	0.03	0	1	1	0	0	0	0	0	0	0	0	0	0	0	9.29
0	0	0	0.01	0	1	1	0	0	0	0	0	0	0	0	0	0	0	9.29
0	0	0	0	0	1	0	0	0	0	0	0	0	0	0	0	0	0	9.29
0	0	0	0.01	0	1	1	0	0	0	0	0	0	0	0	0	0	0	9.29
0	0	0	0.02	0.5	1	4	31	0	0	0	0	0	0	0	0	0	0	0.16
0																		3.04
0																		3.06
0	0	1	0.03	1.7	2	7	1	0	0	0	0	0	0	0	0	0	0	4.69
0																		3.08
0	0	5	0.02	7.1	7	116	5	0	0	0	0.03	0.18	0.45	0	0	0	4.7	0
0	0	5	0.12	11.8	2	128	5	0	0	0	0	0	0.53	0	0	0	0	0
0.2	0	5	0.31	189.6	17	273	33	0.1	0	0.5	0	0.42	12.34	0	0	0	2.4	0
0.2	0	5	0.31	189.6	17	273	33	0.1	0	0.5	0	0.42	12.34	0	0	0	2.4	0
0	0	5	0.11	9	7	82	4	0	0	0	0	0.03	0.5	0	0	0	0	0
0	0	10	0.1	7.2	7	72	5	0	0	0	0	0	0.56	0	0	0	0	0
0.1	0	4	0.06		16	72	65	0	0									0
4.6	26	251	0.64	25.6	205	335	118	0.9	69	0	0.11	0.45	0.35	0.1	1.08	0.1	12.8	0
4.7	25	251	0.9	50.8	254	409	133	1.2	70	0	0.11	0.47	0.39	0.09	1.07	0.1	14.1	0
0	0	120	1	43.5	179	540	228	0.7	36	0.3	0.05	0.28	0.22	0.06	0.33	0.1	2.6	0
0.1	1	300	0.54	27	135	288	180	0.6		0.3	0.06	0.22	0.18	0.05	0.45	0	5.8	0
2.8	0	28	0.5	27.4	71	0	238	0.4		0	0.03	0.12	0.16	0.03	0.1	0	2	0
3.6	20	262	1.2	57.5	262	492	110	1.6	128	0.5	0.1	0.45	0.33	0.1	1.05	0.1	12.5	0
0.9	3	60	0.47	33	118	269	195	0.6	0	0.5	0.04	0.21	0.22	0.04	0.49	0.2	0	0
4.2	0	22	0.5	16.2	58	142	224	0.2		0	0.03	0.12	0.1	0.03	0.12	0	1.1	0
4.9	24	253	0.8	47.9	234	458	154	1.3	70	0.3	0.11	0.48	0.38	0.09	1.06	0.2	13.3	0
5	26	260	0.56	39.8	241	456	159	1.1	70	0.3	0.14	0.49	0.69	0.12	1.11	0.2	23.8	0
5.4	32	310	0.24	45	281	485	209	1.1	87	0.5	0.21	0.64	1.38	0.17	1.22	0.3	21.2	0
5.1	32	293	0.21	31.9	229	370	128	0.9	69	2.4	0.09	0.42	0.22	0.1	0.88	0.3	13.3	0
0	0	18	0.97	7.9	18	312	8	0.1	0	2.4	0.06	0.04	0.26	0.08	0	0	0	0
0	0	14	0.62	12	17	301	17	0.1	0	1.4	0.01	0.04	0.09	0.08	0	0	0	0
0	0	18	0.95	12.6	23	286	8	0.2	166	1.5	0.02	0.04	0.65	0.06	0	0.8	2.5	0
0	0	14	0.58	25.2	14	162	1	0.5	10	13.6	0.01	0.02	0.54	0.03	0	1.1	12	0
0	0	2	0.06		2	25	21			2.7								0
0.1	0	57	1.09	33	99	689	68	0.4	2256	20.1	0.22	0.13	0.91	0.51	0	2.7	9.4	0
	0	13	0.25	8.3	18	148	601	0.1	12	8.3	0.03	0.02	0.38	0.1	0.05	0.2	13.3	0
0	0	8	0.25	2.5	3	35	5	0.1	1	106.9	0	0	0.1	0	0	0.6	0	0

MDA Code	Food Name	Amt	Wt (g)	Ener (kcal)	Prot (g)	Carb (g)	Fiber (g)	Fat (g)	Mono (g)	Poly (g)
20115	Cranberry juice cocktail, from frozen concentrate	1 cup	249.6	137	0	35	0	0	0	0
3275	Cranberry-grape juice	1 cup	244.8	137	0	34	0	0	0	0.1
20024	Fruit punch, w/added nutrients, canned	1 cup	248	117	0	30	0	0	0	0
20035	Fruit punch, from frozen concentrate	1 cup	247.2	114	0	29	0	0	0	0
20101	Grape drink, canned	1 cup	250.4	153	0	39	0	0	0	0
3165	Grapefruit juice, sweetened, canned	1 cup	250	115	1	28	0	0	0	0.1
3052	Grapefruit juice, unsweetened, canned	1 cup	247	94	1	22	0	0	0	0.1
3053	Grapefruit juice, unsweetened, from frozen concentrate	1 cup	247	101	1	24	0	0	0	0.1
20330	Kool-Aid, cherry, sugar free, w/aspartame & vitamin C	1 ea	9.6	28	1	8		0		
20687	Kool-Aid, tropical punch, sweetened, dry mix, serving	1 ea	17	64	0	16	0	0	0	0
3068	Lemon juice, fresh	1 Tbs	15.2	4	0	1	0	0	0	0
20045	Lemonade, prepared from powder	1 cup	266	112	0	29	0	0	0	0
20047	Lemonade, low cal, w/aspartame, prep from powder	1 cup	236.8	5	0	1	0	0	0	0
20117	Lemonade, pink, from frozen concentrate	1 cup	247.2	99	0	26	0	0	0	0
20000	Lemonade, white, from frozen concentrate	1 cup	248	131	0	34	0	0	0	0
3072	Lime juice, fresh	1 Tbs	15.4	4	0	1	0	0	0	0
20002	Limeade, from frozen concentrate	1 cup	247.2	104	0	26	0	0		
20070	Orange drink, w/added vitamin C, canned	1 cup	248	122	0	31	0	0	0	0
20004	Orange breakfast drink, from powder	1 cup	248	122	0	31	0	0	0	0
71108	Orange juice, unsweetened, box	8.45 fl oz	263	110	2	26	1	0	0.1	0.1
3090	Orange juice, fresh	1 cup	248	112	2	26	0	0	0.1	0.1
3091	Orange juice, unsweetened, from frozen concentrate	1 cup	249	112	2	27	0	0	0	0
3170	Orange-grapefruit juice, unsweetened, canned	1 cup	247	106	1	25	0	0	0	0
3095	Papaya nectar, canned	1 cup	250	142	0	36	2	0	0.1	0.1
3200	Passion fruit juice, purple, fresh	1 cup	247	126	1	34	0	0	0	0.1
3101	Peach nectar, w/o added vitamin C, canned	1 cup	249	134	1	35	1	0	0	0
20059	Pineapple-grapefruit juice, canned	1 cup	250.4	118	1	29	0	0	0	0.1
20025	Pineapple-orange juice, canned	1 cup	250.4	125	3	30	0	0	0	0
3120	Pineapple juice, unsweetened, w/o added vitamin C, canned	1 cup	250	132	1	32	1	0	0	0.1
3128	Prune juice, canned	1 cup	256	182	2	45	3	0	0.1	0
20340	Tang, orange, from dry mix	2 Tbs	25	92	0	25	0	0	0	0
3140	Tangerine juice, sweetened, canned	1 cup	249	124	1	30	0	0	0	0.1
5397	Tomato juice, unsalted, canned	1 cup	243	41	2	10	1	0	0	0.1
20849	Vegetable-fruit juice, mixed	4 oz	113.4	33	0	8	0	0		
20080	Vegetable juice, mixed, canned	1 cup	242	46	2	11	2	0	0	0.1
	Soft Drinks									
20006	Club soda	1 cup	236.8	0	0	0	0	0	0	0
20685	Low-calorie cola, with aspartame, caffeine free	12 fl oz	355.2	4	0	1	0	0	0	0
20843	Cola, w/higher caff	12 fl oz	370	152	0	39	0	0	0	0
20028	Cream soda	1 cup	247.2	126	0	33	0	0	0	0
20008	Ginger ale	1 cup	244	83	0	21	0	0	0	0
20031	Grape soda	1 cup	248	107	0	28	0	0	0	0
20032	Lemon-lime soft drink	1 cup	245.6	98	0	25	0	0		
20027	Pepper-type soft drink	1 cup	245.6	101	0	26	0	0	0	0
20009	Root beer	1 cup	246.4	101	0	26	0	0	0	0
	Tea									
20436	Iced tea, lemon flavor	1 cup	240	86	0	22	0	0	0	0
20040	Instant tea mix w/lemon flavor & saccharin	1 cup	236.8	5	0	1	0	0	0	0
20014	Tea, brewed	1 cup	236.8	2	0	1	0	0	0	0
444	Tea, decaffeinated, brewed	1 cup	236.8	2	0	1	0	0	0	0

Sat (g)	Chol (mg)	Calc (mg)	Iron (mg)	Mag (mg)	Phos (mg)	Pota (mg)	Sodi (mg)	Zinc (mg)	Vit A (RAE)	Vit C (mg)	Thia (mg)	Ribo (mg)	Niac (mg)	Vit B_6 (mg)	Vit B_{12} (µg)	Vit E (mg)	Fol (µg)	Alc (g)
0	0	12	0.22	5	2	35	7	0.1	2	24.7	0.02	0.02	0.03	0.03	0	0	0	0
0.1	0	20	0.02	7.3	10	59	7	0.1	1	78.3	0.02	0.04	0.29	0.07	0	0	2.4	0
0	0	20	0.22	7.4	7	77	94	0	5	73.4	0.01	0.06	0.05	0.03	0	0	2.5	0
0	0	10	0.22	4.9	2	32	10	0	1	108.3	0.02	0.03	0.05	0.01	0	0	2.5	0
0	0	130	0.18	2.5	0	30	40	0.3	0	78.6	0	0.01	0.03	0.01	0	0	0	0
0	0	20	0.9	25	28	405	5	0.1	1	67.2	0.1	0.06	0.8	0.05	0	0.1	25	0
0	0	17	0.49	24.7	27	378	2	0.2	1	72.1	0.1	0.05	0.57	0.05	0	0.1	24.7	0
0	0	20	0.35	27.2	35	336	2	0.1	1	83.2	0.1	0.05	0.54	0.11	0	0.1	9.9	0
		0	0			0	41			53.8					0			0
0	0	28	0.01		13	0	2		0	6								0
0	0	1	0	0.9	1	19	0	0	0	7	0	0	0.02	0.01	0	0	2	0
0	0	29	0.05	2.7	3	3	19	0.1	0	34	0	0	0	0	0	0	0	0
0	0	52	0.09	2.4	24	0	5	0	0	5.9	0	0	0	0	0	0	0	0
0	0	7	0.4	4.9	5	37	7	0.1	0	9.6	0.01	0.05	0.04	0.01	0	0	4.9	0
0	0	10	0.52	5	7	50	7	0.1	0	12.9	0.02	0.07	0.05	0.02	0	0	2.5	0
0	0	2	0.01	1.2	2	18	0	0	0	4.6	0	0	0.02	0.01	0	0	1.5	0
	0	7	0.02	2.5	2	22	5	0	0	5.9	0	0.01	0.02	0.01	0	0	2.5	0
0	0	12	0.1	5	2	45	7	0	2	142.1	0	0	0.03	0	0	0	5	0
0	0	126	0.02	2.5	47	60	10	0	191	73.2	0	0.22	2.54	0.25	0	0	0	0
0	0	21	1.16	28.9	37	460	5	0.2	24	90.5	0.16	0.07	0.83	0.23	0	0.5	47.3	0
0.1	0	27	0.5	27.3	42	496	2	0.1	25	124	0.22	0.07	0.99	0.1	0	0.1	74.4	0
0	0	22	0.25	24.9	40	473	2	0.1	12	96.9	0.2	0.04	0.5	0.11	0	0.5	109.6	0
0	0	20	1.14	24.7	35	390	7	0.2	15	71.9	0.14	0.07	0.83	0.06	0	0.3	34.6	0
0.1	0	25	0.85	7.5	0	78	12	0.4	45	7.5	0.02	0.01	0.38	0.02	0	0.6	5	0
0	0	10	0.59	42	32	687	15	0.1	89	73.6	0	0.32	3.61	0.12	0	0	17.3	0
0	0	12	0.47	10	15	100	17	0.2	32	13.2	0.01	0.03	0.72	0.02	0	0.7	2.5	0
0	0	18	0.78	15	15	153	35	0.2	0	115.2	0.08	0.04	0.67	0.11	0	0	22.5	0
0	0	13	0.68	15	10	115	8	0.2	3	56.3	0.08	0.05	0.52	0.12	0	0.1	22.5	0
0	0	32	0.78	30	20	325	5	0.3	1	25	0.14	0.05	0.5	0.25	0	0	45	0
0	0	31	3.02	35.8	64	707	10	0.5	0	10.5	0.04	0.18	2.01	0.56	0	0.3	0	0
0	0	92	0.02	0	42	48	2	0		60	0	0.17	2	0.2	0	2	0	0
0	0	45	0.5	19.9	35	443	2	0.1	32	54.8	0.15	0.05	0.25	0.08	0	0.4	12.4	0
0	0	24	1.04	26.7	44	556	24	0.4	56	44.5	0.11	0.08	1.64	0.27	0	0.8	48.6	0
	0	3	0.05	1.1	2	22	24	0	118	36.9	0	0	0.02	0.01	0	1.8	0	0
0	0	27	1.02	26.6	41	467	653	0.5	189	67	0.1	0.07	1.76	0.34	0	0.8	50.8	0
0	0	12	0.02	2.4	0	5	50	0.2	0	0	0	0	0	0	0	0	0	0
0	0	11	0.07	0	36	25	14	0	0	0	0.02	0.08	0	0	0	0	0	0
0	0	7	0.07	0	41	11	15	0	0	0	0	0	0	0	0	0	0	0
0	0	12	0.12	2.5	0	2	30	0.2	0	0	0	0	0	0	0	0	0	0
0	0	7	0.44	2.4	0	2	17	0.1	0	0	0	0	0	0	0	0	0	0
0	0	7	0.2	2.5	0	2	37	0.2	0	0	0	0	0	0	0	0	0	0
	0	5	0.27	2.5	0	2	22	0.1	0	0	0	0	0.04	0	0	0	0	0
0.2	0	7	0.1	0	27	2	25	0.1	0	0	0	0	0	0	0	0	0	0
0	0	12	0.12	2.5	0	2	32	0.2	0	0	0	0	0	0	0	0	0	0
0		7	0	2.4	86	46	50	0.1										0
0	0	7	0.12	2.4	2	31	9	0	0	0	0	0	0.05	0	0	0	0	0
0	0	0	0.05	7.1	2	88	7	0	0	0	0	0.03	0	0	0	0	11.8	0
0	0	0	0.05	7.1	2	88	7	0	0	0	0	0.03	0	0	0	0	11.8	0

MDA Code	Food Name	Amt	Wt (g)	Ener (kcal)	Prot (g)	Carb (g)	Fiber (g)	Fat (g)	Mono (g)	Poly (g)
20118	Tea, herbal, chamomile, brewed	1 cup	236.8	2	0	0	0	0	0	0
20036	Tea, herbal, not chamomile, brewed	1 cup	236.8	2	0	0	0	0	0	0
	Other									
20983	Bean beverage	1 cup	230	78	6	13	0	0	0	0
17	Eggnog	1 cup	254	343	10	34	0	19	5.7	0.9
20440	Rice milk, original	1 cup	244.8	120	0	25	0	2	1.3	0.3
20033	Soy milk	1 cup	245	127	11	12	3	5	0.9	1.9
21070	Soy milk, plain, lite	1 cup	245	90	4	15	2	2	0.5	1
21064	Soy milk, vanilla	1 cup	245	190	11	25	5	5	1	3
20041	Water, tap, municipal	1 cup	236.6	0	0	0	0	0	0	0
20076	Wine, nonalcoholic	4 fl oz	116	7	1	1	0	0	0	0
	BREAKFAST CEREALS									
40095	All-Bran/Kellogg's	0.5 cup	30	78	4	22	9	1	0.2	0.6
40295	Apple Cinnamon Cheerios/Gen Mills	0.75 cup	30	120	2	25	1	2	1	0.5
40097	Apple Cinnamon Squares cereal/Kellogg's	0.75 cup	55	182	4	44	5	1	0.3	0.5
40098	Apple Jacks/Kellogg's	1 cup	30	117	1	27	1	1	0.2	0.3
40394	Basic 4/Gen Mills	1 cup	55	210	4	44	3	3	1	0.5
40259	Bran Flakes/Post	0.75 cup	30	96	3	24	5	1		
61211	Bran & malted flour cereal	0.33 cup	29	83	4	23	8	1	0.1	0.3
40032	Cap'n Crunch/Quaker	0.75 cup	27	108	1	23	1	2	0.3	0.2
40297	Cheerios/Gen Mills	1 cup	30	110	3	23	3	2	0.7	0.7
40414	Cinnamon Grahams/Gen Mills	0.75 cup	30	113	2	26	1	1	0.3	0.3
40126	Cinnamon Toast Crunch/Gen Mills	0.75 cup	30	130	1	24	1	4	2.5	0.5
40102	Cocoa Krispies/Kellogg's	0.75 cup	31	118	2	27	1	1	0.1	0.1
40425	Cocoa Puffs/Gen Mills	1 cup	30	120	1	26	2	2	1	0
40325	Corn Chex/Gen Mills	1 cup	30	110	2	26	1	1	0.1	0.2
40195	Corn Flakes/Kellogg's	1 cup	28	101	2	24	1	0	0	0.1
40089	Corn Grits, instant, plain, prepared/Quaker	1 ea	137	93	2	21	1	0	0	0.1
92416	Corn grits, white, quick, enriched, cooked w/water & salt	1 cup	242	143	3	31	1	0	0.1	0.2
40206	Corn Pops/Kellogg's	1 cup	31	117	1	28	0	0	0.1	0.1
40205	Cracklin' Oat Bran/Kellogg's	0.75 cup	55	221	4	39	7	8	2.6	1.6
40179	Cream of Rice, prepared w/salt/Kraft	1 cup	244	127	2	28	0	0	0.1	0.1
40104	Crispix/Kellogg's	1 cup	29	109	2	25	0	0	0.1	0.1
40184	Farina, enriched, prepared w/salt	1 cup	233	112	3	24	1	0	0	0.1
40182	Farina, instant, prepared w/salt	1 cup	241	149	4	32	1	1	0.1	0.3
40130	Fiber One/Gen Mills	0.5 cup	30	60	2	25	14	1	0.1	0.4
40218	Froot Loops/Kellogg's	1 cup	30	118	2	26	1	1	0.1	0.2
40217	Frosted Flakes/Kellogg's	0.75 cup	31	114	1	28	1	0	0	0.1
11916	Frosted Mini Wheats, bite size/Kellogg's	1 cup	55	189	6	45	6	1	0.1	0.6
40048	Granola cereal, prep f/recipe	0.5 cup	61	298	9	32	5	15	5.8	5.6
40277	Grape Nuts/Post	0.5 cup	58	208	6	47	5	1		
40292	Honey Bunches of Oats, Honey Roasted/Post	0.75 cup	30	118	2	25	1	2		
40361	Honey Nut Heaven/Quaker	1 cup	49	192	4	38	3	4	1.7	1
40108	Just Right, Crunchy Blends/Kellogg's	1 cup	55	204	4	46	3	1	0.3	1
40010	Kix/Gen Mills	1.33 cup	30	120	2	25	1	1	0.3	0.4
40011	Life, plain/Quaker	0.75 cup	32	120	3	25	2	1	0.5	0.5
40197	Low-Fat Granola, w/raisins/Kellogg's	0.66 cup	55	201	4	44	3	3	1.3	0.5
40300	Lucky Charms/Gen Mills	1 cup	30	120	2	25	1	1	0.5	0.5
40186	Maltex, prep w/water & salt	1 cup	249	189	6	39	2	1	0.1	0.4
38659	Nutri-Grain Cereal, wheat/Kellogg's	1 oz	28.4	102	2	24	2	0	0	0.1

Sat (g)	Chol (mg)	Calc (mg)	Iron (mg)	Mag (mg)	Phos (mg)	Pota (mg)	Sodi (mg)	Zinc (mg)	Vit A (RAE)	Vit C (mg)	Thia (mg)	Ribo (mg)	Niac (mg)	Vit B6 (mg)	Vit B12 (µg)	Vit E (mg)	Fol (µg)	Alc (g)
0	0	5	0.19	2.4	0	21	2	0.1	2	0	0.02	0.01	0	0	0	0	2.4	0
0	0	5	0.19	2.4	0	21	2	0.1	0	0	0.02	0.01	0	0	0	0	2.4	0
0	0	39	2.88	110.4	212	775	5	0.9	0	0	0.35	0.23	1.43	0.23	0	0.6	138	0
11.3	150	330	0.51	48.3	277	419	137	1.2	116	3.8	0.09	0.48	0.27	0.13	1.14	0.5	2.5	0
0.2	0	20	0.2	9.8	34	69	86	0.2	0	1.2	0.08	0.01	1.91	0.04	0	1.8	90.6	0
0.6	0	93	2.7	61.2	135	304	135	1.1	76	0	0.15	0.12	0.71	0.24	2.99	3.3	39.2	0
0	0	300	1.44	32	150	160	90			0	0.42						0	0
0.5	0	300	2.7	60	250	370	85			0	0.42						0	0
0	0	7	0	2.4	0	2	7	0	0	0	0	0	0	0	0	0	0	0
0	0	10	0.46	11.6	17	102	8	0.1	0	0	0	0.01	0.12	0.02	0	0	1.2	0
0.2	0	117	5.28	108.6	345	306	73	3.7	158	6	0.68	0.81	4.44	3.6	5.64	0.4	393	0
0	0	100	4.5	15.9	60	60	120	3.8	149	6	0.38	0.43	5	0.5	1.5	0.2	200.1	0
0.2	0	21	16.23	48.4	154	166	20	1.5	0	0	0.38	0.44	5.01	0.49	1.49	0.3	110	0
0.1	0	8	4.17	16.5	38	36	142	1.5	40	13.8	0.51	0.39	4.62	0.45	1.38	0	93	0
0.5	0	250	4.5	31.9	100	150	320	3.8	150	0	0.37	0.42	5	0.5	1.5	0.6	100.1	0
0.1	0	17	8.1	64.2	152	185	220	1.5	0	0	0.38	0.43	5	0.5	1.5		99.9	0
0.1	0	22	8.1	80.6	236	275	121	3.7	225	0	0.37	0.43	5	0.5	0	0.7	100	0
0.4	0	4	5.16	15.1	45	54	202	4.3	2	0	0.43	0.48	5.71	0.57	0	0.2	420.1	0
0.4	0	100	8.4	39.9	100	200	210	3.8	150	6	0.38	0.43	5	0.5	1.5	0.2	200.1	0
0.2	0	100	4.5	8.1	20	44	237	3.8	150	6	0.38	0.43	5.01	0.5	1.5	0.1	99.9	0
0.5	0	100	4.5	8.1	40	45	210	3.8	150	6	0.38	0.43	5	0.5	1.5	0.9	99.9	0
0.6	0	5	6.88	11.8	32	61	197	1.5	153	15	0.46	0.7	4.96	1.02	2.15	0.1	197.5	0
0	0	100	4.5	8.1	20	60	160	3.8	0	6	0.38	0.43	5	0.5	1.5	0.2	99.9	0
0.1	0	100	9	15	22	45	280	3.8	136	6	0.38	0.43	5	0.5	1.5	0.1	200.1	0
0.1	0	1	8.12	2.5	10	22	202	0.1	128	6.2	0.6	0.74	6.83	0.96	2.65	0	134.4	0
0	0	8	7.96	9.6	29	38	288	0.2	0	0	0.16	0.19	2.21	0.05	0	0	46.6	0
0.1	0	7	1.45	12.1	27	51	540	0.2	0	0	0.2	0.13	1.75	0.05	0	0	79.9	0
0.1	0	5	1.92	2.2	10	26	120	1.5	143	6	0.37	0.43	4.99	0.5	1.52	0	102	0
3.4	0	33	2.04	67.6	179	248	170	1.7	252	17.6	0.44	0.49	5.67	0.56	1.7	0.5	112.8	0
0	0	7	0.49	7.3	41	49	422	0.4	0	0	0	0	0.98	0.07	0	0	7.3	0
0.1	0	4	9.61	7	28	33	222	2.3	262	8.8	1.27	1.25	8.47	0.98	2.09	0	200.1	0
0	0	9	1.16	4.7	28	30	767	0.2	0	0	0.14	0.1	1.14	0.02	0	0	79.2	0
0.1	0	154	11.95	14.5	43	48	364	0.4	559	0	0.56	0.51	7.45	0.74	0	0	149.4	0
0.1	0	100	4.5	39.9	150	180	105	3.8	1	6	0.38	0.43	5	0.5	1.5	0.3	99.9	0
0.5	0	4	6.12	9.9	34	36	150	5.7	140	14.1	0.68	0.58	7.26	1.1	2.12	0.1	105.6	0
0	0	2	4.5	2.5	11	23	148	0.1	160	6.2	0.37	0.46	5.02	0.5	1.55	0	101.4	0
0.2	0	18	15.4	64.9	162	190	4	1.8	0	0	0.41	0.46	5.39	0.54	1.62	0	107.8	0
2.5	0	48	2.58	106.8	278	329	15	2.5	1	0.7	0.45	0.18	1.31	0.18	0	6.8	50	0
0.2	0	20	16.2	58	139	178	354	1.2		0	0.38	0.42	5	0.5	1.5		99.8	0
0.2	0	6	8.1	16.5	48	52	193	0.3		0	0.38	0.43	5	0.5	1.5		99.9	0
0.5	0	133	6.81	60.3	166	181	216	5.4	216	1.5	0.59	0.67	7.18	0.72	0	1.8	436.6	0
0.1	0	14	16.23	34.1	106	121	338	0.9	376	0	0.38	0.44	5.01	0.49	1.49	1.5	102.3	0
0.1	0	150	8.4	8.1	40	40	220	3.8	138	6	0.38	0.43	5	0.5	1.5	0.1	200.1	0
0.3	0	112	8.95	30.7	133	91	164	4.1	1	0	0.4	0.47	5.5	0.55	0	0.2	416	0
0.6	0	23	1.65	41.2	129	165	135	3.5	206	3.3	0.35	0.38	4.57	1.81	5.5	3.1	369.6	0
0	0	100	4.5	15.9	40	50	200	3.8	150	6	0.38	0.43	5	0.5	1.5	0.1	200.1	0
0.2	0	22	1.79	57.3	177	266	189	1.9	0	0	0.26	0.1	2.37	0.08	0	1.1	29.9	0
0.1	0	8	0.8	22.2	106	77	193	3.7	0	15.1	0.37	0.43	5	0.51	1.51	7.5	100.3	0

MDA Code	Food Name	Amt	Wt (g)	Ener (kcal)	Prot (g)	Carb (g)	Fiber (g)	Fat (g)	Mono (g)	Poly (g)
40434	Oat Bran Cereal/Quaker	1.25 cup	57	212	7	43	6	3	0.9	1.2
40430	Oatmeal Squares/Quaker	1 cup	56	212	6	44	4	2	0.8	1
40073	Oatmeal, apple cinnamon, instant, prep w/water/Quaker	1 ea	149	130	3	26	3	1	0.5	0.4
40018	Puffed Rice/Quaker	1 cup	14	54	1	12	0	0	0	0
40242	Puffed Wheat, fortified	1 cup	12	44	2	10	1	0		0
40209	Raisin Bran/Kellogg's	1 cup	61	195	5	47	7	2	0.3	0.9
40343	Reese's Peanut Butter Puffs/Gen Mills	0.75 cup	30	130	2	23	1	4	1.5	1
40333	Rice Chex/Gen Mills	1.25 cup	31	120	2	26	0	0	0.2	0.2
40210	Rice Krispies/Kellogg's	1.25 cup	33	128	2	28	0	0	0.1	0.1
60887	Shredded Wheat, w/o sugar & salt, round biscuits	2 ea	37.8	127	4	30	5	1	0.1	0.5
60879	Smart Start/Kellogg's	1 cup	50	182	4	43	3	1	0.1	0.4
40211	Special K/Kellogg's	1 cup	31	117	7	22	1	0	0.1	0.2
40066	Sweet Crunch/Quisp/Quaker	1 cup	27	109	1	23	1	2	0.3	0.2
40413	Toasty O's/Malt-O-Meal	1 cup	30	121	4	22	3	2	0.6	0.7
40382	Total, raisin bran/Gen Mills	1 cup	55	170	3	42	5	1	0.1	0.5
40021	Total, wheat/Gen Mills	0.75 cup	30	100	2	23	3	1	0.1	0.2
40306	Trix/Gen Mills	1 cup	30	120	1	26	1	2	0.7	0.5
40335	Wheat Chex/Gen Mills	1 cup	30	108	3	24	3	1	0.1	0.2
40307	Wheaties/Gen Mills	1 cup	30	110	3	24	3	1	0.3	0.4

DAIRY AND CHEESE

See Fats and Oils for butter.

MDA Code	Food Name	Amt	Wt (g)	Ener (kcal)	Prot (g)	Carb (g)	Fiber (g)	Fat (g)	Mono (g)	Poly (g)
7	Buttermilk, low fat, cultured	1 cup	245	98	8	12	0	2	0.6	0.1
500	Cream, half & half	2 Tbs	30	39	1	1	0	3	1	0.1
11953	Kefir, peach	1 cup	225	200	7	23	1	7		
218	Milk, 2%, w/added vitamins A & D	1 cup	245	130	8	13	0	5		
21109	Milk, chocolate, reduced fat w/added calcium	1 cup	250	195	7	30	2	5	1.1	0.2
19	Milk, low fat, chocolate	1 cup	250	158	8	26	1	2	0.8	0.1
11	Milk, condensed, sweetened, canned	2 Tbs	38.2	123	3	21	0	3	0.9	0.1
23	Milk, goat	1 cup	244	168	9	11	0	10	2.7	0.4
22	Milk, human breast	1 cup	246	172	3	17	0	11	4.1	1.2
134	Milk, evaporated, w/added vitamin A, canned	2 Tbs	31.5	42	2	3	0	2	0.7	0.1
10	Milk, evaporated, nonfat/skim, canned	2 Tbs	32	25	2	4	0	0	0	0
68	Milk, nonfat/skim, w/added vitamin A, dry	0.5 cup	60	217	22	31	0	0	0.1	0
6	Milk, nonfat/skim, w/added vitamin A	1 cup	245	83	8	12	0	0	0.1	0
1	Milk, whole, 3.25%	1 cup	244	146	8	11	0	8	2	0.5
20	Milk, whole, chocolate	1 cup	250	208	8	26	2	8	2.5	0.3
2834	Yogurt, blueberry, fruit on the bottom	1 ea	227	220	9	41	1	2		
2315	Yogurt, blueberry, low fat	1 ea	113	110	3	23	0	1		
72636	Yogurt, blueberry, nonfat	1 ea	227	120	7	21	0	0	0	0
72639	Yogurt, creamy vanilla, nonfat	1 ea	227	120	7	21	0	0	0	0
2001	Yogurt, fruit, low fat	1 cup	245	250	11	47	0	3	0.7	0.1
72088	Yogurt, fruit, nonfat	1 cup	245	230	11	47	0	0	0.1	0
2096	Yogurt, lemon, nonfat	1 cup	245	223	13	43	0	0	0.1	0

Cheese

MDA Code	Food Name	Amt	Wt (g)	Ener (kcal)	Prot (g)	Carb (g)	Fiber (g)	Fat (g)	Mono (g)	Poly (g)
1287	American cheese, nonfat slice/Kraft	1 pce	21.3	32	5	2	0	0		
47855	Blue, 1" cube	1 ea	17.3	61	4	0	0	5	1.3	0.1
47859	Brie, 1" cube	1 ea	17	57	4	0	0	5	1.4	0.1
47861	Camembert, 1" cube	1 ea	17	51	3	0	0	4	1.2	0.1
48333	Cheddar, fat free, 1" cube	1 ea	16	24	4	2	0	0	0	0
1440	Cheese, fondue	2 Tbs	26.9	62	4	1	0	4	1	0.1

Sat (g)	Chol (mg)	Calc (mg)	Iron (mg)	Mag (mg)	Phos (mg)	Pota (mg)	Sodi (mg)	Zinc (mg)	Vit A (RAE)	Vit C (mg)	Thia (mg)	Ribo (mg)	Niac (mg)	Vit B$_6$ (mg)	Vit B$_{12}$ (μg)	Vit E (mg)	Fol (μg)	Alc (g)
0.5	0	109	17.07	95.8	295	250	207	4	165	6.6	0.41	0.47	5.49	0.55	0	1.4	420.1	0
0.5	0	113	17.07	65.5	206	205	269	4.2	167	6.4	0.39	0.48	5.63	0.55	0	1.4	439.6	0
0.2	0	110	3.84	28.3	94	109	165	0.6	322	0.3	0.29	0.35	4.07	0.43	0	0.1	84.9	0
0	0	1	0.4	4.2	17	16	1	0.2	0	0	0.06	0.04	0.49	0	0	0	21.6	0
0	0	3	3.8	17.4	43	42	0	0.3	0	0	0.31	0.22	4.24	0.02	0	0	3.8	0
0.3	0	29	4.64	83	259	372	362	1.5	155	0.4	0.39	0.44	5.18	0.52	1.55	0.5	103.7	0
0.5	0	100	4.5	8.1	60	65	200	3.8	145	6	0.38	0.43	5	0.5	1.5	0.8	99.9	0
0.1	0	100	9	27.6	35	50	270	3.8	150	6	0.38	0.42	5	0.5	1.5	0.2	200	0
0.1	0	3	2	8.2	33	36	314	0.4	170	7.8	0.73	0.74	7.58	1.08	2.01	0	151.1	0
0.2	0	19	1.12	50.3	140	142	2	1.1	0	3.8	0.1	0.05	1.98	0.44	0	0	16.3	0
0.2	0	17	18	24	80	90	275	15.1	376	15	1.55	1.7	20	2	6	13.5	402.5	0
0.1	0	9	8.37	19.2	68	61	224	0.9	230	21	0.53	0.59	7.13	1.98	6.04	4.7	399.9	0
0.4	0	3	4.96	14.8	45	51	200	4.1	11	2.9	0.41	0.47	5.51	0.55	0	0.2	420.1	0
0.4	0	122	9.81	35.7	112	95	269	4.4	65	6.2	0.47	0.6	5.7	0.72	1.84	0.2	156	0
0.2	0	1000	18	31.9	100	310	240	15	149	0	1.5	1.7	20	2	6	13.5	399.8	0
0.1	0	1000	18	24	80	90	190	15	150	60	1.5	1.7	20	2	6	13.5	399.9	0
0.2	0	100	4.5	3.6	20	30	190	3.8	147	6	0.38	0.43	5	0.5	1.5	0.6	99.9	0
0.1	0	60	8.64	24	90	114	252	2.2	90	3.6	0.22	0.26	3	0.3	0.9	0.2	240	0
0.1	0	20	8.4	32.1	100	105	210	7.5	150	6	0.75	0.85	10	1	3	0.4	200.1	0
1.3	10	284	0.12	27	218	370	257	1	17	2.4	0.08	0.38	0.14	0.08	0.54	0.1	12.2	0
2.1	11	32	0.02	3	28	39	12	0.2	29	0.3	0.01	0.04	0.02	0.01	0.1	0.1	0.9	0
6	35	250	0				110			3.6								0
3	20	250	0				125			1.2		0.45						0
2.9	20	485	0.6	35	190	308	165	1	160	0	0.11	1.41	0.41	0.06	0.83	0.1	5	0
1.5	8	288	0.6	32.5	258	425	152	1	145	2.2	0.09	0.41	0.32	0.1	0.85	0	12.5	0
2.1	13	108	0.07	9.9	97	142	49	0.4	28	1	0.03	0.16	0.08	0.02	0.17	0.1	4.2	0
6.5	27	327	0.12	34.2	271	498	122	0.7	139	3.2	0.12	0.34	0.68	0.11	0.17	0.2	2.4	0
4.9	34	79	0.07	7.4	34	125	42	0.4	150	12.3	0.03	0.09	0.44	0.03	0.12	0.2	12.3	0
1.4	9	82	0.06	7.6	64	95	33	0.2	35	0.6	0.01	0.1	0.06	0.02	0.05	0.1	2.5	0
0	1	93	0.09	8.6	62	106	37	0.3	38	0.4	0.01	0.1	0.06	0.02	0.08	0	2.9	0
0.3	12	754	0.19	66	581	1076	321	2.4	392	4.1	0.25	0.93	0.57	0.22	2.42	0	30	0
0.1	5	306	0.07	27	247	382	103	1	149	0	0.11	0.45	0.23	0.09	1.3	0	12.2	0
4.6	24	276	0.07	24.4	222	349	98	1	69	0	0.11	0.45	0.26	0.09	1.07	0.1	12.2	0
5.3	30	280	0.6	32.5	252	418	150	1	66	2.2	0.09	0.41	0.31	0.1	0.83	0.1	12.5	0
1	10	300	0			440	210		0	0								0
0.5	10	100	0				50		0	0								0
0	5	350	0	16	200	320	110		0	0		0.25						0
0	5	350	0	16	200	320	110		0	0		0.25						0
1.7	10	372	0.17	36.8	292	478	142	1.8	25	1.7	0.09	0.44	0.23	0.1	1.15	0	22	0
0.3	5	372	0.17	36.8	292	475	142	1.8	6	1.7	0.1	0.44	0.25	0.1	1.15	0.1	22	0
0.3	4	436	0.21	41.8	343	559	168	2.1	4	1.9	0.11	0.52	0.27	0.12	1.34	0	26.7	0
0.1	3	152	0.01		197	50	276	0.5		0		0.06						0
3.2	13	91	0.05	4	67	44	241	0.5	34	0	0.01	0.07	0.18	0.03	0.21	0	6.2	0
3	17	31	0.08	3.4	32	26	107	0.4	30	0	0.01	0.09	0.06	0.04	0.28	0	11	0
2.6	12	66	0.06	3.4	59	32	143	0.4	41	0		0.08	0.11	0.04	0.22	0	10.5	0
0.1	2	110	0.04	5.8	150	46	244	0.5	70	0	0.01	0.08	0.03	0.01	0.18	0	4.3	0
2.3	12	128	0.1	6.2	82	28	36	0.5	29	0	0.01	0.05	0.05	0.01	0.22	0.1	2.2	0.08

MDA Code	Food Name	Amt	Wt (g)	Ener (kcal)	Prot (g)	Carb (g)	Fiber (g)	Fat (g)	Mono (g)	Poly (g)
48288	Cheese substitute	1 oz	28.4	40	6	2	0	0	0.1	0
48313	Cheese spread, cream cheese base	1 Tbs	15	44	1	1	0	4	1.2	0.2
13349	Cheez Whiz/Kraft	2 Tbs	33	91	4	3	0	7		
47940	Colby, low fat, 1" cube	1 ea	17.3	30	4	0	0	1	0.4	0
1013	Cottage cheese, creamed, large curd, not packed	0.5 cup	105	108	13	3	0	5	1.3	0.1
1014	Cottage cheese, 2% fat	0.5 cup	113	102	16	4	0	2	0.6	0.1
47867	Cottage cheese, nonfat, small curd, dry	0.5 cup	113	96	20	2	0	0	0.1	0
1015	Cream cheese	2 Tbs	29	101	2	1	0	10	2.9	0.4
1452	Cream cheese, fat free	2 Tbs	29	28	4	2	0	0	0.1	0
1016	Feta, crumbled	0.25 cup	37.5	99	5	2	0	8	1.7	0.2
47874	Fontina, 1 oz slice	1 ea	28.4	110	7	0	0	9	2.5	0.5
1054	Gouda	1 oz	28.4	101	7	1	0	8	2.2	0.2
1442	Mexican, queso anejo, crumbled	0.25 cup	33	123	7	2	0	10	2.8	0.3
47885	Monterey jack, slice	1 ea	28.4	106	7	0	0	9	2.5	0.3
47887	Mozzarella, whole milk, slice	1 ea	34	102	8	1	0	8	2.2	0.3
47892	Muenster, slice	1 ea	28.4	105	7	0	0	9	2.5	0.2
1075	Parmesan, grated	1 Tbs	5	22	2	0	0	1	0.4	0.1
47900	Provolone, slice	1 ea	28.4	100	7	1	0	8	2.1	0.2
1024	Ricotta, part skim	0.25 cup	62	86	7	3	0	5	1.4	0.2
1064	Ricotta, whole milk	0.25 cup	62	108	7	2	0	8	2.2	0.2
EGGS AND EGG SUBSTITUTES										
19524	Egg substitute, frozen	0.25 cup	60	96	7	2	0	7	1.5	3.7
19525	Egg substitute, liquid	0.25 cup	62.8	53	8	0	0	2	0.6	1
19526	Egg substitute, powder	1 oz	28.4	126	16	6	0	4	1.5	0.5
19506	Egg whites, raw, large	1 ea	33.4	17	4	0	0	0		
19509	Egg, whole, large, fried	1 ea	46	90	6	0	0	7	2.9	1.2
19515	Egg, whole, hard boiled	1 ea	37	57	5	0	0	4	1.5	0.5
19521	Egg, whole, poached, small	1 ea	37	53	5	0	0	4	1.4	0.5
19516	Egg, whole, scrambled	1 ea	61	102	7	1	0	7	2.9	1.3
19508	Egg yolk, raw, large	1 ea	16.6	53	3	1	0	4	1.9	0.7
FRUIT										
3512	Apples, Golden Delicious, fresh	1 ea	138	59	0	17	2	0	0	0
71079	Apples, fresh	1 cup	125	65	0	17	3	0	0	0.1
3004	Apples, fresh, peeled, slices	1 cup	110	53	0	14	1	0	0	0
3148	Apples, slices, sweetened, drained, canned	0.5 cup	102	68	0	17	2	0	0	0.1
3331	Applesauce, sweetened, canned, w/salt	0.5 cup	127.5	97	0	25	2	0	0	0.1
3330	Applesauce, unswtnd, w/vitamin C, canned	1 cup	244	105	0	28	3	0	0	0
72101	Apricots, w/heavy syrup, canned, drained	1 cup	182	151	1	39	5	0	0.1	0
3155	Apricots, sweetened, frozen	0.5 cup	121	119	1	30	3	0	0.1	0
3333	Apricots, w/o skin, canned, w/water	0.5 cup	113.5	25	1	6	1	0	0	0
3657	Apricots, raw, sliced	1 cup	165	79	2	18	3	1	0.3	0.1
3210	Avocado, California, fresh	1 ea	173	289	3	15	12	27	17	3.1
71082	Banana, fresh, extra small, 6" or shorter	1 ea	81	72	1	19	2	0	0	0.1
3026	Boysenberries, fresh	0.5 cup	72	31	1	7	4	0	0	0.2
3663	Breadfruit, fresh	1 cup	220	227	2	60	11	1	0.1	0.1
71768	Carambola (starfruit), fresh, small	1 ea	70	22	1	5	2	0	0	0.1
72094	Cherries, maraschino, canned, drained	1 ea	4	7	0	2	0	0	0	0
3403	Cherries, sour, red, canned, w/heavy syrup	0.5 cup	128	116	1	30	1	0	0	0
3159	Cherries, sour, red, frozen, unsweetened	0.5 cup	77.5	36	1	9	1	0	0.1	0.1
3035	Cherries, sour/tart, red, canned in water	0.5 cup	122	44	1	11	1	0	0	0

Sat (g)	Chol (mg)	Calc (mg)	Iron (mg)	Mag (mg)	Phos (mg)	Pota (mg)	Sodi (mg)	Zinc (mg)	Vit A (RAE)	Vit C (mg)	Thia (mg)	Ribo (mg)	Niac (mg)	Vit B_6 (mg)	Vit B_{12} (µg)	Vit E (mg)	Fol (µg)	Alc (g)
0.2	2	157	0.26	9.9	142	95	352	0.9	3	0	0.01	0.14	0.04	0.04	0.35	0	2.3	0
2.7	14	11	0.17	0.9	14	17	101	0.1	51	0	0	0.03	0.14	0.01	0.06	0.1	1.8	0
4.3	25	118	0.06		266	79	541	0.5		0.1		0.08						0
0.8	4	72	0.07	2.8	84	11	106	0.3	10	0	0	0.04	0.01	0.01	0.08	0	1.9	0
3	16	63	0.15	5.2	139	88	425	0.4	46	0	0.02	0.17	0.13	0.07	0.65	0	12.6	0
1.4	9	78	0.18	6.8	171	108	459	0.5	24	0	0.03	0.21	0.16	0.09	0.8	0	14.7	0
0.3	8	36	0.26	4.5	118	36	15	0.5	10	0	0.03	0.16	0.18	0.09	0.94	0	17	0
6.4	32	23	0.35	1.7	30	35	86	0.2	106	0	0	0.06	0.03	0.01	0.12	0.1	3.8	0
0.3	2	54	0.05	4.1	126	47	158	0.3	81	0	0.01	0.05	0.05	0.01	0.16	0	10.7	0
5.6	33	185	0.24	7.1	126	23	418	1.1	47	0	0.06	0.32	0.37	0.16	0.63	0.1	12	0
5.5	33	156	0.07	4	98	18	227	1	74	0	0.01	0.06	0.04	0.02	0.48	0.1	1.7	0
5	32	199	0.07	8.2	155	34	233	1.1	47	0	0.01	0.09	0.02	0.02	0.44	0.1	6	0
6.3	35	224	0.16	9.2	147	29	373	1	18	0	0.01	0.07	0.01	0.02	0.46	0.1	0.3	0
5.4	25	212	0.2	7.7	126	23	152	0.9	56	0	0	0.11	0.03	0.02	0.24	0.1	5.1	0
4.5	27	172	0.15	6.8	120	26	213	1	61	0	0.01	0.1	0.04	0.01	0.78	0.1	2.4	0
5.4	27	204	0.12	7.7	133	38	178	0.8	85	0	0	0.09	0.03	0.02	0.42	0.1	3.4	0
0.9	4	55	0.04	1.9	36	6	76	0.2	6	0	0	0.02	0.01	0	0.11	0	0.5	0
4.9	20	215	0.15	8	141	39	249	0.9	67	0	0.01	0.09	0.04	0.02	0.41	0.1	2.8	0
3.1	19	169	0.27	9.3	113	78	78	0.8	66	0	0.01	0.11	0.05	0.01	0.18	0	8.1	0
5.1	32	128	0.24	6.8	98	65	52	0.7	74	0	0.01	0.12	0.06	0.03	0.21	0.1	7.4	0
1.2	1	44	1.19	9	43	128	119	0.6	7	0.3	0.07	0.23	0.08	0.08	0.2	1	9.6	0
0.4	1	33	1.32	5.7	76	207	111	0.8	11	0	0.07	0.19	0.07	0	0.19	0.2	9.4	0
1.1	162	93	0.9	18.5	136	211	227	0.5	105	0.2	0.06	0.5	0.16	0.04	1	0.4	35.5	0
	0	2	0.03	3.7	5	54	55	0	0	0	0	0.15	0.04	0	0.03	0	1.3	0
2	210	27	0.91	6	96	68	94	0.6	91	0	0.03	0.24	0.04	0.07	0.64	0.6	23.5	0
1.2	157	18	0.44	3.7	64	47	46	0.4	63	0	0.02	0.19	0.02	0.04	0.41	0.4	16.3	0
1.1	156	20	0.68	4.4	70	49	109	0.4	51	0	0.03	0.18	0.03	0.05	0.47	0.4	17.4	0
2.2	215	43	0.73	7.3	104	84	171	0.6	87	0.1	0.03	0.27	0.05	0.07	0.47	0.5	18.3	0
1.6	205	21	0.45	0.8	65	18	8	0.4	63	0	0.03	0.09	0	0.06	0.32	0.4	24.2	0
0	0	4	0.28	5.5		104	3	0.1	2	6.9	0.03	0.01	0.14		0			0
0	0	8	0.15	6.2	14	134	1	0	4	5.7	0.02	0.03	0.11	0.05	0	0.2	3.8	0
0	0	6	0.08	4.4	12	99	0	0.1	2	4.4	0.02	0.03	0.1	0.04	0	0.1	0	0
0.1	0	4	0.23	2	5	69	3	0	3	0.4	0.01	0.01	0.07	0.04	0	0.2	0	0
0	0	5	0.45	3.8	9	78	36	0.1	1	2.2	0.02	0.04	0.24	0.03	0	0.1	1.3	0
0	0	7	0.29	7.3	17	183	5	0.1	2	51.7	0.03	0.06	0.46	0.06	0	0.1	2.4	0
0	0	18	0.55	12.7	24	260	7	0.2	266	5.6	0.04	0.04	0.68	0.1	0	1.6	3.6	0
0	0	12	1.09	10.9	23	277	5	0.1	102	10.9	0.02	0.05	0.97	0.07	0	1.1	2.4	0
0	0	9	0.61	10.2	18	175	12	0.1	103	2	0.02	0.03	0.5	0.06	0	1	2.3	0
0	0	21	0.64	16.5	38	427	2	0.3	158	16.5	0.05	0.07	0.99	0.09	0	1.5	14.8	0
3.7	0	22	1.06	50.2	93	877	14	1.2	12	15.2	0.13	0.25	3.31	0.5	0	3.4	154	0
0.1	0	4	0.21	21.9	18	290	1	0.1	2	7	0.03	0.06	0.54	0.3	0	0.1	16.2	0
0	0	21	0.45	14.4	16	117	1	0.4	8	15.1	0.01	0.02	0.47	0.02	0	0.8	18	0
0.1	0	37	1.19	55	66	1078	4	0.3	0	63.8	0.24	0.07	1.98	0.22	0	0.2	30.8	0
0	0	2	0.06	7	8	93	1	0.1	2	24.1	0.01	0.01	0.26	0.01	0	0.1	8.4	0
0	0	2	0.02	0.2	0	1	0	0	0	0	0	0	0	0	0	0	0	0
0	0	13	1.66	7.7	13	119	9	0.1	46	2.6	0.02	0.05	0.22	0.06	0	0.3	10.2	0
0.1	0	10	0.41	7	12	96	1	0.1	34	1.3	0.03	0.03	0.11	0.05	0	0	3.9	0
0	0	13	1.67	7.3	12	120	9	0.1	46	2.6	0.02	0.05	0.22	0.05	0	0.3	9.8	0

MDA Code	Food Name	Amt	Wt (g)	Ener (kcal)	Prot (g)	Carb (g)	Fiber (g)	Fat (g)	Mono (g)	Poly (g)
3038	Cherries, sweet, canned in heavy syrup	1 cup	253	210	2	54	4	0	0.1	0.1
72103	Cherries, sweet, canned, heavy syrup, drained	1 cup	184	153	1	39	5	0	0.1	0.1
3336	Cherries, sweet, canned in juice	0.5 cup	125	68	1	17	2	0	0	0
71731	Chinese gooseberries, fresh, w/o skin	1 ea	91	56	1	13	3	0	0	0.3
72093	Cranberries, dried, sweetened	0.33 cup	40	123	0	33	2	1	0.1	0.3
3673	Cranberries, raw	1 cup	110	51	0	13	5	0	0	0.1
27019	Cranberry-orange relish, canned	0.25 cup	68.8	122	0	32	0	0	0	0
4900	Currants, red or white, raw	0.25 cup	28	16	0	4	1	0	0	0
3192	Currants, Zante, dried	0.25 cup	36	102	1	27	2	0	0	0.1
3044	Dates, Deglet Noor	5 ea	41.5	117	1	31	3	0	0	0
72111	Dates, medjool	1 ea	24	66	0	18	2	0		
3975	Durian, fresh or frozen	1 ea	602	885	9	163	23	32		
5611	Eggplant, pickled	1 cup	136	67	1	13	3	1	0.1	0.4
3677	Figs, raw	1 ea	40	30	0	8	1	0	0	0.1
3045	Fruit cocktail canned in heavy syrup	1 cup	248	181	1	47	2	0	0	0.1
3164	Fruit cocktail canned in juice	1 cup	237	109	1	28	2	0	0	0
3414	Fruit salad canned in heavy syrup	1 cup	255	186	1	49	3	0	0	0.1
44023	Fruit salad canned in juice	0.5 cup	124.5	62	1	16	1	0	0	0
3203	Gooseberries, raw	0.5 cup	75	33	1	8	3	0	0	0.2
3342	Grapefruit, canned in juice	0.5 cup	124.5	46	1	11	0	0	0	0
71976	Grapefruit, fresh	0.5 ea	154	60	1	16	6	0	0	0
3055	Grapes, Thompson seedless, fresh	0.5 cup	80	55	1	14	1	0	0	0
3634	Guava, raw	0.5 cup	82.5	56	2	12	4	1	0.1	0.3
71732	Kiwifruit (Chinese gooseberry) peeled, raw	1 ea	76	46	1	11	2	0	0	0.2
3252	Kumquat, raw	1 ea	19	13	0	3	1	0	0	0
71979	Lemon, fresh	1 ea	58	15	0	5	1	0	0	0
3071	Limes, peeled, fresh	1 ea	67	20	0	7	2	0	0	0
3033	Loganberries, w/heavy syrup, canned	0.5 cup	128	113	1	29	3	0	0	0.1
71743	Lychee (Litchi), shelled, dried	1 ea	2.5	7	0	2	0	0	0	0
71927	Mango, dried	0.33 cup	40	140	0	34	1	0	0	0
3221	Mango, raw	0.5 ea	103.5	67	1	18	2	0	0.1	0.1
3167	Melon balls (cantaloupe & honeydew), frozen	0.5 cup	86.5	29	1	7	1	0	0	0.1
3642	Melon, cantaloupe, fresh, wedge	1 pce	69	23	1	6	1	0	0	0.1
4488	Melon, casaba, raw	1 pce	164	46	2	11	1	0	0	0.1
3644	Melon, honeydew, fresh	1 ea	1280	461	7	116	10	2	0	0.8
3168	Mixed fruit (prune, apricot & pear), dried	1 oz	28.4	69	1	18	2	0	0.1	0
3216	Nectarine, raw	1 cup	138	61	1	15	2	0	0.1	0.2
27011	Olives, black, pitted, canned	1 ea	3.2	4	0	0	0	0	0.3	0
3228	Orange, California navel, fresh	1 ea	140	69	1	18	3	0	0	0
3230	Orange, Florida, fresh	1 ea	151	69	1	17	4	0	0.1	0.1
3085	Orange, fresh	1 ea	184	86	2	22	4	0	0	0
71990	Orange, mandarin, fresh	1 ea	109	50	1	15	3	0		
3721	Papayas, raw	1 ea	152	59	1	15	3	0	0.1	0
3098	Peach, canned in heavy syrup	1 cup	262	194	1	52	3	0	0.1	0.1
57481	Peach, frozen, sweetened	1 cup	250	235	2	60	4	0	0.1	0.2
3726	Peach, peeled, raw	1 ea	79	31	1	8	1	0	0.1	0.1
3106	Pear, d'anjou, fresh	1 ea	209	121	1	32	6	0	0.1	0.1
3106	Pear, raw	1 ea	209	121	1	32	6	0	0.1	0.1
3194	Persimmon, native, raw	1 ea	25	32	0	8	0	0		
72113	Pineapple, fresh, slice	1 pce	84	38	0	10		0		

Sat (g)	Chol (mg)	Calc (mg)	Iron (mg)	Mag (mg)	Phos (mg)	Pota (mg)	Sodi (mg)	Zinc (mg)	Vit A (RAE)	Vit C (mg)	Thia (mg)	Ribo (mg)	Niac (mg)	Vit B$_6$ (mg)	Vit B$_{12}$ (µg)	Vit E (mg)	Fol (µg)	Alc (g)
0.1	0	23	0.89	22.8	46	367	8	0.3	20	9.1	0.05	0.1	1	0.08	0	0.6	10.1	0
0.1	0	18	0.64	16.6	37	272	6	0.2	22	6.6	0.04	0.08	0.73	0.06	0	0.4	9.2	0
0	0	18	0.72	15	28	164	4	0.1	8	3.1	0.02	0.03	0.51	0.04	0	0.3	5	0
0	7	31	0.28	15.5	31	284	3	0.1	4	84.4	0.02	0.02	0.31	0.06	0	1.3	23	0
0	0	4	0.21	2	3	16	1	0	0	0.1	0	0.01	0.4	0.02	0	0.4	0	0
0	0	9	0.28	6.6	14	94	2	0.1	3	14.6	0.01	0.02	0.11	0.06	0	1.3	1.1	0
0	0	8	0.14	2.8	6	26	22	0.1	3	12.4	0.02	0.01	0.07	0.02	0	0	2.1	0
0	0	9	0.28	3.6	12	77	0	0.1	1	11.5	0.01	0.01	0.03	0.02	0	0	2.2	0
0	0	31	1.17	14.8	45	321	3	0.2	1	1.7	0.06	0.05	0.58	0.11	0	0	3.6	0
0	0	16	0.42	17.8	26	272	1	0.1	0	0.2	0.02	0.03	0.53	0.07	0	0	7.9	0
	0	15	0.22	13	15	167	0	0.1	2	0	0.01	0.01	0.39	0.06			3.6	0
	0	36	2.59	180.6	235	2625	12	1.7	12	119	2.25	1.2	6.47	1.9	0		217	0
0.2	0	34	1.05	8.2	12	16	2277	0.3	4	0	0.07	0.1	0.9	0.19	0	0	27.2	0
0	0	14	0.15	6.8	6	93	0	0.1	3	0.8	0.02	0.02	0.16	0.05	0	0	2.4	0
0	0	15	0.72	12.4	27	218	15	0.2	25	4.7	0.04	0.05	0.93	0.12	0	1	7.4	0
0	0	19	0.5	16.6	33	225	9	0.2	36	6.4	0.03	0.04	0.96	0.12	0	0.9	7.1	0
0	0	15	0.71	12.8	23	204	15	0.2	64	6.1	0.04	0.05	0.88	0.08	0	1	7.6	0
0	0	14	0.31	10	17	144	6	0.2	37	4.1	0.01	0.02	0.44	0.03	0	0.7	3.7	0
0	0	19	0.23	7.5	20	148	1	0.1	11	20.8	0.03	0.02	0.23	0.06	0	0.3	4.5	0
0	0	19	0.26	13.7	15	210	9	0.1	0	42.2	0.04	0.02	0.31	0.02	0	0.1	11.2	0
0		20	0				0		38	66					0			0
0	4	8	0.29	5.6	16	153	2	0.1	2	8.6	0.06	0.06	0.15	0.07	0	0.2	1.6	0
0.2	0	15	0.21	18.2	33	344	2	0.2	26	188.3	0.06	0.03	0.89	0.09	0	0.6	40.4	0
0	0	26	0.24	12.9	26	237	2	0.1	3	70.5	0.02	0.02	0.26	0.05	0	1.1	19	0
0	0	12	0.16	3.8	4	35	2	0	3	8.3	0.01	0.02	0.08	0.01	0	0	3.2	0
0		20	0				5		0	24					0			0
0	3	22	0.4	4	12	68	1	0.1	1	19.5	0.02	0.01	0.13	0.03	0	0.1	5.4	0
0	0	23	0.55	14.1	13	115	4	0.2	3	7.9	0.03	0.04	0.29	0.05	0	0.9	43.5	0
0	0	1	0.04	1	5	28	0	0	0	4.6	0	0.01	0.08	0	0	0	0.3	0
0		80	0.36			10	20	25		1.2					0			0
0.1	0	10	0.13	9.3	11	161	2	0	39	28.7	0.06	0.06	0.6	0.14	0	1.2	14.5	0
0.1	0	9	0.25	12.1	10	242	27	0.1	77	5.4	0.14	0.02	0.55	0.09	0	0.1	22.5	0
0	5	6	0.14	8.3	10	184	11	0.1	117	25.3	0.03	0.01	0.51	0.05	0	0	15	0
0	0	18	0.56	18	8	298	15	0.1	0	35.8	0.02	0.05	0.38	0.27	0	0.1	13.1	0
0.5	77		2.18	128	141	2918	230	1.2	38	230	0.49	0.15	5.35	1.13	0	0.3	243	0
0	0	11	0.77	11.1	22	226	5	0.1	35	1.1	0.01	0.04	0.55	0.05	0	0.2	1.1	0
0	0	8	0.39	12.4	36	277	0	0.2	23	7.5	0.05	0.04	1.55	0.03	0	1.1	6.9	0
0	0	3	0.11	0.1	0	0	28	0	1	0	0	0	0	0	0	0.1	0	0
0	12	60	0.18	15.4	32	232	1	0.1	17	82.7	0.1	0.07	0.6	0.11	0	0.2	48	0
0		65	0.14	15.1	18	255	0	0.1	17	68	0.15	0.06	0.6	0.08	0	0.3	26	0
0		74	0.18	18.4	26	333	0	0.1	20	97.9	0.16	0.07	0.52	0.11	0	0.3	55	0
0		40	0				0		0	30					0			0
0.1	0	36	0.15	15.2	8	391	5	0.1	84	93.9	0.04	0.05	0.51	0.03	0	1.1	57.8	0
0	0	8	0.71	13.1	29	241	16	0.2	45	7.3	0.03	0.06	1.61	0.05	0	1.3	7.9	0
0	0	8	0.93	12.5	28	325	15	0.1	35	235.5	0.03	0.09	1.63	0.04	0	1.6	7.5	0
0	0	5	0.2	7.1	16	150	0	0.1	13	5.2	0.02	0.02	0.64	0.02	0	0.6	3.2	0
0	11	19	0.36	14.6	23	249	2	0.2	2	8.8	0.03	0.05	0.33	0.06	0	0.3	15	0
0	0	19	0.36	14.6	23	249	2	0.2	2	8.8	0.03	0.05	0.33	0.06	0	0.3	14.6	0
	0	7	0.62		6	78	0			16.5					0	0.2	2	0
	0	11	0.21	10.1	8	105	1	0.1	2	14.2	0.07	0.02	0.39	0.09			9.2	0

MDA Code	Food Name	Amt	Wt (g)	Ener (kcal)	Prot (g)	Carb (g)	Fiber (g)	Fat (g)	Mono (g)	Poly (g)
3748	Plantain, cooked, mashed	1 cup	200	232	2	62	5	0	0	0.1
3121	Plums, fresh	1 ea	66	30	0	8	1	0	0.1	0
3197	Pomegranate, fresh	1 ea	154	105	1	26	1	0	0.1	0.1
3263	Quince, fresh	1 ea	92	52	0	14	2	0	0	0
3766	Raisins, seedless	50 ea	26	78	1	21	1	0	0	0
9758	Raisins, golden, seedless	0.25 cup	40	130	1	31	2	0	0	0
71987	Raspberries, fresh	1 cup	125	50	1	17	8	0	0	0
3133	Rhubarb, frozen, cooked w/sugar	0.5 cup	120	139	0	37	2	0	0	0
3767	Rhubarb, fresh, stalk	1 ea	51	11	0	2	1	0	0	0.1
3761	Shaddock (pomelo or grapefruit), fresh, sections	1 cup	190	72	1	18	2	0		
3354	Strawberries, frozen, sweetened, thawed, whole	0.5 cup	127.5	99	1	27	2	0	0	0.1
3135	Strawberries, fresh, sliced	1 cup	166	53	1	13	3	0	0.1	0.3
3792	Tamarindo, Spanish, fresh, pulp	1 cup	120	287	3	75	6	1	0.2	0.1
3717	Tangerines, fresh, large	1 ea	98	52	1	13	2	0	0.1	0.1
3143	Watermelon, fresh, 1/16 melon	1 pce	286	86	2	22	1	0	0.1	0.1

GRAIN PRODUCTS, GRAINS, AND FLOURS
Breads, Rolls, Bread Crumbs, and Croutons

MDA Code	Food Name	Amt	Wt (g)	Ener (kcal)	Prot (g)	Carb (g)	Fiber (g)	Fat (g)	Mono (g)	Poly (g)
71170	Bagel, cinnamon raisin, mini, 2-1/2"	1 ea	26	71	3	14	1	0	0	0.2
71167	Bagel, egg, mini, 2-1/2"	1 ea	26	72	3	14	1	1	0.1	0.2
42744	Bagel, blueberry, 4", Lender's	1 ea	102	264	11	53	2	2	0.4	0.5
71176	Bagel, oat bran, mini, 2-1/2"	1 ea	26	66	3	14	1	0	0.1	0.1
71152	Bagel, sesame, mini, enriched, w/calcium propionate, 2-1/2"	1 ea	26	67	3	13	1	0	0.1	0.2
42039	Banana bread, homemade w/margarine, slice	1 pce	60	196	3	33	1	6	2.7	1.9
42433	Biscuit	1 ea	82	273	5	28	1	16		
47709	Biscuit, buttermilk, refrigerated dough/Pillsbury	1 ea	64	150	4	29	1	2		
42111	Biscuit, mixed grain, refrigerated dough, 2-1/2"	1 ea	44	116	3	21		2	1.3	0.4
71192	Biscuit, plain, lower fat, refrigerated dough, 2-1/4"	1 ea	21	63	2	12	0	1	0.6	0.2
42004	Bread crumbs, plain, grated, dry	1 Tbs	6.8	27	1	5	0	0	0.1	0.1
42144	Bread crumbs, seasoned, grated, dry	1 Tbs	7.5	29	1	5	0	0	0.1	0.2
42090	Bread, egg, slice	1 pce	40	113	4	19	1	2	0.9	0.4
49144	Bread, garlic, crusty Italian	1 pce	50	186	4	21		10	3.9	1.8
70964	Bread, garlic, frozen, Campione	1 pce	28	101	2	12	1	5		
42119	Bread, Irish soda, homemade	1 pce	28	81	2	16	1	1	0.6	0.4
42069	Bread, oat bran, slice	1 pce	30	71	3	12	1	1	0.5	0.5
42076	Bread, oat bran, reduced calorie, slice	1 pce	23	46	2	9	3	1	0.2	0.4
42136	Bread, wheat bran, slice	1 pce	36	89	3	17	1	1	0.6	0.2
42599	Bread, wheat germ, slice	1 pce	28	73	3	14	1	1	0.4	0.2
42095	Bread, wheat, reduced calorie, slice	1 pce	23	46	2	10	3	1	0.1	0.2
71247	Bread, white, soft, w/o crust, thin slice	1 pce	9	24	1	5	0	0	0.1	0.1
42084	Bread, white, reduced calorie, slice	1 pce	23	48	2	10	2	1	0.2	0.1
71259	Breadsticks, plain, small, 4-1/4" long	1 ea	5	21	1	3	0	0	0.2	0.2
26561	Buns, hamburger/Wonder	1 ea	43	117	3	22	1	2	0.4	0.9
42021	Buns, hot dog/frankfurter	1 ea	43	120	4	21	1	2	0.5	0.8
71364	Buns, hot dog/frankfurter, whole wheat	1 ea	43	114	4	22	3	2	0.5	0.9
42115	Cornbread, prepared from dry mix	1 pce	60	188	4	29	1	6	3.1	0.7
49012	Cornbread, hush puppies, homemade	1 ea	22	74	2	10	1	3	0.7	1.6
42016	Croutons, plain, dry	0.25 cup	7.5	31	1	6	0	0	0.2	0.1
71302	Croutons, seasoned, fast food pkg	1 ea	10	46	1	6	0	2	0.9	0.2
71227	Pita bread, white, enriched, small, 4"	1 ea	28	77	3	16	1	0	0	0.1
71228	Pita bread, whole wheat, small, 4"	1 ea	28	74	3	15	2	1	0.1	0.3

Sat (g)	Chol (mg)	Calc (mg)	Iron (mg)	Mag (mg)	Phos (mg)	Pota (mg)	Sodi (mg)	Zinc (mg)	Vit A (RAE)	Vit C (mg)	Thia (mg)	Ribo (mg)	Niac (mg)	Vit B$_6$ (mg)	Vit B$_{12}$ (µg)	Vit E (mg)	Fol (µg)	Alc (g)
0.1	0	4	1.16	64	56	930	10	0.3	90	21.8	0.09	0.1	1.51	0.48	0	0.3	52	0
0	0	4	0.11	4.6	11	104	0	0.1	11	6.3	0.02	0.02	0.28	0.02	0	0.2	3.3	0
0.1	0	5	0.46	4.6	12	399	5	0.2	8	9.4	0.05	0.05	0.46	0.16	0	0.9	9.2	0
0	0	10	0.64	7.4	16	181	4	0	2	13.8	0.02	0.03	0.18	0.04	0	0.5	2.8	0
0	0	13	0.49	8.3	26	195	3	0.1	0	0.6	0.03	0.03	0.2	0.05	0	0	1.3	0
0	0	20	1.08				10		0	0								0
0	0	20	0.36				0		0	24					0			0
0	0	174	0.25	14.4	10	115	1	0.1	5	4	0.02	0.03	0.24	0.02	0	0.3	6	0
0	0	44	0.11	6.1	7	147	2	0.1	3	4.1	0.01	0.02	0.15	0.01	0	0.2	3.6	0
	0	8	0.21	11.4	32	410	2	0.2	1	115.9	0.06	0.05	0.42	0.07	0	0.2	49.4	0
0	0	14	0.6	7.6	15	125	1	0.1	1	50.4	0.02	0.1	0.37	0.04	0	0.3	5.1	0
0	0	27	0.68	21.6	40	254	2	0.2	2	97.6	0.04	0.04	0.64	0.08	0	0.5	39.8	0
0.3	0	89	3.36	110.4	136	754	34	0.1	2	4.2	0.51	0.18	2.33	0.08	0	0.1	16.8	0
0	0	36	0.15	11.8	20	163	2	0.1	33	26.2	0.06	0.04	0.37	0.08	0	0.2	15.7	0
0	0	20	0.69	28.6	31	320	3	0.3	80	23.2	0.09	0.06	0.51	0.13	0	0.1	8.6	0
0.1	0	5	0.99	7.3	26	38	84	0.3	5	0.2	0.1	0.07	0.8	0.02	0	0.1	28.9	0
0.1	6	3	1.03	6.5	22	18	131	0.2	9	0.2	0.14	0.06	0.9	0.02	0.04	0	22.9	0
0.3	0	57	1.84			158	427		0	0	0.27	0.2	4.08	0.06	0		75.5	0
0	0	3	0.8	8.1	29	30	132	0.2	0	0.1	0.09	0.09	0.77	0.01	0	0.1	25.5	0
0.1	0	23	1.57	5.7	23	20	116	0.5	0	0.3	0.16	0.07	1.03	0.02	0	0	37.7	0
1.3	26	13	0.84	8.4	35	80	181	0.2	64	1	0.1	0.12	0.87	0.09	0.06	1.1	19.8	0
3.9	1	30					786			0								0
0.3	0		1.44				570											0
0.6	0	7	1.21	13.2	104	201	295	0.3	0	0	0.17	0.09	1.5	0.03	0	0.4	36.5	0
0.3	0	4	0.65	3.6	98	39	305	0.1	0	0	0.09	0.05	0.72	0.01	0	0	17.4	0
0.1	0	12	0.33	2.9	11	13	50	0.1	0	0	0.07	0.03	0.45	0.01	0.02	0	7.3	0
0.1	0	14	0.37	3.4	13	17	132	0.1	1	0.2	0.07	0.03	0.46	0.01	0	0	8.9	0
0.6	20	37	1.22	7.6	42	46	197	0.3	25	0	0.18	0.17	1.94	0.03	0.04	0.1	42	0
2.4	6		1.18				200											0
0.8			0.3				154											0
0.3	5	23	0.75	6.4	32	74	111	0.2	13	0.2	0.08	0.08	0.67	0.02	0.01	0.3	13.2	0
0.2	0	20	0.94	10.5	42	44	122	0.3	1	0	0.15	0.1	1.45	0.02	0	0.1	24.3	0
0.1	0	13	0.72	12.6	32	23	81	0.2	0	0	0.08	0.05	0.87	0.02	0	0.1	18.6	0
0.3	0	27	1.11	29.2	67	82	175	0.5	0	0	0.14	0.1	1.58	0.06	0	0.1	37.8	0
0.2	0	25	0.97	7.8	34	71	155	0.3	0	0.1	0.1	0.1	1.26	0.02	0.02	0.1	33	0
0.1	0	18	0.68	9	23	28	118	0.3	0	0	0.1	0.07	0.89	0.03	0	0.1	20.9	0
0.1	0	14	0.34	2.1	9	9	61	0.1	0	0	0.04	0.03	0.39	0.01	0	0	10	0
0.1	0	22	0.73	5.3	28	17	104	0.3	0	0.1	0.09	0.07	0.84	0.01	0.06	0	21.8	0
0.1	0	1	0.21	1.6	6	6	33	0	0	0	0.03	0.03	0.26	0	0	0.1	8.1	0
0.4		37	0.95				256											0
0.5	0	59	1.43	9	27	40	206	0.3	0	0	0.17	0.14	1.79	0.03	0.09	0	47.7	0
0.4	0	46	1.04	36.6	96	117	206	0.9	0	0	0.11	0.07	1.58	0.08	0	0.4	12.9	0
1.6	37	44	1.14	12	226	77	467	0.4	26	0.1	0.15	0.16	1.23	0.06	0.1	0.7	33	0
0.5	10	61	0.67	5.3	42	32	147	0.1	9	0	0.08	0.07	0.61	0.02	0.04	0.3	19.6	0
0.1	0	6	0.31	2.3	9	9	52	0.1	0	0	0.05	0.02	0.41	0	0	0	9.9	0
0.5	1	10	0.28	4.2	14	18	124	0.1	1	0	0.05	0.04	0.46	0.01	0.01	0	10.5	0
0	0	24	0.73	7.3	27	34	150	0.2	0	0	0.17	0.09	1.3	0.01	0	0.1	30	0
0.1	0	4	0.86	19.3	50	48	149	0.4	0	0	0.09	0.02	0.8	0.07	0	0.2	9.8	0

MDA Code	Food Name	Amt	Wt (g)	Ener (kcal)	Prot (g)	Carb (g)	Fiber (g)	Fat (g)	Mono (g)	Poly (g)
42159	Rolls, dinner, egg, 2-1/2"	1 ea	35	107	3	18	1	2	1	0.4
71368	Rolls, dinner, homemade w/2% milk, 3-1/2"	1 ea	43	136	4	23	1	3	1.2	0.9
42161	Rolls, French	1 ea	38	105	3	19	1	2	0.7	0.3
71056	Rolls, kaiser, 3-1/2"	1 ea	57	167	6	30	1	2	0.6	1
42297	Tortilla, corn, medium, 6", unsalted	1 ea	26	58	1	12	1	1	0.2	0.3
90645	Taco shells, baked, mini, 3"	1 ea	5	23	0	3	0	1	0.6	0.2
	Crackers									
71277	Cheese crackers, bite size	1 cup	62	312	6	36	1	16	7.5	1.5
43532	Crispbread crackers, rye	1 ea	10	37	1	8	2	0	0	0.1
71451	Goldfish crackers, cheese, low sodium	55 pce	33	166	3	19	1	8	3.9	0.8
43510	Matzoh, whole wheat	1 oz	28.4	100	4	22	3	0	0.1	0.2
71284	Melba toast, plain	1 cup	30	117	4	23	2	1	0.2	0.4
71032	Melba toast, pumpernickel	6 ea	30	117	3	23	2	1	0.3	0.4
43507	Oyster crackers	1 cup	45	193	4	32	1	5	3.2	0.6
43659	Oyster crackers, low sodium	1 cup	45	195	4	32	1	5	2.9	0.8
70963	Ritz crackers, original/Nabisco	5 ea	16	79	1	10	0	4	2.8	0.3
43540	Rusk toast crackers	3 ea	30	122	4	22	1	2	0.8	0.7
43587	Saltine crackers, original/Kraft	5 ea	14	56	1	10	0	1		
43664	Saltines, low sodium, fat free	6 ea	30	118	3	25	1	0	0	0.2
43545	Sandwich crackers, cheese	4 ea	28	134	3	17	1	6	3.2	0.7
43501	Sandwich crackers, cheese, peanut butter	4 ea	28	139	3	16	1	7	3.6	1.4
43546	Sandwich crackers, peanut butter	4 ea	28	138	3	16	1	7	3.9	1.3
44677	Snackwell crackers, wheat/Kraft	1 ea	15	62	1	12	1	2		
43581	Wheat Thins, original/Kraft	16 ea	29	140	3	20	1	6		
43508	Whole-wheat crackers	4 ea	32	142	3	22	3	6	1.9	2.1
43570	Whole-wheat crackers, low sodium	7 ea	28	124	2	19	3	5	1.6	1.8
	Muffins and Baked Goods									
71035	English muffin, granola	1 ea	66	155	6	31	2	1	0.5	0.4
42723	English muffin, plain/Thomas'	1 ea	57	132	5	26		1	0.2	0.5
42060	English muffin, sourdough, w/calcium proprionate	1 ea	57	129	5	25	2	1	0.2	0.3
42153	English muffin, wheat	1 ea	57	127	5	26	3	1	0.2	0.5
62916	Muffin, blueberry, mini, 1-1/4"	1 ea	11	43	1	5	0	2	0.6	1.1
44521	Muffin, corn, 2-1/4" × 2-1/2"	1 ea	57	174	3	29	2	5	1.2	1.8
44514	Muffin, oat bran, 2-1/4" × 2-1/2"	1 ea	57	154	4	28	3	4	1	2.4
44518	Toaster muffin, blueberry	1 ea	33	103	2	18	1	3	0.7	1.8
44522	Toaster muffin, cornmeal	1 ea	33	114	2	19	1	4	0.9	2.1
	Noodles and Pasta									
66103	Angel hair pasta, semolina, dry	1 ea	56	201	7	41	2	1	0.2	0.8
91313	Bow tie pasta, enriched, dry	1.5 cup	56	204	8	42	2	1		
38048	Chow mein noodles, dry	1 cup	45	237	4	26	2	14	3.5	7.8
38047	Egg pasta, enriched, cooked	0.5 cup	80	110	4	20	1	2	0.5	0.4
38251	Egg pasta, enriched, cooked w/salt	0.5 cup	80	110	4	20	1	2	0.5	0.4
91316	Elbow pasta, enriched, dry	0.5 cup	56	204	8	42	2	1		
38356	Fettuccine pasta, frozen/Kraft	70 g	70	200	8	38	2	2		
91293	Fettuccine pasta, spinach, enriched, dry	1.33 cup	56	202	8	40	2	1	0.1	0.6
38102	Macaroni pasta, enriched, cooked	1 cup	140	221	8	43	3	1	0.2	0.4
38110	Macaroni pasta, whole wheat, cooked	1 cup	140	174	7	37	4	1	0.1	0.3
66121	Pasta shells, small, wheat free, low protein, dry	2 oz	56.7	194	0	48	0	0		
92830	Penne pasta, dry	0.25 ea	57	210	7	41	1	1		
38067	Ramen noodles, cooked	0.5 cup	113.5	77	2	10	1	3	0.6	1.7

Sat (g)	Chol (mg)	Calc (mg)	Iron (mg)	Mag (mg)	Phos (mg)	Pota (mg)	Sodi (mg)	Zinc (mg)	Vit A (RAE)	Vit C (mg)	Thia (mg)	Ribo (mg)	Niac (mg)	Vit B$_6$ (mg)	Vit B$_{12}$ (µg)	Vit E (mg)	Fol (µg)	Alc (g)
0.6	18	21	1.23	8.8	35	36	191	0.4	2	0	0.18	0.18	1.15	0.02	0.08	0.1	64.4	0
0.8	15	26	1.27	8.2	54	65	178	0.3	37	0.1	0.17	0.18	1.48	0.03	0.06	0.4	38.7	0
0.4	0	35	1.03	7.6	32	43	231	0.3	0	0	0.2	0.11	1.65	0.01	0	0.1	42.9	0
0.3	0	54	1.87	15.4	57	62	310	0.5	0	0	0.27	0.19	2.42	0.02	0	0.2	54.2	0
0.1	0	46	0.36	16.9	82	40	3	0.2	0	0	0.03	0.02	0.39	0.06	0	0	29.6	0
0.2	0	5	0.09	4.2	11	11	19	0.1	0	0	0.01	0	0.09	0.01	0	0	3.4	0
5.8	8	94	2.96	22.3	135	90	617	0.7	18	0	0.35	0.27	2.9	0.34	0.29	0	94.2	0
0	0	3	0.24	7.8	27	32	26	0.2	0	0	0.02	0.01	0.1	0.02	0	0.1	4.7	0
3.2	4	50	1.57	11.9	72	35	151	0.4	6	0	0.19	0.14	1.54	0.18	0.15	0.1	29.4	0
0.1	0	7	1.32	38.1	87	90	1	0.7	0	0	0.1	0.08	1.54	0.05	0		9.9	0
0.1	0	28	1.11	17.7	59	61	249	0.6	0	0	0.12	0.08	1.23	0.03	0	0.1	37.2	0
0.1	0	23	1.1	11.7	55	58	270	0.4	0	0	0.14	0.09	1.42	0.03	0	0.2	25.5	0
0.7	0	31	2.54	9.9	45	69	482	0.4	0	0	0.04	0.2	2.36	0.04	0	0.4	62.6	0
1.3	0	54	2.43	12.2	47	326	286	0.3	0	0	0.25	0.21	2.36	0.02	0	0.1	55.8	0
0.6	0	24	0.65	3.2	48	15	124	0.2	0	0	0.04	0.05	0.61	0.01	0		9.6	0
0.4	23	8	0.82	10.8	46	74	76	0.3	4	0	0.12	0.12	1.39	0.01	0.05	0.2	26.1	0
0	0	0	0.67				177		0	0								0
0.1	0	7	2.32	7.8	34	34	191	0.3	0	0	0.16	0.18	1.71	0.03	0	0	37.2	0
1.7	1	72	0.67	10.1	114	120	392	0.2	5	0	0.12	0.19	1.05	0.01	0.03	0.1	28	0
1.2	0	14	0.76	15.7	75	61	199	0.3	0	0	0.15	0.08	1.63	0.04	0.08	0.7	26.3	0
1.4	0	23	0.78	15.4	77	60	201	0.3	0	0	0.14	0.08	1.71	0.04	0	0.6	24.1	0
		22	0.59	6.9	50	28	150	0.3	0	0	0.04	0.06				0		0
0.9	0	19	1.01				262		0	0								0
1.1	0	16	0.99	31.7	94	95	211	0.7	0	0	0.06	0.03	1.45	0.06	0	0.3	9	0
1	0	14	0.86	27.7	83	83	69	0.6	0	0	0.06	0.03	1.27	0.05	0	0.2	7.8	0
0.2	0	129	1.99	27.1	53	103	275	0.9	0	0	0.28	0.21	2.36	0.03	0	0	52.8	0
0.2		103	0.8				197		0	0.1					0.21	1	22.8	0
0.4	0	93	2.28	13.7	52	62	242	0.6	0	1	0.27	0.14	2.32	0.03	0.02	0.2	53.6	0
0.2	0	101	1.64	21.1	61	106	218	0.6	0	0	0.25	0.17	1.91	0.05	0	0.3	36.5	0
0.4	4	4	0.22	1.1	14	11	35	0.1	1	0.1	Thia	0.02	0.15	0	0.01	Vit E	5.3	0
0.8	15	42	1.6	18.2	162	39	297	0.3	30	0	0.16	0.19	1.16	0.05	0.05	0.5	45.6	0
0.6	0	36	2.39	89.5	214	289	224	1	0	0	0.15	0.05	0.24	0.09	0.01	0.4	50.7	0
0.5	2	4	0.17	4	19	27	158	0.1	31	0	0.08	0.1	0.67	0.01	0.01	0.3	21.4	0
0.6	4	6	0.49	4.6	50	30	142	0.1	6	0	0.1	0.12	0.76	0.02	0.01	0.5	18.8	0
0.3	0	12	1.61	26.3	90	105	3	0.7	0	0	0.49	0.21	3.34	0.07	0	0.1	111.1	0
0.2	0	10	1.8	30.1	79	81	3	0.6	0	0	0.45	0.25	3				119.8	0
2	0	9	2.13	23.4	72	54	198	0.6	0	0	0.26	0.19	2.68	0.05	0	1.6	40.5	0
0.3	23	10	1.18	16.8	61	30	4	0.5	5	0	0.23	0.11	1.66	0.04	0.07	0.1	67.2	0
0.3	23	10	1.18	16.8	61	30	132	0.5	5	0	0.23	0.11	1.66	0.04	0.07	0.1	67.2	0
0.2	0	10	1.8	30.1	79	81	3	0.6	0	0	0.45	0.25	3				119.8	0
0	0	0	0				140		0	0								0
0.3	1	78	1.8	43.7	117	203	16	0.8	7	0	0.45	0.25	3					0
0.2	0	10	1.79	25.2	81	62	1	0.7	0	0	0.38	0.19	2.36	0.07	0	0.1	102.2	0
0.1	0	21	1.48	42	125	62	4	1.1	0	0	0.15	0.06	0.99	0.11	0	0.4	7	0
0	0	3	0.68			52			0	0.5								0
0	0	0	0.72				0		0	0								0
0.8	0	7	0.2	5.2	12	25	401	0.1	1	0	0.01	0.01	0.13	0.01	0	1.2	1.6	0

MDA Code	Food Name	Amt	Wt (g)	Ener (kcal)	Prot (g)	Carb (g)	Fiber (g)	Fat (g)	Mono (g)	Poly (g)
38551	Rice pasta, cooked	0.5 cup	88	96	1	22	1	0	0	0
38094	Soba noodles, cooked	1 cup	114	113	6	24	1	0	0	0
38118	Spaghetti, enriched, cooked	0.5 cup	70	111	4	22	1	1	0.1	0.2
38066	Spaghetti, spinach, cooked	1 cup	140	182	6	37	5	1	0.1	0.4
38274	Spaghetti, unenriched, cooked w/salt	0.5 cup	70	110	4	21	1	1	0.1	0.2
38060	Spaghetti, whole wheat, cooked	1 cup	140	174	7	37	6	1	0.1	0.3
	Flours									
38071	Arrowroot flour	0.25 cup	32	114	0	28	1	0	0	0
38548	Barley flour	0.25 cup	37	128	4	28	4	1	0.1	0.3
38053	Buckwheat flour, whole groat	0.25 cup	30	100	4	21	3	1	0.3	0.3
38005	Corn flour, masa, white, enriched	0.25 cup	28.5	104	3	22	3	1	0.3	0.5
38054	Semolina flour, enriched	0.25 cup	41.8	150	5	30	2	0	0.1	0.2
7565	Soy flour, full fat, stirred, raw	0.25 cup	21	92	7	7	2	4	1	2.4
38087	Triticale flour, whole grain	0.25 cup	32.5	110	4	24	5	1	0.1	0.3
38033	White flour, all purpose, enriched	0.25 cup	31.2	110	3	23	1	0	0	0.1
38277	White bread flour, enriched	0.25 cup	34.2	123	4	25	1	1	0	0.2
38032	Whole-wheat flour	0.25 cup	30	102	4	22	4	1	0.1	0.2
	Grains									
38003	Barley, pearled, cooked	0.5 cup	78.5	97	2	22	3	0	0	0.2
38028	Bulgur, wheat, cooked	1 cup	182	151	6	34	8	0	0.1	0.2
38252	Corn, white, dry	0.25 cup	41.5	151	4	31		2	0.5	0.9
38279	Corn, yellow, dry	0.25 cup	41.5	151	4	31	3	2	0.5	0.9
38183	Cornmeal, white, degermed, enriched	0.25 cup	34.5	127	3	27	1	1	0.1	0.3
38004	Cornmeal, yellow, degermed, enriched	0.25 cup	34.5	127	3	27	1	1	0.1	0.3
38076	Couscous, cooked	0.5 cup	78.5	88	3	18	1	0	0	0.1
5470	Hominy, yellow, canned	0.5 cup	80	58	1	11	2	1	0.2	0.3
38052	Millet, cooked	0.5 cup	87	104	3	21	1	1	0.2	0.4
38078	Oat bran, cooked	0.5 cup	109.5	44	4	13	3	1	0.3	0.4
38080	Oats, unprocessed whole grain	0.25 cup	39	152	7	26	4	3	0.8	1
38010	Rice, brown, long grain, cooked	1 cup	195	216	5	45	4	2	0.6	0.6
38082	Rice, brown, med grain, cooked	0.5 cup	97.5	109	2	23	2	1	0.3	0.3
38083	Rice, white, glutinous, cooked	1 cup	174	169	4	37	2	0	0.1	0.1
38256	Rice, white, long grain, enriched, cooked w/salt	1 cup	158	205	4	45	1	0	0.1	0.1
38019	Rice, white, long grain, enriched, instant	1 cup	165	193	4	41	1	1	0.1	0
38097	Rice, white, med grain, cooked	0.5 cup	93	121	2	27	0	0	0.1	0.1
38085	Sorghum, whole grain	0.5 cup	96	325	11	72	6	3	1	1.3
38034	Tapioca, pearl, dry	0.25 cup	38	136	0	34	0	0	0	0
38025	Wheat, germ, crude	0.25 cup	28.8	104	7	15	4	3	0.4	1.7
38068	Wheat, sprouted	0.25 cup	27	53	2	11	0	0	0	0.2
	Pancakes, French Toast, and Waffles									
42155	French toast, frozen	1 pce	59	126	4	19	1	4	1.2	0.7
42156	French toast, homemade w/2% milk	1 pce	65	149	5	16	1	7	2.9	1.7
45192	Pancakes, buttermilk, frozen/Eggo	1 ea	42.5	99	3	16	0	3	1.2	0.9
45118	Pancakes, blueberry, homemade, 6"	1 ea	77	171	5	22	1	7	1.8	3.2
45121	Pancakes, buttermilk, homemade, 6"	1 ea	77	175	5	22	1	7	1.8	3.5
45117	Pancakes, plain, homemade, 6"	1 ea	77	175	5	22	1	7	1.9	3.4
45199	Pancakes, buttermilk, frozen, 4"	1 ea	36	81	2	14	1	2	0.7	0.4
45193	Waffles, homestyle, low fat, frozen/Eggo	1 ea	35	83	2	15	0	1	0.4	0.4
45003	Waffles, plain, homemade, round, 7"	1 ea	75	218	6	25	1	11	2.6	5.1
45197	Waffles, buttermilk, frozen, 4"	1 ea	35	100	2	15	1	3	1.8	0.8

Sat (g)	Chol (mg)	Calc (mg)	Iron (mg)	Mag (mg)	Phos (mg)	Pota (mg)	Sodi (mg)	Zinc (mg)	Vit A (RAE)	Vit C (mg)	Thia (mg)	Ribo (mg)	Niac (mg)	Vit B$_6$ (mg)	Vit B$_{12}$ (µg)	Vit E (mg)	Fol (µg)	Alc (g)
0	0	4	0.12	2.6	18	4	17	0.2	0	0	0.02	0	0.06	0.01	0		2.6	0
0	0	5	0.55	10.3	28	40	68	0.1	0	0	0.11	0.03	0.58	0.05	0		8	0
0.1	0	5	0.9	12.6	41	31	1	0.4	0	0	0.19	0.1	1.18	0.03	0	0	51.1	0
0.1	0	42	1.46	86.8	151	81	20	1.5	11	0	0.14	0.14	2.14	0.13	0	0	16.8	0
0.1	0	5	0.35	12.6	41	31	92	0.4	0	0	0.01	0.01	0.28	0.03	0	0	4.9	0
0.1	0	21	1.48	42	125	62	4	1.1	0	0	0.15	0.06	0.99	0.11	0	0.4	7	0
0	0	13	0.11	1	2	4	1	0	0	0	0	0	0	0	0		2.2	0
0.1	0	12	0.99	35.5	110	114	1	0.7	0	0	0.14	0.04	2.32	0.15	0	0.2	3	0
0.2	0	12	1.22	75.3	101	173	3	0.9	0	0	0.13	0.06	1.85	0.17	0	0.1	16.2	0
0.2	0	40	2.05	31.4	64	85	1	0.5	0	0	0.41	0.21	2.81	0.11	0	0	66.4	0
0.1	0	7	1.82	19.6	57	78	0	0.4	0	0	0.34	0.24	2.5	0.04	0	0.1	76.5	0
0.6	0	43	1.34	90.1	104	528	3	0.8	1	0	0.12	0.24	0.91	0.1	0	0.4	72.4	0
0.1	0	11	0.84	49.7	104	151	1	0.9	0	0	0.12	0.04	0.93	0.13	0	0.3	24	0
0	0	105	1.46	5.9	186	39	396	0.2	0	0	0.21	0.13	1.82	0.02	0	0	61.2	0
0.1	0	5	1.51	8.6	33	34	1	0.3	0	0	0.28	0.18	2.58	0.01	0	0.1	62.6	0
0.1	0	10	1.16	41.4	104	122	2	0.9	0	0	0.13	0.06	1.91	0.1	0	0.2	13.2	0
0.1	0	9	1.04	17.3	42	73	2	0.6	0	0	0.07	0.05	1.62	0.09	0	0	12.6	0
0.1	0	18	1.75	58.2	73	124	9	1	0	0	0.1	0.05	1.82	0.15	0	0	32.8	0
0.3	0	3	1.12	52.7	87	119	15	0.9	0	0	0.16	0.08	1.51	0.26	0	0.2		0
0.3	0	3	1.12	52.7	87	119	15	0.9	5	0	0.16	0.08	1.51	0.26	0	0.2	7.9	0
0.1	0	1	1.49	12.1	36	52	2	0.2	0	0	0.21	0.14	1.83	0.07	0	0.1	74.2	0
0.1	0	1	1.49	12.1	36	52	2	0.2	4	0	0.21	0.14	1.83	0.07	0	0.1	74.2	0
0	0	6	0.3	6.3	17	46	4	0.2	0	0	0.05	0.02	0.77	0.04	0	0.1	11.8	0
0.1	0	8	0.5	12.8	28	7	168	0.8	5	0	0	0	0.03	0	0	0.1	0.8	0
0.1	0	3	0.55	38.3	87	54	2	0.8	0	0	0.09	0.07	1.16	0.09	0	0	16.5	0
0.2	0	11	0.96	43.8	130	101	1	0.6	0	0	0.18	0.04	0.16	0.03	0	0.1	6.6	0
0.5	0	21	1.84	69	204	167	1	1.5	0	0	0.3	0.05	0.37	0.05	0	0.3	21.8	0
0.4	0	20	0.82	83.8	162	84	10	1.2	0	0	0.19	0.05	2.98	0.28	0	0.1	7.8	0
0.2	0	10	0.52	42.9	75	77	1	0.6	0	0	0.1	0.01	1.3	0.15	0	0.2	3.9	0
0.1	0	3	0.24	8.7	14	17	9	0.7	0	0	0.03	0.02	0.5	0.05	0	0.1	1.7	0
0.1	0	16	1.9	19	68	55	604	0.8	0	0	0.26	0.02	2.33	0.15	0	0.1	91.6	0
0	0	13	2.92	8.2	61	15	7	0.8	0	0	0.12	0.01	2.87	0.08	0	0	115.5	0
0.1	0	3	1.39	12.1	34	27	0	0.4	0	0	0.16	0.01	1.71	0.05	0	0	53.9	0
0.4	0	27	4.22		276	336	6		0	0	0.23	0.14	2.81		0	0.1		0
0	0	8	0.6	0.4	3	4	0	0	0	0	0	0	0	0	0	0	1.5	0
0.5	0	11	1.8	68.8	242	257	3	3.5	0	0	0.54	0.14	1.96	0.37	0	4	80.9	0
0.1	0	8	0.58	22.1	54	46	4	0.4	0	0.7	0.06	0.04	0.83	0.07	0	0	10.3	0
0.9	48	63	1.3	10	82	79	292	0.5	32	0.2	0.16	0.22	1.61	0.29	0.99	0.4	30.7	0
1.8	75	65	1.09	11	76	87	311	0.4	81	0.2	0.13	0.21	1.06	0.05	0.2	0.7	28	0
0.6	5	15	1.32	7.6	145	44	225	0.3		0.6	0.11	0.12	1.47	0.15	0.44	0	22.1	0
1.5	43	159	1.32	12.3	116	106	317	0.4	38	1.7	0.15	0.21	1.17	0.04	0.15		27.7	0
1.4	45	121	1.31	11.6	107	112	402	0.5	23	0.3	0.16	0.22	1.21	0.03	0.14	1.1	29.3	0
1.6	45	169	1.39	12.3	122	102	338	0.4	42	0.2	0.15	0.22	1.21	0.04	0.17	0.7	29.3	0
0.3	6	26	0.79	5	105	45	182	0.1	23	0.1	0.12	0.18	1.05	0.05	0.03	0.1	25.6	0
0.3	9	20	1.95	23.8	28	50	155		0		0.31	0.26	2.59	0.16	0.55		27	0
2.1	52	191	1.73	14.2	142	119	383	0.5	49	0.3	0.2	0.26	1.55	0.04	0.19	1.7	34.5	0
0.5	5	108	1.96	8	126	44	223	0.2	133	0	0.22	0.22	2.65	0.31	1.03	0.4	23.8	

MEAT AND MEAT SUBSTITUTES

Beef

MDA Code	Food Name	Amt	Wt (g)	Ener (kcal)	Prot (g)	Carb (g)	Fiber (g)	Fat (g)	Mono (g)	Poly (g)
10093	Beef, average of all cuts, cooked, 1/4" trim	3 oz	85.1	260	22	0	0	18	7.8	0.7
10705	Beef, average of all cuts, lean, cooked, 1/4" trim	3 oz	85.1	184	25	0	0	8	3.5	0.3
10108	Beef, brisket, whole, braised, 1/4" trim	3 oz	85.1	328	20	0	0	27	11.8	1
10035	Beef, breakfast strips, cured, cooked	3 ea	34	153	11	0	0	12	5.7	0.5
58239	Beef, brisket, flat half, braised, select, 1/8" trim	3 oz	85.1	238	25	0	0	15	6.4	0.5
58051	Beef, chuck clod roast, roasted, 1/4" trim	3 oz	85.1	206	21	0	0	13	6	0.5
58104	Beef, chuck clod steak, braised, 1/4" trim	3 oz	85.1	231	22	0	0	15	6.8	0.6
58099	Beef, chuck tender steak, broiled, 0" trim	3 oz	85.1	136	22	0	0	5	2.3	0.3
58083	Beef, chuck top blade, broiled, choice, 0" trim	3 oz	85.1	193	22	0	0	11	5.3	0.4
10264	Beef, cured, thin sliced	5 pce	21	37	6	1	0	1	0.4	0
10009	Beef, cured, dried, slices	5 pce	21	32	7	1	0	0	0.2	0
10034	Beef, kidney, cooked	3 oz	85.1	134	23	0	0	4	0.6	0.7
10010	Beef, liver, fried	3 oz	85.1	149	23	4	0	4	0.6	0.5
10624	Beef, short ribs, braised, choice, 1/4" trim	3 oz	85.1	401	18	0	0	36	16.1	1.3
10011	Beef, tongue, cooked	3 oz	85.1	242	16	0	0	19	8.6	0.6
10018	Beef, tripe, raw	4 oz	113.4	96	14	0	0	4	1.7	0.2
10133	Beef, whole rib, roasted, 1/4" trim	3 oz	85.1	305	19	0	0	25	10.6	0.9
10008	Corned beef, cured, canned, slices	3 oz	85.1	213	23	0	0	13	5.1	0.5
57710	Corned beef hash, canned/Hormel	1 cup	236	387	21	22	3	24	12.4	0.7
93273	Corned beef hash, canned	3 oz	85.1	140	7	8	1	9	4.5	0.3
58129	Ground beef, hamburger, pan browned, 25% fat	3 oz	85.1	236	22	0	0	15	7.1	0.4
58124	Ground beef, hamburger, pan browned, 20% fat	3 oz	85.1	231	23	0	0	15	6.5	0.4
58119	Ground beef, hamburger, pan browned, 15% fat	3 oz	85.1	218	24	0	0	13	5.6	0.4
58114	Ground beef, hamburger, pan browned, 10% fat	3 oz	85.1	196	24	0	0	10	4.3	0.4
58109	Ground beef, hamburger, pan browned, 5% fat	3 oz	85.1	164	25	0	0	6	2.7	0.3
10791	Porterhouse steak, broiled, 1/4" trim	3 oz	85.1	280	19	0	0	22	9.8	0.9
11487	Porterhouse steak, broiled, 1/8" trim	3 oz	85.1	253	20	0	0	19	8.2	0.7
58257	Rib eye steak, broiled, 0" trim	3 oz	85.1	210	23	0	0	13	5.1	0.5
58324	Rib steak, lean, broiled, choice, 1/8" trim	3 oz	85.1	172	24	0	0	8	3.1	0.3
57709	Roast beef hash, canned/Hormel	1 cup	236	385	21	23	4	24	11.3	0.6
58094	Skirt steak, broiled, 0" trim	3 oz	85.1	187	22	0	0	10	5.2	0.4
58069	Skirt steak, outside, lean, broiled, 0" trim	3 oz	85.1	198	21	0	0	12	6.3	0.5
58328	Strip steak, top loin, lean, broiled, choice, 1/8" trim	3 oz	85.1	171	25	0	0	7	2.9	0.3
10805	T-bone steak, broiled, 1/4" trim	3 oz	85.1	260	20	0	0	19	8.6	0.7
11491	T-bone steak, broiled, 1/8" trim	3 oz	85.1	238	21	0	0	17	7.3	0.6
58299	Top round steak, lean, broiled, select, 1/8" trim	3 oz	85.1	151	27	0	0	4	1.7	0.2
58098	Tri-tip steak, loin, broiled, 0" trim	3 oz	85.1	226	26	0	0	13	6.6	0.5
58258	Tri-tip roast, sirloin, roasted, 0" trim	3 oz	85.1	177	22	0	0	9	4.7	0.3
11550	Veal tongue, braised	3 oz	85.1	172	22	0	0	9	3.9	0.3
11531	Veal, average of all cuts, cooked	3 oz	85.1	197	26	0	0	10	3.7	0.7
11530	Veal, ground, broiled, 8% fat	3 oz	85.1	146	21	0	0	6	2.4	0.5

Chicken

MDA Code	Food Name	Amt	Wt (g)	Ener (kcal)	Prot (g)	Carb (g)	Fiber (g)	Fat (g)	Mono (g)	Poly (g)
81185	Chicken, breast, mesquite flavor, fat free, sliced	2 pce	42	34	7	1	0	0	0.1	0
81186	Chicken, breast, oven roasted, fat free, sliced	2 pce	42	33	7	1	0	0	0.1	0
15013	Chicken breast, w/skin, batter fried	3 oz	85.1	221	21	8	0	11	4.6	2.6
15057	Chicken breast, w/o skin, fried	3 oz	85.1	159	28	0	0	4	1.5	0.9
15113	Chicken, dark meat, w/skin, batter fried	3 oz	85.1	254	19	8	0	16	6.5	3.8
15080	Chicken, dark meat, w/skin, roasted	3 oz	85.1	215	22	0	0	13	5.3	3

Sat (g)	Chol (mg)	Calc (mg)	Iron (mg)	Mag (mg)	Phos (mg)	Pota (mg)	Sodi (mg)	Zinc (mg)	Vit A (RAE)	Vit C (mg)	Thia (mg)	Ribo (mg)	Niac (mg)	Vit B$_6$ (mg)	Vit B$_{12}$ (µg)	Vit E (mg)	Fol (µg)	Alc (g)
7.3	75	9	2.23	18.7	173	266	53	5	0	0	0.07	0.18	3.1	0.28	2.08	0.2	6	0
3.2	73	8	2.54	22.1	198	306	57	5.9	0	0	0.09	0.2	3.51	0.31	2.25	0.1	6.8	0
10.5	80	7	1.91	15.3	159	197	52	4.3	0	0	0.05	0.15	2.55	0.2	1.94	0.2	5.1	0
4.9	40	3	1.07	9.2	80	140	766	2.2	0	0	0.03	0.09	2.2	0.11	1.17	0.1	2.7	0
5.9	60	14	2.04	16.2	153	202	42	5.9	0	0	0.05	0.13	3.55	0.24	1.63	0.4	7.7	0
4.9	64	7	2.39	17	167	287	57	4.9	0	0	0.07	0.19	2.73	0.22	2.41	0.1	7.7	0
5.7	80	8	2.83	16.2	176	220	49	5.8	0	0	0.06	0.19	2.43	0.21	2.33	0.1	6.8	0
1.6	54	7	2.49	19.6	193	249	60	6.7	0	0	0.09	0.2	3.09	0.27	2.88	0.1	6.8	0
3.5	49	6	2.36	20.4	183	255	58	7.5	0	0	0.09	0.19	3.08	0.27	2.88	0.2	6.8	0
0.3	9	2	0.57	4	35	90	302	0.8	0	0	0.02	0.04	1.11	0.07	0.54	0	2.3	0
0.2	17	1	0.61	4.6	41	61	586	0.8	0	0	0.01	0.05	0.69	0.05	0.5	0	1.7	0
0.9	609	16	4.94	10.2	259	115	80	2.4	0	0	0.14	2.53	3.34	0.33	21.19	0.1	70.6	0
1.3	324	5	5.25	18.7	413	299	66	4.5	6590	0.6	0.15	2.91	14.87	0.87	70.74	0.4	221.3	0
15.1	80	10	1.97	12.8	138	191	43	4.2	0	0	0.04	0.13	2.09	0.19	2.23	0.2	4.3	0
6.9	112	4	2.22	12.8	123	157	55	3.5	0	1.1	0.02	0.25	2.97	0.13	2.66	0.3	6	0
1.5	138	78	0.67	14.7	73	76	110	1.6	0	0	0	0.07	1	0.02	1.58	0.1	5.7	0
10	71	9	1.99	17	149	256	54	4.6	0	0	0.06	0.14	2.9	0.2	2.16	0.2	6	0
5.3	73	10	1.77	11.9	94	116	856	3	0	0	0.02	0.13	2.07	0.11	1.38	0.1	7.7	0
10.2	76	45	2.36	30.7		406	1003	3.3	0	2.1								0
3.7	27	16	0.85	11.1	48	146	362	1.2	0	0.8	0.06	0.04	1.34	0.2	0.35	0	6	0
6	76	29	2.24	18.7	182	301	79	5.3	0	0	0.04	0.16	4.55	0.37	2.5	0.4	10.2	0
5.6	76	24	2.37	19.6	192	323	77	5.4	0	0	0.04	0.16	4.96	0.36	2.43	0.4	9.4	0
5	77	19	2.49	21.3	203	346	76	5.6	0	0	0.04	0.16	5.38	0.36	2.37	0.4	8.5	0
4	76	14	2.62	23	213	368	74	5.8	0	0	0.04	0.16	5.79	0.36	2.31	0.4	6.8	0
2.9	76	8	2.75	23.8	224	391	72	6	0	0	0.04	0.17	6.2	0.36	2.25	0.3	6	0
8.7	61	7	2.28	17	151	217	53	3.5	0	0	0.08	0.18	3.28	0.28	1.8	0.2	6	0
7.2	60	7	2.33	19.6	159	273	54	3.9	0	0	0.09	0.19	3.46	0.3	1.83	0.2	6	0
4.9	94	17	1.49	19.6	180	289	48	4.2	0	0	0.06	0.11	6.18	0.49	1.36	0.4	6.8	0
2.9	72	14	1.63	20.4	186	300	49	4.5	0	0	0.06	0.12	7.1	0.5	1.51	0.4	7.7	0
9.9	73	42	2.36	33		432	793	3.3	0	1.9								0
4	51	9	2.36	20.4	196	246	64	6.2	0	0	0.08	0.16	3.19	0.27	3.17	0.1	6	0
5.1	49	9	2.26	21.3	188	334	80	4.9	0	0	0.1	0.17	3.69	0.42	3.66	0.1	6.8	0
2.7	67	14	1.68	21.3	192	308	51	4.7	0	0	0.07	0.13	7.32	0.52	1.55	0.3	8.5	0
7.6	55	6	2.63	18.7	157	240	57	3.7	0	0	0.08	0.18	3.37	0.29	1.81	0.2	6	0
6.4	53	7	2.41	20.4	164	286	56	4	0	0	0.09	0.19	3.52	0.3	1.85	0.2	6	0
1.4	52	6	2.26	18.7	176	230	37	4.7	0	0	0.06	0.15	4.63	0.35	1.38	0.3	9.4	0
4.9	58	10	3.1	22.1	226	372	61	6	0	0	0.11	0.24	3.6	0.38	2.41	0.1	8.5	0
3.5	71	16	1.41	18.7	171	275	45	4	0	0	0.06	0.11	5.9	0.46	1.3	0.3	6.8	0
3.7	203	8	1.78	15.3	141	138	54	3.8	0	5.1	0.06	0.3	1.25	0.13	4.51	2.1	7.7	0
3.6	97	19	0.98	22.1	203	277	74	4.1	0	0	0.05	0.27	6.78	0.26	1.34	0.3	12.8	0
2.6	88	14	0.84	20.4	185	287	71	3.3	0	0	0.06	0.23	6.83	0.33	1.08	0.1	9.4	0
0.1	15	2	0.13	15.1	108	133	437	0.3	0	0	0.01	0.01	1.15	0.05	0.03	0	0.4	0
0.1	15	3	0.13	3.8	25	28	457	0.1	0	0	0.01	0.01	1.44	0.06	0.04	0	0.4	0
3	72	17	1.06	20.4	157	171	234	0.8	17	0	0.1	0.12	8.96	0.37	0.26	0.9	12.8	0
1.1	77	14	0.97	26.4	209	235	67	0.9	6	0	0.07	0.11	12.58	0.54	0.31	0.4	3.4	0
4.2	76	18	1.23	17	123	157	251	1.8	26	0	0.1	0.19	4.77	0.21	0.23	1	15.3	0
3.7	77	13	1.16	18.7	143	187	74	2.1	51	0	0.06	0.18	5.41	0.26	0.25	0.5	6	0

MDA Code	Food Name	Amt	Wt (g)	Ener (kcal)	Prot (g)	Carb (g)	Fiber (g)	Fat (g)	Mono (g)	Poly (g)
15026	Chicken, dark meat, w/o skin, fried	3 oz	85.1	203	25	2	0	10	3.7	2.4
15030	Chicken drumstick, w/skin, batter fried	3 oz	85.1	228	19	7	0	13	5.5	3.2
15042	Chicken drumstick, w/o skin, fried	3 oz	85.1	166	24	0	0	7	2.5	1.7
58216	Chicken feet, cooked	1 oz	28.4	61	6	0	0	4	1.6	0.8
15105	Chicken giblets, chopped, fried	1 cup	145	402	47	6	0	20	6.4	4.9
15106	Chicken giblets, chopped, simmered	1 cup	145	229	39	1	0	7	1.4	1.2
15025	Chicken gizzard, average, chopped, simmered	3 oz	85.1	124	26	0	0	2	0.4	0.3
15151	Chicken leg, w/skin, batter fried	3 oz	85.1	232	19	7	0	14	5.6	3.3
81432	Chicken leg, skinless, fried	1 ea	94	196	27	1	0	9	3.2	2.1
15111	Chicken, light meat, w/skin, batter fried	3 oz	85.1	236	20	8	0	13	5.4	3.1
15077	Chicken, light meat, w/skin, roasted	3 oz	85.1	189	25	0	0	9	3.6	2
15031	Chicken, light meat, w/o skin, fried	3 oz	85.1	163	28	0	0	5	1.7	1.1
15072	Chicken, whole, w/skin, batter fried	3 oz	85.1	246	19	8	0	15	6	3.5
15214	Chicken, whole, w/o skin, fried	3 oz	85.1	186	26	1	0	8	2.9	1.8
15000	Chicken, whole, w/o skin, roasted	3 oz	85.1	162	25	0	0	6	2.3	1.4
15036	Chicken thigh, w/skin, batter fried	3 oz	85.1	236	18	8	0	14	5.7	3.3
15011	Chicken thigh, w/o skin, fried	3 oz	85.1	186	24	1	0	9	3.3	2.1
15095	Chicken, whole, w/giblet & neck, batter fried	3 oz	85.1	248	19	8	0	15	6.1	3.5
15094	Chicken, whole, w/giblet & neck, raw	4 oz	113.4	242	21	0	0	17	6.9	3.6
15097	Chicken, whole, w/giblet & neck, roasted	3 oz	85.1	199	23	0	0	11	4.4	2.5
15034	Chicken wing, w/skin, batter fried	3 oz	85.1	276	17	9	0	19	7.6	4.3
15048	Chicken wing, w/o skin, fried	3 oz	85.1	180	26	0	0	8	2.6	1.8
15059	Chicken wing, w/o skin, roasted	3 oz	85.1	173	26	0	0	7	2.2	1.5
	Turkey									
13125	Turkey bacon	1 oz	28.4	71	4	0	0	6	2.1	1.3
51151	Turkey bacon, cooked	1 oz	28.4	108	8	1	0	8	3.1	1.9
16073	Turkey giblets, simmered	1 cup	145	289	30	1	0	17	7.2	1.8
51098	Turkey, thick slice, breaded & batter fried, 3" × 2" × 3/8"	1 ea	42	119	6	7	0	8	3.1	2
16308	Turkey, roast, light & dark meat, seasoned, from frozen	1 cup	135	209	29	4	0	8	1.6	2.2
16110	Turkey breast, w/skin, roasted	3 oz	85.1	130	25	0	0	3	1	0.6
16038	Turkey breast, w/o skin, roasted	3 oz	85.1	115	26	0	0	1	0.1	0.2
16101	Turkey, dark meat, w/skin, roasted	3 oz	85.1	155	24	0	0	6	1.9	1.6
16099	Turkey, light meat, w/skin, roasted	3 oz	85.1	140	24	0	0	4	1.4	0.9
16003	Turkey, ground patty, 13% fat, cooked, 4 oz raw	1 ea	82	193	22	0	0	11	4	2.6
	Lamb									
40422	Lamb, Australian, loin, lean, broiled, 1/8" trim	3 oz	85.1	163	23	0	0	7	3	0.3
13604	Lamb, average of all cuts, cooked, choice, 1/4" trim	3 oz	85.1	250	21	0	0	18	7.5	1.3
13616	Lamb, average of all cuts, lean, cooked, choice, 1/4" trim	3 oz	85.1	175	24	0	0	8	3.5	0.5
13669	Lamb, ground, cooked	3 oz	85.1	241	21	0	0	17	7.1	1.2
13522	Lamb, kabob meat, lean, broiled, 1/4" trim	3 oz	85.1	158	24	0	0	6	2.5	0.6
	Pork									
12000	Bacon, broiled/pan fried/roasted, medium slice	3 pce	19	103	7	0	0	8	3.5	0.9
28143	Canadian bacon/Hormel	1 ea	56	68	9	1		3	1.4	0.3
12212	Ham, cured, extra lean, 5% fat, roasted	1 cup	140	203	29	2	0	8	3.7	0.8
12211	Ham, cured, 11% fat, roasted	1 cup	140	249	32	0	0	13	6.2	2
12309	Pork, average of retail cuts, cooked	3 oz	85.1	232	23	0	0	15	6.5	1.2
12097	Pork, ribs, backribs, roasted	3 oz	85.1	315	21	0	0	25	11.5	2
58237	Pork, stomach, cooked	3 oz	85.1	134	18	0	0	6	1.8	0.6
12099	Pork, ground, cooked	3 oz	85.1	253	22	0	0	18	7.9	1.6
12178	Pork, pigs feet, simmered	3 oz	85.1	197	19	0	0	14	6.8	1.3

Sat (g)	Chol (mg)	Calc (mg)	Iron (mg)	Mag (mg)	Phos (mg)	Pota (mg)	Sodi (mg)	Zinc (mg)	Vit A (RAE)	Vit C (mg)	Thia (mg)	Ribo (mg)	Niac (mg)	Vit B$_6$ (mg)	Vit B$_{12}$ (µg)	Vit E (mg)	Fol (µg)	Alc (g)
2.7	82	15	1.27	21.3	159	215	83	2.5	20	0	0.08	0.21	6.02	0.31	0.28	0.5	7.7	0
3.5	73	14	1.15	17	125	158	229	2	22	0	0.1	0.18	4.34	0.23	0.24	1	15.3	0
1.8	80	10	1.12	20.4	158	212	82	2.7	15	0	0.07	0.2	5.23	0.33	0.3	0.4	7.7	0
1.1	24	25	0.26	1.4	24	9	19	0.2	9	0	0.02	0.06	0.11	0	0.13	0.1	24.4	0
5.5	647	26	14.96	36.2	415	478	164	9.1	5194	12.6	0.14	2.21	15.93	0.88	19.3	3.6	549.6	0
1.9	641	20	10.21	20.3	419	325	97	6.1	2542	18.1	0.21	1.53	9.61	0.58	13.69	0.7	372.6	0
0.6	315	14	2.71	2.6	161	152	48	3.8	0	0	0.02	0.18	2.66	0.06	0.89	0.2	4.3	0
3.6	77	15	1.19	17	129	161	237	1.8	23	0	0.1	0.19	4.62	0.23	0.24	1	15.3	0
2.3	93	12	1.32	23.5	181	239	90	2.8	19	0	0.08	0.23	6.29	0.37	0.32		8.5	0
3.5	71	17	1.07	18.7	143	157	244	0.9	20	0	0.1	0.13	7.79	0.33	0.24	0.9	13.6	0
2.6	71	13	0.97	21.3	170	193	64	1	28	0	0.05	0.1	9.48	0.44	0.27	0.3	2.6	0
1.3	77	14	0.97	24.7	197	224	69	1.1	8	0	0.06	0.11	11.37	0.54	0.31	0.3	3.4	0
3.9	74	18	1.17	17.9	132	157	248	1.4	24	0	0.1	0.16	5.99	0.26	0.24	1.1	15.3	0
2.1	80	14	1.15	23	174	219	77	1.9	15	0	0.07	0.17	8.22	0.41	0.29	0.4	6	0
1.7	76	13	1.03	21.3	166	207	73	1.8	14	0	0.06	0.15	7.81	0.4	0.28	0.2	5.1	0
3.8	79	15	1.23	17.9	132	163	245	1.7	25	0	0.1	0.19	4.86	0.22	0.24	1	16.2	0
2.4	87	11	1.24	22.1	169	220	81	2.4	18	0	0.07	0.22	6.06	0.32	0.28	0.5	7.7	0
4	88	18	1.52	17.9	134	162	242	1.6	154	0.3	0.1	0.21	6.03	0.27	0.71	1.1	27.2	0
4.8	102	12	1.49	22.7	169	214	79	1.7	263	2.9	0.07	0.21	7.53	0.39	1.26	0.4	34	0
3.1	91	13	1.41	19.6	155	180	67	1.8	163	0.4	0.05	0.19	6.73	0.32	0.8	0.3	24.7	0
5	67	17	1.1	13.6	103	117	272	1.2	29	0	0.09	0.13	4.48	0.26	0.21	0.9	15.3	0
2.1	71	13	0.97	17.9	140	177	77	1.8	15	0	0.04	0.11	6.16	0.5	0.29	0.3	3.4	0
1.9	72	14	0.99	17.9	141	179	78	1.8	15	0	0.04	0.11	6.22	0.5	0.29	0.2	3.4	0
1.5	26	11	0.41	5.4	57	59	344	0.7	0	0							2.3	0
2.4	28	3	0.6	8.2	131	112	649	0.9	0	0	0.02	0.07	1	0.09	0.1	0.3	2.6	0
5.7	419	9	11.18	26.1	335	392	93	4.5	15569	19.9	0.04	2.18	10.15	0.84	48.21	0.1	485.8	0
2	32	6	0.92	6.3	113	116	336	0.6	4	0	0.04	0.08	0.97	0.08	0.1	0.4	17.2	0
2.6	72	7	2.2	29.7	329	402	918	3.4	0	0	0.06	0.22	8.47	0.36	2.05	0.5	6.8	0
0.7	77	13	1.34	23.8	184	237	45	1.5	0	0	0.03	0.11	5.92	0.43	0.31	0.2	5.1	0
0.2	71	10	1.3	24.7	191	248	44	1.5	0	0	0.04	0.11	6.38	0.48	0.33	0.1	5.1	0
1.8	100	23	1.98	19.6	162	202	65	3.3	0	0	0.04	0.2	2.85	0.28	0.31	0.7	7.7	0
1.1	81	15	1.37	22.1	174	223	49	1.8	0	0	0.03	0.12	5.34	0.42	0.31	0.1	5.1	0
2.8	84	20	1.58	19.7	161	221	88	2.3	0	0	0.04	0.14	3.95	0.32	0.27	0.3	5.7	0
3.1	69	18	1.86	22.1	187	289	68	3			0.15	0.28	6.94	0.44	1.71			0
7.5	83	14	1.6	19.6	160	264	61	3.8	0	0	0.09	0.21	5.67	0.11	2.17	0.1	15.3	0
2.9	78	13	1.74	22.1	179	293	65	4.5	0	0	0.09	0.24	5.38	0.14	2.22	0.2	19.6	0
6.9	83	19	1.52	20.4	171	288	69	4	0	0	0.09	0.21	5.7	0.12	2.22	0.2	16.2	0
2.2	77	11	1.99	26.4	191	285	65	4.9	0	0	0.09	0.26	5.63	0.12	2.58	0.2	19.6	0
2.6	21	2	0.27	6.3	101	107	439	0.7	2	0	0.08	0.05	2.11	0.07	0.23	0.1	0.4	0
1	27	3	0.5	10.6		156	569	1	0	0.8								0
2.5	74	11	2.07	19.6	274	402	1684	4	0	0	1.06	0.28	5.63	0.56	0.91	0.4	4.2	0
4.4	83	11	1.88	30.8	393	573	2100	3.5	0	0	1.02	0.46	8.61	0.43	0.98	0.4	4.2	0
5.3	77	21	0.94	20.4	197	301	53	2.5	2	0.3	0.66	0.28	4.19	0.34	0.66	0.2	5.1	0
9.4	100	38	1.17	17.9	166	268	86	2.9	3	0.3	0.36	0.17	3.02	0.26	0.54	0.4	2.6	0
2.5	269	13	1.05	12.8	110	72	34	2.5	0	0	0.03	0.16	1.17	0.02	0.41	0.1	2.6	0
6.6	80	19	1.1	20.4	192	308	62	2.7	2	0.6	0.6	0.19	3.58	0.33	0.46	0.2	5.1	0
3.7	91	0	0.83	4.3	70	28	62	0.9	0	0	0.01	0.05	0.5	0.03	0.35	0.1	1.7	0

MDA Code	Food Name	Amt	Wt (g)	Ener (kcal)	Prot (g)	Carb (g)	Fiber (g)	Fat (g)	Mono (g)	Poly (g)
	Game Meats									
51147	Dove, whole, cooked	3 oz	85.1	186	20	0	0	11	4.6	2.3
16063	Duck, liver, raw, domesticated	1 ea	44	60	8	2	0	2	0.3	0.3
40567	Deer loin, lean, 1" thick steak, broiled	3 oz	85.1	128	26	0	0	2	0.3	0.1
14009	Bison, roasted	3 oz	85.1	122	24	0	0	2	0.8	0.2
15240	Cornish game hen, whole, w/skin, roasted	3 oz	85.1	221	19	0	0	15	6.8	3.1
15242	Cornish game hen, whole, w/o skin, roasted	3 oz	85.1	114	20	0	0	3	1.1	0.8
16020	Duck breast, w/o skin, raw, wild	4 oz	113.4	139	23	0	0	5	1.4	0.7
16019	Duck, whole, w/skin, raw, wild	4 oz	113.4	239	20	0	0	17	7.7	2.3
51149	Quail, whole, cooked	3 oz	85.1	199	21	0	0	12	4.2	3
16013	Quail, whole, w/skin, raw	4 oz	113.4	218	22	0	0	14	4.7	3.4
14004	Rabbit, domestic, roasted	3 oz	85.1	168	25	0	0	7	1.8	1.3
51111	Pigeon, whole, w/skin, raw	4 oz	113.4	333	21	0	0	27	11	3.5
	Lunchmeats									
13103	Beef, chopped, smoked & cured, 1 oz slice	1 pce	28.4	38	6	1	0	1	0.5	0.1
13335	Beef, smoked, sliced/Carl Buddig	1 pce	71	99	14	0	0	5		0.2
13000	Beef, thin slice	1 oz	28.4	42	5	0	0	2	0.9	0.1
57871	Beerwurst, pork & beef salami, 2-3/4" × 1/16" slice	1 pce	6	17	1	0	0	1	0.6	0.1
58275	Bologna, beef & pork, low fat, 1" cube	1 ea	14	32	2	0	0	3	1.3	0.2
58280	Bologna, beef, low fat, medium slice	1 ea	28	57	3	1	0	4	1.8	0.1
58212	Bologna, beef, reduced sodium, thin slice	1 pce	14	44	2	0	0	4	1.9	0.1
13157	Chicken breast, oven roasted, deluxe/Louis Rich	1 oz	28.4	29	5	1	0	1	0.2	0.1
90737	Chicken salad, lunchmeat spread, canned/Spreadables	1 ea	118	171	6	12		11	3.5	4.2
13306	Corned beef/Carl Buddig	1 ea	71	101	14	1	0	5		0.2
13264	Ham, slices, regular, 11% fat	1 cup	135	220	22	5	2	12	5.9	1.1
13206	Lunchmeat loaf, old fashioned/Oscar Mayer	1 pce	28	65	4	2	0	5	2.2	0.7
13049	Lunchmeat loaf, olive, w/pork, 4" × 4" × 3/32" slice	1 pce	28.4	67	3	3	0	5	2.2	0.5
13337	Pastrami, beef, smoked/Carl Buddig	1 oz	28.4	40	6	0	0	2		0.1
13101	Pastrami, beef, cured, 1 oz slice	1 oz	28.4	41	6	0	0	2	0.6	0.1
13020	Pastrami, turkey, slices	2 pce	56.7	70	9	2	0	2	0.8	0.6
13215	Salami, cotto, beef, slice/Oscar Mayer	1 oz	28.4	59	4	1	0	4	2	0.2
11913	Spam, pork & ham, canned/Spam	1 ea	56.7	176	8	2	0	15	7.8	1.7
13123	Turkey bologna/Louis Rich	1 oz	28.4	52	3	1	0	4	1.5	1
16160	Turkey breast slice, 3-1/2" slice	1 pce	21	22	4	1	0	0	0.1	0.1
57889	Turkey ham, cured thigh meat, 8 oz package	1 ea	227	286	40	5	0	11	4.3	3
58279	Turkey ham, extra lean, package	1 cup	138	163	27	2	0	5	1.2	1.6
13144	Turkey salami/Louis Rich	1 ea	28	41	4	0	0	3	0.9	0.7
	Sausage									
58009	Bacon & beef sticks	2 oz	56.7	293	16	0	0	25	12.4	2.4
58230	Beef sausage, cooked from fresh	2 oz	56.7	188	10	0	0	16	7.2	0.5
58228	Beef sausage, precooked	2 oz	56.7	230	9	0	0	21	9.3	0.6
13077	Blood sausage, 5" × 4-5/8" × 1/16" slice	1 pce	25	95	4	0	0	9	4	0.9
13079	Bratwurst, pork, cooked	1 ea	85	283	12	2	0	25	12.5	2.2
58012	Bratwurst, pork, beef & turkey, light, smoked	3 oz	85.1	158	12	1	0	12	6.1	0.7
13180	Braunschweiger liver sausage, sliced/Oscar Mayer	1 pce	28	93	4	1	0	8	4.2	1
13070	Chorizo, pork & beef sausage, 4" link	1 ea	60	273	14	1	0	23	11	2.1
13190	Frank, beef, bun length/Oscar Mayer	1 ea	57	185	6	2	0	17	8.3	0.5
13250	Frank, beef, fat free/Oscar Mayer	1 ea	50	39	7	3	0	0	0.1	0
13191	Frank, beef/Oscar Mayer	1 ea	45	147	5	1	0	14	6.6	0.6
13129	Frank, turkey & chicken/Louis Rich	1 ea	45	85	5	2	0	6	2.5	1.4

Sat (g)	Chol (mg)	Calc (mg)	Iron (mg)	Mag (mg)	Phos (mg)	Pota (mg)	Sodi (mg)	Zinc (mg)	Vit A (RAE)	Vit C (mg)	Thia (mg)	Ribo (mg)	Niac (mg)	Vit B$_6$ (mg)	Vit B$_{12}$ (µg)	Vit E (mg)	Fol (µg)	Alc (g)
3.2	99	14	5.03	22.1	283	218	49	3.3	24	2.5	0.24	0.3	6.47	0.49	0.35	0.1	5.1	0
0.6	227	5	13.43	10.6	118	101	62	1.4	5273	2	0.25	0.39	2.86	0.33	23.76	0.6	324.7	0
0.7	67	5	3.48	25.5	236	339	49	3.1	0	0	0.24	0.44	9.15	0.64	1.56	0.5	7.7	0
0.8	70	7	2.91	22.1	178	307	49	3.1	0	0	0.09	0.23	3.16	0.34	2.43	0.3	6.8	0
4.3	111	11	0.77	15.3	124	208	54	1.3	27	0.4	0.06	0.17	5.02	0.26	0.24	0.3	1.7	0
0.8	90	11	0.66	16.2	127	213	54	1.3	17	0.5	0.06	0.19	5.34	0.3	0.26	0.2	1.7	0
1.5	87	3	5.11	24.9	211	304	65	0.8	18	7	0.47	0.35	3.91	0.71	0.86	0.3	28.4	0
5.7	91	6	4.72	22.7	191	282	64	0.9	29	5.9	0.4	0.31	3.76	0.6	0.74	0.8		0
3.4	73	13	3.77	18.7	237	184	44	2.6	60	2	0.19	0.26	6.74	0.53	0.31	0.6	5.1	0
3.8	86	15	4.5	26.1	312	245	60	2.7	83	6.9	0.28	0.29	8.55	0.68	0.49	0.8	9.1	0
2	70	16	1.93	17.9	224	326	40	1.9	0	0	0.08	0.18	7.17	0.4	7.06	0.7	9.4	0
9.6	108	14	4.01	24.9	281	226	61	2.5	83	5.9	0.24	0.25	6.86	0.46	0.45	0.1	6.8	0
0.5	13	2	0.81	6	51	107	357	1.1	0	0	0.02	0.05	1.3	0.1	0.49		2.3	0
1.8	48	10	1.6			239	1016				0.06	0.17	2.74					0
0.8	20	3	0.59	5.4	48	122	401	1.1	0	0	0.02	0.05	1.21	0.1	0.73	0.1	3.1	0
0.5	4	2	0.1	1.1	8	15	44	0.1	0	0	0.01	0.01	0.18	0.01	0.07	0	0.3	0
1	5	2	0.09	1.7	25	22	155	0.2	0	0	0.02	0.02	0.36	0.03	0.18	0	0.7	0
1.5	12	3	0.28	3.4	50	41	330	0.5	0	0.3	0.01	0.03	0.7	0.04	0.39	0.1	1.4	0
1.6	8	2	0.2	1.4	11	22	95	0.3	0	0	0.01	0.02	0.37	0.03	0.2	0	0.7	0
0.2	14	2	0.33	6.8	76	75	337	0.2	0	0								0
2.3	31						552		0									0
2	46	12	1.7			250	953				0.06	0.17	2.98					0
4	77	32	1.38	29.7	207	387	1760	1.8	0	5.4	0.85	0.24	3.92	0.44	0.57	0.1	9.4	0
1.6	17	32	0.37	6.4	58	82	332	0.5	0	0								0
1.7	11	31	0.15	5.4	36	84	421	0.4	17	0	0.08	0.07	0.52	0.07	0.36	0.1	0.6	0
0.9	18	5	0.7			104	300				0.03	0.07	1.16					0
0.8	19	3	0.63	5.4	50	67	251	1.4	9	0.4	0.02	0.05	1.21	0.08	0.52	0.1	2	0
0.7	39	6	2.38	7.9	113	196	556	1.2	2	9.1	0.03	0.14	2	0.15	0.14	0.1	2.8	0
1.9	24	2	0.77	4.8	64	59	372	0.6		0								0
5.6	40	8	0.51	7.9		130	776	1	0	0.5							1.7	0
1.1	19	35	0.47	6.2	56	43	306	0.5	0	0							1.7	0
0.1	9	2	0.3	4.4	34	63	213	0.3	2	1.2	0.03	0.07	0.02	0.03	0.02	0	0.8	0
3.5	163	18	5.31	49.9	667	651	2529	5.9	16	0	0.07	0.34	4.81	0.47	0.52	1.5	15.9	0
1.8	92	7	1.86	27.6	420	413	1432	3.3	0	0	0.07	0.34	4.87	0.32	0.36	0.5	8.3	0
0.8	21	11	0.35	6.2	74	60	281	0.6	0	0								0
9.1	58	8	1.05	9.6	81	218	805	1.8	0	0	0.34	0.16	2.76	0.28	1.08	0.2	1.1	0
6.2	46	6	0.89	7.9	80	146	370	2.5	7	0	0.03	0.09	2.04	0.18	1.14	0.1	1.7	0
8.6	47	9	0.87	7.4	105	133	516	1.7	14	0.4	0.02	0.07	1.82	0.11	1.15	0.3	2.8	0
3.3	30	2	1.6	2	6	10	170	0.3	0	0	0.02	0.03	0.3	0.01	0.25	0	1.2	0
8.6	63	24	0.45	17.8	191	220	719	2.1	0	0	0.53	0.22	3.94	0.35	0.68	0	2.6	0
	48	12	0.8	11.9	112	209	836	2.3	0	0	0.08	0.14	1.57	0.18	1.36	0	4.3	0
3	50	3	2.94	3.9	56	57	325	1	1322	2.5	0.06	0.45	2.57	0.09	5.26	0	13.2	0
8.6	53	5	0.95	10.8	90	239	741	2	0	0	0.38	0.18	3.08	0.32	1.2	0.1	1.2	0
7.1	34	7	0.89	8.6	60	90	584	1.3	0	0							6.3	0
0.1	15	10	0.98	9.5	64	234	464	1.2	0	0								0
5.6	25	4	0.6	5.8	63	58	461	1	0	0	0.02	0.05	1.03	0.03	0.73		2.7	0
1.7	41	59	0.98	10.4	66	72	511	0.8	0	0								0

MDA Code	Food Name	Amt	Wt (g)	Ener (kcal)	Prot (g)	Carb (g)	Fiber (g)	Fat (g)	Mono (g)	Poly (g)
57877	Frankfurter, beef, 5" × 3/4"	1 ea	45	148	5	2	0	13	6.4	0.5
58027	Frankfurter, beef, cooked	1 ea	52	170	6	2	0	15	7.4	0.6
13260	Frankfurter, chicken	1 ea	45	116	6	3	0	9	3.8	1.8
13012	Frankfurter, turkey	1 ea	45	102	6	1	0	8	2.5	2.2
57890	Italian sausage, pork, cooked, 1/4 lb	1 ea	83	286	16	4	0	23	9.9	2.7
13043	Kielbasa, beef, pork & nonfat dry milk, slice	1 pce	26	81	3	1	0	7	3.4	0.8
58020	Kielbasa, Polish, turkey & beef, smoked	3 oz	85.1	192	11	3	0	15	7	2
13044	Knockwurst, beef & pork, link, 4" long	1 ea	68	209	8	2	0	19	8.7	2
13019	Liverwurst, pork, 2-1/2" × 1/4" slice	1 pce	18	59	3	0	0	5	2.4	0.5
13021	Pepperoni, beef & pork, slice	1 pce	5.5	26	1	0	0	2	1	0.1
13022	Polish sausage, pork, 10" × 1-1/4"	1 ea	227	740	32	4	0	65	30.7	7
13185	Pork sausage, cooked/Oscar Mayer	2 ea	48	165	8	0	0	15	7.1	1.8
58227	Pork sausage, precooked	3 oz	85	321	12	0	0	30	12.9	4.1
13184	Smokie sausage links/Oscar Mayer	1 ea	43	130	5	1	0	12	5.7	1.2
13200	Summer sausage, Thuringer Cervelat, slice/Oscar Mayer	2 ea	46	140	7	0	0	12	5.6	1
58007	Turkey sausage, breakfast link, mild	2 ea	56	132	9	1	0	10	2.8	1.8
58219	Turkey, pork, and beef sausage, low fat, smoked	2 oz	56	57	4	6	0	1	0.6	0.2
	Meat Substitutes									
27044	Bacon bits, meatless	1 Tbs	7	33	2	2	1	2	0.4	0.9
7509	Bacon strips, meatless	3 ea	15	46	2	1	0	4	1.1	2.3
7558	Beef substitute, fillet	1 ea	85	246	20	8	5	15	3.7	7.9
7561	Beef substitute, patty	1 ea	56	110	12	4	3	5	1.2	2.6
62359	Breakfast patty, vegetarian/Morningstar Farms	1 ea	38	81	10	3	2	3	0.7	1.8
91055	Burger, vegetarian, Grillers Vegan/Morningstar Farms	1 ea	85	114	14	8	5	3	1	1.4
7725	Burger crumbles, vegetarian, Grillers Recipe Crumbles/Morningstar Farms	0.5 cup	55	82	11	5	2	2	0.5	1.4
7547	Chicken, vegetarian	1 cup	168	376	40	6	6	21	4.6	12.2
7722	Garden Veggie Patties, frozen/Morningstar Farms	1 ea	67	111	12	10	3	3	0.7	1.6
7674	Harvest Burger, vegetarian, original, frozen/Gardetto's	1 ea	90	138	18	7	6	4	2.1	0.3
90626	Sausage, vegetarian, slices	1 ea	28	72	5	3	1	5	1.3	2.6
7554	Soy burger	1 ea	70	136	15	5	3	6	1.2	2.5
7726	Spicy Black Bean Burger/Morningstar Farms	1 ea	78	150	12	15	3	5	1.2	2.4
	NUTS AND SEEDS									
4642	Beechnuts, dried	2 oz	56.7	327	4	19	2	28	12.4	11.4
4757	Butternuts, dried	1 ea	3	18	1	0	0	2	0.3	1.3
63195	Cashews, raw	2 oz	56.7	314	10	17	2	25	13.5	4.4
4519	Cashews, dry roasted, salted	0.25 cup	34.2	196	5	11	1	16	9.3	2.7
4645	Chinese chestnuts, dried	1 oz	28.4	103	2	23	1	1	0.3	0.1
63429	Filberts, dry roasted, unsalted	1 oz	28	181	4	5	3	17	13.1	2.4
63081	Flax seeds, whole	1 Tbs	11.2	60	2	3	3	5	0.8	3.2
4728	Macadamia nuts, dry roasted, unsalted	1 cup	134	962	10	18	11	102	79.4	2
4592	Mixed nuts, w/peanuts, dry roasted, salted	0.25 cup	34.2	203	6	9	3	18	10.7	3.7
4626	Peanut butter, chunky	2 Tbs	32	188	8	7	3	16	7.9	4.7
4756	Peanuts, dry roasted, unsalted	30 ea	30	176	7	6	2	15	7.4	4.7
4696	Peanuts, raw	0.25 cup	36.5	207	9	6	3	18	8.9	5.7
4540	Pistachios, dry roasted, salted	0.25 cup	32	182	7	9	3	15	7.7	4.4
4565	Pumpkin seeds/squash kernels, roasted, unsalted	0.25 cup	56.8	296	19	8	2	24	7.4	10.9
4523	Sesame seeds, whole, dried	0.25 cup	36	206	6	8	4	18	6.8	7.8
4551	Sunflower seeds, dry roasted, unsalted	0.25 cup	32	186	6	8	4	16	3	10.5
	SEAFOOD									
19041	Abalone, fried, mixed species	3 oz	85.1	161	17	9	0	6	2.3	1.4

Sat (g)	Chol (mg)	Calc (mg)	Iron (mg)	Mag (mg)	Phos (mg)	Pota (mg)	Sodi (mg)	Zinc (mg)	Vit A (RAE)	Vit C (mg)	Thia (mg)	Ribo (mg)	Niac (mg)	Vit B_6 (mg)	Vit B_{12} (µg)	Vit E (mg)	Fol (µg)	Alc (g)
5.3	24	6	0.68	6.3	72	70	513	1.1	0	0	0.02	0.07	1.07	0.04	0.77	0.1	2.2	0
5.9	29	6	0.81	7.3	89	76	600	1.2	0		0.02	0.07	1.22	0.05	0.86	0.1	3.6	0
2.5	45	43	0.9	4.5	48	38	616	0.5	18	0	0.03	0.05	1.39	0.14	0.11	0.1	1.8	0
2.7	48	48	0.83	6.3	60	81	642	1.4	0	0	0.02	0.08	1.86	0.1	0.13	0.3	3.6	0
7.9	47	17	1.19	14.9	141	252	1002	2	8	0.1	0.52	0.19	3.46	0.27	1.08	0.2	4.2	0
2.6	17	11	0.38	4.2	38	70	280	0.5	0	0	0.06	0.06	0.75	0.05	0.42	0.1	1.3	0
5.3	60		1.06				1021		0	12.6								0
6.9	41	7	0.45	7.5	67	135	632	1.1	0	0	0.23	0.1	1.86	0.12	0.8	0.4	1.4	0
1.9	28	5	1.15	2.2	41	31	155	0.4	1495	0	0.05	0.19	0.77	0.03	2.42	0.1	5.4	0
0.9	6	1	0.08	1	10	17	98	0.2	0	0	0.03	0.01	0.3	0.02	0.09	0	0.3	0
23.4	159	27	3.27	31.8	309	538	1989	4.4	0	2.3	1.14	0.34	7.82	0.43	2.22	0.5	4.5	
5.1	37	8	0.83	8.6	76	114	401	1.2	0	0								0
9.9	63	116	0.78	11	234	261	639	1.3	16	0.6	0.18	0.13	3.44	0.13	0.6	0.5	0.8	
4	27	4	0.5	7.3	103	77	433	0.9	0	0								0
4.9	39	4	1.03	6.9	60	105	658	1		0	0.11	0.13	2.02	0.14	1.73		2.3	0
4.4	34	18	0.6	14	104	110	328	1.2	0	17	0.04	0.1	2.06	0.21	0.24	0.2	4.5	0
0.5	12	6	1.23	9	41	136	446	0.7	0	1.1	0.07	0.04	0.87	0.06	0.16	0.1	3.4	0
0.3	0	7	0.05	6.6	15	10	124	0.1	0	0.1	0.04	0	0.11	0.01	0.08	0.5	8.9	0
0.7	0	3	0.36	2.8	10	26	220	0.1	1	0	0.66	0.07	1.13	0.07	0	1	6.3	0
2.4	0	81	1.7	19.6	382	510	416	1.2	0	0	0.94	0.76	10.2	1.27	3.57	2.9	86.7	0
0.8	0	16	1.18	10.1	193	101	308	1	0	0	0.5	0.34	5.6	0.67	1.34	1	43.7	0
0.4	1	17	2.04	1.1	116	125	255	0.5	0	0	5.53	0.21	3.83	0.31	2.39		0.3	0
0.4	0	31	2.51	16.2	188	423	336	0.7	0	0	0.26	0.55	4.11	0.2	0	0	245.6	0
0.3	0	31	3.05	25.8	111	117	236	0.9	0	0	0.69	0.19	7.83	0.79	4.97	0.3		0
3.1	0	59	5.49	28.6	563	91	1191	1.2	0	0	1.15	0.41	2.44	1.18	3.66	4.5	127.7	0
0.4	1	40	1.47	29.5	110	142	349	0.7	21	0	7.5	0.17	0	0	0	0.5	59	0
1	0	102	3.85	70.2	225	432	411	8.1	0	0	0.31	0.2	6.3	0.39	0	1.6	21.6	0
0.8	0	18	1.04	10.1	63	65	249	0.4	0	0	0.66	0.11	3.13	0.23	0	0.6	7.3	0
0.8	0	20	1.47	12.6	241	126	385	1.3	0	0	0.63	0.42	7	0.84	1.68	1.2	54.6	0
0.6	2	44	3.37	43.7	162	314	458	0.8		0	7.36	0.3	0	0.21	0.07	0.4		0
3.2	0	1	1.39	0	0	577	22	0.2	0	8.8	0.17	0.21	0.5	0.39	0		64.1	0
0	0	2	0.12	7.1	13	13	0	0.1	0	0.1	0.01	0	0.03	0.02	0	0.1	2	0
4.4	0	21	3.79	165.6	336	374	7	3.3	0	0.3	0.24	0.03	0.6	0.24	0	0.5	14.2	0
3.1	0	15	2.05	88.9	168	193	219	1.9	0	0	0.07	0.07	0.48	0.09	0	0.3	23.6	0
0.1	0	8	0.65	38.9	44	206	1	0.4	5	16.6	0.07	0.08	0.37	0.19	0	0.3	31.2	0
1.3	0	34	1.23	48.4	87	211	0	0.7	1	1.1	0.09	0.03	0.57	0.17	0	4.3	24.6	0
0.4	0	29	0.64	43.9	72	91	3	0.5	0	0.1	0.18	0.02	0.34	0.05	0	0	9.7	0
16	0	94	3.55	158.1	265	486	5	1.7	0	0.9	0.95	0.12	3.05	0.48	0	0.8	13.4	0
2.4	0	24	1.27	77	149	204	229	1.3	0	0.1	0.07	0.07	1.61	0.1	0	3.7	17.1	0
2.6	0	14	0.61	51.2	102	238	156	0.9	0	0	0.03	0.04	4.38	0.13	0	2	29.4	0
2.1	0	16	0.68	52.8	107	197	2	1	0	0	0.13	0.03	4.06	0.08	0	2.1	43.5	0
2.5	0	34	1.67	61.3	137	257	7	1.2	0	0	0.23	0.05	4.4	0.13	0	3	87.6	0
1.8	0	35	1.34	38.4	155	333	130	0.7	4	0.7	0.27	0.05	0.46	0.41	0	0.6	16	0
4.5	0	24	8.49	303.3	666	458	10	4.2	11	1	0.12	0.18	0.99	0.05	0	0	32.4	0
2.5	0	351	5.24	126.4	226	168	4	2.8	0	0	0.28	0.09	1.63	0.28	0	0.1	34.9	0
1.7	0	22	1.22	41.3	370	272	1	1.7	0	0.4	0.03	0.08	2.25	0.26	0	8.4	75.8	0
1.4	80	31	3.23	47.7	185	242	503	0.8	2	1.5	0.19	0.11	1.62	0.13	0.59	5.1	11.9	0

MDA Code	Food Name	Amt	Wt (g)	Ener (kcal)	Prot (g)	Carb (g)	Fiber (g)	Fat (g)	Mono (g)	Poly (g)
17029	Bass, freshwater, mixed species, fillet, baked/broiled	3 oz	85.1	124	21	0	0	4	1.6	1.2
17104	Bass, striped, fillet, baked/broiled	3 oz	85.1	106	19	0	0	3	0.7	0.9
50710	Bouillon/fish broth	1 cup	244	39	5	1	0	1	0.3	0.4
71707	Calamari, mixed species, fried	3 oz	85.1	149	15	7	0	6	2.3	1.8
17032	Carp, fillet, raw	4 oz	113.4	144	20	0	0	6	2.6	1.6
17088	Catfish, channel, fillet, breaded, fried	3 oz	85.1	195	15	7	1	11	4.8	2.8
17179	Catfish, channel, farmed, fillet, baked/broiled	3 oz	85.1	129	16	0	0	7	3.5	1.2
19002	Clams, mixed species, canned, drained	3 oz	85.1	126	22	4	0	2	0.1	0.5
71140	Clams, mixed species, raw	4 oz	113.4	84	14	3	0	1	0.1	0.3
17037	Cod, Atlantic, fillet, baked/broiled	3 oz	85.1	89	19	0	0	1	0.1	0.2
17107	Cod, Pacific, fillet, baked/broiled	3 oz	85.1	89	20	0	0	1	0.1	0.3
72116	Conch, baked/broiled	3 oz	85.1	111	22	1	0	1	0.3	0.2
19036	Crab, Alaska king, leg, steamed	3 oz	85.1	83	16	0	0	1	0.2	0.5
19037	Crab, Alaska king, imitation	3 oz	85.1	81	6	13	0	0	0.1	0.1
71722	Crawdads, farmed, mixed species, steamed	3 oz	85.1	74	15	0	0	1	0.2	0.4
17289	Eel, mixed species, fillet, w/o bone, baked/broiled	3 oz	85.1	201	20	0	0	13	7.8	1
7549	Fish sticks, vegetarian	1 ea	28	81	6	3	2	5	1.2	2.6
17090	Haddock, fillet, baked/broiled	3 oz	85.1	95	21	0	0	1	0.1	0.3
17291	Halibut, Atlantic/Pacific, fillet, baked/broiled	3 oz	85.1	119	23	0	0	3	0.8	0.8
17111	Halibut, Greenland, fillet, baked/broiled	3 oz	85.1	203	16	0	0	15	9.1	1.5
17047	Herring, Atlantic, fillet, baked/broiled	3 oz	85.1	173	20	0	0	10	4.1	2.3
17112	Herring, Pacific, fillet, baked/broiled	3 oz	85.1	213	18	0	0	15	7.5	2.6
17049	Mackerel, Atlantic, fillet, baked/broiled	3 oz	85.1	223	20	0	0	15	6	3.7
17115	Mackerel, king, fillet, baked/broiled	3 oz	85.1	114	22	0	0	2	0.8	0.5
19044	Mussels, blue, steamed	3 oz	85.1	146	20	6	0	4	0.9	1
19048	Octopus, steamed	3 oz	85.1	140	25	4	0	2	0.3	0.4
19089	Oysters, eastern, farmed, raw	4 oz	113.4	67	6	6	0	2	0.2	0.7
17094	Perch, mixed species, fillet, baked/broiled	3 oz	85.1	100	21	0	0	1	0.2	0.4
17093	Perch, ocean, Atlantic, fillet, baked/broiled	3 oz	85.1	103	20	0	0	2	0.7	0.5
17095	Pike, northern, fillet, baked/broiled	3 oz	85.1	96	21	0	0	1	0.2	0.2
17118	Pike, walleye, fillet, baked/broiled	3 oz	85.1	101	21	0	0	1	0.3	0.5
17096	Pollock, walleye, fillet, baked/broiled	3 oz	85.1	96	20	0	0	1	0.1	0.4
17073	Pompano, Florida, fillet, baked/broiled	3 oz	85.1	180	20	0	0	10	2.8	1.2
17074	Rockfish, Pacific, mixed species, fillet, baked/broiled	3 oz	85.1	103	20	0	0	2	0.4	0.5
17035	Roe, black/red, granular	1 Tbs	16	40	4	1	0	3	0.7	1.2
17120	Roe, mixed species, baked/broiled	3 oz	85.1	174	24	2	0	7	1.8	2.9
17121	Orange roughy, fillet, baked/broiled	3 oz	85.1	89	19	0	0	1	0.4	0.2
17181	Salmon, Atlantic, farmed, fillet, baked/broiled	3 oz	85.1	175	19	0	0	11	3.8	3.8
17123	Salmon, Atlantic, fillet, baked/broiled, wild	3 oz	85.1	155	22	0	0	7	2.3	2.8
17099	Salmon, sockeye, fillet, baked/broiled	3 oz	85.1	184	23	0	0	9	4.5	2.1
17086	Sea bass, mixed species, fillet, baked/broiled	3 oz	85.1	106	20	0	0	2	0.5	0.8
17023	Sea trout, mixed species, fillet, baked/broiled	3 oz	85.1	113	18	0	0	4	1	0.8
17076	Shark, mixed species, batter dipped, fried	3 oz	85.1	194	16	5	0	12	5.1	3.1
17100	Smelt, rainbow, baked/broiled	3 oz	85.1	106	19	0	0	3	0.7	1
17022	Snapper, mixed species, fillet, baked/broiled	3 oz	85.1	109	22	0	0	1	0.3	0.5
71139	Sturgeon, mixed species, baked/broiled, 4.5 × 2-1/8 × 7/8	3 oz	85.1	115	18	0	0	4	2.1	0.8
17079	Sturgeon, mixed species, smoked	3 oz	85.1	147	27	0	0	4	2	0.4
17066	Swordfish, fillet, baked/broiled	3 oz	85.1	132	22	0	0	4	1.7	1
17185	Trout, rainbow, farmed, fillet, baked/broiled	3 oz	85.1	144	21	0	0	6	1.8	2
17082	Trout, rainbow, wild, fillet, baked/broiled	3 oz	85.1	128	20	0	0	5	1.5	1.6

Sat (g)	Chol (mg)	Calc (mg)	Iron (mg)	Mag (mg)	Phos (mg)	Pota (mg)	Sodi (mg)	Zinc (mg)	Vit A (RAE)	Vit C (mg)	Thia (mg)	Ribo (mg)	Niac (mg)	Vit B_6 (mg)	Vit B_{12} (µg)	Vit E (mg)	Fol (µg)	Alc (g)
0.9	74	88	1.63	32.3	218	388	77	0.7	30	1.8	0.07	0.08	1.3	0.12	1.97	0.6	14.5	0
0.6	88	16	0.92	43.4	216	279	75	0.4	26	0	0.1	0.03	2.18	0.29	3.75	0.5	8.5	0
0.3	0	73	0.51	2.4	73	210	776	0.2	2	0	0	0.07	3.34	0.02	0.24	0.4	9.8	0
1.6	221	33	0.86	32.3	214	237	260	1.5	9	3.6	0.05	0.39	2.21	0.05	1.05	1.6	11.9	0
1.2	75	46	1.41	32.9	471	378	56	1.7	10	1.8	0.13	0.06	1.86	0.22	1.74	0.7	17	0
2.8	69	37	1.22	23	184	289	238	0.7	7	0	0.06	0.11	1.94	0.16	1.62	1.1	25.5	0
1.5	54	8	0.7	22.1	208	273	68	0.9	13	0.7	0.36	0.06	2.14	0.14	2.38	1.1	6	0
0.2	57	78	23.79	15.3	288	534	95	2.3	154	18.8	0.13	0.36	2.85	0.09	84.16	0.5	24.7	0
0.1	39	52	15.85	10.2	192	356	64	1.6	102	14.7	0.09	0.24	2	0.07	56.06	0.4	18.1	0
0.1	47	12	0.42	35.7	117	208	66	0.5	12	0.9	0.07	0.07	2.14	0.24	0.89	0.7	6.8	0
0.1	40	8	0.28	26.4	190	440	77	0.4	9	2.6	0.02	0.04	2.11	0.39	0.89	0.3	6.8	0
0.3	55	83	1.2	202.5	185	139	130	1.5	6	0	0.05	0.07	0.89	0.05	4.47	5.4	152.3	0
0.1	45	50	0.65	53.6	238	223	912	6.5	8	6.5	0.05	0.05	1.14	0.15	9.79	0.8	43.4	0
0.1	17	11	0.33	36.6	240	77	716	0.3	0	0	0.03	0.07	0.53	0.11	0.49	0.1	0	0
0.2	117	43	0.94	28.1	205	203	83	1.3	13	0.4	0.04	0.07	1.42	0.11	2.64	0.8	9.4	0
2.6	137	22	0.54	22.1	236	297	55	1.8	968	1.5	0.16	0.04	3.82	0.07	2.46	4.3	14.5	0
0.8	0	27	0.56	6.4	126	168	137	0.4	0	0	0.31	0.25	3.36	0.42	1.18	1.1	28.6	0
0.1	63	36	1.15	42.6	205	340	74	0.4	16	0	0.03	0.04	3.94	0.29	1.18	0.4	11.1	0
0.4	35	51	0.91	91.1	243	490	59	0.5	46	0	0.06	0.08	6.06	0.34	1.17	0.9	11.9	0
2.6	50	3	0.72	28.1	179	293	88	0.4	15	0	0.06	0.09	1.64	0.41	0.82	1.1	0.9	0
2.2	66	63	1.2	34.9	258	357	98	1.1	31	0.6	0.1	0.25	3.51	0.3	11.18	1.2	10.2	0
3.6	84	90	1.23	34.9	248	461	81	0.6	30	0	0.06	0.22	2.4	0.44	8.19	1.1	5.1	0
3.6	64	13	1.34	82.5	237	341	71	0.8	46	0.3	0.14	0.35	5.83	0.39	16.17	1.6	1.7	0
0.4	58	34	1.94	34.9	271	475	173	0.6	214	1.4	0.1	0.49	8.9	0.43	15.32	1.5	7.7	0
0.7	48	28	5.72	31.5	243	228	314	2.3	77	11.6	0.26	0.36	2.55	0.09	20.42	1.2	64.7	0
0.4	82	90	8.12	51.1	237	536	391	2.9	77	6.8	0.05	0.06	3.22	0.55	30.64	1	20.4	0
0.5	28	50	6.55	37.4	105	141	202	43	9	5.3	0.12	0.07	1.44	0.07	18.37	0.8	20.4	0
0.2	98	87	0.99	32.3	219	293	67	1.2	9	1.4	0.07	0.1	1.62	0.12	1.87	1.3	5.1	0
0.3	46	117	1	33.2	236	298	82	0.5	12	0.7	0.11	0.11	2.07	0.23	0.98	1.4	8.5	0
0.1	43	62	0.6	34	240	282	42	0.7	20	3.2	0.06	0.07	2.38	0.11	1.96	0.2	14.5	0
0.3	94	120	1.42	32.3	229	425	55	0.7	20	0	0.27	0.17	2.38	0.12	1.97	0.2	14.5	0
0.2	82	5	0.24	62.1	410	329	99	0.5	21	0	0.06	0.06	1.4	0.06	3.57	0.7	3.4	0
3.8	54	37	0.57	26.4	290	541	65	0.6	31	0	0.58	0.13	3.23	0.2	1.02	0.2	14.5	0
0.4	37	10	0.45	28.9	194	443	66	0.5	60	0	0.04	0.07	3.34	0.23	1.02	1.3	8.5	0
0.6	94	44	1.9	48	57	29	240	0.2	90	0	0.03	0.1	0.02	0.05	3.2	1.1	8	0
1.6	408	24	0.66	22.1	438	241	100	1.1	77	14	0.24	0.81	1.87	0.16	9.82	7.2	78.3	0
0	68	9	0.96	15.3	87	154	59	0.3	20	0	0.04	0.05	1.55	0.06	0.4	1.6	4.3	0
2.1	54	13	0.29	25.5	214	327	52	0.4	13	3.1	0.29	0.11	6.85	0.55	2.38	0.8	28.9	0
1.1	60	13	0.88	31.5	218	534	48	0.7	11	0	0.23	0.41	8.58	0.8	2.6	1.1	24.7	0
1.6	74	6	0.47	26.4	235	319	56	0.5	54	0	0.18	0.15	5.68	0.19	4.94	1.1	4.3	0
0.6	45	11	0.31	45.1	211	279	74	0.4	54	0	0.11	0.13	1.62	0.39	0.26	0.5	5.1	0
1.1	90	19	0.3	34	273	372	63	0.5	30	0	0.06	0.18	2.49	0.39	2.94	0.2	5.1	0
2.7	50	43	0.94	36.6	165	132	104	0.4	46	0	0.06	0.08	2.37	0.26	1.03	0.9	12.8	0
0.5	77	66	0.98	32.3	251	317	66	1.8	14	0	0.01	0.12	1.5	0.14	3.38	0.5	4.3	0
0.3	40	34	0.2	31.5	171	444	49	0.4	30	1.4	0.05	0	0.29	0.39	2.98	0.5	5.1	0
1	66	14	0.77	38.3	231	310	59	0.5	224	0	0.07	0.08	8.6	0.2	2.13	0.5	14.5	0
0.9	68	14	0.79	40	239	323	629	0.5	238	0	0.08	0.08	9.45	0.23	2.47	0.4	17	0
1.2	43	5	0.89	28.9	287	314	98	1.3	35	0.9	0.04	0.1	10.03	0.32	1.72	0.5	1.7	0
1.8	58	73	0.28	27.2	226	375	36	0.4	73	2.8	0.2	0.07	7.48	0.34	4.23	0	20.4	0
1.4	59	73	0.32	26.4	229	381	48	0.4	13	1.7	0.13	0.08	4.91	0.29	5.36	0.4	16.2	0

MDA Code	Food Name	Amt	Wt (g)	Ener (kcal)	Prot (g)	Carb (g)	Fiber (g)	Fat (g)	Mono (g)	Poly (g)
56007	Tuna salad, lunchmeat spread	2 Tbs	25.6	48	4	2	0	2	0.7	1.1
17101	Tuna, bluefin, fillet, baked/broiled	3 oz	85.1	157	25	0	0	5	1.7	1.6
17177	Tuna, yellowfin, fillet, baked/broiled	3 oz	85.1	118	26	0	0	1	0.2	0.3
17151	Tuna, white, w/water, drained, can	3 oz	85.1	109	20	0	0	3	0.7	0.9
17083	Tuna, white, canned, w/oil, drained	3 oz	85.1	158	23	0	0	7	2.8	2.5
17162	Whitefish, mixed species, fillet, baked/broiled	3 oz	85.1	146	21	0	0	6	2.2	2.3
17164	Yellowtail, mixed species, fillet, baked/broiled	3 oz	85.1	159	25	0	0	6		

VEGETABLES AND LEGUMES

Beans

MDA Code	Food Name	Amt	Wt (g)	Ener (kcal)	Prot (g)	Carb (g)	Fiber (g)	Fat (g)	Mono (g)	Poly (g)
92132	Baked beans, unsalted, canned	1 cup	253	266	12	52	14	1	0.1	0.4
7038	Baked beans, plain/vegetarian, canned	1 cup	254	239	12	54	10	1	0.2	0.3
56101	Baked beans, w/franks, canned	0.5 cup	129.5	184	9	20	9	9	3.7	1.1
5197	Bean sprouts, mung, mature, canned, drained	1 cup	125	15	2	3	1	0	0	0
7012	Black beans, mature, cooked	1 cup	172	227	15	41	15	1	0.1	0.4
92152	Chili beans, ranch style bbq, cooked	1 cup	253	245	13	43	11	3	0.2	1.4
9574	Black eyed peas, immature, cooked w/salt	1 cup	165	155	5	33	8	1	0.1	0.3
90018	Cowpeas, mature, cooked w/salt	1 cup	171	198	13	35	11	1	0.1	0.4
7057	Cowpeas, mature, w/pork, canned	0.5 cup	120	100	3	20	4	2	0.8	0.3
9583	Fava beans (broadbeans), mature, cooked w/salt	1 cup	170	187	13	33	9	1	0.1	0.3
7913	Fava beans, immature, in pod	1 cup	126	111	10	22		1	0.1	0.4
7219	Golden gram beans, mature, cooked	1 cup	202	212	14	39	15	1	0.1	0.3
7217	Golden gram beans, mature	1 cup	207	718	49	130	34	2	0.3	0.8
7081	Hummus, garbanzo or chick pea spread, homemade	1 Tbs	15.4	27	1	3	1	1	0.8	0.3
7087	Kidney beans, all types, mature, canned	1 cup	256	215	13	37	11	2	0.7	0.5
7047	Kidney beans, red, mature, cooked	1 cup	177	225	15	40	13	1	0.1	0.5
7006	Lentils, mature, cooked	1 cup	198	230	18	40	16	1	0.1	0.3
90021	Lima beans, baby, cooked w/salt	1 cup	182	229	15	42	14	1	0.1	0.3
7010	Lima beans, large, mature, cooked	1 cup	188	216	15	39	13	1	0.1	0.3
7011	Lima beans, large, mature, canned	1 cup	241	190	12	36	12	0	0	0.2
5850	Lima beans, baby, immature, cooked from frozen w/salt	0.5 cup	90	94	6	18	5	0	0	0.1
7022	Navy beans, mature, cooked	1 cup	182	255	15	47	19	1	0.2	0.8
7122	Navy beans, mature, canned	1 cup	262	296	20	54	13	1	0.1	0.5
7051	Pinto beans, mature, canned	1 cup	240	206	12	37	11	2	0.4	0.7
5854	Pinto beans, immature, cooked from frozen w/salt	3 oz	85.1	138	8	26	7	0	0	0.2
5856	Snap beans, green, cooked w/salt	1 cup	125	44	2	10	4	0	0	0.2
6748	Snap beans, green, fresh, 4" long	10 ea	55	17	1	4	2	0	0	0
5857	Snap beans, yellow, cooked w/salt	1 cup	125	44	2	10	4	0	0	0.2
5320	Snap beans, yellow, fresh	0.5 cup	55	17	1	4	2	0	0	0
90026	Peas, green, split, mature, cooked w/salt	0.5 cup	98	114	8	20	8	0	0.1	0.2
7053	White beans, mature, cooked	1 cup	179	249	17	45	11	1	0.1	0.3
7054	White beans, mature, canned	1 cup	262	299	19	56	13	1	0.1	0.3
7052	Yellow beans, mature, cooked	1 cup	177	255	16	45	18	2	0.2	0.8

Fresh Vegetables

MDA Code	Food Name	Amt	Wt (g)	Ener (kcal)	Prot (g)	Carb (g)	Fiber (g)	Fat (g)	Mono (g)	Poly (g)
90542	Arrowroot, fresh	1 ea	33	21	1	4	0	0	0	0
9577	Artichokes, French, cooked w/salt, medium	1 ea	20	10	1	2	1	0	0	0
5723	Artichokes, globe, frozen	3 oz	85.1	32	2	7	3	0	0	0.2
6033	Arugula greens, chopped, fresh	1 cup	20	5	1	1	0	0	0	0.1
5841	Asparagus, cooked w/salt	0.5 cup	90	20	2	4	2	0	0	0.1
90406	Asparagus spears, tips, fresh, 2" long or less	10 ea	35	9	1	1	1	0	0	0
5863	Beet greens, cooked w/salt, drained, 1" pieces	1 cup	144	39	4	8	4	0	0.1	0.1

Sat (g)	Chol (mg)	Calc (mg)	Iron (mg)	Mag (mg)	Phos (mg)	Pota (mg)	Sodi (mg)	Zinc (mg)	Vit A (RAE)	Vit C (mg)	Thia (mg)	Ribo (mg)	Niac (mg)	Vit B$_6$ (mg)	Vit B$_{12}$ (µg)	Vit E (mg)	Fol (µg)	Alc (g)
0.4	3	4	0.26	4.9	46	46	103	0.1	6	0.6	0.01	0.02	1.72	0.02	0.31	0.2	2	0
1.4	42	9	1.11	54.5	277	275	43	0.7	644	0	0.24	0.26	8.97	0.45	9.26	1.1	1.7	0
0.3	49	18	0.8	54.5	208	484	40	0.6	17	0.9	0.43	0.05	10.16	0.88	0.51	0.5	1.7	0
0.7	36	12	0.83	28.1	185	202	321	0.4	5	0	0.01	0.04	4.93	0.18	1	0.7	1.7	0
1.1	26	3	0.55	28.9	227	283	337	0.4	4	0	0.01	0.07	9.95	0.37	1.87	2	4.3	0
1	66	28	0.4	35.7	294	346	55	1.1	33	0	0.15	0.13	3.27	0.29	0.82	0.2	14.5	0
	60	25	0.54	32.3	171	458	43	0.6	26	2.5	0.15	0.04	7.42	0.16	1.06	0.2	3.4	0
0.3	0	126	0.73	81	263	749	3	3.5	13	7.8	0.38	0.15	1.09	0.33	0	1.3	60.7	0
0.2	0	86	3.02	68.6	188	569	871	5.8	13	0	0.24	0.1	1.09	0.21	0	0.4	30.5	0
3	8	62	2.24	36.3	135	304	557	2.4	5	3	0.08	0.07	1.17	0.06	0.44	0.6	38.8	0
0	0	18	0.54	11.2	40	34	175	0.4	1	0.4	0.04	0.09	0.27	0.04	0	0	12.5	0
0.2	0	46	3.61	120.4	241	611	2	1.9	0	0	0.42	0.1	0.87	0.12	0	0.1	256.3	0
0.4	0	78	4.71	113.8	390	1138	1834	5.1	3	4.3	0.1	0.38	0.91	0.68	0.03	0.5	65.8	0
0.2	0	211	1.85	85.8	84	690	396	1.7	66	3.6	0.17	0.24	2.31	0.11	0	0.4	209.6	0
0.2	0	41	4.29	90.6	267	475	410	2.2	2	0.7	0.35	0.09	0.85	0.17	0	0.5	355.7	0
0.7	8	20	1.7	51.6	115	214	420	1.2	0	0.2	0.08	0.06	0.52	0.05	0	0.6	61.2	0
0.1	0	61	2.55	73.1	212	456	410	1.7	2	0.5	0.16	0.15	1.21	0.12	0	0	176.8	0
0.1	0	47	1.95	41.6	163	418	32	1.3	21	4.7	0.17	0.37	2.83	0.13	0		186.5	0
0.2	0	55	2.83	97	200	537	4	1.7	2	2	0.33	0.12	1.17	0.14	0	0.3	321.2	0
0.7	0	273	13.95	391.2	760	2579	31	5.5	12	9.9	1.29	0.48	4.66	0.79	0	1.1	1293.8	0
0.2	0	8	0.24	4.5	17	27	37	0.2	0	1.2	0.01	0.01	0.06	0.06	0	0.1	9.1	0
0.3	0	87	3	69.1	230	607	758	1.2	0	3.1	0.3	0.13	1.05	0.19	0	0.1	92.2	0
0.1	0	50	5.2	79.6	251	713	4	1.9	0	2.1	0.28	0.1	1.02	0.21	0	1.5	230.1	0
0.1	0	38	6.59	71.3	356	731	4	2.5	1	3	0.33	0.14	2.1	0.35	0	0.2	358.4	0
0.2	0	53	4.37	96.5	231	730	435	1.9	0	0	0.29	0.1	1.2	0.14	0	0.3	273	0
0.2	0	32	4.49	80.8	209	955	4	1.8	0	0	0.3	0.1	0.79	0.3	0	0.3	156	0
0.1	0	51	4.36	94	178	530	810	1.6	0	0	0.13	0.08	0.63	0.22	0	0.2	120.5	0
0.1	0	25	1.76	50.4	101	370	238	0.5	7	5.2	0.06	0.05	0.69	0.1	0	0.6	14.4	0
0.2	0	126	4.3	96.5	262	708	0	1.9	0	1.6	0.43	0.12	1.18	0.25	0	0	254.8	0
0.3	0	123	4.85	123.1	351	755	1174	2	0	1.8	0.37	0.14	1.28	0.27	0	2	162.4	0
0.4	0	103	3.5	64.8	221	583	706	1.7	0	2.2	0.24	0.15	0.7	0.18	0	1.4	144	0
0	3	44	2.31	46	85	550	271	0.6	0	0.6	0.23	0.09	0.54	0.17		0.3	28.9	0
0.1	0	55	0.81	22.5	36	182	299	0.3	44	12.1	0.09	0.12	0.77	0.07	0	0.6	41.2	0
0	0	20	0.57	13.8	21	115	3	0.1	19	9	0.05	0.06	0.41	0.04	0	0.2	20.4	0
0.1	0	58	1.6	31.2	49	374	299	0.5	5	12.1	0.09	0.12	0.77	0.07	0	0.6	41.2	0
0	0	20	0.57	13.8	21	115	3	0.1	3	9	0.05	0.06	0.41	0.04	0	0.1	20.4	0
0.1	0	14	1.26	35.3	97	355	233	1	0	0.4	0.19	0.05	0.87	0.05	0	0	63.7	0
0.2	0	161	6.62	112.8	202	1004	11	2.5	0	0	0.21	0.08	0.25	0.17	0	1.7	145	0
0.2	0	191	7.83	133.6	238	1189	13	2.9	0	0	0.25	0.1	0.3	0.2	0	2.1	170.3	0
0.5	0	110	4.39	131	324	575	9	1.9	0	3.2	0.33	0.18	1.25	0.23	0	0.9	143.4	0
0	0	2	0.73	8.2	32	150	9	0.2	0	0.6	0.05	0.02	0.56	0.09	0		111.5	0
0	0	9	0.26	12	17	71	66	0.1	2	2	0.01	0.01	0.2	0.02	0	0	10.2	0
0.1	0	16	0.43	23	49	211	40	0.3	7	4.5	0.05	0.12	0.73	0.07	0	0.1	107.2	0
0	0	32	0.29	9.4	10	74	5	0.1	24	3	0.01	0.02	0.06	0.01	0	0.1	19.4	0
0	0	21	0.82	12.6	49	202	216	0.5	45	6.9	0.15	0.13	0.98	0.07	0	1.4	134.1	0
0	0	8	0.75	4.9	18	71	1	0.2	13	2	0.05	0.05	0.34	0.03	0	0.4	18.2	0
0	0	164	2.74	97.9	59	1309	687	0.7	552	35.9	0.17	0.42	0.72	0.19	0	2.6	20.2	0

MDA Code	Food Name	Amt	Wt (g)	Ener (kcal)	Prot (g)	Carb (g)	Fiber (g)	Fat (g)	Mono (g)	Poly (g)
5312	Beet greens, fresh	0.5 cup	19	4	0	1	1	0	0	0
5862	Beets, cooked w/salt, drained, slices	0.5 cup	85	37	1	8	2	0	0	0.1
6755	Beets, canned, drained, slices	1 cup	170	53	2	12	3	0	0	0.1
5573	Beets, fresh, slices	0.5 cup	68	29	1	7	2	0	0	0
9160	Belgian endive, fresh, head	0.5 cup	45	8	0	2	1	0	0	0
5558	Broccoli, stalk, fresh	1 ea	114	32	3	6	4	0	0	0.2
6091	Broccoli, cooked w/salt, drained, chopped	0.5 cup	78	22	2	4	3	0	0	0.1
7909	Broccoli, Chinese, cooked	1 cup	88	19	1	3	2	1	0	0.3
9542	Broccoli raab, cooked	3 oz	85.1	28	3	3	2	0	0	0.1
9541	Broccoli raab, fresh, stalk	3 oz	85.1	19	3	2	2	0	0	0.1
5870	Brussels sprouts, cooked w/salt, drained	0.5 cup	78	32	2	7	2	0	0	0.2
5036	Cabbage, fresh, shredded	1 cup	70	18	1	4	2	0	0	0
5878	Cabbage, cooked w/salt, drained, shredded	0.5 cup	75	17	1	4	1	0	0	0
5608	Cabbage, pickled, Japanese style	0.5 cup	75	22	1	4	2	0	0	0
5609	Cabbage, mustard, salted	1 cup	128	36	1	7	4	0	0	0.1
9591	Cabbage, pak choi, shredded, cooked w/salt, drained	0.5 cup	85	10	1	2	1	0	0	0.1
5040	Cabbage, petsai, fresh, chopped	1 cup	76	12	1	2	1	0	0	0.1
5880	Cabbage, red, cooked w/salt, drained, shredded	0.5 cup	75	22	1	5	2	0	0	0
5042	Cabbage, red, fresh, shredded	0.5 cup	35	11	1	3	1	0	0	0
9550	Carrots, dehydrated	1 Tbs	4.6	16	0	4	1	0	0	0
90605	Carrots, fresh, baby, large	1 ea	15	5	0	1	0	0	0	0
5887	Carrots, cooked w/salt, slices	0.5 cup	78	27	1	6	2	0	0	0.1
5199	Carrots, canned, drained, slices	0.5 cup	73	18	0	4	1	0	0	0.1
5045	Carrots, fresh, whole, 7-1/2" long	1 ea	72	30	1	7	2	0	0	0.1
5049	Cauliflower, fresh	0.5 cup	50	12	1	3	1	0	0	0
5891	Cauliflower, cooked w/salt, drained, 1" pces	0.5 cup	62	14	1	3	1	0	0	0.1
5894	Celery, cooked w/salt, drained, diced	0.5 cup	75	14	1	3	1	0	0	0.1
90436	Celery, stalk, small, 5" long, fresh	1 ea	17	3	0	1	0	0	0	0
9203	Chicory, red leafed, fresh, shredded	1 cup	40	9	1	2	0	0	0	0
6093	Collard greens, chopped, cooked w/salt, drained	1 cup	190	49	4	9	5	1	0	0.3
5060	Collard greens, chopped, fresh	1 cup	36	11	1	2	1	0	0	0.1
6801	Corn, yellow, sweet, ear, fresh, small, 5.5"-6.5" long	1 ea	73	63	2	14	2	1	0.3	0.4
7202	Corn, white, sweet, kernels from small ear, fresh	1 ea	73	63	2	14	2	1	0.3	0.4
5900	Corn, yellow, sweet, kernels, cooked w/salt, drained	0.5 cup	82	89	3	21	2	1	0.3	0.5
5241	Dandelion greens, fresh	1 cup	55	25	1	5	2	0	0	0.2
9221	Dasheen, cooked w/salt, slices	0.5 cup	66	94	0	23	3	0	0	0
5908	Eggplant, cooked w/salt, drained, 1" cubes	1 cup	99	35	1	9	2	0	0	0.1
5202	Endive greens, fresh, chopped	0.5 cup	25	4	0	1	1	0	0	0
5450	Fennel, bulb, fresh, slices	0.5 cup	43.5	13	1	3	1	0		
5373	Garden cress greens, fresh, sprigs	20 ea	20	6	1	1	0	0	0	0
7270	Hearts of palm, canned	0.5 cup	73	20	2	3	2	0	0.1	0.1
9182	Jicama, fresh, slices	1 cup	120	46	1	11	6	0	0	0.1
5915	Kale, cooked w/salt, drained, chopped	0.5 cup	65	18	1	4	1	0	0	0.1
9191	Kale, borecole, fresh, chopped	1 cup	67	34	2	7	1	0	0	0.2
5918	Kohlrabi, cooked w/salt, drained, slices	1 cup	165	48	3	11	2	0	0	0.1
5078	Kohlrabi, fresh	0.5 cup	67.5	18	1	4	2	0	0	0
90182	Ladies fingers, fresh, pods, 3" long	8 ea	95	29	2	7	3	0	0	0
5205	Leeks, bulb & lower leaf, fresh, chopped	0.5 cup	44.5	27	1	6	1	0	0	0.1
5920	Leeks, bulb & lower leaf, cooked w/salt, chopped	1 ea	124	38	1	9	1	0	0	0.1
90445	Lettuce, butterhead, fresh, leaf, small	1 pce	5	1	0	0	0	0	0	0

Sat (g)	Chol (mg)	Calc (mg)	Iron (mg)	Mag (mg)	Phos (mg)	Pota (mg)	Sodi (mg)	Zinc (mg)	Vit A (RAE)	Vit C (mg)	Thia (mg)	Ribo (mg)	Niac (mg)	Vit B_6 (mg)	Vit B_{12} (µg)	Vit E (mg)	Fol (µg)	Alc (g)
0	0	22	0.49	13.3	8	145	43	0.1	60	5.7	0.02	0.04	0.08	0.02	0	0.3	2.8	0
0	0	14	0.67	19.6	32	259	242	0.3	2	3.1	0.02	0.03	0.28	0.06	0	0	68	0
0	0	26	3.09	28.9	29	252	330	0.4	2	7	0.02	0.07	0.27	0.1	0	0.1	51	0
0	0	11	0.54	15.6	27	221	53	0.2	1	3.3	0.02	0.03	0.23	0.05	0	0	74.1	0
0	0	9	0.11	4.5	12	95	1	0.1	0	1.3	0.03	0.01	0.07	0.02	0		16.6	0
0.1	0	55	1	28.5	75	370	31	0.5	23	106.2	0.07	0.14	0.73	0.18	0	0.5	80.9	0
0	0	31	0.52	16.4	52	229	204	0.4	76	32.8	0.05	0.1	0.43	0.16	0	1.1	84.2	0
0.1	0	88	0.49	15.8	36	230	6	0.3	72	24.8	0.08	0.13	0.38	0.06	0	0.4	87.1	0
0	0	100	1.08	23	70	292	48	0.5	193	31.5	0.14	0.12	1.71	0.19		2.2	60.4	0
0	0	92	1.82	18.7	62	167	28	0.7	112	17.2	0.14	0.11	1.04	0.15		1.4	70.6	0
0.1	0	28	0.94	15.6	44	247	200	0.3	30	48.4	0.08	0.06	0.47	0.14	0	0.3	46.8	0
0	0	28	0.33	8.4	18	119	13	0.1	4	25.6	0.04	0.03	0.16	0.09	0	0.1	30.1	0
0	0	36	0.13	11.2	25	147	191	0.2	3	28.1	0.05	0.03	0.19	0.08	0	0.1	22.5	0
0	0	36	0.37	9	32	640	208	0.2	7	0.5	0	0.03	0.14	0.08	0	0.1	31.5	0
0	0	86	0.9	19.2	35	315	918	0.4	63	0	0.05	0.12	0.92	0.38	0	0	92.2	0
0	0	79	0.88	9.4	25	315	230	0.1	180	22.1	0.03	0.05	0.36	0.14	0	0.1	34.8	0
0	0	59	0.24	9.9	22	181	7	0.2	12	20.5	0.03	0.04	0.3	0.18	0	0.1	60	0
0	0	32	0.5	12.8	25	196	183	0.2	2	8.1	0.05	0.04	0.29	0.17	0	0.1	18	0
0	0	16	0.28	5.6	10	85	9	0.1	20	20	0.02	0.02	0.15	0.07	0	0	6.3	0
0	0	10	0.18	5.4	16	117	13	0.1	249	0.7	0.02	0.02	0.3	0.05	0	0.3	2.5	0
0	0	5	0.13	1.5	4	36	12	0	104	0.4	0	0.01	0.08	0.02	0	0.1	4	0
0	0	23	0.27	7.8	23	183	236	0.2	671	2.8	0.05	0.03	0.5	0.12	0	0.8	1.6	0
0	0	18	0.47	5.8	18	131	177	0.2	407	2	0.01	0.02	0.4	0.08	0	0.5	6.6	0
0	0	24	0.22	8.6	25	230	50	0.2	606	4.2	0.05	0.04	0.71	0.1	0	0.5	13.7	0
0	0	11	0.22	7.5	22	152	15	0.1	0	23.2	0.03	0.03	0.26	0.11	0	0	28.5	0
0	0	10	0.2	5.6	20	88	150	0.1	1	27.5	0.03	0.03	0.25	0.11	0	0	27.3	0
0	0	32	0.31	9	19	213	245	0.1	22	4.6	0.03	0.04	0.24	0.06	0	0.3	16.5	0
0	0	7	0.03	1.9	4	44	14	0	4	0.5	0	0.01	0.05	0.01	0	0	6.1	0
0	0	8	0.23	5.2	16	121	9	0.2	0	3.2	0.01	0.01	0.1	0.02	0	0.9	24	0
0.1	0	266	2.2	38	57	220	479	0.4	771	34.6	0.08	0.2	1.09	0.24	0	1.7	176.7	0
0	0	52	0.07	3.2	4	61	7	0	120	12.7	0.02	0.05	0.27	0.06	0	0.8	59.8	0
0.1	0	1	0.38	27	65	197	11	0.3	7	5	0.15	0.04	1.24	0.04	0	0.1	33.6	0
0.1	0	1	0.38	27	65	197	11	0.3	0	5	0.15	0.04	1.24	0.04	0	0.1	33.6	0
0.2	0	2	0.5	26.2	84	204	207	0.4	11	5.1	0.18	0.06	1.32	0.05	0	0.1	37.7	0
0.1	0	103	1.7	19.8	36	218	42	0.2	136	19.2	0.1	0.14	0.44	0.14	0	2.6	14.8	0
0	0	12	0.48	19.8	50	319	166	0.2	3	3.3	0.07	0.02	0.34	0.22	0	1.9	12.5	0
0	0	6	0.25	10.9	15	122	237	0.1	2	1.3	0.08	0.02	0.59	0.09	0	0.4	13.9	0
0	0	13	0.21	3.8	7	78	6	0.2	27	1.6	0.02	0.02	0.1	0	0	0.1	35.5	0
	0	21	0.32	7.4	22	180	23	0.1	3	5.2	0	0.01	0.28	0.02	0		11.7	0
0	0	16	0.26	7.6	15	121	3	0	69	13.8	0.02	0.05	0.2	0.05	0	0.1	16	0
0.1	0	42	2.28	27.7	47	129	311	0.8	0	5.8	0.01	0.04	0.32	0.02	0		28.5	0
0	0	14	0.72	14.4	22	180	5	0.2	1	24.2	0.02	0.03	0.24	0.05	0	0.6	14.4	0
0	0	47	0.58	11.7	18	148	168	0.2	443	26.6	0.03	0.05	0.32	0.09	0	0.6	8.4	0
0.1	0	90	1.14	22.8	38	299	29	0.3	515	80.4	0.07	0.09	0.67	0.18	0	0.5	19.4	0
0	0	41	0.66	31.4	74	561	424	0.5	3	89.1	0.07	0.03	0.64	0.25	0	0.9	19.8	0
0	0	16	0.27	12.8	31	236	14	0	1	41.8	0.03	0.01	0.27	0.1	0	0.3	10.8	0
0	0	77	0.76	54.2	60	288	8	0.6	18	20	0.19	0.06	0.95	0.2	0	0.3	83.6	0
0	0	26	0.93	12.5	16	80	9	0.1	37	5.3	0.03	0.01	0.18	0.1	0	0.4	28.5	0
0	0	37	1.36	17.4	21	108	305	0.1	2	5.2	0.03	0.02	0.25	0.14	0	0.8	29.8	0
0	0	2	0.06	0.6	2	12	0	0	8	0.2	0	0	0.02	0	0	0	3.6	0

MDA Code	Food Name	Amt	Wt (g)	Ener (kcal)	Prot (g)	Carb (g)	Fiber (g)	Fat (g)	Mono (g)	Poly (g)
5089	Lettuce, romaine, fresh, inner leaf	2 pce	20	3	0	1	0	0	0	0
5087	Lettuce, green leaf, fresh, leaf	2 pce	20	3	0	1	0	0	0	0
9545	Lettuce, red leaf, fresh, shredded	1 cup	28	4	0	1	0	0		
7949	Mushrooms, oyster, fresh, small	1 ea	15	5	0	1	0	0	0	0
5926	Mushrooms, shiitake, cooked w/salt, pieces	1 cup	145	78	2	20	3	0	0.1	0
51069	Mushrooms, crimini, fresh	2 ea	28	8	1	1	0	0	0	0
90457	Mushrooms, canned, drained, caps	8 ea	47	12	1	2	1	0	0	0.1
51067	Mushrooms, portabella, fresh, small	1 oz	28	7	1	1	0	0	0	0
5927	Mustard greens, cooked w/salt, drained, chopped	0.5 cup	70	10	2	1	1	0	0.1	0
5207	Mustard greens, fresh, chopped	1 cup	56	15	2	3	2	0	0.1	0
6971	Okra, cooked w/salt, drained, slices	0.5 cup	80	18	1	4	2	0	0	0
6074	Onion, cooked w/salt, drained	0.5 cup	105	44	1	10	1	0	0	0.1
90472	Onion, yellow, fresh, small, whole	1 ea	70	28	1	7	1	0	0	0
90487	Onion, spring, tops & bulb, fresh, small, 3" long	1 ea	5	2	0	0	0	0	0	0
9548	Onion, sweet, fresh	1 oz	28	9	0	2	0	0		
9547	Onion, green, tops only, fresh, stalk	1 Tbs	6	2	0	0	0	0	0	0
5936	Parsnips, cooked w/salt, drained, slices	0.5 cup	78	55	1	13	3	0	0.1	0
5211	Parsnips, fresh, slices	0.5 cup	66.5	50	1	12	3	0	0.1	0
5281	Peas & carrots, canned, w/liquid	0.5 cup	127.5	48	3	11	3	0	0	0.2
6096	Pea pods, cooked w/salt, drained	1 cup	160	64	5	10	4	0	0	0.2
6836	Pea pods, fresh, chopped	1 cup	98	41	3	7	3	0	0	0.1
5938	Peas, green, cooked w/salt, drained	0.5 cup	80	67	4	13	4	0	0	0.1
5116	Peas, green, fresh	1 cup	145	117	8	21	7	1	0.1	0.3
9611	Peppers, green chili, canned	0.5 cup	69.5	15	1	3	1	0	0	0.1
7932	Peppers, jalapeno, fresh, sliced	1 cup	90	27	1	5	2	1	0	0.3
9632	Peppers, serrano, fresh	1 cup	105	34	2	7	3	0	0	0.2
90493	Peppers, bell, green, sweet, fresh, strips	10 pce	27	5	0	1	0	0	0	0
9549	Peppers, bell, green, sweet, sauteed	1 oz	28	36	0	1	1	3	0.7	1.7
6990	Peppers, bell, red, sweet, fresh, ring, 3" × 1/4" thick	1 ea	10	3	0	1	0	0	0	0
9551	Peppers, bell, red, sweet, sauteed	1 oz	28	37	0	2	1	4	0.6	1.6
9300	Peppers, bell, yellow, sweet, fresh, med	1 ea	119	32	1	8	1	0		
90589	Pickles, sweet, spear	1 ea	20	16	0	4	0	0	0	0
92209	Pickles, bread & butter	1 ea	8	6	0	2	0	0	0	0
5228	Pimentos, canned, slices	20 pce	20	5	0	1	0	0	0	0
9251	Potatoes, red, w/skin, baked, small, 1-3/4" to 2-1/2"	1 ea	138	123	3	27	2	0	0	0.1
9245	Potatoes, russet, w/skin, baked, small, 1-3/4" to 2-1/2"	1 ea	138	134	4	30	3	0	0	0.1
90564	Potatoes, peeled, cooked w/salt, large, 3" to 4-1/4"	1 ea	299.6	258	5	60	6	0	0	0.1
5950	Potatoes, skin, baked w/salt	1 ea	58	115	2	27	5	0	0	0
5964	Pumpkin, canned, w/salt	0.5 cup	122.5	42	1	10	4	0	0	0
90505	Radishes, fresh, small	10 ea	20	3	0	1	0	0	0	0
5969	Rutabaga, cooked w/salt, drained, mashed	0.5 cup	120	47	2	10	2	0	0	0.1
6859	Seaweed, oarweed, fresh, Laminaria spp.	0.5 cup	40	17	1	4	1	0	0	0
5260	Seaweed, spirulina, dried	0.5 cup	59.5	173	34	14	2	5	0.4	1.2
5427	Shallots, chopped, fresh	1 Tbs	10	7	0	2	0	0	0	0
9212	Silverbeet greens, cooked w/salt, drained, chopped	0.5 cup	87.5	18	2	4	2	0		
5972	Spinach, cooked w/salt, drained	0.5 cup	90	21	3	3	2	0	0	0.1
5149	Spinach, canned, drained	0.5 cup	107	25	3	4	3	1	0	0.2
5146	Spinach, fresh, chopped	1 cup	30	7	1	1	1	0	0	0
5982	Squash, acorn, baked w/salt, cubes	0.5 cup	102.5	57	1	15	5	0	0	0.1
5984	Squash, butternut, baked w/salt, cubes	0.5 cup	102.5	41	1	11	3	0	0	0

Sat (g)	Chol (mg)	Calc (mg)	Iron (mg)	Mag (mg)	Phos (mg)	Pota (mg)	Sodi (mg)	Zinc (mg)	Vit A (RAE)	Vit C (mg)	Thia (mg)	Ribo (mg)	Niac (mg)	Vit B$_6$ (mg)	Vit B$_{12}$ (µg)	Vit E (mg)	Fol (µg)	Alc (g)
0	0	7	0.19	2.8	6	49	2	0	58	4.8	0.01	0.01	0.06	0.01	0	0	27.2	0
0	0	7	0.17	2.6	6	39	6	0	74	3.6	0.01	0.02	0.08	0.02	0	0.1	7.6	0
		9	0.34	3.4	8	52	7	0.1	105	1	0.02	0.02	0.09	0.03		0	10.1	
0	0	0	0.2	2.7	18	63	3	0.1	0	0	0.02	0.05	0.74	0.02	0	0	4	0
0.1	0	4	0.64	20.3	42	170	348	1.9	0	0.4	0.05	0.25	2.17	0.23	0	0	30.4	0
0	0	5	0.11	2.5	34	125	2	0.3	0	0	0.03	0.14	1.06	0.03	0.03	0	3.9	0
0	0	5	0.37	7	31	61	200	0.3	0	0	0.04	0.01	0.75	0.03	0	0	5.6	0
0	0	2	0.17	3.1	36	136	2	0.2	0	0	0.02	0.13	1.26	0.03	0.01	0	6.2	0
0	0	52	0.49	10.5	29	141	176	0.1	221	17.7	0.03	0.04	0.3	0.07	0	0.8	51.1	0
0	0	58	0.82	17.9	24	198	14	0.1	294	39.2	0.04	0.06	0.45	0.1	0	1.1	104.7	0
0	0	62	0.22	28.8	26	108	193	0.3	11	13	0.11	0.04	0.7	0.15	0	0.2	36.8	0
0	0	23	0.25	11.6	37	174	251	0.2	0	5.5	0.04	0.02	0.17	0.14	0	0	15.8	0
0	0	16	0.15	7	20	102	3	0.1	0	5.2	0.03	0.02	0.08	0.08	0	0	13.3	0
0	0	4	0.07	1	2	14	1	0	2	0.9	0	0	0.03	0	0	0	3.2	0
	0	6	0.07	2.5	8	33	2	0	0	1.3	0.01	0.01	0.04	0.04		0	6.4	
0	0	4	0.12	1.2	2	16	0	0	12	2.7	0	0.01	0.01	0	0	0	0.8	0
0	0	29	0.45	22.6	54	286	192	0.2	0	10.1	0.06	0.04	0.56	0.07	0	0.8	45.2	0
0	0	24	0.39	19.3	47	249	7	0.4	0	11.3	0.06	0.03	0.47	0.06	0	1	44.6	0
0.1	0	29	0.96	17.8	59	128	332	0.7	368	8.4	0.09	0.07	0.74	0.11	0	0.2	23	0
0.1	0	67	3.15	41.6	88	384	384	0.6	83	76.6	0.2	0.12	0.86	0.23	0	0.6	46.4	0
0	0	42	2.04	23.5	52	196	4	0.3	53	58.8	0.15	0.08	0.59	0.16	0	0.4	41.2	0
0	0	22	1.23	31.2	94	217	191	1	32	11.4	0.21	0.12	1.62	0.17	0	0.1	50.4	0
0.1	0	36	2.13	47.8	157	354	7	1.8	55	58	0.39	0.19	3.03	0.25	0	0.2	94.2	0
0	0	25	0.92	2.8	8	79	276	0.1	4	23.8	0.01	0.02	0.44	0.08	0		37.5	0
0.1	0	9	0.63	17.1	28	194	1	0.2	36	39.9	0.13	0.05	1.01	0.46	0	0.4	42.3	0
0.1	0	12	0.9	23.1	42	320	10	0.3	49	47.1	0.06	0.09	1.61	0.53	0	0.7	24.2	0
0	0	3	0.09	2.7	5	47	1	0	5	21.7	0.02	0.01	0.13	0.06	0	0.1	2.7	0
0.4	0	2	0.08	2.2	4	38	5	0	4	49.6	0.01	0.01	0.16	0.05	0	0.4	0.6	0
0	0	1	0.04	1.2	3	21	0	0	16	12.8	0.01	0.01	0.1	0.03	0	0.2	4.6	0
0.4	0	2	0.13	3.4	6	54	6	0	39	45.6	0.02	0.03	0.27	0.1	0	0.9	0.6	0
0	0	13	0.55	14.3	29	252	2	0.2	12	218.4	0.03	0.03	1.06	0.2	0	0.8	30.9	0
0	0	12	0.05	1.4	4	20	91	0	8	0.1	0.01	0.01	0.02	0	0	0.1	0.2	0
0	0	3	0.03	0.2	2	16	54	0	1	0.7	0	0	0	0	0	0	0.3	0
0	0	1	0.34	1.2	3	32	3	0	27	17	0	0.01	0.12	0.04	0	0.1	1.2	0
0	0	12	0.97	38.6	99	752	17	0.6	1	17.4	0.1	0.07	2.2	0.29	0	0.1	37.3	0
0	0	25	1.48	41.4	98	759	19	0.5	1	17.8	0.09	0.07	1.86	0.49	0	0.1	35.9	0
0.1	0	24	0.93	59.9	120	983	722	0.8	0	22.2	0.29	0.06	3.93	0.81	0	0	27	0
0	0	20	4.08	24.9	59	332	149	0.3	1	7.8	0.07	0.06	1.78	0.36	0	0	12.8	0
0.2	0	32	1.7	28.2	43	252	295	0.2	953	5.1	0.03	0.07	0.45	0.07	0	1.3	14.7	0
0	0	5	0.07	2	4	47	8	0.1	0	3	0	0.01	0.05	0.01	0	0	5	0
0	0	58	0.64	27.6	67	391	305	0.4	0	22.6	0.1	0.05	0.86	0.12	0	0.4	18	0
0.1	0	67	1.14	48.4	17	36	93	0.5	2	1.2	0.02	0.06	0.19	0	0	0.3	72	0
1.6	0	71	16.96	116	70	811	624	1.2	17	6	1.42	2.18	7.63	0.22	0	3	55.9	0
0	0	4	0.12	2.1	6	33	1	0	6	0.8	0.01	0	0.02	0.03	0	0	3.4	0
	0	51	1.98	75.2	29	480	363	0.3	268	15.8	0.03	0.08	0.32	0.07	0	1.7	7.9	0
0	0	122	3.21	78.3	50	419	275	0.7	472	8.8	0.09	0.21	0.44	0.22	0	1.9	131.4	0
0.1	0	136	2.46	81.3	47	370	29	0.5	524	15.3	0.02	0.15	0.42	0.11	0	2.1	104.9	0
0	0	30	0.81	23.7	15	167	24	0.2	141	8.4	0.02	0.06	0.22	0.06	0	0.6	58.2	0
0	0	45	0.95	44.1	46	448	246	0.2	22	11.1	0.17	0.01	0.9	0.2	0	0.1	19.5	0
0	0	42	0.62	29.7	28	291	246	0.1	572	15.5	0.07	0.02	0.99	0.13	0	1.3	19.5	0

MDA Code	Food Name	Amt	Wt (g)	Ener (kcal)	Prot (g)	Carb (g)	Fiber (g)	Fat (g)	Mono (g)	Poly (g)
6922	Squash, spaghetti, cooked w/salt, drained	0.5 cup	77.5	21	1	5	1	0	0	0.1
5975	Squash, summer, all types, cooked w/salt, drained	0.5 cup	90	18	1	4	1	0	0	0.1
5981	Squash, winter, all types, baked w/salt, cubes	0.5 cup	102.5	40	1	9	3	1	0	0.3
5989	Succotash, cooked w/salt, drained	0.5 cup	96	107	5	23	5	1	0.1	0.4
6924	Sweet potatoes, dark orange, baked in skin w/salt	0.5 cup	100	90	2	21	3	0	0	0.1
5555	Sweet potatoes, dark orange, canned, w/syrup, drained	1 cup	196	212	3	50	6	1	0	0.3
5445	Tomatillo, fresh, medium	1 ea	34	11	0	2	1	0	0.1	0.1
5476	Tomato puree, canned	0.5 cup	125	48	2	11	2	0	0	0.1
5180	Tomato sauce, canned	0.5 cup	122.5	29	2	7	2	0	0	0.1
5474	Tomatoes, red, stewed, canned	0.5 cup	127.5	33	1	8	1	0	0	0.1
6887	Tomato, red, whole, w/tomato juice, canned	1 ea	190	32	1	8	2	0	0	0.1
90532	Tomato, red, fresh, year round avg, small/thin slices	1 pce	15	3	0	1	0	0	0	0
5447	Tomatoes, sun dried	10 pce	20	52	3	11	2	1	0.1	0.2
9299	Tomato, yellow, cherry, fresh	1 ea	17	3	0	1	0	0	0	0
6949	Tung sun, slices, cooked w/salt, drained, 1/2" slices	1 cup	120	13	2	2	1	0	0	0.1
6737	Tung sun, slices, fresh	1 cup	151	41	4	8	3	0	0	0.2
6004	Turnip greens, cooked w/salt, drained, chopped	0.5 cup	72	14	1	3	3	0	0	0.1
6002	Turnips, cooked w/salt, drained, mashed	0.5 cup	115	25	1	6	2	0	0	0
7955	Wasabi, root, fresh	1 ea	169	184	8	40	13	1		
5388	Water chestnuts, Chinese, canned, w/liquid	4 ea	28	14	0	3	1	0	0	0
5223	Watercress greens, fresh, sprig	10 ea	25	3	1	0	0	0	0	0
6010	Yams, tropical, cooked/baked w/salt, drained, cubes	0.5 cup	68	78	1	18	3	0	0	0
5306	Yams, tropical, fresh, cubes	0.5 cup	75	88	1	21	3	0	0	0.1
9197	Yuca, fresh	1 cup	206	330	3	78	4	1	0.2	0.1
90525	Zucchini, w/skin, fresh, small	1 ea	118	19	1	4	1	0	0	0.1
6921	Zucchini, w/skin, cooked w/salt, drained, mashed	0.5 cup	120	19	1	5	2	0	0	0
	Soy and Soy Products									
7503	Miso	1 Tbs	17.2	34	2	5	1	1	0.2	0.6
7508	Natto, fermented soybeans	1 cup	175	371	31	25	9	19	4.3	10.9
7564	Tempeh	0.5 cup	83	160	15	8		9	2.5	3.2
7015	Soybeans, mature, cooked	1 cup	172	298	29	17	10	15	3.4	8.7
7014	Soybeans, mature, dry	0.25 cup	46.5	193	17	14	4	9	2	5.2
4707	Soybeans, mature, roasted, salted	0.25 cup	43	203	15	14	8	11	2.4	6.2
7585	Soymeal, defatted, raw	0.5 cup	61	207	27	24		1	0.2	0.6
71584	Soy yogurt, peach/Silk	1 ea	170.1	170	4	32	1	2		
7542	Tofu, firm, silken, 1" slice/Mori-Nu	3 oz	85.1	53	6	2	0	2	0.5	1.3
7799	Tofu, firm, silken, light, 1" slice/Mori-Nu	3 oz	85.1	31	5	1	0	1	0.1	0.4
7541	Tofu, soft, silken, 1" slice/Mori-Nu	3 oz	85.1	47	4	2	0	2	0.4	1.3
7546	Tofu yogurt, tofu	1 cup	262	246	9	42	1	5	1	2.7
	MEALS AND DISHES									
	Homemade									
57482	Coleslaw	0.5 cup	60	47	1	7	1	2	0.4	0.8
56102	Falafel patty, 2-1/4"	1 ea	17	57	2	5		3	1.7	0.7
53125	Mole poblano	2 Tbs	30.3	50	1	4	1	3		
56005	Potato salad	0.5 cup	125	179	3	14	2	10	3.1	4.7
5786	Potatoes au gratin, w/butter	1 cup	245	323	12	28	4	19	5.3	0.7
56076	Spinach souffle	1 cup	136	233	11	8	1	18	4.1	0.8
92216	Tortellini pasta, cheese filled	1 cup	108	332	15	51	2	8	2.2	0.5
	Packaged or Canned Meals or Dishes									
57705	Egg noodles, w/creamy alfredo sauce, dry mix/Lipton	1 ea	124	518	19	77		15	4.8	1.5

Sat (g)	Chol (mg)	Calc (mg)	Iron (mg)	Mag (mg)	Phos (mg)	Pota (mg)	Sodi (mg)	Zinc (mg)	Vit A (RAE)	Vit C (mg)	Thia (mg)	Ribo (mg)	Niac (mg)	Vit B$_6$ (mg)	Vit B$_{12}$ (µg)	Vit E (mg)	Fol (µg)	Alc (g)
0	0	16	0.26	8.5	11	91	197	0.2	5	2.7	0.03	0.02	0.63	0.08	0	0.1	6.2	0
0.1	0	24	0.32	21.6	35	173	213	0.4	10	5	0.04	0.04	0.46	0.06	0	0.1	18	0
0.1	0	14	0.34	8.2	20	448	243	0.3	268	9.8	0.09	0.02	0.72	0.07	0	0.1	28.7	0
0.1	0	16	1.46	50.9	112	394	243	0.6	14	7.9	0.16	0.09	1.27	0.11	0	0.3	31.7	0
0.1	0	38	0.69	27	54	475	246	0.3	961	19.6	0.11	0.11	1.49	0.29	0	0.7	6	0
0.1	0	33	1.86	23.5	49	378	76	0.3	898	21.2	0.05	0.07	0.67	0.12	0	2.3	15.7	0
0	0	2	0.21	6.8	13	91	0	0.1	2	4	0.01	0.01	0.63	0.02	0	0.1	2.4	0
0	0	22	2.22	28.8	50	549	499	0.5	32	13.3	0.03	0.1	1.83	0.16	0	2.5	13.8	0
0	0	16	1.25	19.6	32	405	642	0.2	21	8.6	0.03	0.08	1.19	0.12	0	1.7	13.5	0
0	0	43	1.7	15.3	26	264	282	0.2	11	10.1	0.06	0.04	0.91	0.02	0	1.1	6.4	0
0	0	59	1.84	20.9	36	357	272	0.3	11	17.7	0.09	0.1	1.35	0.21	0	1.3	15.2	0
0	0	2	0.04	1.6	4	36	1	0	6	1.9	0.01	0	0.09	0.01	0	0.1	2.2	0
0.1	0	22	1.82	38.8	71	685	419	0.4	9	7.8	0.11	0.1	1.81	0.07	0	0	13.6	0
0	0	2	0.08	2	6	44	4	0	0	1.5	0.01	0.01	0.2	0.01	0		5.1	0
0.1	0	14	0.29	3.6	24	640	288	0.6	0	0	0.02	0.06	0.36	0.12	0	0.8	2.4	0
0.1	0	20	0.76	4.5	89	805	6	1.7	2	6	0.23	0.11	0.91	0.36	0	1.5	10.6	0
0	0	99	0.58	15.8	21	146	191	0.1	274	19.7	0.03	0.05	0.3	0.13	0	1.4	85	0
0	0	25	0.25	9.2	22	155	329	0.2	0	13.3	0.03	0.03	0.34	0.08	0	0	10.4	0
	0	216	1.74	116.6	135	960	29	2.7	3	70.8	0.22	0.19	1.26	0.46	0		30.4	0
0	0	1	0.24	1.4	5	33	2	0.1	0	0.4	0	0.01	0.1	0.04	0	0.1	1.7	0
0	0	30	0.05	5.2	15	82	10	0	59	10.8	0.02	0.03	0.05	0.03	0	0.2	2.2	0
0	0	10	0.35	12.2	33	456	166	0.1	4	8.2	0.06	0.02	0.38	0.16	0	0.3	10.9	0
0	0	13	0.41	15.8	41	612	7	0.2	5	12.8	0.08	0.02	0.41	0.22	0	0.3	17.2	0
0.2	0	33	0.56	43.3	56	558	29	0.7	2	42.4	0.18	0.1	1.76	0.18	0	0.4	55.6	0
0	0	18	0.41	20.1	45	309	12	0.3	12	20.1	0.06	0.17	0.57	0.26	0	0.1	34.2	0
0	0	16	0.42	26.4	48	304	287	0.2	67	5.5	0.05	0.05	0.51	0.09	0	0.1	20.4	0
0.2	0	10	0.43	8.3	27	36	641	0.4	1	0	0.02	0.04	0.16	0.03	0.01	0	3.3	0
2.8	0	380	15.05	201.2	304	1276	12	5.3	0	22.8	0.28	0.33	0	0.23	0	0	14	0
1.8	0	92	2.24	67.2	221	342	7	0.9	0	0	0.06	0.3	2.19	0.18	0.07	0	19.9	0
2.2	0	175	8.84	147.9	421	886	2	2	4	2.9	0.27	0.49	0.69	0.4	0	0.6	92.9	0
1.3	0	129	7.3	130.2	327	836	1	2.3	0	2.8	0.41	0.4	0.75	0.18	0	0.4	174.4	0
1.6	0	59	1.68	62.4	156	632	70	1.4	4	0.9	0.04	0.06	0.61	0.09	0	0.4	90.7	0
0.2	0	149	8.36	186.7	428	1519	2	3.1	1	0	0.42	0.15	1.58	0.35	0		184.8	0
0	0	500	0				20			0								0
0.3	0	27	0.88	23	77	165	31	0.5	0	0	0.09	0.03	0.21	0.01	0	0.2		0
0.1	0	31	0.64	8.5	69	54	72	0.3	0	0	0.03	0.02	0.09	0	0	0.1		0
0.3	0	26	0.7	24.7	53	153	4	0.4	0	0	0.09	0.03	0.26	0.01	0	0.2		0
0.7	0	309	2.78	104.8	100	123	92	0.8	5	6.6	0.16	0.05	0.63	0.05	0	0.8	15.7	0
0.2	5	27	0.35	6	19	109	14	0.1	32	19.6	0.04	0.04	0.16	0.08	0	0.1	16.2	0
0.4	0	9	0.58	13.9	33	99	50	0.3	0	0.3	0.02	0.03	0.18	0.02	0	0.2	15.8	0
	0	7	0.56	9.7	25	99	41	0.1	45	0	0.01	0	0.5	0.08	0.01	0.4	8.5	0
1.8	85	24	0.81	18.8	65	318	661	0.4	40	12.5	0.1	0.07	1.11	0.18	0	2.3	8.8	0
11.6	56	292	1.57	49	277	970	1061	1.7	157	24.3	0.16	0.28	2.43	0.43	0	0.5	27	0
8.3	160	224	1.62	40.8	192	318	770	1.2	325	9.9	0.11	0.36	0.66	0.13	0.53	1.3	99.3	0
3.9	45	164	1.62	22.7	229	96	372	1.1	41	0	0.34	0.33	2.91	0.05	0.17	0.2	79.9	0
5.7	139	157	3.74				2195											0

MDA Code	Food Name	Amt	Wt (g)	Ener (kcal)	Prot (g)	Carb (g)	Fiber (g)	Fat (g)	Mono (g)	Poly (g)
90098	Beef ravioli, w/tomato & meat sauce, canned, svg/Chef Boyardee	1 ea	244	224	8	33	1	7	2.7	0.3
25279	Beefaroni, w/tomato sauce, canned, svg/Chef Boyardee	1 ea	212.6	196	7	29	1	6	2.4	0.3
56976	Sweet Sue chicken & dumplings, canned/Bryan Foods	1 cup	240	218	15	23	3	7	3	1.6
57658	Chili con carne, w/beans, canned	1 cup	222	269	16	25	9	12	4.8	0.9
56001	Chili w/beans, canned	1 cup	256	287	15	30	11	14	6	0.9
57700	Chili w/o beans, canned/Hormel	1 cup	236	194	17	18	3	7	2.2	0.8
57703	Chili, vegetarian, w/beans, canned/Hormel	1 cup	247	205	12	38	10	1	0.1	0.4
50317	Chili w/beans, canned/Chef-Mate	1 cup	253	420	18	34	8	24	10.7	1.4
90738	Cheeseburger macaroni pasta/Hamburger Helper	1.5 oz	42.5	168	5	27		4		
57068	Macaroni & cheese, original, dry mix, svg/Kraft	1 ea	70	259	11	48	1	3		
90103	Mini beef ravioli, w/tomato sauce, canned, svg/Chef Boyardee	1 ea	252	232	8	31	3	8	3.4	0.4
90508	Sauerkraut, canned, drained	0.5 cup	71	13	1	3	2	0	0	0
47708	Spaghetti, w/meatballs & tomato sauce, canned/Chef Boyardee	1 ea	240	240	10	29	3	9	3.9	0.8
57484	Scalloped potatoes, from dry w/whole milk & butter	1 ea	822	764	17	105	9	35	10	1.6
42147	Stuffing, cornbread, from dry mix	0.5 cup	100	179	3	22	3	9	3.9	2.7
42037	Stuffing, plain, from dry mix	0.5 cup	100	177	3	22	3	9	3.8	2.6
57701	Turkey chili w/beans, canned/Hormel	1 cup	247	203	19	26	6	3	0.4	1.2
90739	Macaroni & cheese, whole wheat, dry mix, svg/Hodgson Mill	1 ea	70	263	10	48	5	3		
	Frozen Meals or Dishes									
50	Beef, sliced, w/gravy & vegetables/Freezer Queen	1 ea	255	207	15	26	4	5	1.2	1.7
70943	Beef & bean burrito, svg/Las Campanas	1 ea	114	296	9	38	1	12	5.5	0.8
70961	Beef & bean chimichanga/Fiesta Café	1 ea	227	422	24	56	6	12	3.9	3.5
70948	Beef enchilada & tamale, w/beans & rice/Patio	1 ea	376	508	14	68	8	20	7.7	2.7
11112	Beef macaroni, svg	1 ea	226.8	200	13	32	4	2	1.1	0.3
70893	Beef pot pie	1 ea	198	449	13	44	2	24	9.7	2.7
83051	Beef pot roast w/whipped potatoes, homestyle/Stouffer's	1 ea	255	184	13	21	3	5	2.6	1
83027	Beef stir fry w/rice, vegetables & sauce, svg/Tyson	1 ea	405	433	26	71		5		
57474	Beef stroganoff, w/peas & carrots/Marie Callender's	1 ea	368	420	25	40	7	18	5.5	4.1
56915	Broccoli w/cheese flavored sauce/Gardetto's	0.5 cup	84	56	2	7		2	0.8	0.2
56738	Cabbage, stuffed, w/whipped potato/Lean Cuisine	1 ea	269	196	11	24	4	6	3	0.9
16310	Chicken, French recipe, w/potato, vegetables, sauce/Budget Gourmet	1 ea	255	178	23	9	6	6	2.7	0.5
70949	Chicken, roasted, w/garlic sauce, pasta, vegetables/Tyson	1 ea	255	214	17	22	4	7	2.3	2.1
1746	Chicken, thigh, fried, w/mashed potatoes & corn/Banquet	1 ea	228	388	22	30	4	20	8.1	5.3
15974	Chicken & noodles, escalloped/Stouffer's	1 ea	283	419	17	31		25	7	12.3
16195	Chicken & vegetables w/vermicelli/Lean Cuisine	1 ea	297	232	20	26	4	5	1.8	1.1
15965	Chicken a l'orange w/broccoli & rice/Lean Cuisine	1 ea	255	268	24	39		2	0.5	0.4
83052	Chicken alfredo, fettuccine/Stouffer's Lunch Express	1 ea	272	373	19	33	4	18	6.3	2.4
16220	Chicken, BBQ glazed, w/sauce & vegetables/Weight Watchers	1 ea	209	217	19	26		4	1.6	1.1
83053	Chicken cacciatore, w/pasta & vegetables/Healthy Choice	1 ea	354	266	22	36	5	4	2.4	0.6
70945	Chicken cordon bleu, svg/Barber Food	1 ea	168	344	26	15		20	8.2	3.2
16198	Chicken enchilada w/rice & cheese sauce/Stouffer's	1 ea	283	424	15	61	4	13	2.7	0.9
83028	Chicken fajita kit, svg/Tyson	1 ea	107	128	7	17	2	4	1.1	1.6
70931	Chicken mesquite BBQ, w/corn & potato/Tyson	1 ea	255	321	18	45	4	8	2.7	0.5
70582	Chicken nuggets w/mac & cheese, corn, pudding	1 ea	257	457	19	51	7	20	7.9	4.9
70899	Chicken pot pie	1 ea	217	484	13	43	2	29	12.5	4.5
16266	Chicken teriyaki w/rice medley & broccoli/Healthy Choice	1 ea	312	250	16	36	9	5	1.7	1.4
6247	Creamed spinach/Stouffer's	0.5 cup	125	169	3	9	2	13	2.8	4.5
70918	Croissant Pockets chicken broccoli cheddar sandwich	1 ea	128	301	11	39	1	11	4.4	1.7
70895	Egg, scrambled, & sausage, w/hashbrowns	1 ea	177	361	13	17	1	27	12.7	3.6
90565	French fries, heated w/salt	10 ea	50	100	2	16	2	4	2.4	0.4

Sat (g)	Chol (mg)	Calc (mg)	Iron (mg)	Mag (mg)	Phos (mg)	Pota (mg)	Sodi (mg)	Zinc (mg)	Vit A (RAE)	Vit C (mg)	Thia (mg)	Ribo (mg)	Niac (mg)	Vit B$_6$ (mg)	Vit B$_{12}$ (µg)	Vit E (mg)	Fol (µg)	Alc (g)
2.8	7	27	1.63			354	910			0								0
2.5	6	23	1.42				793			0								0
1.8	36		2.57				946		0									0
3.9	29	84	5.79	64.4	215	608	941	2.3		3.1	0.12	0.22	2.16	0.28	1.44	0.3	57.7	0
6	44	120	8.78	115.2	394	934	1336	5.1	44	4.4	0.12	0.27	0.92	0.34	0	1.5	58.9	0
2.2	35	50	2.6	37.8		349	970	2.6		0								0
0.1	0	96	3.46	81.5		803	778	1.7		1.2								0
10.1	40	71	3.8	45.5	167	511	1280	3.9		0	0.11	0.2	3.48	0.23	1.44	1.2		0
1.2	4						863											0
1.3	10	92	2.56	40	265	296	561			0.4	0.67	0.41	4.54				65.1	0
3.5	8	30	2.57				935		50	0								0
0	0	21	1.04	9.2	14	121	469	0.1	1	10.4	0.01	0.02	0.1	0.09	0	0.1	17	0
3.8	17	26	1.97				864		0	1.4								0
21.6	90	296	3.12	115.1	460	1669	2803	2.1	288	27.1	0.16	0.46	8.46	0.35	0	1.2	82.2	0
1.8	0	26	0.94	13	34	62	455	0.2	78	0.8	0.12	0.09	1.25	0.04	0.01	0.9	97	0
1.7	0	32	1.09	12	42	74	543	0.3	118	0	0.14	0.11	1.48	0.04	0.01	1.4	39	0
0.7	35	116	3.46	69.2		682	1198	2.7		1.5								0
1	6	80	1.83				428											0
																		0
1.3	31						648		529									0
4.2	13		3.11				579		0									0
2.2	36		6.81				804		0	5.9								0
6.8	26	241	2.86				1812		30	4.9								0
0.6	14	43	2.56	34	127	345	420	1.2	52	54.9	0.26	0.15	2.94	0.18	0.11	1.6	99.8	0
8.5	38						737		51									0
1.4	20	71	1.58			895	768			3.3	0.18	0.15	3.03					0
							1584			25.1								0
7.2	63	77	2.06				1343			0								0
0.4		45	0.54			403		29.7										0
1.7	13	89	1.51		732	710		0.5	0.22	1			2.58					0
1.4	26						864	115										0
1.3	28		1.56				467											0
4.4	68	135	1.62				604			2.7								0
6	76	116	1.13		329	1211		0	0									0
1.9	30	163	1.43		692	633				2.7	0.27	0.24	6.62					0
0.4	46	20	0.36		430	360	1			18.1								0
7	57	147				588				24.2								0
1	48		1.09			405		0		21.5								0
1	32	53	2.23		255	750	552											0
5.7	81	144					754											0
7.4	51	300	2.18			243	855			4								0
0.9	12	21	1.13				368			20								0
2.6	26						793			0								0
5.6	57	85	2.78				843			0								0
9.7	41	33	2.06	23.9	119	256	857	1	256	1.5	0.25	0.36	4.13	0.2	0.15	3.8	41.2	0
1.6	22	31	0.59		225	424	596			43.7								0
3.7	16	141	1.06			245	335			5.9					0			0
3.4	37		3.8				652			6.3								0
7.3	283		1.66				772		0									0
0.6	0	4	0.62	11	41	209	133	0.2	0	5.1	0.06	0.01	1.04	0.15	0	0.1	6	0

MDA Code	Food Name	Amt	Wt (g)	Ener (kcal)	Prot (g)	Carb (g)	Fiber (g)	Fat (g)	Mono (g)	Poly (g)
56762	Green peppers, stuffed w/beef, w/tomato sauce/Stouffer's	0.5 ea	219.5	160	8	19	3	6	2.2	0.4
70917	Hot Pockets beef cheddar pocket sandwich	1 ea	142	403	16	39		20	6.7	1.2
70434	Italian sausage lasagne/The Budget Gourmet	1 ea	298	456	21	40	3	24	9.8	2
56757	Lasagna w/meat sauce, fzn, svg	1 ea	215	249	17	27	2	8	2.8	0.5
70921	Lean Pockets, chicken supreme	1 ea	128	233	10	34		6	2.5	1
11029	Macaroni, w/beef & tomato sauce/Lean Cuisine	1 ea	283	258	17	37	5	4	1.7	0.6
5587	Mashed potatoes, granules w/milk, prep w/water & margarine	0.5 cup	105	122	2	17	1	5	2.1	1.4
11107	Meatloaf w/sauce, potato, carrot/Banquet	1 ea	453	612	29	34	6	40	17.3	7.2
90491	Onion rings, breaded, pan-fried	1 cup	48	195	3	18	1	13	5.2	2.5
70898	Pizza, pepperoni, cooked, svg	1 ea	146	432	16	42	3	22	10	3.4
81146	Sausage w/biscuit sandwich/Jimmy Dean	1 ea	48	192	5	12	1	14		
70935	Salisbury steak w/red potato & vegetables/Budget Gourmet	1 ea	311	261	18	34	7	6	1.8	0.9
56703	Spaghetti, w/meat sauce/Lean Cuisine	1 ea	326	284	14	49	5	4	1.3	0.9
70960	Spaghetti w/meatballs & pomodoro sauce, low fat/Michelina's	1 ea	284	312	14	49	6	7	2.6	1.1
70959	Spinach, au gratin, frozen/The Budget Gourmet	1 ea	155	222	7	11	2	17		
70958	Stir fry rice & vegetables w/soy sauce/Hanover	1 cup	137	130	5	27	2	0		
11099	Swedish meatballs w/pasta/Lean Cuisine	1 ea	258	273	22	31	3	7	2.6	0.9
16930	Turkey, country roast, w/gravy mushroom & rice/Healthy Choice	1 ea	240	223	19	28	3	4	1.8	0.9
70892	Turkey pot pie	1 ea	397	699	26	70	4	35	13.7	5.5
16306	Turkey w/gravy, 5 oz pkg	1 ea	141.8	95	8	7	0	4	1.4	0.7
70936	Turkey w/gravy dressing & broccoli/Marie Callender's	1 ea	397	504	31	52		19	8.2	1.7
6999	Vegetables, mixed, from frozen w/salt, drained, 10 oz pkg	1 ea	275	165	8	36	12	0	0	0.2

SNACK FOODS AND GRANOLA BARS

MDA Code	Food Name	Amt	Wt (g)	Ener (kcal)	Prot (g)	Carb (g)	Fiber (g)	Fat (g)	Mono (g)	Poly (g)
3307	Banana chips	1 oz	28.4	147	1	17	2	10	0.6	0.2
10051	Beef jerky, large piece	1 ea	19.8	81	7	2	0	5	2.2	0.2
10052	Beef meat stick, smoked	1 ea	19.8	109	4	1		10	4.1	0.9
63331	Breakfast bar w/oats, raisins & coconut	1 ea	43	200	4	29	1	8	0.8	0.7
53227	Cereal bar, mixed berry/Kellogg's	1 ea	37	137	2	27	1	3	1.8	0.4
61251	Cheese puffs & twists, corn based, low fat	1 oz	28.4	123	2	21	3	3	1	1.6
44032	Chex snack mix, traditional	1 cup	42.5	181	5	28	2	7		
44034	Corn Nuts, BBQ	1 oz	28.4	124	3	20	2	4	2.1	0.9
44031	Corn Nuts, original	1 oz	28.4	127	2	20	2	4	2.7	0.9
44212	Fruit leather, bar	1 ea	23	81	0	18	1	1	0.1	0
11594	Fruit leather, berry, w/vitamin C/Fruit Roll-Ups	2 ea	28	104	0	24		1	0.5	0
44214	Fruit leather pieces, 0.75 oz package	1 ea	21.3	76	0	18	0	1	0.3	0.1
23404	Fruit leather, roll, large	1 ea	21	78	0	18	0	1	0.3	0.1
23103	Granola bar, peanut butter, hard	1 ea	23.6	114	2	15	1	6	1.7	2.9
23059	Granola bar, plain, hard	1 ea	24.5	115	2	16	1	5	1.1	3
23101	Granola bar, chocolate chip, hard	1 ea	23.6	103	2	17	1	4	0.6	0.3
23096	Granola bar, chocolate chip, chocolate coated, soft, 1.25 oz	1 ea	35.4	165	2	23	1	9	2.8	0.6
23107	Granola bar, nut & raisin, uncoated, soft	1 oz	28.4	129	2	18	2	6	1.2	1.6
23104	Granola bar, plain, uncoated, soft	1 ea	28.4	126	2	19	1	5	1.1	1.5
44036	Oriental mix, rice based	1 oz	28.4	144	5	15	4	7	2.8	3
44022	Popcorn cake	1 ea	10	38	1	8	0	0	0.1	0.1
44012	Popcorn, air popped	1 cup	8	31	1	6	1	0	0.1	0.2
44014	Popcorn, caramel coated, w/o peanuts	1 oz	28.4	122	1	22	1	4	0.8	1.3
44038	Popcorn, cheese flavored	1 cup	11	58	1	6	1	4	1.1	1.7
44066	Popcorn, low fat, low sodium, microwave	1 cup	8	34	1	6	1	1	0.3	0.3
44013	Popcorn, oil popped, microwaved	1 cup	11	64	1	5	1	5	1.1	2.6
61252	Popcorn, sugar syrup/caramel, fat free	1 cup	37.3	142	1	34	1	1	0.1	0.2

Sat (g)	Chol (mg)	Calc (mg)	Iron (mg)	Mag (mg)	Phos (mg)	Pota (mg)	Sodi (mg)	Zinc (mg)	Vit A (RAE)	Vit C (mg)	Thia (mg)	Ribo (mg)	Niac (mg)	Vit B$_6$ (mg)	Vit B$_{12}$ (µg)	Vit E (mg)	Fol (µg)	Alc (g)
2.2	18	37	1.49			347	623			25.7	0.13	0.11	1.4					0
8.8	53	337	2.93				906		0									0
8.2	48	316	2.68				903											0
4.1	28	148	1.31			340	671			1.3	0.13	0.11	1.38					0
1.9	23	122					562		38									0
1.7	17	85	1.78			773	569			2.3	0.2	0.08	3.28					0
1.3	2	36	0.21	21	67	165	180	0.3	49	6.8	0.09	0.09	0.91	0.17	0.11	0.5	8.4	0
15.5	113	77	3.94				1943			7.7								0
4.1	0	15	0.81	9.1	39	62	180	0.2	5	0.7	0.13	0.07	1.73	0.04	0	0.3	31.7	0
7.1	22	220	3.52	35	302	289	902	2.2	0	2.8	0.33	0.34	3.61	0.14	0.83	1.6	68.6	0
4.3	16	38	0.79				441											0
2	44		3.05				494		72	51								0
1.1	13	101	2.38			574	548			2.9	0.33	0.2	3.88					0
2.2	14		2.93				1011		26	8.8								0
7.6	42	243	1.95				654			27.1								0
							636			16.3								0
2.8	49	114	2.58	43.9	206	560	614	3.7	0	0	0.23	0.28	4.21	0.31	1.01	0.3	31.9	0
1.2	26	22	1.03				437											0
11.4	64		3.97				1390		351									0
1.2	26	20	1.32	11.3	115	86	786	1	18	0	0.03	0.18	2.55	0.14	0.34	0.5	5.7	0
9.1	79	131	4.37				2037			23.8								0
0.1	0	69	2.25	60.5	140	465	745	1.3	588	8.8	0.2	0.33	2.34	0.2	0	1.2	52.2	0
8.2	0	5	0.36	21.6	16	152	2	0.2	1	1.8	0.02	0	0.2	0.07	0	0.1	4	0
2.1	10	4	1.07	10.1	81	118	438	1.6	0	0	0.03	0.03	0.34	0.04	0.2	0.1	26.5	0
4.1	26	13	0.67	4.2	36	51	293	0.5	3	1.3	0.03	0.09	0.9	0.04	0.2	0.1	0	0
5.5	0	26	1.37	43.4	119	140	120	0.7	3	0.4	0.12	0.05	0.75	0.15	0	0.4	34.8	0
0.6	0	14	1.81	9.6	36	70	110	1.5		0	0.37	0.41	5	0.52	0	0	40	0
0.6	0	101	0.36	11.6	101	81	365	0.6	12	6.1	0.15	0.17	2.03	0.2	0.61	1.2	27.5	0
2.4	0	15	10.5	26.8	79	114	432	0.9	3	20.2	0.66	0.21	7.16	0.66	5.27	0.1	21.2	0
0.7	0	5	0.48	31	80	81	277	0.5	5	0.1	0.1	0.04	0.43	0.05	0	0.3	0	0
0.7	0	3	0.47	32.1	78	79	156	0.5	0	0	0.01	0.04	0.48	0.07	0	0.6	0	0
0.9	0	7	0.18	5.1	13	32	18	0	1	16.1	0.01	0.01	0.02	0.07	0	0.1	0.9	0
0.3	0						89			33.6								0
0.1	0	4	0.16	3	5	35	86	0	1	11.9	0.01	0.02	0.02	0.06	0	0.1	0.9	0
0.1	0	7	0.21	4.2	7	62	67	0	1	25.2	0.02	0	0.02	0.06	0	0.1	0.4	0
0.8	0	10	0.57	13	33	69	67	0.3	0	0	0.05	0.02	0.46	0.02	0	0.3	4.2	0
0.6	0	15	0.72	23.8	68	82	72	0.5	2	0.2	0.06	0.03	0.39	0.02	0	0.3	5.6	0
2.7	0	18	0.72	17	48	59	81	0.5	0	0	0.04	0.02	0.13	0.01	0	0.2	3.1	0
5	2	36	0.82	23.4	70	111	71	0.5	2	0	0.03	0.09	0.25	0.04	0.2	0.4	9.2	0
2.7	0	24	0.62	25.8	68	111	72	0.5	1	0	0.05	0.05	0.74	0.03	0.07	0.3	8.5	0
2.1	0	30	0.73	21	65	92	79	0.4	0	0	0.08	0.05	0.15	0.03	0.11	0.3	6.8	0
1.1	0	15	0.69	33.5	74	93	117	0.8	0	0.1	0.09	0.04	0.88	0.02	0	1.6	10.8	0
0	0	1	0.19	15.9	28	33	29	0.4	0	0	0.01	0.02	0.6	0.02	0	0	1.8	0
0	0	1	0.26	11.5	29	26	1	0.2	1	0	0.01	0.01	0.18	0.01	0	0	2.5	0
1	1	12	0.49	9.9	24	31	59	0.2	1	0	0.02	0.02	0.62	0.01	0	0.3	1.4	0
0.7	1	12	0.25	10	40	29	98	0.2	4	0.1	0.01	0.03	0.16	0.03	0.06	0	1.2	0
0.1	0	1	0.18	12.1	21	19	39	0.3	1	0	0.03	0.01	0.17	0.01	0	0.4	1.4	0
0.8	0	0	0.22	8.7	22	20	116	0.3	1	0	0.01	0.01	0.13	0.01	0	0.3	2.8	0
0.1	0	7	0.3	10.1	21	41	107	0.2	1	0	0.01	0.02	0.13	0.02	0	0	1.5	0

MDA Code	Food Name	Amt	Wt (g)	Ener (kcal)	Prot (g)	Carb (g)	Fiber (g)	Fat (g)	Mono (g)	Poly (g)
12080	Pork skins, plain	1 oz	28	153	17	0	0	9	4.1	1
61249	Potato chips, fat free, w/olestra	1 oz	28	77	2	17	2	0	0	0.1
44043	Potato chips, reduced fat	1 oz	28.4	134	2	19	2	6	1.4	3.1
44076	Potato chips, unsalted, plain	1 oz	28.4	152	2	15	1	10	2.8	3.5
5437	Potato chips, sour cream & onion	1 oz	28.4	151	2	15	1	10	1.7	4.9
61257	Potato chips, reduced fat, unsalted	1 oz	28.4	138	2	19	2	6	1.4	3.1
44015	Pretzels, hard	5 pce	30	114	3	24	1	1	0.4	0.2
44079	Pretzels, hard, unsalted, w/enriched flour	10 ea	60	229	5	48	2	2	0.8	0.7
61182	Pretzels, soft, medium	1 ea	115	389	9	80	2	4	1.2	1.1
44053	Rice cake, brown rice & sesame seed	2 ea	18	71	1	15	1	1	0.2	0.2
44021	Rice cake, brown rice, plain	1 ea	9	35	1	7	0	0	0.1	0.1
44020	Taro chips	1 oz	28.4	141	1	19	2	7	1.3	3.7
44058	Trail mix, regular	0.25 cup	37.5	173	5	17	2	11	4.7	3.6
44059	Trail mix, w/chocolate chips, salted nuts & seeds	0.25 cup	36.2	175	5	16	2	12	4.9	4.1

SOUPS

MDA Code	Food Name	Amt	Wt (g)	Ener (kcal)	Prot (g)	Carb (g)	Fiber (g)	Fat (g)	Mono (g)	Poly (g)
92160	Bean & ham, canned, reduced sodium, prepared w/water	0.5 cup	128	95	5	17	5	1	0.5	0.3
50151	Bean & bacon, dehydrated, prepared w/water	1 cup	265	106	5	16	9	2	0.9	0.2
92192	Beef & mushroom, canned, chunky, low sodium	1 cup	251	173	11	24	1	6	1	0.2
50398	Beef barley, canned, ready-to-serve/Progresso	1 cup	241	142	11	20	3	2	0.7	0.3
50198	Beef mushroom, canned, prepared w/water	1 cup	244	73	6	6	0	3	1.2	0.1
57659	Beef stew, canned, serving	1 ea	232	220	11	16	3	12	5.5	0.5
50155	Cauliflower, dehydrated, prepared w/water	1 cup	256.1	69	3	11		2	0.7	0.6
50077	Chicken gumbo, canned, prepared w/water	1 cup	244	56	3	8	2	1	0.7	0.3
50080	Chicken mushroom, canned, prepared w/water	1 cup	244	132	4	9	0	9	4	2.3
50081	Chicken noodle, canned, chunky, ready-to-serve	1 cup	240	175	13	17	4	6	2.7	1.5
50085	Chicken rice, canned, chunky, ready-to-serve	1 cup	240	127	12	13	1	3	1.4	0.7
50088	Chicken vegetable, canned, chunky, ready-to-serve	1 cup	240	166	12	19	0	5	2.2	1
90238	Chicken, canned, chunky	1 cup	240	170	12	17	1	6	2.8	1.3
50021	Clam chowder, Manhattan style, canned, prepared w/water	1 cup	244	78	2	12	1	2	0.4	1.3
50402	Cream of broccoli, canned/Progresso Healthy Classics	1 cup	244	88	2	13	2	3	0.9	0.6
50016	Cream of celery, canned, prepared w/water	1 cup	244	90	2	9	1	6	1.3	2.5
50049	Cream of mushroom, canned, prepared w/water	1 cup	244	129	2	9	0	9	1.7	4.2
50197	Cream of potato, canned, prepared w/water	1 cup	244	73	2	11	0	2	0.6	0.4
50697	Cup of Noodles, ramen noodle soup, chicken flavor, dry	1 ea	64	296	6	37		14		
50050	Green pea, canned, prepared w/water	1 cup	250	165	9	27	5	3	1	0.4
50009	Minestrone, canned, prepared w/water	1 cup	241	82	4	11	1	3	0.7	1.1
92163	Ramen noodle soup, any flavor, dry	0.5 cup	38	172	4	25	1	6	2.4	1
50690	Shark fin soup, restaurant prepared	1 cup	216	99	7	8	0	4	1.3	0.7
50025	Split pea soup, w/ham, canned, prepared w/water	1 cup	253	190	10	28	2	4	1.8	0.6
50689	Stock, fish, homemade	1 cup	233	40	5	0	0	2	0.5	0.3
50043	Tomato vegetable, from dry mix, w/water	1 cup	253	56	2	10	1	1	0.3	0.1
50028	Tomato, canned, prepared w/water	1 cup	244	85	2	17	0	2	0.4	1
50014	Vegetable beef, canned, prepared w/water	1 cup	244	78	6	10	0	2	0.8	0.1
92189	Vegetable chicken, low sodium	1 cup	241	166	12	21	1	5	2.2	1
7559	Vegetarian stew	1 cup	247	304	42	17	3	7	1.8	3.8
50013	Vegetable, vegetarian, canned, prepared w/water	1 cup	241	72	2	12	0	2	0.8	0.7

BABY FOODS

MDA Code	Food Name	Amt	Wt (g)	Ener (kcal)	Prot (g)	Carb (g)	Fiber (g)	Fat (g)	Mono (g)	Poly (g)
61234	Infant cereal, brown rice, instant	1 Tbs	3.7	15	0	3	0	0	0	0
60619	Infant cereal, rice, dry	1 Tbs	2.5	10	0	2	0	0	0	0.1
60844	Infant cookie, banana/Gerber	1 ea	8	34	1	6	0	1		

Sat (g)	Chol (mg)	Calc (mg)	Iron (mg)	Mag (mg)	Phos (mg)	Pota (mg)	Sodi (mg)	Zinc (mg)	Vit A (RAE)	Vit C (mg)	Thia (mg)	Ribo (mg)	Niac (mg)	Vit B$_6$ (mg)	Vit B$_{12}$ (µg)	Vit E (mg)	Fol (µg)	Alc (g)
3.2	27	8	0.25	3.1	24	36	515	0.2	3	0.1	0.03	0.08	0.43	0.01	0.18	0.1	0	0
0.1	0	10	0.67	19.3	49	325	155	1	0	7.9	0.09	0.01	1.22	0.04	0	0	23.2	0
1.2	0	6	0.38	25.3	55	495	140	0	0	7.3	0.06	0.08	1.99	0.19	0	1.6	7.7	0
3.1	0	7	0.46	19	47	362	2	0.3	0	8.8	0.05	0.06	1.09	0.19	0	2.6	12.8	0
2.5	2	20	0.45	21	50	378	178	0.3	4	10.6	0.05	0.06	1.14	0.19	0.28	1.4	17.6	0
1.2	0	6	0.38	25.3	55	495	2	0.3	0	7.3	0.06	0.08	1.99	0.19	0	1.6	2.8	0
0.1	0	5	1.56	8.7	34	41	407	0.4	0	0	0.15	0.1	1.54	0.01	0	0.1	55.8	0
0.4	0	22	2.59	21	68	88	173	0.5	0	0	0.28	0.37	3.15	0.07	0	0.2	102.6	0
0.8	3	26	4.51	24.2	91	101	1615	1.1	0	0	0.47	0.33	4.91	0.02	0	0.6	27.6	0
0.1	0	2	0.28	24.5	68	52	41	0.5	0	0.5	0.01	0.02	1.3	0.03	0	0	3.2	0
0.1	0	1	0.13	11.8	32	26	29	0.3	0	0	0.01	0.01	0.7	0.01	0	0.1	1.9	0
1.8	0	17	0.34	23.9	37	214	97	0.1	2	1.4	0.05	0.01	0.15	0.12	0	3.2	5.7	0
2.1	0	29	1.14	59.2	129	257	86	1.2	0	0.5	0.17	0.07	1.77	0.11	0	1.3	26.6	0
2.2	1	39	1.23	58.3	140	235	44	1.1	1	0.5	0.15	0.08	1.59	0.09	0	3.9	23.5	0
0.3	3	49	1.31	24.3	17	202	239	0.7	45	1.4	0.07	0.04	0.41	0.06	0.04	0.5	37.1	0
1	3	56	1.32	29.2	90	326	928	0.7	3	1.1	0.05	0.27	0.4	0.03	0.03	0.6	8	0
4.1	15	33	2.43	5	126	351	63	2.8	246	7.5	0.1	0.28	2.84	0.15	0.65	0.6	12.6	0
0.7	19	29	1.86	31.3	118	366	470	1.5		3.6	0.13	0.13	2.92	0.19	0.36	0.3	24.1	0
1.5	7	5	0.88	9.8	34	154	942	1.5	0	4.6	0.04	0.06	0.95	0.05	0.2		9.8	0
5.2	37	28	1.65	32.5	128	404	947	1.9	204	10.2	0.17	0.14	2.86	0.3	0.86	0.3	25.5	0
0.3	0	10	0.51	2.6	51	105	843	0.3	0	2.6	0.08	0.08	0.51	0.03	0.18		2.6	0
0.3	5	24	0.9	4.9	24	76	954	0.4	7	4.9	0.02	0.05	0.66	0.06	0.02	0.4	4.9	0
2.4	10	29	0.88	9.8	27	154	942	1	56	0	0.02	0.11	1.63	0.05	0.05	1.2	0	0
1.4	19	24	1.44	9.6	72	108	850	1	67	0	0.07	0.17	4.32	0.05	0.31	0.3	38.4	0
1	12	34	1.87	9.6	72	108	888	1	293	3.8	0.02	0.1	4.1	0.05	0.31	0.6	4.8	0
1.4	17	26	1.46	9.6	106	367	1068	2.2	300	5.5	0.04	0.17	3.29	0.1	0.24	0.1	12	0
1.9	29	24	1.66	7.2	108	168	850	1	65	1.2	0.08	0.17	4.22	0.05	0.24	0.3	4.8	0
0.4	2	27	1.63	12.2	41	188	578	1	56	3.9	0.03	0.04	0.82	0.1	4.05	0.3	9.8	0
0.7	5	41	1.22	14.6	39	161	578	0.3		5.9	0.03	0.06	0.32	0.07	0	0.4	29.3	0
1.4	15	39	0.63	7.3	37	122	949	0.1	56	0.2	0.03	0.05	0.33	0.01	0.24	0.9	2.4	0
2.4	2	46	0.51	4.9	49	100	881	0.6	15	1	0.05	0.09	0.72	0.01	0.05	1	4.9	0
1.2	5	20	0.49	2.4	46	137	1000	0.6	71	0	0.03	0.04	0.54	0.04	0.05	0	2.4	0
6.3			2.18				1434		20									0
1.4	0	28	1.95	40	125	190	918	1.7	10	1.7	0.11	0.07	1.24	0.05	0	0.4	2.5	0
0.6	2	34	0.92	7.2	55	313	911	0.7	118	1.2	0.05	0.04	0.94	0.1	0	0.1	36.2	0
2.9	0	6	1.62	9.1	41	46	441	0.2	0	0	0.25	0.17	2.05	0.02	0	0.8	55.9	0
1.1	4	22	2.03	15.1	45	114	1082	1.8	0	0.2	0.06	0.08	1.06	0.06	0.41	6.9	19.4	0
1.8	8	23	2.28	48.1	213	400	1007	1.3	23	1.5	0.15	0.08	1.47	0.07	0.25	0.2	2.5	0
0.5	2	7	0.02	16.3	130	336	363	0.1	5	0.2	0.08	0.18	2.76	0.09	1.61	0.4	4.7	0
0.4	0	8	0.63	20.2	30	104	1146	0.2	10	6.1	0.06	0.05	0.79	0.05	0	0.4	10.1	0
0.4	0	12	1.76	7.3	34	264	695	0.2	24	66.4	0.09	0.05	1.42	0.11	0	2.3	14.6	0
0.9	5	17	1.12	4.9	41	173	791	1.5	95	2.4	0.04	0.05	1.03	0.08	0.32	0.4	9.8	0
1.4	17	27	1.47	9.6	106	369	84	2.2	333	5.5	0.05	0.17	3.3	0.1	0.24	0.7	43.4	0
1.2	0	77	3.21	313.7	543	296	988	2.7	116	0	1.73	1.48	29.64	2.72	5.43	1.2	254.4	0
0.3	0	22	1.08	7.2	34	210	822	0.5	116	1.4	0.05	0.05	0.92	0.06	0	0.4	9.6	0
0	0	2	1.76	1	10	14	0	0	0	0	0.03	0.01	0.59	0.04	0	0	0.6	0
0	0	21	1.19	5.2	15	10	1	0	0	0.1	0.07	0.06	0.78	0.01	0	0.1	0.6	0
0.2		120	3	2.8	14	33	1	2.4	122	0.1	0.03	0.03	1.35	0.02		2		0

MDA Code	Food Name	Amt	Wt (g)	Ener (kcal)	Prot (g)	Carb (g)	Fiber (g)	Fat (g)	Mono (g)	Poly (g)
60419	Infant dessert, apricot tapioca—Nature's Goodness	6.25 Tbs	100	66	0	16	0	0		
60192	Infant dessert, vanilla custard pudding/3rd Foods	1 ea	170	163	4	31		3		
60778	Infant dinner, beef & carrots, strained/Heinz	1 ea	113.4	64	4	4	2	4		
60871	Infant dinner, broccoli chicken, strained	1 ea	113.4	48	4	4	2	2	0.6	0.4
60793	Infant vegetable, peas, strained/Nature's Goodness	1 ea	113.4	65	5	11	4	0		
62354	Infant formula, Lactofree, w/iron/Mead Johnson	0.125 cup	30.5	19	0	2	0	1	0.4	0.2
60135	Infant formula, low iron/Similac	1 fl-oz	31	20	0	2	0	1	0.4	0.2
60299	Infant formula, soy, w/iron/Isomil	1 fl-oz	30.5	20	0	2	0	1	0.4	0.3
62586	Child formula, soy, preppowder/Enfamil	1 fl-oz	30.5	20	1	2	0	1	0.3	0.2

DESSERTS, CANDIES, AND PASTRIES

Brownies and Fudge

MDA Code	Food Name	Amt	Wt (g)	Ener (kcal)	Prot (g)	Carb (g)	Fiber (g)	Fat (g)	Mono (g)	Poly (g)
62904	Brownie, square, large, 2-3/4" × 7/8"	1 ea	56	227	3	36	1	9	5	1.3
47019	Brownie, homemade, 2" square	1 ea	24	112	1	12	1	7	2.6	2.3
23127	Fudge, chocolate marshmallow, w/nuts, homemade	1 pce	22	104	1	15	0	5	1.2	0.9
23026	Fudge, chocolate, w/nuts, homemade	1 pce	19	88	1	13	0	4	0.7	1.4
23025	Fudge, chocolate, homemade	1 pce	17	70	0	13	0	2	0.5	0

Cakes, Pies, and Donuts

MDA Code	Food Name	Amt	Wt (g)	Ener (kcal)	Prot (g)	Carb (g)	Fiber (g)	Fat (g)	Mono (g)	Poly (g)
46062	Cake, chocolate, homemade, w/o frosting, 9"	1 pce	95	340	5	51	2	14	5.7	2.6
46092	Coffee cake, w/cheese, 1/6 of 16 oz	1 pce	76	258	5	34	1	12	5.4	1.3
46096	Coffee cake, creme filled, w/chocolate frosting, 1/6 of 19 oz	1 pce	90	298	4	48	2	10	5.1	1.3
46003	Cake, white, w/coconut frosting, homemade, 1/12 of 9"	1 pce	112	399	5	71	1	12	4.1	2.4
46085	Cake, white, w/o frosting, homemade, 9"	1 pce	74	264	4	42	1	9	3.9	2.3
46091	Cake, yellow, w/o frosting, homemade, 8"	1 pce	68	245	4	36	0	10	4.2	2.4
49001	Cheesecake, no bake, from dry mix, 1/12 of 9"	1 pce	99	271	5	35	2	13	4.5	0.8
46426	Cupcake, chocolate, w/frosting, low fat	1 ea	43	131	2	29	2	2	0.8	0.2
46011	Cupcake, snack, chocolate, w/frosting & cream filling	1 ea	50	200	2	30	2	8	4.3	0.9
42721	Ding Dongs, w/cream filling/Hostess	1 ea	80	368	3	45	2	19	4	1.2
71338	Doughnut, chocolate, glazed/sugared, 3-3/4"	1 ea	60	250	3	34	1	12	6.8	1.5
71337	Doughnut, w/chocolate icing, large, 3-1/2"	1 ea	57	258	3	29	1	14	4.9	1.1
45525	Doughnut, glazed/sugared, medium, 3"	1 ea	45	192	2	23	1	10	5.7	1.3
71335	Doughnut holes	1 ea	14	59	1	6	0	3	1.8	0.4
45527	Doughnut, French crullers, glazed, 3"	1 ea	41	169	1	24	0	8	4.3	0.9
45563	Doughnut, creme filled, 3-1/2" oval	1 ea	85	307	5	26	1	21	10.3	2.6
46000	Gingerbread, homemade, 1/9 of 8" square	1 pce	74	263	3	36	1	12	5.3	3.1
46001	Sponge cake, 1/12 of 16 oz	1 pce	38	110	2	23	0	1	0.4	0.2
48044	Pie filling, pumpkin, canned	0.5 cup	135	140	1	36	11	0	0	0

Candy

MDA Code	Food Name	Amt	Wt (g)	Ener (kcal)	Prot (g)	Carb (g)	Fiber (g)	Fat (g)	Mono (g)	Poly (g)
51150	Candied fruit	1 oz	28.4	91	0	23	0	0	0	0
23074	Candy, hard, dietetic/low calorie	1 pce	3	11	0	3	0	0	0	0
4148	Candy, Bit O Honey/Nestle	6 pce	40	150	1	32	0	3	0.4	0.1
23115	Candy, butterscotch	5 pce	30	117	0	27	0	1	0.3	0
23015	Candy, caramels	1 pce	10.1	39	0	8	0	1	0.2	0.4
92202	Candy, caramel, w/nuts, chocolate covered	1 ea	14	66	1	8	1	3	1.3	0.8
90671	Candy, jellybeans, large	10 ea	28.4	106	0	27	0	0		
90690	Candy, M & M's milk chocolate peanut, 1.67-oz pkg	1 ea	47.3	244	5	29	2	12	3.8	1.6
90691	Candy, M & M's milk chocolate, 1.48-oz box	1 ea	42	207	2	30	1	9	1.4	0.2
92212	Candy, milk chocolate covered coffee beans	1 oz	28.4	146	2	18	2	7	1.7	0.2
23419	Candy, milk chocolate covered peanuts	10 pce	40	208	5	20	2	13	5.2	1.7
23022	Candy, milk chocolate covered raisins	1.5 oz	42.5	166	2	29	2	6	2	0.2
90682	Candy, milk chocolate w/almonds, 1.55-oz bar	1 ea	43.9	231	4	23	3	15	5.9	1

Sat (g)	Chol (mg)	Calc (mg)	Iron (mg)	Mag (mg)	Phos (mg)	Pota (mg)	Sodi (mg)	Zinc (mg)	Vit A (RAE)	Vit C (mg)	Thia (mg)	Ribo (mg)	Niac (mg)	Vit B6 (mg)	Vit B12 (µg)	Vit E (mg)	Fol (µg)	Alc (g)
0		9	0.25		6	63	9	0		61.6	0.02	0.01	0.14	0.01				0
		95	0.51	9.9	114	112	42	0.7			0.03	0.15	0.12	0.05				0
		27	0.54		39	164	16			0.3	0.02	0.05	0.83	0.08				0
0.5	7	46	0.65	13.6	67	192	22	0.7	26	21.5	0.02	0.1	0.88	0.1	0.01	1	51	0
0.1		22	1		78	136	2		23	0	0.11	0.09	1.35					0
0.5	0	16	0.36	1.5	11	22	6	0.2	18	2.4	0.02	0.03	0.2	0.01	0.06	0.3	3.4	0
0.4	1	16	0.04	1.2	9	21	5	0.2	18	1.8	0.02	0.03	0.21	0.01	0.05	0.4	3.1	0
0.4	0	21	0.36	1.5	15	22	9	0.1	18	1.8	0.01	0.02	0.27	0.01	0.09	0.4	3	0
0.4	0	39	0.4	2.1	26	24	7	0.2	18	2.4	0.02	0.02	0.2	0.01	0.06	0.3	3.4	0
2.4	10	16	1.26	17.4	57	83	175	0.4	11	0	0.14	0.12	0.96	0.02	0.04	0.1	26.3	0
1.8	18	14	0.44	12.7	32	42	82	0.2	42	0.1	0.03	0.05	0.24	0.02	0.04	0.7	7	0
2.3	5	11	0.24	10.1	19	37	17	0.2	15	0.1	0.01	0.02	0.05	0.01	0.01	0.2	2.4	0
1.1	2	10	0.37	10.4	21	34	8	0.3	7	0	0.01	0.02	0.06	0.02	0.01	0	3	0
1	2	8	0.3	6.1	12	22	8	0.2	7	0	0	0.01	0.03	0	0.02	0	0.7	0
5.2	55	57	1.53	30.4	101	133	299	0.7	38	0.2	0.13	0.2	1.08	0.04	0.15	1.5	25.6	0
4.1	65	45	0.49	11.4	77	220	258	0.4	65	0.1	0.08	0.1	0.52	0.04	0.26	1.2	29.6	0
2.5	62	34	0.46	13.5	68	70	291	0.4	33	0.1	0.07	0.07	0.76	0.04	0.18	1.6	36.9	0
4.4	1	101	1.3	13.4	78	111	318	0.4	14	0.1	0.14	0.21	1.19	0.03	0.07	0.1	34.7	0
2.4	1	96	1.12	8.9	69	70	242	0.2	11	0.1	0.14	0.18	1.13	0.02	0.06	0.1	28.1	0
2.7	37	99	1.12	8.2	80	62	233	0.3	27	0.1	0.12	0.16	0.99	0.02	0.11	0.8	23.1	0
6.6	29	170	0.47	18.8	232	209	376	0.5	95	0.5	0.12	0.26	0.49	0.05	0.31	1.1	29.7	0
0.5	0	15	0.66	10.8	79	96	178	0.2	0	0	0.02	0.06	0.31	0	0	0.8	6.4	0
2.4	0	58	1.8	18	44	88	194	0.5	0	0.9	0.02	0.04	0.46	0.07	0.03	0.5	13	0
11	14	3	1.84				241											0
3.1	34	128	1.36	20.4	97	64	204	0.3	7	0.1	0.03	0.04	0.28	0.02	0.06	0.1	27	0
7.7	11	14	2.28	17.1	120	115	235	0.6	2	0.7	0.09	0.07	0.91	0.01	0.06	1.2	37	0
2.7	14	27	0.48	7.6	53	46	181	0.2	1	0	0.1	0.09	0.68	0.01	0.11	0.4	20.7	0
1	1	4	0.42	2.2	37	16	78	0.1	0	0.2	0.03	0.02	0.28	0	0.01	0.3	11.2	0
1.9	5	11	0.99	4.9	50	32	141	0.1	1	0	0.07	0.09	0.87	0.01	0.02	0.1	17.2	0
4.6	20	21	1.56	17	65	68	263	0.7	10	0	0.29	0.13	1.91	0.06	0.12	0.2	59.5	0
3.1	24	53	2.13	51.8	40	325	242	0.3	10	0.1	0.14	0.12	1.29	0.14	0.04	1.8	24.4	0
0.3	39	27	1.03	4.2	52	38	93	0.2	17	0	0.09	0.1	0.73	0.02	0.09	0.1	17.9	0
0.1	0	50	1.43	21.6	61	186	281	0.4	560	4.7	0.02	0.16	0.5	0.21	0	1.1	47.2	0
0	0	5	0.05	1.1	1	16	28	0	0	0	0	0	0	0	0	0	0	0
0	0	0	0	0	0	0	0	0	0	0	0	0	0	0	0	0	0	0
2.2	0	14	0.08	2.8	11	18	118	0.2	0	0.3	0.02	0.02	0.03	0	0.02	0.1	0.8	0
0.6	3	1	0	0	0	1	117	0	8	0	0	0	0	0	0	0	0	0
0.3	1	14	0.01	1.7	12	22	25	0	1	0	0.01	0.03	0.01	0.01	0.03	0	0.4	0
0.7	0	11	0.24	11.3	23	62	3	0.3	6	0.2	0.01	0.02	0.67	0.02	0	0.2	12.9	0
	0	1	0.04	0.6	1	11	14	0	0	0	0	0	0	0	0	0	0	0
4.8	4	48	0.55	32.6	90	164	24	0.8	10	0	0.03	0.05	1.59	0.04	0.15	1.3	26	0
5.5	6	44	0.47	18.9	62	112	26	0.6	24	0.2	0.03	0.09	0.12	0.01	0.18	0.6	3.4	0
3.5	6	48	0.65	18.2	53	117	20	0.5	12	0	0.03	0.09	0.09	0.01	0.15	0.5	2.8	0
5.8	4	42	0.52	38.4	85	201	16	1	14	0	0.05	0.07	1.7	0.08	0.18	1.4	3.2	0
3.7	1	37	0.73	19.1	61	218	15	0.3	10	0.1	0.04	0.07	0.17	0.03	0.08	0.4	3	0
7.5	8	98	0.72	39.5	116	195	32	0.6	19	0.1	0.03	0.19	0.33	0.02	0.14	2	6.1	0

MDA Code	Food Name	Amt	Wt (g)	Ener (kcal)	Prot (g)	Carb (g)	Fiber (g)	Fat (g)	Mono (g)	Poly (g)
91509	Candy, milk chocolate, w/almonds, bites/Hershey's Bites	17 pce	39	214	4	20	1	14	5.6	0.9
92201	Candy, nougat w/almonds	1 ea	14	56	0	13	0	0	0	0
23081	Candy, peanut brittle, homemade	1.5 oz	42.5	207	3	30	1	8	3.4	1.9
90698	Candy, Rolo, caramels in milk chocolate, 1.74-oz roll	1 ea	49.3	234	3	33	0	10	1	0.1
23142	Candy, sesame crunch	20 pce	35	181	4	18	3	12	4.4	5.1
90702	Candy, Starburst, fruit chews, original	1 oz	28.4	116	0	23	0	2	0	0
92198	Candy, Twizzlers strawberry twists	4 pce	45	158	1	36	0	1		
90661	Candy, York peppermint patty, small, .6 oz	1 ea	17	65	0	14	0	1	0.1	0
90681	Candy bar, milk chocolate, mini	1 ea	7	37	1	4	0	2	0.9	0.1
90685	Candy bar, milk chocolate, w/crisped rice, mini	1 ea	10	50	1	6	0	3	0.9	0.1
23145	Candy bar, sweet chocolate, 1.45-oz bar	1 ea	41.1	208	2	24	2	14	4.6	0.4
90704	Candy bar, 3 Musketeers, 0.8-oz bar	1 ea	22.7	97	1	18	0	3	0.5	0.1
23405	Candy bar, Almond Joy, fun size, .7 oz	1 ea	19.8	95	1	12	1	5	1	0.2
90679	Candy bar, Baby Ruth, 2.28-oz bar	1 ea	64.6	297	3	42	1	14	3.6	1.7
90653	Candy bar, Butterfinger, 1.6-oz bar	1 ea	45.4	208	2	33	1	9	2.3	1.4
23116	Candy bar, Caramello, 1.6-oz bar	1 ea	45.4	210	3	29	1	10	2.4	0.3
23060	Candy bar, Kit Kat, 1.5-oz bar	1 ea	42.5	220	3	27	0	11	2.5	0.4
23061	Candy bar, Krackel, 1.5-oz bar	1 ea	42.5	218	3	27	1	11	2.7	0.2
23037	Candy bar, Mars almond, 1.76-oz bar	1 ea	50	234	4	31	1	12	5.3	2
90688	Candy bar, Milky Way, 2.05-oz bar	1 ea	58.1	263	2	41	1	10	1.3	0.2
23062	Candy bar, Mr. Goodbar, 1.75-oz bar	1 ea	49.6	267	5	27	2	16	4.1	2.2
23135	Candy bar, Oh Henry!, 2-oz bar	1 ea	56.7	262	4	37	1	13	3.1	1.5
23036	Candy bar, Skor, toffee bar, 1.4-oz bar	1 ea	39.7	212	1	25	1	13	3.7	0.5
23057	Candy bar, Special Dark, sweet chocolate, 1.45-oz bar	1 ea	41.1	218	2	24	3	13	2.1	0.2
23149	Candy bar, Twix, caramel, 2-oz pkg	1 ea	56.7	285	3	37	1	14	1.2	0.2
90712	Chewing gum, small pieces	10 pce	16	40	0	11	0	0	0	0
	Cookies									
47026	Animal crackers	10 ea	12.5	56	1	9	0	2	1	0.2
90636	Chocolate chip cookie, enriched, higher fat, large 3.5" to 4"	1 ea	40	196	2	26	1	10	5.3	0.6
47037	Chocolate chip cookie, homemade w/butter, 2-1/4"	2 ea	32	156	2	19	1	9	2.6	1.5
47032	Chocolate chip cookie, lower fat	3 ea	30	136	2	22	1	5	1.8	1.4
47001	Chocolate chip cookie, soft	2 ea	30	137	1	18	1	7	3.9	1
43527	Chocolate coated graham crackers, 2-1/2" square	2 ea	28	136	2	19	1	6	2.2	0.3
47006	Chocolate sandwich cookie, creme filled	3 ea	30	140	2	21	1	6	3.2	0.7
47042	Coconut macaroon, homemade, 2"	1 ea	24	97	1	17	0	3	0.1	0
62905	Fig bar	1 ea	56.7	197	2	40	3	4	1.7	1.6
47043	Fortune cookie	3 ea	24	91	1	20	0	1	0.3	0.1
90638	Gingersnap, large, 3-1/2" to 4"	1 ea	32	133	2	25	1	3	1.7	0.4
71272	Graham crackers, cinnamon, small rectangle pieces	4 ea	14	59	1	11	0	1	0.6	0.5
45787	Little Debbie Nutty Bars wafer, w/peanut butter, chocolate covered	1 ea	57	312	5	31		19		
90639	Molasses cookie, large, 3-1/2" to 4"	1 ea	32	138	2	24	0	4	2.3	0.6
47706	Molasses cookie, home style/Archway	1 ea	26	105	1	18	0	3	1.3	0.3
90640	Oatmeal cookie, big, 3-1/2" to 4"	1 ea	25	112	2	17	1	5	2.5	0.6
47003	Oatmeal raisin cookie, homemade, 2-5/8"	1 ea	15	65	1	10	0	2	1	0.8
47010	Peanut butter cookie, homemade, 3"	1 ea	20	95	2	12	0	5	2.2	1.4
47549	Peanut butter cookie, home style/Archway	1 ea	21	101	2	12	1	5	2.1	0.9
47059	Peanut butter sandwich cookie	2 ea	28	134	2	18	1	6	3.1	1.1
47062	Shortbread pecan cookie, 2"	2 ea	28	152	1	16	1	9	5.2	1.2
47007	Shortbread cookie, plain, 1-5/8" square	4 ea	32	161	2	21	1	8	4.3	1
47559	Sugar cookie, home style/Archway	1 ea	24	99	1	17	0	3	1.2	0.3

Sat (g)	Chol (mg)	Calc (mg)	Iron (mg)	Mag (mg)	Phos (mg)	Pota (mg)	Sodi (mg)	Zinc (mg)	Vit A (RAE)	Vit C (mg)	Thia (mg)	Ribo (mg)	Niac (mg)	Vit B$_6$ (mg)	Vit B$_{12}$ (µg)	Vit E (mg)	Fol (µg)	Alc (g)
6.8	7	86	0.58	23	89	184	29	0.5		0.7	0.03	0.15	0.24	0.03			0.2	6.2	0
0.2	0	4	0.08	4.5	8	15	5	0.1	0	0	0	0.02	0.07	0		0	0.4	0.7	0
1.8	5	11	0.52	17.8	45	71	189	0.4	17	0	0.06	0.02	1.12	0.03		0	1.1	19.6	0
7.2	6	71	0.21	0	35	93	93	0	17	0.4	0.01	0.06	0.02	0	0.16	0.5	0	0	
1.6	0	229	1.49	87.8	148	113	58	1.3	0	0	0.19	0.06	1.3	0.19		0	0.1	18.2	0
2.2	0	0	0	0.3	1	1	1	0		16.7	0	0	0	0		0	0.1	0.3	0
0	0	0	0.23				129		0	0									0
0.7	0	2	0.16	10.7	0	19	5	0.1		0	0.01	0.02	0.14			0	0	0	0
1	2	13	0.16	4.4	15	26	6	0.1	3	0	0.01	0.02	0.03	0		0.04	0.1	0.8	0
1.6	2	17	0.08	4.9	19	34	14	0.1	6	0	0.01	0.03	0.05	0.01		0.06	0.2	1.5	0
8.3	0	10	1.13	46.4	60	119	7	0.6	0	0	0.01	0.1	0.28	0.02		0	0.1	1.2	0
2	1	12	0.15	6.6	16	30	44	0.1	5	0	0.01	0.01	0.05	0		0.04	0.2	0.9	0
3.5	1	13	0.25	13.1	22	50	28	0.2		0.1	0.01	0.03	0.09	0.01		0.02	0		0
7.8	0	30	0.41	27.8	61	161	149	0.5	0	0	0.04	0.08	0.81	0.03		0.04	0.6	7.8	0
4.3	0	16	0.36	21.8	44	100	104	0.5	0	0	0.05	0.03	1.2	0.03		0.02	0.8	12.7	0
5.8	12	97	0.49	19.1	68	155	55	0.4		0.8	0.02	0.18	0.52	0.02		0.29	0.1		0
7.6	5	53	0.42	15.7	57	98	23	0	10	0	0.05	0.09	0.21	0.01		0.24	0.1	6	0
6.8	5	67	0.45	5.5	52	138	83	0.2		0.3	0.02	0.08	0.11	0.02		0.25	0	2.6	0
3.6	8	84	0.55	36	117	162	85	0.6	8	0.3	0.02	0.16	0.47	0.03		0.18	3.9	4.5	0
7	5	67	0.28	11.6	39	72	97	0.4	19	0.4	0.03	0.06	0.09	0.01		0.1	0.5	2.3	0
7	5	55	0.69	23.3	81	195	20	0.5	17	0.4	0.07	0.07	1.71	0.03		0.16	1.6	18.8	0
5.4	4	39	0.28	28.9	79	147	109	0.7	0	0	0.08	0.07	1.44	0.05		0.11	1.3	24.9	0
7.5	21	52	0.23	4	24	61	126	0.1		0.2	0.01	0.04	0.05	0.01		0.11	0	1.2	0
	2	12	0.88	12.7	21	206	2	0	0	0	0	0	0	0		0.1	0	0	0
10.8	4	60	0.46	15.3	60	105	112	0.5	12	0.3	0.09	0.12	0.63	0.01		0.16	0.7	14.7	0
0	0	0	0	0	0	0	0	0	0	0	0	0	0	0	0	0	0	0	0
0.4	0	5	0.34	2.2	14	12	49	0.1	0	0	0.04	0.04	0.43	0		0.01	0	12.9	0
3.1	0	14	1.43	19.2	46	59	119	0.3	0	0	0.1	0.09	0.96	0.02		0	0.6	25.2	0
4.5	22	12	0.79	17.6	32	71	109	0.3	44	0.1	0.06	0.06	0.44	0.03		0.03	0.3	10.6	0
1.1	0	6	0.92	8.4	25	37	113	0.2	0	0	0.09	0.08	0.83	0.08		0	0.5	21	0
2.2	0	4	0.72	10.5	15	28	98	0.1	0	0	0.03	0.06	0.49	0.05		0	0.9	11.7	0
3.7	0	16	1	16.2	38	59	81	0.3	1	0	0.04	0.06	0.61	0.02		0	0.1	5.6	0
1.1	0	6	1.18	14.4	28	56	145	0.3	0	0	0.05	0.04	0.8	0		0.01	0.5	15.9	0
2.7	0	2	0.18	5	10	37	59	0.2	0	0	0	0.03	0.03	0.02		0.01	0	1	0
0.6	0	36	1.64	15.3	35	117	198	0.2	5	0.2	0.09	0.12	1.06	0.04		0.05	0.4	19.8	0
0.2	0	3	0.35	1.7	8	10	66	0	0	0	0.04	0.03	0.44	0		0	0	15.8	0
0.8	0	25	2.05	15.7	27	111	209	0.2	0	0	0.06	0.09	1.04	0.03		0	0.3	27.8	0
0.2	0	3	0.52	4.2	15	19	85	0.1	0	0	0.03	0.04	0.58	0.01		0	0	6.4	0
3.6							127			1.1									0
1	0	24	2.06	16.6	30	111	147	0.1	0	0	0.11	0.08	0.97	0.03		0	0	28.5	0
0.7	6	8	1.22			30	150			0	0.08	0.06	0.7					17.9	0
1.1	0	9	0.64	8.2	34	36	96	0.2	1	0.1	0.07	0.06	0.56	0.02		0	0.1	14.8	0
0.5	5	15	0.4	6.3	24	36	81	0.1	21	0.1	0.04	0.02	0.19	0.01		0.01	0.4	4.5	0
0.9	6	8	0.45	7.8	23	46	104	0.2	27	0	0.04	0.04	0.7	0.02		0.02	0.8	11	0
1.1	8	7	0.57			44	85			0	0.05	0.04	0.92						0
1.4	0	15	0.73	13.7	53	54	103	0.3	0	0	0.09	0.07	1.05	0.04		0.06	0.5	17.1	0
2.3	9	8	0.68	5	24	20	79	0.2	0	0	0.08	0.06	0.69	0.01		0	1.1	17.6	0
2	6	11	0.88	5.4	35	32	146	0.2	6	0	0.11	0.11	1.07	0.03		0.03	0.1	22.4	0
0.7	4	6	0.59			21	154			0	0.08	0.06	0.62					18.7	0

MDA Code	Food Name	Amt	Wt (g)	Ener (kcal)	Prot (g)	Carb (g)	Fiber (g)	Fat (g)	Mono (g)	Poly (g)
47690	Sugar cookie, fat free, home style/Archway	1 ea	20	71	1	17	0	0	0	0.1
62907	Sugar cookie, from refrigerated dough, pre-sliced	1 ea	23	111	1	15	0	5	3	0.7
90642	Sugar wafer cookie, creme filled, small, 2-1/2" × 3/4" × 1/4"	1 ea	3.5	18	0	2	0	1	0.4	0.3
90643	Vanilla sandwich cookie, creme filled, oval 3-1/8" × 1-1/4"	2 ea	30	145	1	22	0	6	2.5	2.3
47072	Vanilla wafer, higher fat	4 ea	24	114	1	17	0	5	2.7	0.6
	Custards, Gelatin, and Puddings									
2622	Custard, egg, from dry mix w/2% milk	0.5 cup	133	148	5	23	0	4	1.1	0.3
2613	Custard, egg, from dry mix w/whole milk	0.5 cup	133	161	5	23	0	5	1.6	0.3
57896	Custard, flan, dry mix, serving	1 ea	21	73	0	19	0	0	0	0
23052	Gelatin dessert, from dry mix w/water	0.5 cup	135	84	2	19	0	0	0	0
23360	Gelatin dessert, Jell-O, strawberry, sugar free, low calorie w/aspartame, dry mix serving	1 ea	2.5	8	1	0	0	0		
2632	Pudding, banana, ready-to-eat, 5 oz can	1 ea	141.8	180	3	30	0	5	2.2	1.9
57894	Pudding, chocolate, ready-to-eat, snack can	1 ea	113.4	158	3	26	1	5	1.9	1.6
2612	Pudding, vanilla, ready-to-eat, snack can	1 ea	113.4	147	3	25	0	4	1.7	0.5
2764	Pudding, Jell-O, vanilla, fat free, snack cup	1 ea	113	104	2	23	0	0		
2757	Pudding, Jell-O, vanilla, sugar free, reduced calorie, instant, serving	1 ea	8	26	0	6	0	0		
2651	Pudding, rice, ready-to-eat, 5 oz can	1 ea	141.8	231	3	31	0	11	4.6	4
57902	Pudding, tapioca, ready-to-eat, snack can	1 ea	113.4	135	2	22	0	4	2.6	0.4
	Ice Cream and Frozen Desserts									
71819	Frozen yogurt, chocolate, nonfat, w/artificial sweetener	1 cup	186	199	8	37	2	1	0.4	0.1
72124	Frozen yogurt, all flavors, not chocolate	1 cup	174	221	5	38	0	6	1.7	0.2
49111	Ice cream cone, wafer/cake type, large	1 ea	29	121	2	23	1	2	0.5	0.9
49014	Ice cream cone, sugar, rolled type	1 ea	10	40	1	8	0	0	0.1	0.1
52152	Ice cream bar, Eskimo Pie, vanilla, dark chocolate coated	1 ea	50	166	2	12		12		
2010	Ice cream, vanilla, light, soft serve	0.5 cup	88	111	4	19	0	2	0.7	0.1
90723	Popsicle, 2 fl oz bar	1 ea	59	47	0	11	0	0	0	0
	Pastries									
45788	Apple turnover, frozen/Pepperidge Farm	1 ea	89	284	4	31	2	16		
42264	Cinnamon rolls, w/icing, refrigerated dough/Pillsbury	1 ea	44	145	2	23	0	5		
45675	Éclair shell, homemade, 5" × 2" × 1-3/4"	1 ea	48	174	4	11	0	12	5.3	3.5
71299	Croissant, butter, large	1 ea	67	272	5	31	2	14	3.7	0.7
71301	Croissant, cheese, large	1 ea	67	277	6	31	2	14	4.4	1.6
45572	Danish, cheese	1 ea	71	266	6	26	1	16	8	1.8
71330	Danish, cinnamon nut, 15 oz ring	1 pce	53.2	229	4	24	1	13	7.3	2.3
70913	Crust, pie, Nilla, ready to use/Nabisco	1 ea	28	144	1	18	0	8	5.2	0.4
49015	Strudel, apple	1 pce	71	195	2	29	2	8	2.3	3.8
42164	Sweet roll, cheese	1 ea	66	238	5	29	1	12	6	1.3
42166	Sweet roll, cinnamon, frosted, from refrigerated dough	1 ea	30	109	2	17	1	4	2.2	0.5
71367	Sweet roll, cinnamon raisin, large	1 ea	83	309	5	42	2	14	4	6.2
45683	Toaster pastry, brown sugar & cinnamon	1 ea	50	206	3	34	0	7	4	0.9
45593	Toaster pastry, Pop Tarts, apple cinnamon	1 ea	52	205	2	37	1	5	3.1	1.4
45763	Toaster pastry, Pop Tarts, apple cinnamon, frosted, low fat	1 ea	52	191	2	40	1	3	1.5	0.8
45768	Toaster pastry, Pop Tarts, chocolate fudge, frosted, low fat	1 ea	52	190	3	40	1	3	1.2	0.9
45601	Toaster pastry, Pop Tarts, chocolate fudge, frosted	1 ea	52	201	3	37	1	5	2.7	1.1
	Toppings and Frostings									
23000	Apple butter	1 Tbs	18	31	0	8	0	0	0	0
23070	Caramel topping	2 Tbs	41	103	1	27	0	0	0	0
23014	Chocolate fudge topping	2 Tbs	38	133	2	24	1	3	1.5	0.1
46039	Cream cheese frosting, 16 oz can	1 oz	28.4	118	0	19	0	5	1.1	1.7

Sat (g)	Chol (mg)	Calc (mg)	Iron (mg)	Mag (mg)	Phos (mg)	Pota (mg)	Sodi (mg)	Zinc (mg)	Vit A (RAE)	Vit C (mg)	Thia (mg)	Ribo (mg)	Niac (mg)	Vit B$_6$ (mg)	Vit B$_{12}$ (µg)	Vit E (mg)	Fol (µg)	Alc (g)
0.1	0	3	0.44			12	80		0	0	0.06	0.04	0.5				15.2	0
1.4	7	21	0.42	1.8	43	37	108	0.1	3	0	0.04	0.03	0.55	0.01	0.02	0	16.1	0
0.1	0	1	0.07	0.4	2	2	5	0	0	0	0	0.01	0.09	0	0	0.1	1.8	0
0.9	0	8	0.66	4.2	22	27	105	0.1	0	0	0.08	0.07	0.81	0.01	0	0.5	15	0
1.2	0	6	0.53	2.9	15	26	73	0.1	0	0	0.09	0.05	0.71	0.01	0.01	0.3	10.3	0
1.8	64	193	0.47	25.3	184	298	118	0.7	81	1.1	0.07	0.28	0.17	0.09	0.6	0.3	12	0
2.8	70	190	0.47	25.3	181	294	117	0.7	49	1.1	0.07	0.28	0.17	0.09	0.59	0.1	12	0
0	0	5	0.02	0	0	32	91	0	0	0	0	0	0	0	0	0	0	0
0	0	4	0.03	1.4	30	1	101	0	0	0	0	0.01	0	0	0	0	1.4	0
0	0	1	0.03		34	0	57		0	0								0
0.8	0	121	0.18	11.3	98	156	278	0.4	9	0.7	0.03	0.21	0.23	0.03	0.26	0	2.8	0
0.8	3	102	0.58	23.8	91	204	146	0.5	12	2	0.03	0.18	0.39	0.03	0	0.3	3.4	0
1.7	8	100	0.15	9.1	77	128	153	0.3	7	0	0.02	0.16	0.29	0.01	0.11	0	0	0
0.2	2	86	0.05		115	123	241			0.3								0
0	0	12	0.01		189	2	332		0	0								0
1.7	1	74	0.43	11.3	96	85	121	0.7	35	0.7	0.03	0.1	0.23	0.04	0.3	2	4.3	0
1.1	1	95	0.26	9.1	90	109	180	0.3	0	0.8	0.02	0.11	0.35	0.02	0.24	0.3	3.4	0
0.9	7	296	0.07	74.4	240	631	151	0.9	4	1.3	0.07	0.33	0.37	0.07	0.91	0.1	22.3	0
4	23	174	0.8	17.4	155	271	110	0.5	85	1.2	0.07	0.31	0.12	0.07	0.12	0.2	7	0
0.4	0	7	1.04	7.5	28	32	41	0.2	0	0	0.07	0.1	1.28	0.01	0	0.2	50.2	0
0.1	0	4	0.44	3.1	10	14	32	0.1	0	0	0.05	0.04	0.51	0.01	0	0	14	0
7.2	14	60					34											0
1.4	11	138	0.05	12.3	106	194	62	0.5	26	0.8	0.05	0.17	0.1	0.04	0.44	0.1	4.4	0
0	0	0	0.32	0.6	0	9	4	0.1	0	0.4	0	0	0	0	0	0	0	0
4			1.22				176			0								0
1.5	0		0.72				340											0
2.7	94	17	0.97	5.8	57	47	267	0.4	133	0	0.1	0.17	0.75	0.04	0.19	1.3	25.4	0
7.8	45	25	1.36	10.7	70	79	498	0.5	138	0.1	0.26	0.16	1.47	0.04	0.11	0.6	59	0
7.1	38	36	1.44	16.1	87	88	372	0.6	137	0.1	0.35	0.22	1.45	0.05	0.21	1	49.6	0
4.8	11	25	1.14	10.6	77	70	320	0.5	25	0.1	0.13	0.18	1.42	0.03	0.12	0.2	42.6	0
3.1	24	50	0.96	17	59	51	193	0.5	5	0.9	0.12	0.13	1.22	0.06	0.11	0.4	44.2	0
1.4	3	11	0.5	2.2	23	19	63	0.1			0.05	0.05	0.7	0.01	0.03		8.4	0
1.5	4	11	0.3	6.4	23	106	191	0.1	5	1.2	0.03	0.02	0.23	0.03	0.16	1	19.9	0
4	50	78	0.5	12.5	65	90	236	0.4		0.1	0.1	0.09	0.55	0.05	0.2	1.3	28.4	0
1	0	10	0.8	3.6	104	19	250	0.1	0	0.1	0.12	0.07	1.09	0.01	0.02	0.5	16.5	0
2.6	55	60	1.33	14.1	63	92	318	0.5	51	1.7	0.27	0.22	1.98	0.09	0.12	1.7	59.8	0
1.8	0	17	2.02	12	66	57	212	0.3	148	0.1	0.19	0.29	2.29	0.21	0.11	0.9	14.5	0
0.9	0	12	1.82	5.7	28	47	174	0.3		0	0.15	0.17	1.98	0.2	0	0	41.6	0
0.6	0	6	1.82	4.7	21	28	206	0.2		0	0.16	0.16	1.98	0.21	0	0	52	0
0.5	0	14	1.82	14.6	40	62	249	0.3		0	0.16	0.16	1.98	0.21	0	0	52	0
1	0	20	1.82	15.1	44	82	203	0.3		0	0.16	0.16	1.98	0.21	0	0	52	0
0	0	3	0.06	0.9	1	16	3	0	0	0.2	0	0	0.01	0.01	0	0	0.2	0
0	0	22	0.08	2.9	19	34	143	0.1	11	0.1	0	0.04	0.02	0.01	0.04	0	0.8	0
1.5	1	38	0.6	24.3	64	171	131	0.3	2	0	0.03	0.11	0.14	0.03	0.11	0.9	1.9	0
1.3	0	1	0.05	0.6	1	10	54	0	0	0	0	0	0	0	0	1.2	0	0

MDA Code	Food Name	Amt	Wt (g)	Ener (kcal)	Prot (g)	Carb (g)	Fiber (g)	Fat (g)	Mono (g)	Poly (g)
54334	Hazelnut spread, chocolate flavored	1 oz	28	151	2	17	2	8	4.6	1.9
23164	Strawberry topping	2 Tbs	42.5	108	0	28	0	0	0	0
510	Whipped cream, pressurized	2 Tbs	7.5	19	0	1	0	2	0.5	0.1
514	Whipped topping, pressurized	2 Tbs	8.8	23	0	1	0	2	0.2	0
508	Whipped topping, semi-solid, frozen	2 Tbs	9.4	30	0	2	0	2	0.2	0
54387	Whipped topping, low fat, frozen	2 Tbs	9.4	21	0	2	0	1	0.1	0
FATS AND OILS										
44469	Butter, light, salted	1 Tbs	13	65	0	0	0	7	2.1	0.3
44470	Butter, light, unsalted	1 Tbs	13	65	0	0	0	7	2.1	0.3
44952	Butter, salted, organic	1 Tbs	14	100	0	0	0	11		
90210	Butter, unsalted, stick	1 Tbs	14	100	0	0	0	11	2.9	0.4
90209	Butter, salted, whipped, stick	1 Tbs	9.4	67	0	0	0	8	2.2	0.3
8003	Fat, bacon grease	1 tsp	4.3	39	0	0	0	4	1.9	0.5
8005	Fat, chicken	1 Tbs	12.8	115	0	0	0	13	5.7	2.7
8107	Fat, lard	1 Tbs	12.8	115	0	0	0	13	5.8	1.4
8135	Margarine & butter, blend, w/soybean oil	1 Tbs	14.2	101	0	0	0	11	4.3	3.4
44476	Margarine, 80% fat, tub	1 Tbs	14.2	102	0	0	0	11	5.1	4
8067	Oil, fish, cod liver	1 Tbs	13.6	123	0	0	0	14	6.4	3.1
8084	Oil, canola	1 Tbs	14	124	0	0	0	14	8.2	4.1
8008	Oil, olive, salad or cooking	1 Tbs	13.5	119	0	0	0	14	9.8	1.4
8111	Oil, safflower, salad or cooking, greater than 70% oleic	1 Tbs	13.6	120	0	0	0	14	10.2	2
8027	Oil, sesame, salad or cooking	1 Tbs	13.6	120	0	0	0	14	5.4	5.7
44483	Shortening, household, vegetable	1 Tbs	12.8	113	0	0	0	13	5.3	3.6
8007	Shortening, household, hydrogenated soybean & cottonseed oil	1 Tbs	12.8	113	0	0	0	13	5.7	3.3
CONDIMENTS, SAUCES, AND SYRUPS										
53382	Sauce, barbecue, hickory smoke/Kraft	2 Tbs	34	39	0	9	0	0		
1708	Sauce, barbecue, original/Bull's Eye	2 Tbs	36	63	0	15		0		
27001	Catsup	1 ea	6	6	0	2	0	0	0	0
53523	Cheese sauce, ready-to-serve	0.25 cup	63	110	4	4	0	8	2.4	1.6
54388	Cream substitute, light, powder	1 Tbs	5.9	25	0	4	0	1	0.7	0
63334	Dietetic syrup	1 Tbs	15	6	0	7	0	0	0	0
53636	Enchilada sauce/La Victoria	0.25 cup	60.3	20	0	3	0	1		
53474	Fish sauce	2 Tbs	36	13	2	1	0	0	0	0
50939	Gravy, brown, homestyle, savory, canned/Heinz	0.25 cup	60	25	1	3		1	0.3	0
53472	Hoisin sauce	2 Tbs	32	70	1	14	1	1	0.3	0.5
9533	Hollandaise sauce, w/butter fat, from dehydrated w/water, packet	1 ea	204	188	4	11	1	16	4.7	0.7
27004	Horseradish	1 tsp	5	2	0	1	0	0	0	0
92174	Hot sauce, chili, from immature green peppers	1 Tbs	15	3	0	1	0	0	0	0
92173	Hot sauce, chili, from mature red peppers	1 Tbs	15	3	0	1	0	0	0.1	0
23003	Jelly	1 Tbs	19	51	0	13	0	0	0	0
25002	Maple syrup	1 Tbs	20	52	0	13	0	0	0	0
23005	Marmalade, orange	1 Tbs	20	49	0	13	0	0	0	0
44697	Mayonnaise, light	1 Tbs	15	49	0	1	0	5	1.2	2.7
8145	Mayonnaise, soybean & safflower oil	1 Tbs	13.8	99	0	0	0	11	1.8	7.6
8502	Miracle Whip, light	1 Tbs	16	37	0	2	0	3		
435	Mustard, yellow	1 tsp	5	3	0	0	0	0	0.1	0
53656	Nacho cheese sauce w/jalapenos, medium/La Victoria	0.25 cup	71.6	122	1	7	0	10	4.5	1.8
53473	Oyster sauce	2 Tbs	8	4	0	1	0	0	0	0
23042	Pancake syrup	1 Tbs	20	47	0	12	0	0	0	0
23172	Pancake syrup, reduced calorie	1 Tbs	15	25	0	7	0	0	0	0

Sat (g)	Chol (mg)	Calc (mg)	Iron (mg)	Mag (mg)	Phos (mg)	Pota (mg)	Sodi (mg)	Zinc (mg)	Vit A (RAE)	Vit C (mg)	Thia (mg)	Ribo (mg)	Niac (mg)	Vit B$_6$ (mg)	Vit B$_{12}$ (µg)	Vit E (mg)	Fol (µg)	Alc (g)
1.5	0	30	1.23	17.9	43	114	11	0.3	0	0	0.03	0.05	0.12	0.02	0.08	1.4	3.9	0
0	0	3	0.12	1.7	2	22	9	0	0	5.8	0	0.01	0.07	0.01	0	0	2.6	0
1	6	8	0	0.8	7	11	10	0	14	0	0	0	0.01	0	0.02	0	0.2	0
1.7	0	0	0	0.1	2	2	5	0	0	0	0	0	0	0	0	0.1	0	0
2	0	1	0.01	0.2	1	2	2	0	1	0	0	0	0	0	0	0.1	0	0
1.1	0	7	0.01	0.7	7	9	7	0	0	0	0	0.01	0.01	0	0.02	0	0.3	0
4.5	14	6	0.14	0.6	4	9	58	0	60	0	0	0.01	0	0	0.02	0.2	0.1	0
4.5	14	6	0.14	0.6	4	9	5	0	60	0	0	0.01	0	0	0.02	0.2	0.1	0
7	30	0	0				75			0								0
7.2	30	3	0	0.3	3	3	2	0	96	0	0	0	0.01	0	0.02	0.3	0.4	0
4.7	21	2	0.02	0.2	2	2	78	0	64	0	0	0	0	0	0.01	0.2	0.3	0
1.7	4	0	0	0	0	0	6	0	0	0	0	0	0	0	0	0	0	0
3.8	11	0	0	0	0	0	0	0	0	0	0	0	0	0	0	0.3	0	0
5	12	0	0	0	0	0	0	0	0	0	0	0	0	0	0	0.1	0	0
2	2	1	0.01	0.1	1	3	90	0	116	0	0	0	0	0	0	0.6	0.3	0
1.8	0	4	0	0.3	3	5	153	0	116	0	0	0	0	0	0.01	0.7	0.1	0
3.1	78	0	0	0	0	0	0	0	4080	0	0	0	0	0	0	0.4	0	0
1	0	0	0	0	0	0	0	0	0	0	0	0	0	0	0	2.4	0	0
1.9	0	0	0.08	0	0	0	0	0	0	0	0	0	0	0	0	1.9	0	0
0.8	0	0	0	0	0	0	0	0	0	0	0	0	0	0	0	4.6	0	0
1.9	0	0	0	0	0	0	0	0	0	0	0	0	0	0	0	0.2	0	0
3.2	0	0	0.01	0	0	0	1	0	0	0	0	0	0	0	0	0.1	0	0
3.2	0	0	0	0	0	0	0	0	0	0	0	0	0	0	0	0.1	0	0
0	0	5	0.21		3	28	418			0.1								0
							302											0
0	0	1	0.03	1.1	2	23	67	0	3	0.9	0	0.01	0.09	0.01	0	0.1	0.6	0
3.8	18	116	0.13	5.7	99	19	522	0.6	50	0.3	0	0.07	0.02	0.01	0.09	0.2	2.5	0
0.2	0	0	0	0	8	53	14	0	0	0	0	0	0	0	0	0	0.1	0
0	0	0	0	0	0	0	3	0	0	0	0	0	0	0	0	0	0	0
	0	7	0.07				397		70	2.7								0
0	0	15	0.28	63	3	104	2779	0.1	1	0.2	0	0.02	0.83	0.14	0.17	0	18.4	0
0.3	2						352											0
0.2	1	10	0.32	7.7	12	38	517	0.1	0	0.1	0	0.07	0.37	0.02	0	0.1	7.4	0
9.1	41	98	0.71	6.1	100	98	1232	0.6	120	0.2	0.04	0.14	0.04	0.41	0.61	0.6	10.2	0
0	0	3	0.02	1.4	2	12	16	0	0	1.2	0	0	0.02	0	0	0	2.8	0
0	0	1	0.06	1.8	2	85	4	0	4	10.2	0	0	0.1	0.02	0	0.1	1.8	0
0	0	1	0.08	1.8	2	85	4	0	3	4.5	0	0.01	0.09	0.02	0	0.1	1.6	0
0	0	1	0.04	1.1	1	10	6	0	0	0.2	0	0	0.01	0	0	0	0.4	0
0	0	13	0.24	2.8	0	41	2	0.8	0	0	0	0	0.01	0	0	0	0	0
0	0	8	0.03	0.4	1	7	11	0	1	1	0	0.01	0.01	0	0	0	1.8	0
0.8	5	1	0.05	0.3	5	6	101	0	3	0	0	0	0	0	0	0.5	0.6	0
1.2	8	2	0.07	0.1	4	5	78	0	12	0	0	0	0	0.08	0.04	3	1.1	0
0.5	4	1	0.03		2	4	131			0						0.1		0
0	0	3	0.08	2.4	5	7	57	0	0	0.1	0.02	0	0.03	0	0	0	0.4	0
2.7	4	64	0.86				548			1.1								0
0	0	3	0.01	0.3	2	4	219	0	0	0	0	0.01	0.12	0	0.03	0	1.2	0
0	0	1	0.01	0.4	2	3	16	0	0	0	0	0	0	0	0	0	0	0
0	0	0	0	0	6	0	30	0	0	0	0	0	0	0	0	0	0	0

MDA Code	Food Name	Amt	Wt (g)	Ener (kcal)	Prot (g)	Carb (g)	Fiber (g)	Fat (g)	Mono (g)	Poly (g)
23090	Pancake syrup, w/butter	1 Tbs	19.7	58	0	15	0	0	0.1	0
53650	Pasta sauce, smooth, jar, Old World Style/Ragu	0.5 cup	125	80	2	12	3	3	0.5	1.3
53524	Pasta sauce, spaghetti/marinara, ready-to-serve	0.5 cup	125	92	2	14	1	3	1	1.3
53470	Pepper/hot sauce, ready-to-serve	1 tsp	4.7	1	0	0	0	0	0	0
53461	Plum sauce, ready-to-serve	2 Tbs	38.1	70	0	16	0	0	0.1	0.2
92229	Preserves	1 Tbs	20	56	0	14	0	0	0	0
90594	Relish, pickle, sweet, packet	1 ea	10	13	0	4	0	0	0	0
53651	Salsa, chili, chunky, canned/La Victoria	2 Tbs	30	9	0	2	0	0		
53642	Salsa, green chili, mild/La Victoria	2 Tbs	30.5	8	0	1	0	0		
53638	Salsa, green, Jalapena/La Victoria	2 Tbs	30.2	10	0	1	0	0		
53637	Salsa, red, Jalapena/La Victoria	2 Tbs	30.5	12	0	2	0	0		
90280	Salsa, ready-to-serve, packet	1 ea	8.9	2	0	1	0	0	0	0
53646	Salsa, picante, mild/La Victoria	2 Tbs	30.5	8	0	1	0	0		
504	Sour cream, cultured	2 Tbs	28.8	62	1	1	0	6	1.7	0.2
54383	Sour cream, fat free	1 oz	28	21	1	4	0	0	0	0
505	Sour cream, imitation, cultured	2 Tbs	28.8	60	1	2	0	6	0.2	0
54381	Sour cream, light	1 oz	28	38	1	2	0	3	0.9	0.1
515	Sour cream, reduced fat, cultured	2 Tbs	30	40	1	1	0	4	1	0.1
516	Sour dressing, non-butterfat, cultured, filled cream-type	1 Tbs	14.7	26	0	1	0	2	0.3	0.1
53063	Soy sauce, tamari	1 Tbs	18	11	2	1	0	0	0	0
90035	Soy sauce, low sodium	1 Tbs	18	10	1	2	0	0	0	0
53357	Sweet & sour sauce/Nestle	2 Tbs	33	40	0	8	0	1	0.2	0.4
91056	Taco sauce, green, medium/La Victoria	1 Tbs	15.1	5	0	1	0	0		
53652	Taco sauce, red, mild/La Victoria	1 Tbs	15.7	7	0	1	0	0		
4655	Tahini, from roasted & toasted kernels	1 Tbs	15	89	3	3	1	8	3	3.5
53004	Teriyaki sauce	1 Tbs	18	15	1	3	0	0	0	0
53468	White sauce, medium, homemade	1 cup	250	368	10	23	1	27	11.1	7.2
53099	Worcestershire sauce	1 Tbs	17	11	0	3	0	0	0	0
27175	Yeast extract spread	1 tsp	6	9	2	1	0	0	0	0
	Salad Dressing									
44497	Thousand island, fat free	1 Tbs	16	21	0	5	1	0	0.1	0.1
8024	Thousand island	1 Tbs	15.6	58	0	2	0	5	1.2	2.8
8013	Blue cheese	2 Tbs	30.6	154	1	2	0	16	3.8	8.5
92511	Caesar	2 Tbs	30	150	1	1	0	16		
90232	French, packet	1 ea	12.3	56	0	2	0	6	1	2.6
44467	French, fat free	1 Tbs	16	21	0	5	0	0	0	0
8255	French, reduced fat, unsalted	1 Tbs	16.3	38	0	5	0	2	1	0.8
92510	Italian	2 Tbs	30	140	0	2	0	15		
44498	Italian, fat free	1 Tbs	14	7	0	1	0	0	0	0
44499	Ranch, fat free	1 oz	28.4	34	0	8	0	1		
44696	Ranch, reduced fat	1 Tbs	15	33	0	2	0	3	0.8	0.7
8022	Russian	1 Tbs	15.3	54	0	5	0	4	0.9	2.3
8144	Sesame seed	2 Tbs	30.6	136	1	3	0	14	3.6	7.7
8035	Vinegar & oil, homemade	2 Tbs	31.2	140	0	1	0	16	4.6	7.5
	SPICES, FLAVORS, AND SEASONINGS									
26000	Allspice, ground	1 tsp	1.9	5	0	1	0	0	0	0
26106	Anise seed	1 tsp	2.1	7	0	1	0	0	0.2	0.1
26001	Basil, dried	1 tsp	1.4	4	0	1	1	0	0	0
26107	Bay leaf, crumbled	1 tsp	0.6	2	0	0	0	0	0	0
9518	Celery flakes, dried	0.5 oz	14.2	45	2	9	4	0	0.1	0.1

Sat (g)	Chol (mg)	Calc (mg)	Iron (mg)	Mag (mg)	Phos (mg)	Pota (mg)	Sodi (mg)	Zinc (mg)	Vit A (RAE)	Vit C (mg)	Thia (mg)	Ribo (mg)	Niac (mg)	Vit B$_6$ (mg)	Vit B$_{12}$ (µg)	Vit E (mg)	Fol (µg)	Alc (g)
0.2	1	0	0.02	0.4	2	1	19	0	3	0	0	0	0	0	0	0	0	0
0.4	0		1.02				756		32									0
0.5	0	34	1.06	26.2	45	470	601	0.7	34	3.9	0.03	0.08	4.9	0.22	0	2.5	13.8	0
0	0	0	0.02	0.2	1	7	124	0	0	3.5	0	0	0.01	0.01	0	0	0.3	0
0.1	0	5	0.54	4.6	8	99	205	0.1	1	0.2	0.01	0.03	0.39	0.03	0	0.1	2.3	0
0	0	4	0.1	0.8	4	15	6	0	0	1.8	0	0.02	0.01	0	0	0	2.2	0
0	0	0	0.09	0.5	1	2	81	0	4	0.1	0	0	0.02	0	0	0	0.1	0
		4	0.01				148		3	3.2								0
		5	0.28				175		7	4.1								0
	0	5	0.12				181		4	3.6								0
	0	6	0.05				149		43	9.8								0
0	0	2	0.04	1.3	3	26	53	0	1	0.2	0	0	0.01	0.02	0	0.1	0.4	0
	0	5	0.03				182		6	1.9								0
3.8	13	33	0.02	3.2	24	41	15	0.1	51	0.3	0.01	0.04	0.02	0	0.09	0.2	3.2	0
0	3	35	0	2.8	27	36	39	0.1	20	0	0.01	0.04	0.02	0.01	0.08	0	3.1	0
5.1	0	1	0.11	1.7	13	46	29	0.3	0	0	0	0	0	0	0	0.2	0	0
1.8	10	39	0.02	2.8	20	59	20	0.1	25	0.3	0.01	0.03	0.02	0.01	0.12	0.1	3.1	0
2.2	12	31	0.02	3	28	39	12	0.2	31	0.3	0.01	0.04	0.02	0	0.09	0.1	3.3	0
2	1	17	0	1.5	13	24	7	0.1	0	0.1	0.01	0.02	0.01	0	0.05	0.2	1.8	0
0	0	4	0.43	7.2	23	38	1005	0.1	0	0	0.01	0.03	0.71	0.04	0	0	3.2	0
0	0	3	0.36	6.1	20	32	600	0.1	0	0	0.01	0.02	0.6	0.03	0	0	2.9	0
0.1	0	6	0.28	2.3	3	22	116	0		0	0.01	0	0.07	0.01	0	0.1	0.7	0
	0	1	0.01				96		1	0.7								0
	0	3	0.03				103		13	2.8								0
1.1	0	64	1.34	14.2	110	62	17	0.7	0	0	0.18	0.07	0.82	0.02	0	0	14.7	0
0	0	4	0.31	11	28	40	690	0	0	0	0.01	0.01	0.23	0.02	0	0	3.6	0
7.1	18	295	0.83	35	245	390	885	1	225	2	0.17	0.46	1.01	0.1	0.7	0.7	20	0
0	0	18	0.9	2.2	10	136	167	0	1	2.2	0.01	0.02	0.12	0	0	0	1.4	0
0	0	5	0.22	10.8	6	156	216	0.1	0	0	0.58	0.86	5.82	0.08	0.03	0	60.6	0
0	1	2	0.04	0.6	0	20	117	0	0	0	0.04	0.01	0.04	0	0	0.1	1.9	0
0.8	4	3	0.18	1.2	4	17	135	0	2	0	0.23	0.01	0.07	0	0	0.6	0	0
3	5	25	0.06	0	23	11	335	0.1	21	0.6	0	0.03	0.03	0.01	0.08	1.8	8.6	0
3	5	0	0.36				280		0	0								0
0.7	0	3	0.1	0.6	2	8	103		3	0		0.01	0.02	0	0.02	0.6	0	0
0	0	1	0.09	0.5	0	13	128	0	1	0	0	0	0.02	0	0	0	2.2	0
0.2	0	2	0.14	1.3	3	17	5	0	4	0	0	0.01	0.08	0.01	0	0.5	0.3	0
2.5	0	0	0				360		0	0								0
0	0	4	0.06	0.7	15	14	158	0.1	1	0.1	0	0.01	0.02	0	0.04	0.1	1.7	0
	2	14	0.3	2.3	32	32	214	0.1	0	0	0.01	0.01	0	0.01	0	0.1	1.7	0
0.2	3	19	0.13	0.9	29	20	140	0.1	3	0.1	0	0	0	0	0	0.2	0.6	0
0.6	0	3	0.11	1.5	3	26	144	0	7	0.7	0	0.01	0.09	0.01	0	0.5	0.8	0
1.9	0	6	0.18	0	11	48	306	0	1	0	0	0	0	0	0	1.5	0	0
2.8	0	0	0	0	0	2	0	0	0	0	0	0	0	0	0	1.4	0	0
0	0	13	0.13	2.6	2	20	1	0	1	0.7	0	0	0.05	0	0	0	0.7	0
0	0	14	0.78	3.6	9	30	0	0.1	0	0.4	0.01	0.01	0.06	0.01	0	0	0.2	0
0	0	30	0.59	5.9	7	48	0	0.1	7	0.9	0	0	0.1	0.03	0	0.1	3.8	0
0	0	5	0.26	0.7	1	3	0	0	2	0.3	0	0	0.01	0.01	0	0	1.1	0
0.1	0	83	1.11	27.8	57	623	204	0.4	14	12.3	0.06	0.07	0.66	0.07	0	0.8	15.2	0

MDA Code	Food Name	Amt	Wt (g)	Ener (kcal)	Prot (g)	Carb (g)	Fiber (g)	Fat (g)	Mono (g)	Poly (g)
26040	Celery seeds	1 tsp	2	8	0	1	0	1	0.3	0.1
26002	Chili pepper, powdered	1 tsp	2.6	8	0	1	1	0	0.1	0.2
26003	Cinnamon, ground	1 tsp	2.3	6	0	2	1	0	0	0
26019	Clove, ground	1 tsp	2.1	7	0	1	1	0	0	0.1
26041	Coriander seeds	1 tsp	1.8	5	0	1	1	0	0.2	0
26036	Cumin seeds	1 tsp	2.1	8	0	1	0	0	0.3	0.1
26004	Curry blend, powder	1 tsp	2	6	0	1	1	0	0.1	0.1
26109	Dill seed	1 tsp	2.1	6	0	1	0	0	0.2	0
26105	Fennel seed	1 tsp	2	7	0	1	1	0	0.2	0
26007	Garlic powder	1 tsp	2.8	9	0	2	0	0	0	0
26023	Ginger, ground	1 tsp	1.8	6	0	1	0	0	0	0
90442	Ginger root, fresh	1 tsp	2	2	0	0	0	0	0	0
3067	Lemon peel, fresh	1 Tbs	6	3	0	1	1	0	0	0
26110	Mustard seed, yellow	1 tsp	3.3	15	1	1	0	1	0.7	0.2
26026	Nutmeg, ground	1 tsp	2.2	12	0	1	0	1	0.1	0
26008	Onion powder	1 tsp	2.1	7	0	2	0	0	0	0
26010	Paprika	1 tsp	2.1	6	0	1	1	0	0	0.2
26035	Parsley, dried	1 tsp	0.3	1	0	0	0	0	0	0
90212	Pepper, black, dash	1 ea	0.1	0	0	0	0	0	0	0
26015	Poppy seed	1 tsp	2.8	15	1	1	0	1	0.2	0.9
26030	Rosemary, dried	1 tsp	1.2	4	0	1	1	0	0	0
26111	Saffron	1 tsp	0.7	2	0	0	0	0	0	0
26014	Salt, table	0.25 tsp	1.5	0	0	0	0	0	0	0
26033	Thyme, ground	1 tsp	1.4	4	0	1	1	0	0	0
26034	Turmeric, ground	1 tsp	2.2	8	0	1	0	0	0	0
26624	Vanilla extract	1 tsp	4.3	12	0	1	0	0	0	0
BAKING INGREDIENTS										
28001	Baker's yeast, dry active, package	1 ea	7	21	3	3	1	0	0.2	0
28003	Baking soda	1 tsp	4.6	0	0	0	0	0	0	0
25005	Brown sugar, packed	1 tsp	4.6	17	0	4	0	0	0	0
23010	Baking chocolate, unsweetened, square	1 ea	28.4	142	4	8	5	15	4.6	0.4
23418	Baking chocolate, Mexican, square	1 ea	20	85	1	15	1	3	1	0.2
90657	Chocolate chips, semi sweet, mini	0.25 cup	43.2	207	2	27	3	13	4.3	0.4
4649	Coconut cream, canned	1 Tbs	18.5	36	0	2	0	3	0.1	0
4527	Coconut water, fresh	1 cup	240	46	2	9	3	0	0	0
4574	Coconut, dried, flaked, sweetened, package	2 Tbs	9.2	42	0	5	1	3	0.1	0
4510	Coconut, dried, unsweetened	2 Tbs	9.2	61	1	2	1	6	0.3	0.1
25203	Corn syrup, high fructose	1 Tbs	19.4	55	0	15	0	0	0	0
25000	Corn syrup, light	1 Tbs	20.5	58	0	16	0	0		
26017	Cream of tartar	1 tsp	3	8	0	2	0	0	0	0
25006	Granulated white sugar	1 tsp	4.2	16	0	4	0	0	0	0
25001	Honey, strained/extracted	1 Tbs	21.2	64	0	17	0	0	0	0
25202	Maple sugar	1 tsp	3	11	0	3	0	0	0	0
25003	Molasses	1 Tbs	20.5	59	0	15	0	0	0	0
25111	Sorghum syrup	1 Tbs	21	61	0	16	0	0	0	0
27007	Vinegar, cider	1 Tbs	15	3	0	0	0	0	0	0
92153	Vinegar, distilled	1 Tbs	17	3	0	0	0	0	0	0
92129	Wheat gluten, vital	1 oz	28.4	105	21	4	0	1	0	0.2

Sat (g)	Chol (mg)	Calc (mg)	Iron (mg)	Mag (mg)	Phos (mg)	Pota (mg)	Sodi (mg)	Zinc (mg)	Vit A (RAE)	Vit C (mg)	Thia (mg)	Ribo (mg)	Niac (mg)	Vit B$_6$ (mg)	Vit B$_{12}$ (µg)	Vit E (mg)	Fol (µg)	Alc (g)
0	0	35	0.9	8.8	11	28	3	0.1	0	0.3	0.01	0.01	0.06	0.02	0	0	0.2	0
0.1	0	7	0.37	4.4	8	50	26	0.1	39	1.7	0.01	0.02	0.21	0.1	0	0.8	2.6	0
0	0	28	0.88	1.3	1	12	1	0	0	0.7	0	0	0.03	0.01	0	0	0.7	0
0.1	0	14	0.18	5.5	2	23	5	0	1	1.7	0	0.01	0.03	0.01	0	0.2	2	0
0	0	13	0.29	5.9	7	23	1	0.1	0	0.4	0	0.01	0.04			0		0
0	0	20	1.39	7.7	10	38	4	0.1	1	0.2	0.01	0.01	0.1	0.01	0	0.1	0.2	0
0	0	10	0.59	5.1	7	31	1	0.1	1	0.2	0.01	0.01	0.07	0.02	0	0.4	3.1	0
0	0	32	0.34	5.4	6	25	0	0.1	0	0.4	0.01	0.01	0.06	0.01	0	0	0.2	0
0	0	24	0.37	7.7	10	34	2	0.1	0	0.4	0.01	0.01	0.12	0.01	0			0
0	0	2	0.08	1.6	12	31	1	0.1	0	0.5	0.01	0	0.02	0.08	0	0	0.1	0
0	0	2	0.21	3.3	3	24	1	0.1	0	0.1	0	0	0.09	0.02	0	0.3	0.7	0
0	0	0	0.01	0.9	1	8	0	0	0	0.1	0	0	0.02	0	0	0	0.2	0
0	0	8	0.05	0.9	1	10	0	0	0	7.7	0	0	0.02	0.01	0	0	0.8	0
0	0	17	0.33	9.8	28	23	0	0.2	0	0.1	0.02	0.01	0.26	0.01	0	0.1	2.5	0
0.6	0	4	0.07	4	5	8	0	0	0	0.1	0.01	0	0.03	0	0	0	1.7	0
0	0	8	0.05	2.6	7	20	1	0	0	0.3	0.01	0	0.01	0.03	0	0	3.5	0
0	0	4	0.5	3.9	7	49	1	0.1	55	1.5	0.01	0.04	0.32	0.08	0	0.6	2.2	0
0	0	4	0.29	0.7	1	11	1	0	2	0.4	0	0	0.02	0	0	0	0.5	0
0	0	0	0.03	0.2	0	1	0	0	0	0	0	0	0	0	0	0	0	0
0.1	0	41	0.26	9.3	24	20	1	0.3	0	0.1	0.02	0	0.03	0.01	0	0	1.6	0
0.1	0	15	0.35	2.6	1	11	1	0	2	0.7	0.01	0.01	0.01	0.02	0	0	3.7	0
0	0	1	0.08	1.8	2	12	1	0	0	0.6	0	0	0.01	0.01	0	0	0.7	0
0	0	0	0	0	0	0	581	0	0	0	0	0	0	0	0	0	0	0
0	0	26	1.73	3.1	3	11	1	0.1	3	0.7	0.01	0.01	0.07	0.01	0	0.1	3.8	0
0.1	0	4	0.91	4.2	6	56	1	0.1	0	0.6	0	0.01	0.11	0.04	0	0.1	0.9	0
0	0	0	0.01	0.5	0	6	0	0	0	0	0	0	0.02	0	0	0	0	1.48
0	0	4	1.16	6.9	90	140	4	0.4	0	0	0.17	0.38	2.78	0.11	0	0	163.8	0
0	0	0	0	0	0	0	1259	0	0	0	0	0	0	0	0	0	0	0
0	0	4	0.09	1.3	1	16	2	0	0	0	0	0	0	0	0	0	0	0
9.2	0	29	4.94	92.9	114	236	7	2.7	0	0	0.04	0.03	0.38	0.01	0	0.1	8	0
1.7	0	7	0.44	19	28	79	1	0.3	0	0	0.01	0.02	0.37	0.01	0	0.1	1	0
7.7	0	14	1.35	49.7	57	158	5	0.7	0	0	0.02	0.04	0.18	0.02	0	0.1	5.6	0
2.9	0	0	0.09	3.1	4	19	9	0.1	0	0.3	0	0.01	0.01	0.01	0	0	2.6	0
0.4	0	58	0.7	60	48	600	252	0.2	0	5.8	0.07	0.14	0.19	0.08	0	0	7.2	0
2.4	0	1	0.14	4.7	9	33	26	0.1	0	0	0	0	0.06	0	0	0	0.3	0
5.3	0	2	0.31	8.3	19	50	3	0.2	0	0.1	0.01	0.01	0.06	0.03	0	0	0.8	0
0	0	0	0.01	0	0	0	0	0	0	0	0	0	0	0	0	0	0	0
	0	3	0	0.2	0	0	13	0.1	0	0	0.01	0	0	0	0	0	0	0
0	0	0	0.11	0.1	0	495	2	0	0	0	0	0	0	0	0	0	0	0
0	0	0	0	0	0	0	0	0	0	0	0	0	0	0	0	0	0	0
0	0	1	0.09	0.4	1	11	1	0	0	0.1	0	0.01	0.03	0.01	0	0	0.4	0
0	0	3	0.05	0.6	0	8	0	0.2	0	0	0	0	0	0	0	0	0	0
0	0	42	0.97	49.6	6	300	8	0.1	0	0	0.01	0	0.19	0.14	0	0	0	0
0	0	32	0.8	21	12	210	2	0.1	0	0	0.02	0.03	0.02	0.14	0	0	0	0
0	0	1	0.03	0.8	1	11	1	0	0	0	0	0	0	0	0	0	0	0
0	0	1	0.01	0.2	1	0	0	0	0	0	0	0	0	0	0	0	0	0
0.1	0	40	1.48	7.1	74	28	8	0.2	0	0	0	0	0	0	0	0	0	0

MDA Code	Food Name	Amt	Wt (g)	Ener (kcal)	Prot (g)	Carb (g)	Fiber (g)	Fat (g)	Mono (g)	Poly (g)
	FAST FOOD									
	Generic Fast Food									
6178	Baked potatoes w/cheese sauce & bacon	1 ea	299	451	18	44		26	9.7	4.8
6177	Baked potatoes w/cheese sauce	1 ea	296	474	15	47		29	10.7	6
6181	Baked potatoes w/sour cream & chives	1 ea	302	393	7	50		22	7.9	3.3
66025	Burrito, bean	1 ea	108.5	224	7	36	4	7	2.4	0.6
56629	Burrito, bean & cheese	1 ea	93	189	8	27		6	1.2	0.9
66024	Burrito, beef	1 ea	110	262	13	29	1	10	3.7	0.4
66023	Burrito, beef, bean & cheese	1 ea	101.5	165	7	20	2	7	2.2	0.5
56600	Breakfast biscuit w/egg sandwich	1 ea	136	373	12	32	1	22	9.1	6.4
56601	Breakfast biscuit w/egg & bacon	1 ea	150	458	17	29	1	31	13.4	7.5
56602	Breakfast biscuit w/egg & ham	1 ea	192	461	20	35	1	27	11	7.7
66028	Breakfast biscuit w/egg & sausage	1 ea	180	581	19	41	1	39	16.4	4.4
66029	Breakfast biscuit w/egg, cheese & bacon	1 ea	144	461	18	33	1	29	14.1	3.5
56604	Biscuit w/ham sandwich	1 ea	113	386	13	44	1	18	4.8	1
66030	Biscuit w/sausage sandwich	1 ea	124	485	12	40	1	32	12.8	3
66013	Cheeseburger, double, w/condiments & vegetables	1 ea	166	417	21	35		21	7.8	2.7
66016	Cheeseburger, double	1 ea	155	477	27	32	1	27	9	0.9
56651	Cheeseburger w/bacon & condiments	1 ea	195	550	31	37	3	31	10.6	1.3
56649	Cheeseburger w/condiments & vegetables	1 ea	219	453	25	37	3	23	7.7	0.7
15063	Chicken drumstick & thigh, dark meat, breaded & fried	3 oz	85.1	248	17	9	1	15	6.3	3.6
15064	Chicken breast & wing, white meat, breaded & fried	3 oz	85.1	258	19	10	1	15	6.4	3.5
56656	Chicken fillet sandwich w/cheese	1 ea	228	632	29	42		39	13.7	9.9
56000	Chicken fillet sandwich, plain	1 ea	182	515	24	39		29	10.4	8.4
50312	Chili con carne	1 cup	253	256	25	22		8	3.4	0.5
56635	Chimichanga, beef & cheese	1 ea	183	443	20	39		23	9.4	0.7
19110	Clams, breaded & fried	3 oz	85.1	334	9	29		20	8.5	5
5461	Cole slaw	0.75 cup	99	147	1	13		11	2.4	6.4
6175	Corn cob w/butter	1 ea	146	155	4	32		3	1	0.6
56668	Corn dog	1 ea	175	460	17	56		19	9.1	3.5
56606	Croissant sandwich w/egg & cheese	1 ea	127	368	13	24		25	7.5	1.4
56607	Croissant sandwich w/egg, cheese & bacon	1 ea	129	413	16	24		28	9.2	1.8
56608	Croissant sandwich w/egg, cheese & ham	1 ea	152	474	19	24		34	11.4	2.4
45588	Danish, cheese	1 ea	91	353	6	29		25	15.6	2.4
45513	Danish, fruit	1 ea	94	335	5	45		16	10.1	1.6
66021	Enchilada, cheese	1 ea	163	319	10	29		19	6.3	0.8
66022	Enchilada, beef & cheese	1 ea	192	323	12	30		18	6.1	1.4
66020	Enchirito, beef, bean & cheese	1 ea	193	344	18	34		16	6.5	0.3
42064	English muffin w/butter	1 ea	63	189	5	30	2	6	1.5	1.3
66031	English muffin sandwich, w/cheese & sausage	1 ea	115	393	15	29	1	24	10.1	2.7
66032	English muffin sandwich, w/egg, cheese & bacon	1 ea	146	308	18	28	2	13	5	1.7
66010	Fish sandwich, w/tartar sauce	1 ea	158	431	17	41	0	23	7.7	8.2
66011	Fish sandwich, w/cheese & tartar sauce	1 ea	183	523	21	48	0	29	8.9	9.4
90736	French fries, fried in vegetable oil, medium	1 ea	134	427	5	50	5	23	13.3	4
42354	French toast sticks	5 pce	141	513	8	58	3	29	12.6	9.9
42353	French toast w/butter	2 pce	135	356	10	36	0	19	7.1	2.4
56638	Frijoles (beans) w/cheese	0.5 cup	83.5	113	6	14		4	1.3	0.3
56664	Ham & cheese sandwich	1 ea	146	352	21	33		15	6.7	1.4
56665	Ham, egg & cheese sandwich	1 ea	143	347	19	31		16	5.7	1.7
69150	Hamburger w/condiments	1 ea	171.5	439	27	38	2	20	9	2.1

Sat (g)	Chol (mg)	Calc (mg)	Iron (mg)	Mag (mg)	Phos (mg)	Pota (mg)	Sodi (mg)	Zinc (mg)	Vit A (RAE)	Vit C (mg)	Thia (mg)	Ribo (mg)	Niac (mg)	Vit B$_6$ (mg)	Vit B$_{12}$ (µg)	Vit E (mg)	Fol (µg)	Alc (g)
10.1	30	308	3.14	68.8	347	1178	972	2.2	188	28.7	0.27	0.24	3.98	0.75	0.33		29.9	0
10.6	18	311	3.02	65.1	320	1166	382	1.9	252	26	0.24	0.21	3.34	0.71	0.18		26.6	0
10	24	106	3.11	69.5	184	1383	181	0.9	266	33.8	0.27	0.18	3.71	0.79	0.21		33.2	0
3.4	2	56	2.26	43.4	49	327	493	0.8	8	1	0.31	0.3	2.03	0.15	0.54	0.9	43.4	0
3.4	14	107	1.13	40	90	248	583	0.8	49	0.8	0.11	0.35	1.79	0.12	0.45		37.2	0
5.2	32	42	3.05	40.7	87	370	746	2.4	7	0.6	0.12	0.46	3.22	0.15	0.98	0.6	64.9	0
3.6	62	65	1.87	25.4	70	205	495	1.2	75	2.5	0.15	0.36	1.93	0.11	0.55	0.4	37.6	0
4.7	245	82	2.9	19	388	238	891	1	180	0.1	0.3	0.49	2.15	0.11	0.63	3.3	57.1	0
8	352	189	3.74	24	238	250	999	1.6	108	2.7	0.14	0.23	2.4	0.14	1.03	2	60	0
5.9	300	221	4.55	30.7	317	319	1382	2.2	236	0	0.67	0.6	2	0.27	1.19	2.3	65.3	0
15	302	155	3.96	25.2	490	320	1141	2.2	160	0	0.5	0.45	3.6	0.2	1.37	2.8	64.8	0
11.1	252	157	2.94	20.2	459	230	1250	1.5		2.3	0.34	0.52	2.57	0.1	1.05	1.4	105.1	0
11.4	25	160	2.72	22.6	554	197	1433	1.6	31	0.1	0.51	0.32	3.48	0.14	0.03	1.7	38.4	0
14.2	35	128	2.58	19.8	446	198	1071	1.6	13	0.1	0.4	0.29	3.27	0.11	0.51	1.4	45.9	0
8.7	60	171	3.42	29.9	242	335	1051	3.5	71	1.7	0.35	0.28	8.05	0.18	1.93		61.4	0
11	85	279	3.67	32.6	284	335	963	4.3	99	0	0.29	0.44	6.79	0.29	2.14	1.2	77.5	0
11.9	98	267	4.04	44.8	353	464	1314	5.2	82	1.4	0.34	0.68	8.25	0.47	2.44		95.6	0
8.5	74	208	4.07	41.6	261	460	843	4.8		4.2	0.32	0.62	7.29		2.21		102.9	0
4.1	95	20	0.92	21.3	138	256	434	1.9	38	0	0.08	0.25	4.14	0.19	0.48	0.8	14.5	0
4.1	77	31	0.77	19.6	160	295	509	0.8	30	0	0.08	0.15	6.25	0.3	0.35	0.8	15.3	0
12.4	78	258	3.63	43.3	406	333	1238	2.9	164	3	0.41	0.46	9.07	0.41	0.46		109.4	0
8.5	60	60	4.68	34.6	233	353	957	1.9	31	8.9	0.33	0.24	6.81	0.2	0.38		100.1	0
3.4	134	68	5.19	45.5	197	691	1007	3.6	83	1.5	0.13	1.14	2.48	0.33	1.14	1.6	45.5	0
11.2	51	238	3.84	60.4	187	203	957	3.4	132	2.7	0.38	0.86	4.67	0.22	1.3		91.5	0
4.9	65	15	2.26	23	176	197	617	1.2	27	0	0.15	0.2	2.12	0.03	0.82		31.5	0
1.6	5	34	0.72	8.9	36	177	267	0.2	36	8.3	0.04	0.03	0.08	0.11	0.18	4	38.6	0
1.6	6	4	0.88	40.9	108	359	29	0.9	34	6.9	0.25	0.1	2.18	0.32	0		43.8	0
5.2	79	102	6.18	17.5	166	262	973	1.3	60	0	0.28	0.7	4.17	0.09	0.44	0.7	103.2	0
14.1	216	244	2.2	21.6	348	174	551	1.8	277	0.1	0.19	0.38	1.51	0.1	0.77		47	0
15.4	215	151	2.19	23.2	276	201	889	1.9	142	2.2	0.35	0.34	2.19	0.12	0.86		45.2	0
17.5	213	144	2.13	25.8	336	272	1081	2.2	131	11.4	0.52	0.3	3.19	0.23	1		45.6	0
5.1	20	70	1.85	15.5	80	116	319	0.6	45	2.6	0.26	0.21	2.55	0.05	0.23		54.6	0
3.3	19	22	1.4	14.1	69	110	333	0.5	25	1.6	0.29	0.21	1.8	0.06	0.24	0.8	31	0
10.6	44	324	1.32	50.5	134	240	784	2.5	99	1	0.08	0.42	1.91	0.39	0.75	1.5	65.2	0
9	40	228	3.07	82.6	167	574	1319	2.7	98	1.3	0.1	0.4	2.52	0.27	1.02	1.5	67.2	0
7.9	50	218	2.39	71.4	224	560	1251	2.8	89	4.6	0.17	0.69	2.99	0.21	1.62	1.5	94.6	0
2.4	13	103	1.59	13.2	85	69	386	0.4	32	0.8	0.25	0.32	2.61	0.04	0.02	0.1	56.7	0
9.9	59	168	2.25	24.2	186	215	1036	1.7	101	1.3	0.7	0.25	4.14	0.15	0.68	1.3	66.7	0
5	250	161	2.6	24.8	288	212	777	1.7	188	1.9	0.53	0.48	3.55	0.16	0.72	0.6	73	0
5.2	55	84	2.61	33.2	212	340	615	1	33	2.8	0.33	0.22	3.4	0.11	1.07	0.9	85.3	0
8.1	68	185	3.5	36.6	311	353	939	1.2	130	2.7	0.46	0.42	4.23	0.11	1.08	1.8	91.5	0
5.3	0	17	1.84	45.6	185	737	260	1	0	3.6	0.23	0.09	3.35	0.51	0	1	40.2	0
4.7	75	78	2.96	26.8	123	127	499	0.9	0	0	0.23	0.25	2.96	0.25	0.07	2.3	197.4	0
7.7	116	73	1.89	16.2	146	177	513	0.6	136	0.1	0.58	0.5	3.92	0.05	0.36		72.9	0
2	18	94	1.12	42.6	88	302	441	0.9	18	0.8	0.07	0.17	0.74	0.1	0.34		55.9	0
6.4	58	130	3.24	16.1	152	291	771	1.4	96	2.8	0.31	0.48	2.69	0.2	0.54	0.3	75.9	0
7.4	246	212	3.1	25.7	346	210	1005	2	166	2.7	0.43	0.56	4.2	0.16	1.23	0.6	75.8	0
8.6	69	149	2.97	41.2	208	386	641	5.2		0.5	0.27	0.34	7.97	0.25	2.85	0.1	37.7	0

MDA Code	Food Name	Amt	Wt (g)	Ener (kcal)	Prot (g)	Carb (g)	Fiber (g)	Fat (g)	Mono (g)	Poly (g)
56662	Hamburger, double, w/condiments & vegetables	1 ea	226	540	34	40		27	10.3	2.8
56661	Hamburger, w/condiments & vegetables	1 ea	218	429	25	38	3	20	7.2	0.5
56659	Hamburger, w/condiments & vegetables	1 ea	110	279	13	27		13	5.3	2.6
66007	Hamburger, plain	1 ea	90	266	13	30	1	10	3.5	0.2
5463	Hash browns	0.5 cup	72	235	2	23	2	16		
56667	Hot dog w/chili & bun	1 ea	114	296	14	31		13	6.6	1.2
66004	Hot dog, plain	1 ea	98	242	10	18		15	6.9	1.7
56666	Hush puppies, cornbread	5 pce	78	257	5	35	3	12	7.8	0.4
2032	Hot fudge sundae	1 ea	158	284	6	48	0	9	2.3	0.8
6185	Mashed potatoes	0.5 cup	121	100	3	20		1	0.4	0.4
90214	Mayonnaise, soybean oil, packet	1 ea	10	72	0	0	0	8	2	4.3
71129	Milk shake, chocolate, small, 12 fl oz	1 ea	249.6	317	8	51	5	9	2.7	0.3
71132	Milk shake, vanilla, small, 12 fl oz	1 ea	249.6	369	8	49	2	16	4.5	0.8
56639	Nachos, w/cheese	7 pce	113	346	9	36		19	8	2.2
56641	Nachos w/cheese, beans, beef & peppers	7 pce	225	502	17	49		27	9.7	5
6176	Onion rings	8 pce	78.1	259	3	29		15	6.3	0.6
19109	Oysters, breaded & battered, fried	3 oz	85.1	226	8	24	0	11	4.2	2.8
45122	Pancakes, w/butter & syrup	1 ea	116	260	4	45	1	7	2.6	1
6173	Potato salad	0.333 cup	95	108	1	13		6	1.6	2.9
56619	Pizza, pepperoni, frozen, 12" or 1/8 pce	1 pce	108	275	15	30		11	4.8	1.8
56669	Roast beef sandwich, w/cheese	1 ea	176	473	32	45		18	3.7	3.5
66003	Roast beef sandwich, plain	1 ea	139	346	22	33		14	6.8	1.7
56643	Taco salad	1.5 cup	198	279	13	24		15	5.2	1.7
56644	Taco salad, w/chili con carne	1.5 cup	261	290	17	27		13	4.5	1.5
19115	Shrimp, breaded & fried	4 ea	93.7	260	11	23		14	9.9	0.4
56670	Steak sandwich	1 ea	204	459	30	52		14	5.3	3.3
56671	Submarine sandwich, w/cold cuts	1 ea	228	456	22	51	2	19	8.2	2.3
56673	Submarine sandwich, w/tuna salad	1 ea	256	584	30	55		28	13.4	7.3
57531	Taco, small	1 ea	171	371	21	27		21	6.6	1
66017	Tostada, bean & cheese	1 ea	144	223	10	27		10	3.1	0.7
56645	Tostada, beef & cheese	1 ea	163	315	19	23		16	3.3	1

Arby's

MDA Code	Food Name	Amt	Wt (g)	Ener (kcal)	Prot (g)	Carb (g)	Fiber (g)	Fat (g)	Mono (g)	Poly (g)
6429	Baked potato w/broccoli & cheese	1 ea	384	517	12	69	8	21		
8988	Beef melt sandwich, w/cheddar	1 ea	150	320	16	36	2	14		
9014	Breakfast sandwich, bacon, egg & cheese, w/biscuit	1 ea	144	420	15	27	1	25		
9008	Cheese sticks, mozzarella, breaded & fried	1 ea	137	426	18	38	2	28		
9011	Chicken tenders, 5 piece serving	1 ea	192	555	37	41	3	27		
69043	French dip submarine sandwich, w/au jus	1 ea	285	453	29	49	3	18		
8987	French fries, curly, large	1 ea	198	631	8	73	7	37		
9006	French fries, homestyle, large	1 ea	212.6	565	6	82	6	37		
8998	Grilled chicken caesar salad	1 ea	338	230	33	8	3	8		
69046	Grilled chicken sandwich, deluxe	1 ea	252	450	29	37	2	22		
9001	Grilled chicken sandwich, grilled	1 ea	174	280	29	30	3	5		
8991	Ham & swiss submarine sandwich, hot	1 ea	278	501	28	46	2	18		
69055	Philly beef & swiss submarine sandwich	1 ea	311	678	35	47	4	36		
56336	Roast beef sandwich, regular	1 ea	157	326	20	35	1	14		
53256	Sauce, Arby's, packet	1 ea	14	15	0	4	0	0		
9018	Sauce, barbecue, dipping, svg	1 serving	28.4	45	0	11	0	0		

Source: Arby's

Sat (g)	Chol (mg)	Calc (mg)	Iron (mg)	Mag (mg)	Phos (mg)	Pota (mg)	Sodi (mg)	Zinc (mg)	Vit A (RAE)	Vit C (mg)	Thia (mg)	Ribo (mg)	Niac (mg)	Vit B$_6$ (mg)	Vit B$_{12}$ (µg)	Vit E (mg)	Fol (µg)	Alc (g)
10.5	122	102	5.85	49.7	314	570	791	5.7	5	1.1	0.36	0.38	7.57	0.54	4.07		76.8	0
6.9	68	150	4.29	41.4	222	462	676	4.8		4.4	0.33	0.6	7.72		2.2		106.8	0
4.1	26	63	2.63	22	124	227	504	2.1	4	1.6	0.23	0.2	3.68	0.12	0.88	0.8	51.7	0
3.2	30	124	2.74	18.9	110	174	396	2	0	0	0.26	0.25	4.81	0.13	0.9	0.5	66.6	0
	0	12	0.48	13.7	79	256	373	0.2	0	2.1	0.1	0.06	1.21	0.16	0	0.7	14.4	0
4.9	51	19	3.28	10.3	192	166	480	0.8	3	2.7	0.22	0.4	3.74	0.05	0.3		73	0
5.1	44	24	2.31	12.7	97	143	670	2	0	0.1	0.24	0.27	3.65	0.05	0.51	0.3	48	0
2.7	135	69	1.43	16.4	190	188	965	0.4	9	0	0	0.02	2.03	0.1	0.17		57.7	0
5	21	207	0.58	33.2	228	395	182	0.9	58	2.4	0.06	0.3	1.07	0.13	0.65	0.7	9.5	0
0.6	2	25	0.57	21.8	67	356	275	0.4	13	0.5	0.11	0.06	1.45	0.28	0.06		9.7	0
1.2	4	2	0.05	0.1	3	3	57	0	8	0	0	0	0	0.06	0.03	0.5	0.8	0
5.8	32	282	0.77	42.4	255	499	242	1	65	1	0.14	0.61	0.4	0.12	0.85	0.3	12.5	0
9.9	57	287	1.15	32.4	245	414	202	1.4	227	0	0.06	1.65	0.53	0.15	0.55	0.6	0	0
7.8	18	272	1.28	55.4	276	172	816	1.8	149	1.2	0.19	0.37	1.54	0.2	0.82		10.2	0
11	18	340	2.45	85.5	342	398	1588	3.2	385	4.3	0.2	0.61	2.95	0.36	0.9		33.8	0
6.5	13	69	0.8	14.8	81	122	405	0.3	1	0.5	0.08	0.09	0.87	0.05	0.12	0.3	51.5	0
2.8	66	17	2.73	14.5	120	111	414	9.6	66	2.6	0.19	0.21	2.71	0.02	0.62		18.7	0
2.9	29	64	1.31	24.4	238	125	552	0.5	41	1.7	0.2	0.28	1.69	0.06	0.12	0.7	25.5	0
1	57	13	0.69	7.6	53	256	312	0.2	28	1	0.07	0.1	0.26	0.14	0.11		23.8	0
3.4	22	98	1.43	13	114	232	406	0.8	80	2.5	0.21	0.36	4.63	0.09	0.28		56.2	0
9	77	183	5.05	40.5	401	345	1633	5.4	58	0	0.39	0.46	5.9	0.33	2.06		63.4	0
3.6	51	54	4.23	30.6	239	316	792	3.4	11	2.1	0.38	0.31	5.87	0.26	1.22	0.2	57	0
6.8	44	192	2.28	51.5	143	416	762	2.7	71	3.6	0.1	0.36	2.46	0.22	0.63		83.2	0
6	5	245	2.66	52.2	154	392	885	3.3	258	3.4	0.16	0.5	2.53	0.52	0.73		91.4	0
3.1	114	48	1.69	22.5	197	105	826	0.7	21	0	0.12	0.52	0	0.04	0.08		57.2	0
3.8	73	92	5.16	49	298	524	798	4.5	20	5.5	0.41	0.37	7.3	0.37	1.57		89.8	0
6.8	36	189	2.51	68.4	287	394	1651	2.6	71	12.3	1	0.8	5.49	0.14	1.09		86.6	0
5.3	49	74	2.64	79.4	220	335	1293	1.9	46	3.6	0.46	0.33	11.34	0.23	1.61		102.4	0
11.4	56	221	2.41	70.1	203	474	802	3.9	108	2.2	0.15	0.44	3.21	0.24	1.04	1.9	68.4	0
5.4	30	210	1.89	59	117	403	543	1.9	45	1.3	0.1	0.33	1.32	0.16	0.69	1.2	43.2	0
10.4	41	217	2.87	63.6	179	572	896	3.7	51	2.6	0.1	0.55	3.15	0.23	1.17		75	0
10.9	46	174	3.82				756			82.2								0
	645	80	2.7				850			0								0
7.3	153	137	0.82				1318			0								0
12.9	45	380	0.99				1370			0.6								0
4.8	61	330	2.63				1742			0.9								0
7.2	59	61	4.38				2843		0	0.6								0
6.8	0	80	3.24				1476			9.6								0
6.7	0	50	1.62				1027			12.6								0
3.5	80	200	1.8				920			42								0
4	110	60	2.7			722	1050			1.2	0.34	0.32	14.9					0
1.5	55	80	1.8				1170			0								0
4.2	55	282	3.26				1840			10.3								0
10.9	91	314	4.56				1968			9.1								0
5.5	45	61	3.67				972		0	0								0
0	0	0	0				177		0	1.2								0
0	0	10	0.18				348			0.6								0

MDA Code	Food Name	Amt	Wt (g)	Ener (kcal)	Prot (g)	Carb (g)	Fiber (g)	Fat (g)	Mono (g)	Poly (g)
	Burger King									
56352	Cheeseburger	1 ea	133	380	19	32	4	20	7.6	2
56355	Cheeseburger, Whopper	1 ea	316	790	35	53	3	48	16	12
56357	Cheeseburger, Whopper, double	1 ea	399	1061	58	54	6	68	25.1	11.9
9087	Chicken tenders, 4 piece serving	1 ea	62	179	11	11	1	10	5.9	1.3
9065	French fries, large	1 ea	160	530	6	64	5	28	17.7	1.8
56351	Hamburger	1 ea	121	333	17	33	2	15	6.4	1.5
56354	Hamburger, Whopper	1 ea	291	678	31	54	5	37	13.6	9.9
9071	Hash browns, rounds, medium	1 ea	128	472	4	44	4	31	17.6	4.1
2127	Milk shake, chocolate, medium	1 ea	397	440	13	80	4	8		
2129	Milk shake, vanilla, medium	1 ea	397	667	13	76	0	35	9.8	1.7
9041	Onion rings, large	1 ea	137	480	7	60	5	23		
69071	Sandwich, breakfast, bacon, egg & cheese, w/biscuit	1 ea	189	692	27	51	1	61		
57002	Sandwich, Chicken Broiler	1 ea	258	550	30	52	3	25		
9084	Sandwich, croissant w/sausage & cheese	1 ea	107	402	15	25	1	27	12.9	3.3
	Source: Burger King Corporation									
	Chik-Fil-A									
69185	Chicken breast fillet, chargrilled	1 ea	79	100	20	1	0	2		
15263	Chicken nuggets, 8 piece serving	1 ea	113	260	26	12	1	12		
15262	Chick-N-Strips, 4 piece serving	1 ea	108	250	25	12	0	11		
52138	Cole slaw, small	1 ea	105	210	1	14	2	17		
48214	Pie, lemon, slice	1 pce	113	320	7	51	3	10		
52134	Salad, garden, chicken, chargrilled	1 ea	278	180	23	8	3	6		
52137	Salad, side	1 ea	164	80	5	6	2	5		
69155	Sandwich, chicken salad, w/whole wheat	1 ea	153	350	20	32	5	15		
69189	Sandwich, chicken deluxe	1 ea	208	420	28	39	2	16		
69176	Sauce, honey mustard, dipping, packet	1 ea	28	45	0	10	0	0	0	0
69182	Wrap, chicken, spicy	1 ea	225	390	31	51	3	7		
	Source: Chik-Fil-A									
	Dairy Queen									
56372	Cheeseburger, double, homestyle	1 ea	219	540	35	30	2	31		
72142	Frozen dessert, banana split, large	1 ea	527	810	17	134	2	23		
71693	Frozen dessert, Brownie Earthquake	1 ea	304	740	10	112	0	27		
72139	Frozen dessert, chocolate cookie dough, large	1 ea	560	1320	21	193	0	52		
72134	Frozen dessert, sundae, chocolate, large	1 ea	333	580	11	100	1	15		
72138	Frozen dessert, Oreo, large	1 ea	500	1010	19	148	2	37		
72135	Frozen dessert, sundae, strawberry, large	1 ea	333	500	10	83	1	15		
72137	Frozen dessert, Triple Chocolate Utopia	1 ea	284	770	12	96	5	39		
2222	Ice cream cone, chocolate, medium	1 ea	198	340	8	53	0	11		
2136	Ice cream cone, dipped, medium	1 ea	220	490	8	59	1	24		
2143	Ice cream cone, vanilla, medium	1 ea	213	355	9	57	0	10		
2134	Ice cream sandwich	1 ea	85	200	4	31	1	6		
72129	Milk shake, chocolate malt, large	1 ea	836	1320	29	222	2	35		
	Source: International Dairy Queen, Inc.									
	Domino's Pizza									
91365	Breadsticks	1 ea	37.2	116	3	18	1	4		
91369	Chicken, buffalo wings	1 ea	24.9	50	6	2	0	2		
56386	Pizza, cheese, hand tossed, 12"	2 pce	159	375	15	55	3	11		
91356	Pizza, Deluxe Feast, hand tossed, 12"	2 pce	200.8	465	19	57	3	18		
91358	Pizza, MeatZZa Feast, hand tossed, 12"	2 pce	216.2	560	26	57	3	26		

Sat (g)	Chol (mg)	Calc (mg)	Iron (mg)	Mag (mg)	Phos (mg)	Pota (mg)	Sodi (mg)	Zinc (mg)	Vit A (RAE)	Vit C (mg)	Thia (mg)	Ribo (mg)	Niac (mg)	Vit B6 (mg)	Vit B12 (µg)	Vit E (mg)	Fol (µg)	Alc (g)
9.1	60	124	3.32	31.9	190	237	801	3.2		0.3	0.4	0.32	4.52	0.12		0.1		0
18.3	114	259	6.32	56.9	357	534	1431	5.1		0.6	0.67	0.63	8.09	0.23		0.3	161.2	0
27.9	188	311	21.15	75.8	511	754	1544	14		0.8	1.07	0.84	11.97	0.45		0.2	107.7	0
2.6	32	9	0.38	15.5	141	163	447	0.4		0.4	0.08	0.07	4.64	0.22		0.5	4.3	0
7		14	2.06	48	229	757	728	1.8		1.1	0.28	0.05	3.75	0.28		1.2		0
6.1	42	62	3.05	29	144	220	551	2.6		0.2	0.4	0.27	4.78	0.12		0	77.4	0
12.4	87	113	12.72	52.4	262	492	911	8.2		0.6	0.63	0.51	8.36	0.26		0.4	136.8	0
7.6	0	20	0.88	24.3	141	467	654	0.4	0	2	0.2	0.11	2.31	0.29	0	1.4		0
5	35	350	1.8				270			0								0
21.2	123	413	1.67	47.6	385	607	397	2.7		0	0	0.71	0.36	0.12	1.43	1.3		0
6	0	150	0				690		0	0								0
18.6	253	200	3.59				2130			0								0
5	105	60	3.6				1110			6								0
9.2	46	114	2	20.3	169	219	837	1.5		0	0.35	0.34	4.38	0.19	0.59	1		0
0	60	0	0.36				690		0	0								0
2.5	70	40	1.08				1090		0	0								0
2.5	70	40	1.08				570		0	0								0
2.5	20	40	0.36				180			27								0
3.5	110	150	0				220			4.8								0
3	70	150	0.36				730			6								0
2.5	15	150	0				110			4.8								0
3	65	150	1.8				880		0	0								0
3.5	60	100	2.7				1300			2.4								0
0	0	0	0				150		0	0								0
3.5	70	200	3.6				1150			4.8								0
16	115	250	4.5				1130			3.6								0
15	70	600	2.7				360			12								0
16	50	250	1.8				350			0								0
26	90	600	4.5				670			2.4								0
10	45	350	1.8				260			1.2								0
18	70	600	4.5				770			2.4								0
9	45	400	1.8				230			18								0
17	55	300	1.8				390			1.2								0
7	30	250	1.8				160			1.2								0
13	30	250	1.8				190			2.4								0
6.5	32	269	1.94				172			2.6								0
3	10	80	1.08				140			0								0
22	110	900	3.6				670			4.8								0
0.8	0	6	0.87				152			0.1								0
0.6	26	6	0.32				175			0.1								0
4.8	23	187	2.99				776			0								0
7.7	40	199	3.56				1063			1.4								0
11.4	64	282	3.72				1463			0.1								0

MDA Code	Food Name	Amt	Wt (g)	Ener (kcal)	Prot (g)	Carb (g)	Fiber (g)	Fat (g)	Mono (g)	Poly (g)
91361	Pizza, Pepperoni Feast, hand tossed, 12"	2 pce	196.1	534	24	56	3	25		
91357	Pizza, Veggie Feast, hand tossed, 12"	2 pce	203.2	439	19	57	4	16		
	Source: Domino's Pizza Incorporated									

Hardee's

9295	Apple turnover	1 ea	91	270	4	38		12		
42330	Biscuit, cinnamon 'n raisin	1 ea	75	250	2	42		8		
15201	Chicken wing, serving	1 ea	66	200	10	23	0	8		
9278	Hot dog, w/chili	1 ea	160	451	15	24	2	32		
9284	Chicken strips, breaded & fried, 5 piece serving	1 ea	92	201	18	13	0	8		
9277	Hamburger, Monster	1 ea	278	949	53	35	2	67		
9275	Hamburger, Six Dollar	1 ea	353	911	41	50	2	61		
2247	Ice cream cone, twist	1 ea	118	180	4	34		2		
6147	French fries, large	1 ea	150	440	5	59	0	21		
9281	Sandwich, chicken, bbq, grilled	1 ea	171	268	24	34	2	3		
56423	Sandwich, fish, Fisherman's Fillet	1 ea	221	530	25	45		28		
	Source: Hardee's Food Systems, Inc.									

Jack in the Box

56437	Cheeseburger, Jumbo Jack	1 ea	296	714	26	56	3	43		
62547	Cheeseburger, bacon ultimate	1 ea	302	974	41	47	2	69		
57014	Chicken teriyaki bowl	1 ea	502	670	26	128	3	4		
56445	Egg roll, 3 piece serving	1 ea	170	400	14	44	6	19		
6425	French fries, curly, medium	1 ea	125	404	6	44	4	23		
6150	French fries, natural cut, small	1 ea	113	306	5	40	3	14		
62558	French toast, original, sticks, serving	1 ea	120	466	7	58	4	23		
56433	Hamburger	1 ea	104	273	14	26	1	12		
62560	Milk shake, cappuccino, medium	1 ea	419	630	11	80	0	29		
2964	Milk shake, Oreo cookie, medium	1 ea	419	941	15	112	1	46		
2165	Milk shake, vanilla, medium	1 ea	332	664	13	75	1	34		
56446	Onion rings, serving	1 ea	120	504	6	51	3	30		
62551	Potato wedges, bacon cheddar, serving	1 ea	268	692	21	53	6	44		
8368	Salad dressing, blue cheese, packet	1 ea	57	210	1	11	0	15		
8449	Salad dressing, Italian, low cal, serving	1 ea	57	25	0	2	0	2		
52088	Salad, garden chicken	1 ea	253	200	23	8	3	9		
56441	Sandwich, chicken fajita pita	1 ea	230	317	24	33	3	11		
56431	Sandwich, breakfast, sausage w/croissant	1 ea	181	603	22	38	2	41		
56377	Taco, beef, regular	1 ea	90	189	6	18	2	9		
	Source: Jack in the Box									

KFC

42331	Biscuit, buttermilk	1 ea	57	190	2	23	0	10		
15169	Chicken breast, extra crispy	1 ea	162	460	34	19	0	28		
15185	Chicken breast, hot & spicy	1 ea	179	460	33	20	0	27		
15163	Chicken breast, original recipe	1 ea	161	380	40	11	0	19		
81292	Chicken breast, original recipe, w/o skin or breading	1 ea	108	140	29	0	0	3		
81293	Chicken, drumstick, original recipe	1 ea	59	140	14	4	0	8		
15166	Chicken thigh, original recipe	1 ea	126	360	22	12	0	25		
416	Chicken wing, pieces, honey bbq	6 ea	157	540	25	36	1	33		
56451	Cole slaw, serving	1 ea	130	190	1	22	3	11		
9535	Corn, cob, small	1 ea	82	76	3	13	4	2		
2897	Dessert, strawberry shortcake, Lil Bucket	1 ea	99	200	2	34	0	6		
56681	Macaroni & cheese	1 ea	287	130	5	15	1	6		

Sat (g)	Chol (mg)	Calc (mg)	Iron (mg)	Mag (mg)	Phos (mg)	Pota (mg)	Sodi (mg)	Zinc (mg)	Vit A (RAE)	Vit C (mg)	Thia (mg)	Ribo (mg)	Niac (mg)	Vit B6 (mg)	Vit B12 (µg)	Vit E (mg)	Fol (µg)	Alc (g)
10.9	57	279	3.4				1349			0.1								0
7.1	34	279	3.44				987			1.3								0
4	0						250											0
2	0						350											0
2	30						740											0
12	55						1238											0
1.7	25						736											0
25	185						1573											0
27	137						1584											0
1	10						120											0
3	0						520											0
1	60						697											0
7	75						1280											0
16.6	72					424	1356											0
26.8	125					482	1823											0
1	15	100	4.5			620	1730			24								0
6	15					430	920											0
4.4	0					581	882											0
3.5	0					715	502											0
5	25					119	446											0
5.3	35					220	529											0
17	90	350	0			710	320			0								0
25.8	157					913	488											0
21	134					734	256											0
6.1	0					141	424											0
14.8	49					951	1581											0
2.5	25	20	0			40	750	0		0								0
0	0	10	0			40	670	0		0								0
4	65	200	0.72			560	420			12								0
4.7	69					475	928											0
13.5	265					270	801											0
3.6	18					225	320											0
2	0	0	0.72				580	0		0								0
8	135	0	1.44				1230	0		0								0
8	130	0	1.14				1450	0		0								0
6	145	0	1.8				1150	0		0								0
1	95	0	0.72				410	0		0								0
2	75	0	0.72				440	0		0								0
7	165	0	1.14				1060	0		0								0
7	150	60	2.7				1130			4.8								0
2	5	40	0				300			24								0
0.5	0	30	0.55				5	0		3								0
4	20	20	0				110	0		0								0
2	5	100	0.72				610			24								0

MDA Code	Food Name	Amt	Wt (g)	Ener (kcal)	Prot (g)	Carb (g)	Fiber (g)	Fat (g)	Mono (g)	Poly (g)
56453	Mashed potatoes w/gravy, serving	1 ea	136	130	2	18	1	4		
45166	Pecan pie, Colonel's Pies, slice	1 pce	95	370	4	55	2	15		
81090	Pot pie, chicken, chunky	1 ea	423	770	29	70	5	40		
56454	Potato salad, serving	1 ea	128	180	2	22	1	9		
49148	Sandwich, chicken, honey bbq flavor, w/sauce	1 ea	147	300	21	41	4	6		
81301	Sandwich, chicken, tender roasted, w/o sauce	1 ea	177	260	31	23	1	5		
81093	Sandwich, chicken, tender roasted, w/sauce	1 ea	196	390	31	24	1	19		
81302	Sandwich, chicken, Twister	1 ea	252	670	27	55	3	38		
	Source: Yum! Brands, Inc.									

Long John Silver's

MDA Code	Food Name	Amt	Wt (g)	Ener (kcal)	Prot (g)	Carb (g)	Fiber (g)	Fat (g)	Mono (g)	Poly (g)
91388	Cheese sticks, breaded, fried	3 ea	45	140	4	12	1	8		
91390	Clam chowder, serving	1 ea	227	220	9	23	1	10		
56477	Cornbread, hush puppies, serving	1 ea	23	60	1	9	1	2		
56461	Fish, batter dipped, regular	1 pce	92	230	11	16	0	13		
92415	Fish, cod, baked, serving	1 ea	100.7	120	21	0	0	5		
91392	Sandwich, fish, batter dipped, ultimate	1 ea	199	500	20	48	3	25		
92290	Shrimp, battered, 4 piece serving	1 ea	65.8	197	7	14	0	13		
92292	Shrimp, crunchy, breaded, fried, basket	1 ea	114	340	12	32	2	19		
	Source: Yum! Brands, Inc.									

McDonald's

MDA Code	Food Name	Amt	Wt (g)	Ener (kcal)	Prot (g)	Carb (g)	Fiber (g)	Fat (g)	Mono (g)	Poly (g)
81465	Breakfast, big, w/eggs, sausage, hashbrowns, biscuit	1 ea	266	742	27	46	3	52	22.9	7.5
56675	Burrito, sausage, breakfast	1 ea	113	296	13	24	1	17	6.5	2.4
69010	Cheeseburger, Big Mac	1 ea	219	563	26	44	4	33	7.6	0.7
81458	Cheeseburger, double	1 ea	173	458	26	34	1	26	8.6	0.8
69012	Cheeseburger, Quarter Pounder	1 ea	199	513	29	40	3	28	9.2	0.9
49152	Chicken McNuggets, 6 piece serving	6 pce	100	264	16	16	0	15	6.2	5
42334	Croutons, serving	1 ea	12	50	1	9	1	1		
42335	Danish, apple	1 ea	105	340	5	47	2	15		
72902	Dessert, apple dipper, w/low fat caramel sauce	1 ea	89	99	0	23		1	0.2	0
81440	French fries, large	1 ea	171	576	6	70	7	31	13.8	8
2171	Hot fudge sundae	1 ea	179	333	7	54	1	11	1.9	0.4
69008	Hamburger	1 ea	105	265	13	32	1	10	3.3	0.2
69011	Hamburger, Quarter Pounder	1 ea	171	417	24	38	3	20	7.2	0.5
6155	Hash browns	1 ea	53	136	1	13	2	9	3.9	2.2
1747	McFlurry, frozen dessert, Butterfinger	1 ea	348	620	16	90	1	22		
72913	Milk shake, chocolate, triple thick, large	1 ea	713	1162	26	199	1	32	8	1.5
81453	Pancakes, hotcake, w/2 pats margarine & syrup	1 ea	221	601	9	102	2	18	1.9	4.6
81154	Parfait, fruit n' yogurt, w/o granola	1 ea	142	128	4	25	1	2	0	0
48136	Pie, apple	1 ea	77	249	2	34	2	12	7.1	0.8
69218	Salad, bacon ranch, w/crispy chicken	1 ea	316	335	27	21	3	18	6.2	4
608	Salad, caesar, w/chicken, shaker	1 ea	163	100	17	3	2	2		
61674	Salad, California cobb, w/grilled chicken	1 ea	325	273	34	11	3	11	3.8	1.4
57764	Salad, chef, shaker	1 ea	206	150	17	5	2	8		
61667	Salad, fruit & walnut	1 ea	264	312	5	44		13	2.1	8.5
81466	Sandwich, breakfast, McGriddle w/bacon, egg & cheese	1 ea	168	457	20	44	1	22	7.9	3
69013	Sandwich, Filet-O-Fish	1 ea	141	400	15	40	1	20	4.3	7
81456	Sandwich, Filet-O-Fish, w/o tartar sauce	1 ea	123	289	15	40	1	11	2.2	1.8
53176	Sauce, barbecue, packet	1 ea	28	46	0	10	0	0	0.1	0.1
53177	Sauce, sweet & sour, packet	1 ea	28	48	0	11	0	0	0.1	0.1
12230	Sausage, pork, serving	1 ea	43	170	6	0	0	16		
42747	Sweet roll, cinnamon	1 ea	105	418	8	56	2	19	9.5	3
	Source: McDonald's Nutrition Information Center									

Sat (g)	Chol (mg)	Calc (mg)	Iron (mg)	Mag (mg)	Phos (mg)	Pota (mg)	Sodi (mg)	Zinc (mg)	Vit A (RAE)	Vit C (mg)	Thia (mg)	Ribo (mg)	Niac (mg)	Vit B6 (mg)	Vit B12 (µg)	Vit E (mg)	Fol (µg)	Alc (g)
1	0	0	0.36				380			2.4								0
2.5	40	0	1.44				190			0								0
15	115	0	3.6				1680			0								0
1.5	5	0	0.36				470		0	6								0
1.5	50	60	2.7				640			2.4								0
1.5	65	40	1.8				690		0	0								0
4	70	40	1.8				810		0	0								0
7	60	150	2.7				1650			4.8								0
2	10	100	0.72				320			0								0
4	25	150	0.72				810			0								0
0.5	0	20	0.36				200		0	0								0
4	30	20	1.8				700		0	4.8								0
1	90	20	0.72				240			0								0
8	50	150	3.6				1310			9								0
4.1	64	23	0.83				579		0	2.8								0
5	105	500	1.8				720		0	0								0
13.6	466	130	5	37.2	684	545	1463	2.6	189	1.6	0.61	0.94	6.04	0.46	1.54	3.3	196.8	0
6.1	173	203	1.84	19.2	247	155	763	1.3	97	0.9	0.18	0.33	1.92	0.41	0.61	0.2	70.1	0
8.3	79	254	4.38	43.8	267	396	1007	4.2		0.9	0.39	0.46	7.41	0.37	1.93	0.1	100.7	0
10.5	83	277	3.68	34.6	280	375	1137	4.2		0.7	0.28	0.43	6.68		2.04		77.8	0
11.2	94	287	4.18	43.8	320	436	1152	5.2		1.6	0.33	0.7	7.66	0.19	2.51	0.4	101.5	0
3.3	39	14	0.78	22	332	251	699	0.6		1	0.16	0.11	7.4	0.4	0.33		28	0
0	0	20	0.36	3.9	18	26	105	0.1	0	0.2	0.08	0.05	0.57	0.02	0.02		5.1	0
3	20	60	1.44		0	113	340			15	0.3	0.17	2					0
0.4	3	57	0.1				36	0.1	11	188.3	0.02	0.03	0	0.01	0	0.1	0	0
6.1	0	27	1.76	54.7	226	958	332	0.8	0	8.4	0.56	0.06	4.72	0.89		3.5	102.6	0
6.4	23	249	1.49	34	229	440	168	1	145		0.08	0.4	0.27	0.09	0.98	0.3	0	0
3.1	28	127	2.77	21	112	213	532	2		0.6	0.26	0.25	4.77	0.1	0.87	0.1	67.2	0
6.9	67	144	4.12	37.6	212	388	730	4.6		1.5	0.31	0.59	7.61	0.25	2.19	0.1	95.8	0
1.6	0	10	0.4	11.1	57	207	289	0.2	0	1.6	0.06	0.01	1.19	0.13		1	20.1	0
14	70	450	0.36				260			2.4								0
16.4	100	870	3.85	114.1	749	1611	506	3.6	649		0.28	1.53	0.94	0.36	3.85	0	7.1	0
1.8	20	126	2.83	28.7	391	276	625	0.6		0	0.45	0.4	3.24	0.11	0.02		143.6	0
0	7	124	0.51	17	101	234	54	0.4		20.6	0.05	0.17	0.27		0.28		15.6	0
3.1		15	1.53	5.4	28	49	153	0.2		24.9	0.23	0.16	2.03	0.04		1.5	87	0
5	70	149	2.05				1112			31.6	0.19	0.22	9.56		0.41		154.8	0
1.5	40	100	1.08				240			12								0
4.8	143	143	2.21				1079			31.9	0.18	0.33	11.67				149.5	0
3.5	95	150	1.44				740			15								0
1.8	5	172	0.9	34.3	129		84	0.7		383.6	0.1	0.15	0.27	0.25	0.16		13.2	0
7.1	247	183	2.77				1263	3		0.21	0.5	2.22					89	0
3.7	39	164	2.07	28.2	166	247	633	0.7		0	0.36	0.26	3.4	0.06	1.03	1.6	70.5	0
2.1	31	159	2	28.3	161	237	520	0.7		0	0.35	0.25	3.41		0.98		70.1	0
0		3	0.11	3.6	8	55	255	0	3	0	0.01	0.01	0.19	0.02		0.3	2.2	0
0		2	0.18	1.7	4	28	156	0	2	0.3	0.05	0.01	0.11	0.01		0.2	0	0
5	35	7	0.36	6.6	59	102	290	0.8	0	0	0.18	0.06	1.7	0.09	0.35	0.3		0
4.7	61	60	1.81	20	109	147	397	0.9	132	0	0.32	0.28	2.53	0.11		1.9	108.2	0

MDA Code	Food Name	Amt	Wt (g)	Ener (kcal)	Prot (g)	Carb (g)	Fiber (g)	Fat (g)	Mono (g)	Poly (g)
	Pizza Hut									
92497	Breadsticks, cheese	1 ea	67	200	7	21	1	10		
92526	Dessert pizza, cherry, slice	1 pce	102	240	4	47	1	4		
92519	Pasta Bakes, primavera w/chicken, serving	1 ea	540	1050	52	97	6	50		
57394	Pizza, beef, med, 12"	1 pce	91	230	11	21	2	11		
56489	Pizza, cheese, med, 12"	1 pce	96	260	11	30	2	10	2.8	1.8
56481	Pizza, cheese, pan, med, 12"	1 pce	100	280	12	30	2	13	3.2	2.8
57781	Pizza, chicken supreme, med, 12"	1 pce	120	230	14	30	2	6		
830	Pizza, super supreme, med, 12"	1 pce	127	309	14	33	3	14	5	2.2
92483	Pizza, green pepper onion & tomato, med, 12"	1 pce	104	150	6	24	2	4		
92482	Pizza, ham pine & tomato, med, 12"	1 pce	99	160	8	24	2	4		
57810	Pizza, Meat Lover's, med, 12"	1 pce	169	450	21	43	3	21		
56486	Pizza, pepperoni, med, 12"	1 pce	77	210	10	21	1	10		
57811	Pizza, Veggie Lover's, med, 12"	1 pce	172	360	16	45	3	14		
	Source: Yum! Brands, Inc.									
	Subway									
47658	Cookie, chocolate chip, M & M's	1 ea	45	220	2	30	1	10		
52119	Salad, chicken breast, roasted	1 ea	303	140	16	12	3	3		
52115	Salad, club	1 ea	322	150	17	12	3	4		
52118	Salad, tuna, w/light mayonnaise	1 ea	314	240	13	10	3	16		
52113	Salad, veggie delite	1 ea	233	50	2	9	3	1		
91761	Sandwich, chicken teriyaki, w/sweet onion, on white bread, 6"	1 ea	269	380	26	59	4	5		
69117	Sandwich, club, on white bread, 6"	1 ea	255	320	24	46	4	6		
69113	Sandwich, cold cut trio, on white bread, 6"	1 ea	257	440	21	47	4	21		
91763	Sandwich, ham w/honey mustard, on white bread, 6"	1 ea	232	310	18	52	4	5		
69139	Sandwich, Italian BMT, on white bread, 6"	1 ea	248	480	23	46	4	24		
69129	Sandwich, meatball, on white bread, 6"	1 ea	287	530	24	53	6	26		
69103	Sandwich, roast beef, deli style	1 ea	151	220	13	35	3	4		
69143	Sandwich, tuna, w/light mayonnaise, on white bread, 6"	1 ea	255	450	20	46	4	22		
69101	Sandwich, turkey, deli style	1 ea	151	220	13	36	3	4		
69109	Sandwich, veggie delite, on white bread, 6"	1 ea	166	230	9	44	4	3		
91778	Soup, chicken noodle, roasted	1 cup	240	90	7	7	1	4		
91791	Soup, cream of broccoli	1 cup	240	130	5	15	2	6		
91783	Soup, minestrone	1 cup	240	70	3	11	2	1		
91788	Soup, rice, brown & wild, w/chicken	1 cup	240	190	6	17	2	11		
	Source: Subway International									
	Taco Bell									
92107	Border Bowl, chicken, zesty	1 ea	417	730	23	65	12	42		
56519	Burrito, bean	1 ea	198	404	16	55	8	14	5.9	1.7
56522	Burrito, beef, supreme	1 ea	248	469	20	52	8	20	8.1	2
57668	Burrito, chicken, fiesta	1 ea	184	370	18	48	3	12		
56691	Burrito, seven layer	1 ea	283	530	18	67	10	22		
92113	Burrito, steak, grilled, Stuft	1 ea	325	680	31	76	8	28		
92118	Chalupa, beef, nacho cheese	1 ea	153	380	12	33	3	22		
92120	Chalupa, chicken, Baja	1 ea	153	400	17	30	2	24		
92122	Chalupa, steak, supreme	1 ea	153	370	15	29	2	22		
45585	Cinnamon twists, serving	1 ea	35	160	1	28	0	5		
57666	Gordita, beef, Baja	1 ea	153	350	14	31	4	19		
57669	Gordita, chicken, Baja	1 ea	153	320	17	29	2	15		
57662	Gordita, steak, Baja	1 ea	153	320	15	29	2	16		

Sat (g)	Chol (mg)	Calc (mg)	Iron (mg)	Mag (mg)	Phos (mg)	Pota (mg)	Sodi (mg)	Zinc (mg)	Vit A (RAE)	Vit C (mg)	Thia (mg)	Ribo (mg)	Niac (mg)	Vit B$_6$ (mg)	Vit B$_{12}$ (µg)	Vit E (mg)	Fol (µg)	Alc (g)
3.5	15	100	3.6				340			0								0
0.5	0	20	1.08				250			6								0
12	75	800	5.4				2760			6								0
5	25	150	1.8				710			3.6								0
4.8	23	201	1.87	21.1	239	166	658	1.6	71	0	0.25	0.25	3.16	0.11	0.67	0.7		0
5.2	21	208	1.86	21	241	168	624	1.6	74	0	0.24	0.25	3.91	0.11	0.64	1.1		0
3	25	150	1.8				550			6								0
5.8	25	164	2.54	29.2	254	296	875	1.8	46	0	0.34	0.31	4.55	0.19	0.79	1		0
1.5	10	80	1.44				360			21								0
2	15	80	1.44				470			12								0
10	55	250	2.7				1250			9								0
4.5	25	150	1.44				550			2.4								0
7	35	250	2.7				980			9								0
4	15	0	1.08				105	0	0									0
1	45	40	1.08				800			30								0
1.5	35	40	18				1110			30								0
4	40	100	1.08				880			30								0
0	0	40	1.08				310			30								0
1.5	50	80	3.6				1100			27								0
2	35	60	5.4				1300			21								0
7	55	150	5.4				1680			24								0
1.5	25	60	3.6				1260			24								0
9	55	150	3.6				1900			24								0
10	55	150	5.4				1360			27								0
2	15	60	5.4				660			12								0
6	40	15	3.6				1190			24								0
1.5	15	60	3.6				730			12								0
1	0	60	3.6				510			21								0
1	20	20	0				1180			3.6								0
0	10	150	0				860			12								0
0	10	40	0				1030			6								0
4.5	20	300	0				990			24								0
9	45	150	3.6				1640			9								0
4.8	18	232	4.57	61.4	337	533	1216	1.7	6		0.4	0.3	3.39	0.24	0	1	99	0
7.6	40	231	5.6	62	337	608	1424	2.6	10		0.38	0.37	4.33	0.26	1.24	1.1	111.6	0
3.5	30	200	2.7				1090			3.6								0
8	25	300	3.6				1360			4.8								0
8	55	300	4.5				1940			3.6								0
7	20	100	1.44				740			6								0
6	40	100	1.08				690			3.6								0
8	35	100	1.44				520			3.6								0
1	0	0	0.36				150	0	0									0
5	30	150	2.7				750			4.8								0
3.5	40	100	1.8				690			3.6								0
4	30	100	1.8				680			3.6								0

MDA Code	Food Name	Amt	Wt (g)	Ener (kcal)	Prot (g)	Carb (g)	Fiber (g)	Fat (g)	Mono (g)	Poly (g)
56530	Guacamole, serving	1 ea	21	35	0	2	1	3		
38561	Mexican rice, serving	1 ea	131	210	6	23	3	10		
56534	Nachos, BellGrande, svg	1 ea	308	780	20	80	12	43		
56536	Pintos & cheese, serving	1 ea	128	180	10	20	6	7		
56531	Pizza, Mexican	1 ea	216	550	21	46	7	31		
57689	Quesadilla, chicken	1 ea	184	540	28	40	3	30		
92098	Salsa, fiesta	1 ea	21	5	0	1		0	0	0
53186	Sauce, border, hot, packet	1 ea	11	4	0	0	0	0	0	0
92105	Southwest steak bowl	1 ea	443	700	30	73	13	32		
56524	Taco, beef	1 ea	78	184	8	14	3	11	4.2	1.6
57671	Taco, Double Decker, supreme	1 ea	191	380	15	40	6	18		
56693	Taco, soft, steak	1 ea	127	286	15	22	2	15	5	4.4
56537	Salad, taco, w/salsa & shell	1 ea	533	906	36	80	16	49	21.2	4
56528	Tostada	1 ea	170	250	11	29	7	10		
	Source: Taco Bell/Yum! Brands, Inc.									

Wendy's

MDA Code	Food Name	Amt	Wt (g)	Ener (kcal)	Prot (g)	Carb (g)	Fiber (g)	Fat (g)	Mono (g)	Poly (g)
56579	Baked potato bacon cheese	1 ea	380	580	18	79	7	22		
56582	Baked potato, w/sour cream & chives	1 ea	312	370	7	73	7	6		
81445	Cheeseburger, classic single	1 ea	236	522	35	34	3	27	10.4	3.3
56571	Cheeseburger, w/bacon, jr	1 ea	165	380	20	34	2	19		
15176	Chicken nuggets, 5 piece serving	1 ea	75	250	12	12	0	17	8.5	4.3
50311	Chili, small	1 ea	227	200	17	21	5	6		
6169	French fries, Biggie	1 ea	159	507	6	63	6	26	13.5	5.9
2177	Frozen dessert, dairy, medium	1 ea	298	393	10	70	10	8	2.1	0.3
56574	Hamburger, Big Bacon Classic	1 ea	282	570	34	46	3	29		
56566	Hamburger, classic single	1 ea	218	464	28	37	3	23	8.9	3.4
8457	Salad dressing, blue cheese, packet	1 ea	71	290	2	3	0	30		
8461	Salad dressing, French, fat free, packet	1 ea	71	90	0	21	1	0	0	0
71595	Salad dressing, Oriental sesame, packet	1 ea	71	280	2	21	0	21		
81444	Sandwich, chicken fillet, homestyle	1 ea	230	492	32	50	3	19	6.7	7.1
81443	Sandwich, chicken, Ultimate Grill	1 ea	225	403	33	42	2	11	3.3	4.1
52080	Salad, caesar, w/o dressing, side	1 ea	99	70	7	2	1	4		
71592	Salad, chicken, mandarin, w/o dressing	1 ea	348	150	20	17	3	2		
52083	Salad, garden, w/o dressing, side	1 ea	167	35	2	7	3	0	0	0
	Source: Wendy's Foods International									

Sat (g)	Chol (mg)	Calc (mg)	Iron (mg)	Mag (mg)	Phos (mg)	Pota (mg)	Sodi (mg)	Zinc (mg)	Vit A (RAE)	Vit C (mg)	Thia (mg)	Ribo (mg)	Niac (mg)	Vit B$_6$ (mg)	Vit B$_{12}$ (µg)	Vit E (mg)	Fol (µg)	Alc (g)
0	0	0	0				100		0	0								0
4	15	100	1.8				740			4.8								0
13	35	200	2.7				1300			6								0
3.5	15	150	1.08				700			3.6								0
11	45	350	3.6				1030			6								0
13	80	500	1.8				1380			2.4								0
0	0	0	0				60		5	2.4								0
0	0	0	0				102			0								0
8	55	200	6.3				2050			9								0
3.6	24	62	1.47	25.7	139	168	349	1.7	3		0.07	0.15	1.5	0.11	0.75	0.5	14.8	0
8	40	150	2.7				820			4.8								0
4.3	39	149	2.82	26.7	197	232	700	2.7	1		0.39	0.25	3.78	0.11	1.22	0.5	47	0
15.9	101	506	9.43	143.9	549	1221	1935	6.2	16		0.8	0.56	8.02	0.55	2.13	2.9	229.2	0
4	15	150	1.44				710			4.8								0
6	40	200	3.6			1410	950			42								0
4	15	60	3.6			1230	40			36								0
12.3	90	177	5.52	44.8	297	441	1123	6.1		1.2	0.61	0.6	7.53	0.25	3.63			0
7	55	150	3.6			320	890			9								0
3.7	38	18	0.56	18	215	177	509	0.5		1	0.06	0.09	4.53	0.19	0.25			0
2.5	35	80	1.8			470	870			2.4								0
5.1		24	3.07	54.1	218	914	273	0.8		8.1	0.28	0.1	3.95	0.62			27	0
4.9	48	381	3.1	59.6	334	551	292	1.3		0	0.18	2.15	1.04	0	1.76			0
12	100	200	5.4			580	1460			15								0
8	76	74	5.95	39.2	225	425	861	5.4		1.1	0.6	0.45	7.03	0.25	3.16			0
6	45	60	1.08			25	870			0								0
0	0	0	0.72			10	240		0	0								0
3	0	20	0.72			40	620		0	0								0
3.7	71	53	3.45	55.2	370	524	922	1.4		0.7	0.68	0.3	7.59	0.43	0.76			0
2.3	90	56	3.49	54	378	497	961	1.3		2.5	0.88	0.58	9.36	0.32	0.74			0
2	15	150	1.08			280	250			21								0
0	10	60	1.8			420	650			30								0
0	0	40	0.72			350	20		350	18								0

APPENDIX B CALCULATIONS & CONVERSIONS

Calculation and Conversion Aids

Commonly Used Metric Units

millimeter (mm): one-thousandth of a meter (0.001)

centimeter (cm): one-hundredth of a meter (0.01)

kilometer (km): one-thousand times a meter (1000)

kilogram (kg): one-thousand times a gram (1000)

milligram (mg): one-thousandth of a gram (0.001)

microgram (μg): one-millionth of a gram (0.000001)

milliliter (ml): one-thousandth of a liter (0.001)

International Units

Some vitamin supplements may report vitamin content as International Units (IU).

To convert IU to:

- Micrograms of vitamin D (cholecalciferol), divide the IU value by 40 or multiply by 0.025.
- Milligrams of vitamin E (alpha-tocopherol), divide the IU value by 1.5 if vitamin E is from natural sources. Divide the IU value by 2.22 if vitamin E is from synthetic sources.
- Vitamin A: 1 IU = 0.3 μg retinol or 3.6 μg beta-carotene

Retinol Activity Equivalents

Retinol Activity Equivalents (RAE) are a standardized unit of measure for vitamin A. RAE account for the various differences in bioavailability from sources of vitamin A. Many supplements will report vitamin A content in IU, as shown above, or Retinol Equivalents (RE).

1 RAE = 1 μg retinol
        12 μg beta-carotene
        24 μg other vitamin A carotenoids

To calculate RAE from the RE value of vitamin carotenoids in foods, divide RE by 2.

For vitamin A supplements and foods fortified with vitamin A, 1 RE = 1 RAE.

Folate

Folate is measured as Dietary Folate Equivalents (DFE). DFE account for the different factors affecting bioavailability of folate sources.

1 DFE = 1 μg food folate
        0.6 μg folate from fortified foods
        0.5 μg folate supplement taken on an
          empty stomach
        0.6 μg folate as a supplement consumed
          with a meal

To convert micrograms of synthetic folate, such as that found in supplements or fortified foods, to DFE:

$$\mu\text{g synthetic folate} \times 1.7 = \mu\text{g DFE}$$

For naturally occurring food folate, such as spinach, each microgram of folate equals 1 microgram DFE:

$$\mu\text{g folate} = \mu\text{g DFE}$$

Conversion Factors

Use the following table to convert U.S. measurements to metric equivalents:

Original Unit	Multiply by	To Get
ounces avdp	28.3495	grams
ounces	0.0625	pounds
pounds	0.4536	kilograms
pounds	16	ounces
grams	0.0353	ounces
grams	0.002205	pounds
kilograms	2.2046	pounds
liters	1.8162	pints (dry)
liters	2.1134	pints (liquid)
liters	0.9081	quarts (dry)
liters	1.0567	quarts (liquid)
liters	0.2642	gallons (U.S.)
pints (dry)	0.5506	liters
pints (liquid)	0.4732	liters
quarts (dry)	1.1012	liters
quarts liquid	0.9463	liters
gallons (U.S.)	3.7853	liters
millimeters	0.0394	inches
centimeters	0.3937	inches
centimeters	0.03281	feet
inches	25.4000	millimeters
inches	2.5400	centimeters
inches	0.0254	meters
feet	0.3048	meters
meters	3.2808	feet
meters	1.0936	yards
cubic feet	0.0283	cubic meters
cubic meters	35.3145	cubic feet
cubic meters	1.3079	cubic yards
cubic yards	0.7646	cubic meters

Length: U.S. and Metric Equivalents

¼ inch = 0.6 centimeters
1 inch = 2.54 centimeters
1 foot = 0.3048 meter
         30.48 centimeters
1 yard = 0.91144 meter
1 millimeter = 0.03937 inch
1 centimeter = 0.3937 inch
1 decimeter = .937 inches
1 meter = 39.37 inches
         1.094 yards
1 micron = 0.00003937 inch

Weights and Measures

Food Measurement Equivalencies from U.S. to Metric

Capacity

⅛ teaspoon = 1 milliliter
¼ teaspoon = 1.25 milliliters
½ teaspoon = 2.5 milliliters
1 teaspoon = 5 milliliters
1 tablespoon = 15 milliliters
1 fluid ounce = 28.4 milliliters
¼ cup = 60 milliliters
⅓ cup = 80 milliliters
½ cup = 120 milliliters
1 cup = 225 milliliters
1 pint (2 cups) = 473 milliliters
1 quart (4 cups) = 0.95 liter
1 liter (1.06 quarts) = 1,000 milliliters
1 gallon (4 quarts) = 3.84 liters

Weight

0.035 ounce = 1 gram
1 ounce = 28 grams
¼ pound (4 ounces) = 114 grams
1 pound (16 ounces) = 454 grams
2.2 pounds (35 ounces) = 1 kilogram

U.S. Food Measurement Equivalents

3 teaspoons = 1 tablespoon
½ tablespoon = 1½ teaspoons
2 tablespoons = ⅛ cup
4 tablespoons = ¼ cup
5 tablespoons + 1 teaspoon = ⅓ cup
8 tablespoons = ½ cup
10 tablespoons + 2 teaspoons = ⅔ cup
12 tablespoons = ¾ cup
16 tablespoons = 1 cup
2 cups = 1 pint
4 cups = 1 quart
2 pints = 1 quart
4 quarts = 1 gallon

Volumes and Capacities

1 cup = 8 fluid ounces
½ liquid pint
1 milliliter = 0.061 cubic inches
1 liter = 1.057 liquid quarts
0.908 dry quart
61.024 cubic inches
1 U.S. gallon = 231 cubic inches
3.785 liters
0.833 British gallon
128 U.S. fluid ounces

1 British Imperial gallon = 277.42 cubic inches
1.201 U.S. gallons
4.546 liters
160 British fluid ounces
1 U.S. ounce, liquid or fluid = 1.805 cubic inches
29.574 milliliters
1.041 British fluid ounces
1 pint, dry = 33.600 cubic inches
0.551 liter
1 pint, liquid = 28.875 cubic inches
0.473 liter
1 U.S. quart, dry = 67.201 cubic inches
1.101 liters
1 U.S. quart, liquid = 57.75 cubic inches
0.946 liter
1 British quart = 69.354 cubic inches
1.032 U.S. quarts, dry
1.201 U.S. quarts, liquid

Energy Units

Commonly Used Energy Units

1 kilocalorie (kcal) = 4.2 kilojoules
1 millijoule (MJ) = 240 kilocalories
1 kilojoule (kJ) = 0.24 kcal
1 gram carbohydrate = 4 kcal
1 gram fat = 9 kcal
1 gram protein = 4 kcal

Temperature Standards

	°Fahrenheit	°Celsius
Body temperature	98.6°	37°
Comfortable room temperature	65–75°	18–24°
Boiling point of water	212°	100°
Freezing point of water	32°	0°

Temperature Scales

To Convert Fahrenheit to Celsius:

$[(°F - 32) \times 5]/9$

1. Subtract 32 from °F
2. Multiply (°F − 32) by 5, then divide by 9

To Convert Celsius to Fahrenheit:

$[(°C \times 9)/5] + 32$

1. Multiply °C by 9, then divide by 5
2. Add 32 to (°C × 9/5)

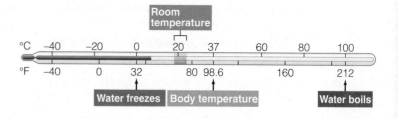

APPENDIX C FOODS CONTAINING CAFFEINE

Source: Values are obtained from the USDA Nutrient Database for Standard Reference, Release 18.

Beverages

Food Name	Serving	Caffeine/serving (mg)
Beverage mix, chocolate flavor, dry mix, prep w/milk	1 cup (8 fl. oz)	7.98
Beverage mix, chocolate malt powder, fortified, prepared w/milk	1 cup (8 fl. oz)	5.3
Beverage mix, chocolate malted milk powder, no added nutrients, prepared w/milk	1 cup (8 fl. oz)	7.95
Beverage, chocolate syrup w/o added nutrients, prepared w/milk	1 cup (8 fl. oz)	5.64
Beverage, chocolate syrup, fortified, mixed w/milk	1 cup milk and 1 tbsp syrup	2.63
Cocoa mix w/aspartame and calcium and phosphorus, no sodium or vitamin A, low kcal, dry, prepared	6 fl. oz water and 0.53 oz packet	5
Cocoa mix w/aspartame, dry, low kcal, prepared w/water	1 packet dry mix with 6 fl. oz H_2O	1.92
Cocoa mix, dry mix	1 serving (3 heaping tsp or 1 envelope)	5.04
Cocoa mix, dry, w/o added nutrients, prepared w/water	1 oz packet with 6 fl. oz H_2O	4.12
Cocoa mix, fortified, dry, prepared w/water	6 fl. oz H_2O and 1 packet	6.27
Cocoa, dry powder, hi-fat or breakfast, plain	1 piece	6.895
Cocoa, hot, homemade w/who!e milk	1 cup	5
Coffee liqueur 53 proof	1 fl. oz	9.048
Coffee liqueur 63 proof	1 fl. oz	9.048
Coffee w/cream liqueur, 34 proof	1 fl. oz	2.488
Coffee mix w/sugar (cappuccino), dry, prepared w/water	6 fl. oz H_2O and 2 rounded tsp mix	74.88
Coffee mix w/sugar (French), dry, prepared w/water	6 fl. oz H_2O and 2 rounded tsp mix	51.03
Coffee mix w/sugar (mocha), dry, prepared w/water	6 fl. oz H_2O and 2 rounded tsp mix	33.84
Coffee, brewed	1 cup (8 fl. oz)	85.32
Coffee, brewed, prepared with tap water, decaffeinated	1 cup (8 fl. oz)	2.37
Coffee, instant, prepared	1 fl. oz	7.748
Coffee, instant, regular, powder, half the caffeine	1 cup (8 fl. oz)	3723.27
Coffee, instant powder, decaffeinated, prepared	6 fl. oz	1.79
Coffee and cocoa (mocha) powder, with whitener and low-calorie sweetener	1 cup	405.48
Coffee, brewed, espresso, restaurant-prepared	1 fl. oz	60.081
Coffee, brewed, espresso, restaurant-prepared, decaffeinated	1 cup (8 fl.oz)	2.37
Energy drink, with caffeine, niacin, pantothenic acid, vitamin B_6	1 fl. oz	9.517
Milk beverage mix, dairy drink w/aspartame, low kcal, dry, prep	6 fl. oz	4.08
Milk, lowfat, 1% fat, chocolate	1 cup	5
Milk, whole, chocolate	1 cup	5
Soft drink, cola w/caffeine	1 fl. oz	2
Soft drink, cola, w/higher caffeine	1 fl. oz	8.37
Soft drink, cola or pepper type, low kcal w/saccharin and caffeine	1 fl. oz	3.256
Soft drink, cola, low kcal w/saccharin and aspartame, w/caffeine	1 fl. oz	4.144
Soft drink, lemon-lime soda, w/caffeine	1 fl. oz	4.605
Soft drink, low kcal, not cola or pepper, with aspartame and caffeine	1 fl. oz	4.44
Soft drink, pepper type	1 fl. oz	3.07
Tea mix, instant w/lemon flavor, w/saccharin, dry, prepared	1 cup (8 fl. oz)	16.59
Tea mix, instant w/lemon, unsweetened, dry, prepared	1 cup (8 fl. oz)	26.18
Tea mix, instant w/sugar and lemon, dry, no added vitamin C, prepared	1 cup (8 fl. oz)	28.49
Tea mix, instant, unsweetened, dry, prepared	1 cup (8 fl. oz)	30.81
Tea, brewed	1 cup (8 fl. oz)	47.4
Tea, brewed, prepared with tap water, decaffeinated	1 cup (8 fl. oz)	2.37
Tea, instant, unsweetened, powder, decaffeinated	1 tsp	1.183
Tea, instant, w/sugar, lemon-flavored, w/added vitamin C, dry prepared	1 cup (8 fl. oz)	28.49
Tea, instant, with sugar, lemon-flavored, decaffeinated, no added vitamin	1 cup	9.1

Cake, Cookies, and Desserts

Food Name	Serving	Caffeine/serving (mg)
Brownies, commercially prepared, Little Debbie	1 oz	0.567
Cake, chocolate pudding, dry mix	1 oz	1.701
Cake, chocolate, dry mix, regular	1 oz	3.118
Cake, German chocolate pudding, dry mix	1 oz	1.985
Cake, marble pudding, dry mix	1 oz	1.985
Candies, chocolate covered, caramel with nuts	1 cup	3.534
Candies, chocolate covered, dietetic or low calorie	1 cup	16.74
Candy, milk chocolate w/almonds	1 bar (1.45 oz)	9.02
Candy, milk chocolate w/rice cereal	1 bar (1.4 oz)	9.2
Candy, raisins, milk chocolate coated	1 cup	45
Chocolate chips, semisweet	1 cup chips (6 oz package)	104.16
Chocolate, baking, unsweetened, square	1 cup, grated	105.6
Chocolate, baking, Mexican, squares	1 tablet	2.8
Chocolate, sweet	1 oz	18.711
Cookie cake, Snackwell's Fat Free Devil's Food, Nabisco	1 serving	1.28
Cookie, Snackwell's Caramel Delights, Nabisco	1 serving	1.44
Cookie, chocolate chip, enriched, commercially prepared	1 oz	3.118
Cookie, chocolate chip, homemade w/margarine	1 oz	4.536
Cookie, chocolate chip, lower fat, commercially prepared	1 oz	1.985
Cookie, chocolate chip, refrigerated dough	1 portion, dough spoon from roll	2.61
Cookie, chocolate chip, soft, commercially prepared	1 oz	1.985
Cookie, chocolate wafers	1 cup, crumbs	7.84
Cookie, graham crackers, chocolate coated	1 oz	13.041
Cookie, sandwich, chocolate, cream filled	1 oz	3.686
Cookie, sandwich, chocolate, cream filled, special dietary	1 oz	0.85
Cupcakes, chocolate w/frosting, low-fat	1 oz	0.567
Donut, cake, chocolate w/sugar or glaze	1 oz	0.284
Donut, cake, plain w/chocolate icing	1 oz	0.567
Fast food, ice cream sundae, hot fudge	1 sundae	1.58
Fast food, milk beverage, chocolate shake	1 cup (8 fl. oz)	1.66
Frosting, chocolate, creamy, ready to eat	2 tbsp creamy	0.82
Frozen yogurts, chocolate	1 cup	5.58
Fudge, chocolate w/nuts, homemade	1 oz	1.984
Granola bar, soft, milk chocolate coated, peanut butter	1 oz	0.85
Granola bar, with coconut, chocolate coated	1 cup	5.58
Ice cream, chocolate	1 individual (3.5 fl. oz)	1.74
Ice cream, chocolate, light	1 oz	0.85
Ice cream, chocolate, rich	1 cup	5.92
M&M's Peanut Chocolate	1 cup	18.7
M&M's Plain Chocolate	1 cup	22.88
Milk chocolate	1 cup chips	33.6
Milk chocolate coated coffee beans	1 NLEA serving	48
Milk dessert, frozen, fat-free milk, chocolate	1 oz	0.85
Milk shake, thick, chocolate	1 fl. oz	0.568
Pastry, eclair/cream puff, homemade, custard filled w/chocolate	1 oz	0.567
Pie crust, chocolate wafer cookie type, chilled	1 crust, single 9"	11.15
Pie, chocolate mousse, no bake mix	1 oz	0.284
Pudding, chocolate, instant dry mix prep w/reduced fat (2%) milk	1 oz	0.283
Pudding, chocolate, regular dry mix prep w/reduced fat (2%) milk	1 oz	0.567
Pudding, chocolate, ready-to-eat, fat-free	1 oz	0.567
Syrups, chocolate, genuine chocolate flavor, lite, Hershey	2 tbsp	1.05
Topping, chocolate-flavored hazelnut spread	1 oz	1.984
Yogurt, chocolate, nonfat milk	1 oz	0.567
Yogurt, frozen, chocolate, soft serve	0.5 cup (4 fl. oz)	2.16

APPENDIX D U.S. EXCHANGE LISTS FOR MEAL PLANNING

Source: From *Choose Your Foods: Exchange Lists For Diabetes.* © 2008 by the American Diabetes Association and the American Dietetic Association. Reproduced with permission.

Starch List

1 starch choice = 15 g carbohydrate, 0–3 g protein, 0–1 g fat, and 80 cal

Icon Key

☺ = More than 3 g of dietary fiber per serving.

❢ = Extra fat, or prepared with added fat. (Count as 1 starch + 1 fat.)

🧂 = 480 mg or more of sodium per serving.

Food	Serving Size	Food	Serving Size
Bread		Grits, cooked	½ c
Bagel, 4 oz	¼ (1 oz)	Kasha	½ c
❢ Biscuit, 2½" across	1	Millet, cooked	⅓ c
Bread		Muesli	¼ c
☺ reduced-calorie	2 slices (1½ oz)	Pasta, cooked	⅓ c
white, whole-grain, pumpernickel, rye,		Polenta, cooked	⅓ c
unfrosted raisin	1 slice (1 oz)	Quinoa, cooked	⅓ c
Chapatti, small, 6" across	1	Rice, white or brown, cooked	⅓ c
❢ Cornbread, 1¾" cube	1 (1½ oz)	Tabbouleh (tabouli), prepared	½ c
English muffin	½	Wheat germ, dry	3 tbs
Hot dog bun or hamburger bun	½ (1 oz)	Wild rice, cooked	½ c
Naan, 8" by 2"	¼	**Starchy Vegetables**	
Pancake, 4" across, ¼" thick	1	Cassava	⅓ c
Pita, 6" across	½	Corn	½ c
Roll, plain small	1 (1 oz)	on cob, large	½ cob (5 oz)
❢ Stuffing, bread	⅓ cup	☺ Hominy, canned	¾ c
❢ Taco shell, 5" across	2	☺ Mixed vegetables with corn, peas, or pasta	1 c
Tortilla		☺ Parsnips	½ c
Corn, 6" across	1	☺ Peas, green	½ c
Flour, 6" across	1	Plantain, ripe	⅓ c
Flour, 10" across	⅓ tortilla	Potato	
❢ Waffle, 4"-square or 4" across	1	baked with skin	¼ large (3 oz)
Cereals and Grains		boiled, all kinds	½ c or ½ medium (3 oz)
Barley, cooked	⅓ cup	❢ mashed, with milk and fat	½ c
Bran, dry		French fried (oven-baked)	1 cup (2 oz)
☺ oat	¼ c	☺ Pumpkin, canned, no sugar added	1 c
☺ wheat	½ c	Spaghetti/pasta sauce	½ c
☺ Bulgur (cooked)	½ c	☺ Squash, winter (acorn, butternut)	1 c
Cereals	½ c	☺ Succotash	½ c
☺ bran	½ c	Yam, sweet potato, plain	½ c
cooked (oats, oatmeal)	½ c	**Crackers and Snacks**	
puffed	1½ c	Animal crackers	8
shredded wheat, plain	½ c	Crackers	
sugar-coated	½ c	❢ round-butter type	6
unsweetened, ready-to-eat	¾ c	saltine-type	6
Couscous	⅓ c	❢ sandwich-style, cheese or peanut butter filling	3
Granola		❢ whole-wheat regular	2–5 (¾ oz)
low-fat	¼ c	☺ whole-wheat lower fat or crispbreads	2–5 (¾ oz)
❢ regular	¼ c	Graham crackers, 2½" square	3

Food	Serving Size	Food	Serving Size
Matzoh	¾ oz	**Beans, Peas, and Lentils**	
Melba toast, about 2" by 4" piece	4 pieces	*(Count as 1 starch + 1 lean meat)*	
Oyster crackers	20	☺ Baked beans	⅓ c
Crackers and Snacks		☺ Beans, cooked (black, garbanzo, kidney, lima, navy, pinto, white)	½ c
Popcorn	3 c	☺ Lentils, cooked (brown, green, yellow)	½ c
! ☺ with butter	3 c	☺ Peas, cooked (black-eyed, split)	½ c
☺ no fat added	3 c	🧂 ☺ Refried beans, canned	½ c
☺ lower fat	3 c		
Pretzels	¾ oz		
Rice cakes, 4" across	2		
Snack chips			
fat-free or baked (tortilla, potato),			
baked pita chips	15–20 (¾ oz)		
! regular (tortilla, potato)	9–13 (¾ oz)		

Fruit List

1 fruit choice = 15 g carbohydrate, 0 g protein, 0 g fat, and 60 cal
Weight includes skin, core, seeds, and rind.

Icon Key

☺ = More than 3 g of dietary fiber per serving.

! = Extra fat, or prepared with added fat.

🧂 = 480 mg or more of sodium per serving.

Food	Serving Size	Food	Serving Size
Apples		Grapes, small	17 (3 oz)
unpeeled, small	1 (4 oz)	Honeydew melon	1 slice or 1 c cubed (10 oz)
dried	4 rings	☺ Kiwi	1 (3½ oz)
Applesauce, unsweetened	½ c	Mandarin oranges, canned	¾ c
Apricots		Mango, small	½ fruit (5½ oz) or ½ c
canned	½ c	Nectarine, small	1 (5 oz)
dried	8 halves	☺ Orange, small	1 (6½ oz)
☺ fresh	4 whole (5½ oz)	Papaya	½ fruit or 1 c cubed (8 oz)
Banana, extra small	1 (4 oz)	Peaches	
☺ Blackberries	¾ c	canned	½ c
Blueberries	¾ c	fresh, medium	1 (6 oz)
Cantaloupe, small	⅓ melon or 1 c cubed (11 oz)	Pears	
Cherries		canned	½ c
sweet, canned	½ c	fresh, large	½ (4 oz)
sweet, fresh	12 (3 oz)	Pineapple	
Dates	3	canned	½ c
Dried fruits (blueberries, cherries, cranberries,		fresh	¾ c
mixed fruit, raisins)	2 tbs	Plums	
Figs		canned	½ c
dried	1½	dried (prunes)	3
☺ fresh	1½ large or 2 medium (3½ oz)	small	2 (5 oz)
Fruit cocktail	½ c	☺ Raspberries	1 c
Grapefruit		☺ Strawberries	1¼ c whole berries
large	½ (11 oz)		
sections, canned	¾ c		

Food	Serving Size	Food	Serving Size
☺ Tangerines, small	2 (8 oz)	Grape juice	½ c
Watermelon	1 slice or 1¼ c cubes (13½ oz)	Grapefruit juice	½ c
		Orange juice	½ c
Fruit Juice		Pineapple juice	½ c
Apple juice/cider	½ c	Prune juice	⅓ c
Fruit juice blends, 100% juice	⅓ c		

Milk and Yogurts

1 milk choice = 12 g carbohydrate and 8 g protein

Food	Serving Size	Count as
Fat-free or Low-Fat (1%)		
(0–3 g fat per serving, 100 calories per serving)		
Milk, buttermilk, acidophilus milk, Lactaid	1 c	1 fat-free milk
Evaporated milk	½ c	1 fat-free milk
Yogurt, plain or flavored with an artificial sweetener	⅔ c (6 oz)	1 fat-free milk
Reduced-fat (2%)		
(5 g fat per serving, 120 calories per serving)		
Milk, acidophilus milk, kefir, Lactaid	1 c	1 reduced-fat milk
Yogurt, plain	⅔ c (6 oz)	1 reduced-fat milk
Whole		
(8 g fat per serving, 160 calories per serving)		
Milk, buttermilk, goat's milk	1 c	1 whole milk
Evaporated milk	½ c	1 whole milk
Yogurt, plain	8 oz	1 whole milk
Dairy-Like Foods		
Chocolate milk		
fat-free	1 c	1 fat-free milk + 1 carbohydrate
whole	1 c	1 whole milk + 1 carbohydrate
Eggnog, whole milk	½ c	1 carbohydrate + 2 fats
Rice drink		
flavored, low-fat	1 c	2 carbohydrates
plain, fat-free	1 c	1 carbohydrate
Smoothies, flavored, regular	10 oz	1 fat-free milk + 2½ carbohydrates
Soy milk		
light	1 c	1 carbohydrate + ½ fat
regular, plain	1 c	1 carbohydrate + 1 fat
Yogurt		
and juice blends	1 c	1 fat-free milk + 1 carbohydrate
low carbohydrate (less than 6 g carbohydrate per choice)	⅔ c (6 oz)	½ fat-free milk
with fruit, low-fat	⅔ c (6 oz)	1 fat-free milk + 1 carbohydrate

Sweets, Desserts, and Other Carbohydrates List

1 other carbohydrate choice = 15 g carbohydrate and variable protein, fat, and calories.

Icon Key

🧂 = 480 mg or more of sodium per serving.

Food	Serving Size	Count as
Beverages, Soda, and Energy/Sports Drinks		
Cranberry juice cocktail	½ c	1 carbohydrate
Energy drink	1 can (8.3 oz)	2 carbohydrates
Fruit drink or lemonade	1 c (8 oz)	2 carbohydrates
Hot chocolate		
regular	1 envelope added to 8 oz water	1 carbohydrate + 1 fat
sugar-free or light	1 envelope added to 8 oz water	1 carbohydrate
Soft drink (soda), regular	1 can (12 oz)	2½ carbohydrates
Sports drink	1 cup (8 oz)	1 carbohydrate
Brownies, Cake, Cookies, Gelatin, Pie, and Pudding		
Brownie, small, unfrosted	1¼" square, ⅞" high (about 1 oz)	1 carbohydrate + 1 fat
Cake		
angel food, unfrosted	1⁄12 of cake (about 2 oz)	2 carbohydrates
frosted	2" square (about 2 oz)	2 carbohydrates + 1 fat
unfrosted	2" square (about 2 oz)	1 carbohydrate + 1 fat
Cookies		
chocolate chip	2 cookies (2¼" across)	1 carbohydrate + 2 fats
gingersnap	3 cookies	1 carbohydrate
sandwich, with creme filling	2 small (about ⅔ oz)	1 carbohydrate + 1 fat
sugar-free	3 small or 1 large (¾ oz–1oz)	1 carbohydrate + 1–2 fats
vanilla wafer	5 cookies	1 carbohydrate + 1 fat
Cupcake, frosted	1 small (about 1¾ oz)	2 carbohydrates + 1–1½ fats
Fruit cobbler	½ c (3½ oz)	3 carbohydrates + 1 fat
Gelatin, regular	½ c	1 carbohydrate
Pie		
commercially prepared fruit, 2 crusts	⅙ of 8" pie	3 carbohydrates + 2 fats
pumpkin or custard	⅛ of 8" pie	1½ carbohydrates + 1½ fats
Pudding		
regular (made with reduced-fat milk)	½ c	2 carbohydrates
sugar-free, or sugar-free and fat-free (made with fat-free milk)	½ c	1 carbohydrate
Candy, Spreads, Sweets, Sweeteners, Syrups, and Toppings		
Candy bar, chocolate/peanut	2 "fun size" bars (1 oz)	1½ carbohydrates + 1½ fats
Candy, hard	3 pieces	1 carbohydrate
Chocolate "kisses"	5 pieces	1 carbohydrate + 1 fat
Coffee creamer		
dry, flavored	4 tsp	½ carbohydrate + ½ fat
liquid, flavored	2 tbsp	1 carbohydrate
Fruit snacks, chewy (pureed fruit concentrate)	1 roll (¾ oz)	1 carbohydrate
Fruit spreads, 100% fruit	1½ tbs	1 carbohydrate
Honey	1 tbsp	1 carbohydrate

Food	Serving Size	Count as
Jam or jelly, regular	1 tbs	1 carbohydrate
Sugar	1 tbs	1 carbohydrate
Syrup		
chocolate	2 tbs	2 carbohydrates
light (pancake type)	2 tbs	1 carbohydrate
regular (pancake type)	1 tbs	1 carbohydrate

Condiments and Sauces

Barbeque sauce	3 tbs	1 carbohydrate
Cranberry sauce, jellied	¼ c	1½ carbohydrates
Gravy, canned or bottled	½ c	½ carbohydrate + ½ fat
Salad dressing, fat-free, low-fat, cream-based	3 tbs	1 carbohydrate
Sweet and sour sauce	3 tbs	1 carbohydrate

Doughnuts, Muffins, Pastries, and Sweet Breads

Banana nut bread	1" slice (1 oz)	2 carbohydrates + 1 fat
Doughnut		
cake, plain	1 medium, (1½ oz)	1½ carbohydrates + 2 fats
yeast type, glazed	3¾" across (2 oz)	2 carbohydrates + 2 fats
Muffin (4 oz)	¼ muffin (1 oz)	1 carbohydrate + ½ fat
Sweet roll or Danish	1 (2½ oz)	2½ carbohydrates + 2 fats

Frozen Bars, Frozen Dessert, Frozen Yogurt, and Ice Cream

Frozen pops	1	½ carbohydrate
Fruit juice bars, frozen, 100% juice	1 bar (3 oz)	1 carbohydrate
Ice cream		
fat-free	½ c	1-½ carbohydrates
light	½ c	1 carbohydrate + 1 fat
no sugar added	½ c	1 carbohydrate + 1 fat
regular	½ c	1 carbohydrate + 2 fats
Sherbet, sorbet	½ c	2 carbohydrates
Yogurt, frozen		
fat-free	⅓ c	1 carbohydrate
regular	½ c	1 carbohydrate + 0–1 fat

Granola Bars, Meal Replacement Bars/Shakes, and Trail Mix

Granola or snack bar, regular or low-fat	1 bar (1 oz)	1½ carbohydrates
Meal replacement bar	1 bar (1⅓ oz)	1½ carbohydrates + 0–1 fat
Meal replacement bar	1 bar (2 oz)	2 carbohydrates + 1 fat
Meal replacement shake, reduced-calorie	1 can (10–11 oz)	1½ carbohydrates + 0–1 fat
Trail mix		
candy/nut-based	1 oz	1 carbohydrates + 2 fats
dried-fruit-based	1 oz	1 carbohydrate + 1 fat

Nonstarchy Vegetable List

1 vegetable choice = 5 g carbohydrate, 2 g protein, 0 g fat, 25 cal

Icon Key

☺ = More than 3 g of dietary fiber per serving.

🧂 = 480 mg or more of sodium per serving.

Amaranth or Chinese spinach

Artichoke

Artichoke hearts

Asparagus

Baby corn

Bamboo shoots

Beans (green, wax, Italian)

Bean sprouts

Beets

🧂 Borscht

Broccoli

☺ Brussels sprouts

Cabbage (green, bok choy, Chinese)

☺ Carrots

Cauliflower

Celery

☺ Chayote

Coleslaw, packaged, no dressing

Cucumber

Eggplant

Gourds (bitter, bottle, luffa, bitter melon)

Green onions or scallions

Greens (collard, kale, mustard, turnip)

Hearts of palm

Jicama

Kohlrabi

Leeks

Mixed vegetables (without corn, peas, or pasta)

Mung bean sprouts

Mushrooms, all kinds, fresh

Okra

Onions

Oriental radish or daikon

Pea pods

☺ Peppers (all varieties)

Radishes

Rutabaga

🧂 Sauerkraut

Soybean sprouts

Spinach

Squash (summer, crookneck, zucchini)

Sugar pea snaps

☺ Swiss chard

Tomato

Tomatoes, canned

🧂 Tomato sauce

🧂 Tomato/vegetable juice

Turnips

Water chestnuts

Yard-long beans

Meat and Meat Substitutes List

Icon Key

! = Extra fat, or prepared with added fat. (Add an additional fat choice to this food.)

🧂 = 480 mg or more of sodium per serving (based on the sodium content of a typical 3-oz serving of meat, unless 1 or 2 is the normal serving size).

Food	Amount
Lean Meats and Meat Substitutes	
(1 lean meat choice = 7 g protein, 0–3 g fat, 100 calories)	
Beef: Select or Choice grades trimmed of fat: ground round, roast (chuck, rib, rump), round, sirloin, steak (cubed, flank, porterhouse, T-bone), tenderloin	1 oz
🧂 Beef jerky	1 oz
Cheeses with 3 g of fat or less per oz	1 oz
Cottage cheese	¼ cup
Egg substitutes, plain	¼ cup
Egg whites	2

Food	Amount
Fish, fresh or frozen, plain: catfish, cod, flounder, haddock, halibut, orange roughy, salmon, tilapia, trout, tuna	1 oz
🧂 *Fish, smoked:* herring or salmon (lox)	1 oz
Game: buffalo, ostrich, rabbit, venison	1 oz
🧂 Hot dog with 3 g of fat or less per oz (8 dogs per 14 oz package) (*Note: May be high in carbohydrate.*)	1
Lamb: chop, leg, or roast	1 oz
Organ meats: heart, kidney, liver (*Note: May be high in cholesterol*)	1 oz

Food	Amount	Food	Amount
Oysters, fresh or frozen	6 medium	*Poultry:* chicken with skin; dove, pheasant, wild duck, or goose; fried chicken; ground turkey	1 oz
Pork, lean		Ricotta cheese	2 oz or ¼ c
🧂 Canadian bacon	1 oz	🧂 Sausage with 4–7 g fat per oz	1 oz
rib or loin chop/roast, ham, tenderloin	1 oz	*Veal:* Cutlet (no breading)	1 oz

High-Fat Meat and Substitutes[a]
(1 high-fat meat choice = 7 g protein, 8+ g fat, 150 calories)

Food	Amount
Poultry without skin: Cornish hen, chicken, domestic duck or goose (well drained of fat), turkey	1 oz
Processed sandwich meats with 3 g of fat or less per oz: chipped beef, deli thin-sliced meats, turkey ham, turkey kielbasa, turkey pastrami	1 oz
Salmon, canned	1 oz
Sardines, canned	2 medium
🧂 Sausage with 3 g or less fat per oz	1 oz
Shellfish: clams, crab, imitation shellfish, lobster, scallops, shrimp	1 oz
Tuna, canned in water or oil, drained	1 oz
Veal: Lean chop, roast	1 oz

Bacon

Food	Amount
🧂 pork	2 slices (16 slices per lb or 1 oz each, before cooking)
🧂 turkey	3 slices (½ oz each before cooking)
Cheese, regular: American, bleu, brie, cheddar, hard goat, Monterey Jack, queso, Swiss	1 oz
🧂 ❗ *Hot dog:* beef, pork, or combination (10 per lb-sized package)	1
🧂 *Hot dog:* turkey or chicken (10 per lb-sized package)	1
Pork: ground, sausage, spareribs	1 oz
Processed sandwich meats with 8 g of fat or more per oz: bologna, pastrami, hard salami	1 oz
🧂 *Sausage with 8 g of fat or more per oz:* bratwurst, chorizo, Italian, knockwurst, Polish, smoked, summer	1 oz

Medium-Fat Meat and Meat Substitutes
(1 medium-fat meat choice = 7 g protein, 4–7 g fat, and 130 calories)

Food	Amount
Beef: corned beef, ground beef, meatloaf, Prime grades trimmed of fat (prime rib), short ribs, tongue	1 oz
Cheeses with 4–7 g of fat per oz: feta, mozzarella, pasteurized processed cheese spread, reduced-fat cheeses, string	1 oz
Egg (*Note:* High in cholesterol, limit to 3 per week.)	1
Fish, any fried product	1 oz
Lamb: ground, rib roast	1 oz
Pork: cutlet, shoulder roast	1 oz

[a]These foods are high in saturated fat, cholesterol, and calories and may raise blood cholesterol levels if eaten on a regular basis. Try to eat 3 or fewer servings from this group per week.

Plant-Based Proteins

Because carbohydrate content varies among plant-based proteins, you should read the food label.

Icon Key

😊 = More than 3 g of dietary fiber per serving.

🧂 = 480 mg or more of sodium per serving (based on the sodium content of a typical 3-oz serving of meat, unless 1 or 2 oz is the normal serving size).

Food	Amount	Count as
"Bacon" strips, soy-based	3 strips	1 medium-fat meat
😊 Baked beans	⅓ c	1 starch + 1 lean meat
😊 *Beans, cooked:* black, garbanzo, kidney, lima, navy, pinto, white	½ c	1 starch + 1 lean meat
😊 "Beef" or "sausage" crumbles, soy-based	2 oz	½ carbohydrate + 1 lean meat
"Chicken" nuggets, soy-based	2 nuggets (1½ oz)	½ carbohydrate + 1 medium-fat meat
😊 Edamame	½ c	½ carbohydrate + 1 lean meat
Falafel (spiced chickpea and wheat patties)	3 patties (about 2 inches across)	1 carbohydrate + 1 high-fat meat
Hot dog, soy-based	1 (1½ oz)	½ carbohydrate + 1 lean meat
😊 Hummus	⅓ c	1 carbohydrate + 1 high-fat meat

Food	Amount	Count as
😊 Lentils, brown, green, or yellow	½ c	1 carbohydrate + 1 lean meat
😊 Meatless burger, soy-based	3 oz	½ carbohydrate + 2 lean meats
😊 Meatless burger, vegetable- and starch-based	1 patty (about 2½ oz)	1 carbohydrate + 2 lean meats
Nut spreads: almond butter, cashew butter, peanut butter, soy nut butter	1 tbs	1 high-fat meat
😊 *Peas, cooked:* black-eyed and split peas	½ c	1 starch + 1 lean meat
🧂😊 Refried beans, canned	½ c	1 starch + 1 lean meat
"Sausage" patties, soy-based	1 (1½ oz)	1 medium-fat meat
Soy nuts, unsalted	¾ oz	½ carbohydrate + 1 medium-fat meat
Tempeh	¼ cup	1 medium-fat meat
Tofu	4 oz (½ cup)	1 medium-fat meat
Tofu, light	4 oz (½ cup)	1 lean meat

Fat List

Icon Key

1 fat choice = 5 g fat, 45 cal

🧂 = 480 mg or more of sodium per serving.

Food	Serving Size	Food	Serving Size
Unsaturated Fats—		Nuts	
Monounsaturated Fats		Pignolia (pine nuts)	1 tbs
Avocado, medium	2 tbs (1 oz)	walnuts, English	4 halves
Nut butters (trans fat-free): almond butter,		*Oil:* corn, cottonseed, flaxseed, grape seed,	
cashew butter, peanut butter (smooth or crunchy)	1½ tsp	safflower, soybean, sunflower	1 tsp
Nuts		*Oil:* made from soybean and canola oil—Enova	1 tsp
almonds	6 nuts	Plant stanol esters	
Brazil	2 nuts	light	1 tbs
cashews	6 nuts	regular	2 tsp
filberts (hazelnuts)	5 nuts	Salad dressing	
macadamia	3 nuts	🧂 reduced-fat (*Note: May be high*	
mixed (50% peanuts)	6 nuts	*in carbohydrate.*)	2 tbs
peanuts	10 nuts	🧂 regular	1 tbs
pecans	4 halves	Seeds	1 tbs
pistachios	16 nuts	flaxseed, whole	1 tbs
Oil: canola, olive, peanut	1 tsp	pumpkin, sunflower	1 tbs
Olives		sesame seeds	1 tbs
black (ripe)	8 large	Tahini or sesame paste	2 tsp
green, stuffed	10 large	**Saturated Fats**	
Polyunsaturated Fats		Bacon, cooked, regular or turkey	1 slice
Margarine: lower-fat spread (30% to 50% vegetable		Butter	
oil, *trans* fat-free)	1 tbs	reduced-fat	1 tbs
Margarine: stick, tub (*trans* fat-free), or squeeze		stick	1 tsp
(*trans* fat-free)	1 tsp	whipped	2 tsp
Mayonnaise		Butter blends made with oil	
reduced-fat	1 tbs	reduced-fat or light	1 tbs
regular	1 tsp	regular	1½ tsp
Mayonnaise-style salad dressing		Chitterlings, boiled	2 tbs (½ oz)
reduced-fat	1 tbs	Coconut, sweetened, shredded	2 tbs
regular	2 tsp		

Food	Serving Size	Food	Serving Size
Coconut milk		Lard	1 tsp
light	⅓ c	*Oil:* coconut, palm, palm kernel	1 tsp
regular	1½ tbs	Salt pork	¼ oz
Cream		Shortening, solid	1 tsp
half and half	2 tbs	Sour cream	
heavy	1 tbs	reduced-fat or light	3 tbs
light	1½ tbs	regular	2 tbs
whipped	2 tbs		
whipped, pressurized	¼ c		
Cream cheese			
reduced-fat	1½ tbs (¾ oz)		
regular	1 tbs (½ oz)		

Free Foods List

A *free food* is any food or drink that has less than 20 calories and 5 g or less of carbohydrate per serving. Foods with a serving size listed should be limited to three servings per day. Foods listed without a serving size can be eaten as often as you like.

Icon Key

🧂 = 480 mg or more of sodium per serving.

Food	Serving Size	Food	Serving Size
Low Carbohydrate Foods		Salad dressing	
Cabbage, raw	½ c	fat-free or low-fat	1 tbs
Candy, hard (regular or sugar-free)	1 piece	fat-free, Italian	2 tbs
Carrots, cauliflower, or green beans, cooked	¼ c	Sour cream, fat-free, reduced-fat	1 tbs
Cranberries, sweetened with sugar substitute	½ c	Whipped topping	
Cucumber, sliced	½ c	light or fat-free	2 tbs
Gelatin		regular	1 tbs
dessert, sugar-free		**Condiments**	
unflavored		Barbecue sauce	2 tsp
Gum		Catsup (ketchup)	1 tbs
Jam or jelly, light or no sugar added	2 tsp	Honey mustard	1 tbs
Rhubarb, sweetened with sugar substitute	½ c	Horseradish	
Salad greens		Lemon juice	
Sugar substitutes (artificial sweeteners)		Miso	1½ tsp
Syrup, sugar-free	2 tbs	Mustard	
Modified Fat Foods		Parmesan cheese, freshly grated	1 tbs
with Carbohydrate		Pickle relish	1 tbs
Cream cheese, fat-free	1 tbs (½ oz)	Pickles	
Creamers		🧂 dill	1½ medium
nondairy, liquid	1 tbs	sweet, bread and butter	2 slices
nondairy, powdered	2 tsp	sweet, gherkin	¾ oz
Margarine spread		Salsa	¼ c
fat-free	1 tbs	🧂 Soy sauce, regular or light	1 tbs
reduced-fat	1 tsp	Sweet and sour sauce	2 tsp
Mayonnaise		Sweet chili sauce	2 tsp
fat-free	1 tbs	Taco sauce	1 tbs
reduced-fat	1 tsp	Vinegar	
Mayonnaise-style salad dressing		Yogurt, any type	2 tbs
fat-free	1 tbs		
reduced-fat	1 tsp		

Drinks/Mixes

Any food on this list—without serving size listed—can be consumed in any moderate amount.

Icon Key

🧂 = 480 mg or more of sodium per serving.

🧂 Bouillon, broth, consommé	Diet soft drinks, sugar-free
Bouillon or broth, low sodium	Drink mixes, sugar-free
Carbonated or mineral water	Tea, unsweetened or with sugar substitute
Club soda	Tonic water, diet
Cocoa powder, unsweetened (1 tbs)	Water
Coffee, unsweetened or with sugar substitute	Water, flavored, carbohydrate free

Seasonings

Any food on this list can be consumed in any moderate amount.

Flavoring extracts (for example, vanilla, almond, peppermint)	Spices
Garlic	Hot pepper sauce
Herbs, fresh or dried	Wine, used in cooking
Nonstick cooking spray	Worcestershire sauce
Pimento	

Combination Foods List

Icon Key

☺ = More than 3 g of dietary fiber per serving.

🧂 = 600 mg or more of sodium per serving (for combination food main dishes/meals).

Food	Serving Size	Count as
Entrées		
🧂 Casserole type (tuna noodle, lasagna, spaghetti with meatballs, chili with beans, macaroni and cheese)	1 c (8 oz)	2 carbohydrates + 2 medium-fat meats
🧂 Stews (beef/other meats and vegetables)	1 c (8 oz)	1 carbohydrate + 1 medium-fat meat + 0–3 fats
Tuna salad or chicken salad	½ c (3½ oz)	½ carbohydrate + 2 lean meats + 1 fat
Frozen Meals/Entrées		
🧂☺ Burrito (beef and bean)	1 (5 oz)	3 carbohydrates + 1 lean meat + 2 fats
🧂 Dinner-type meal	generally 14–17 oz	3 carbohydrates + 3 medium-fat meats + 3 fats
🧂 Entrée or meal with less than 340 calories	about 8–11 oz	2–3 carbohydrates + 1–2 lean meats
Pizza		
🧂 cheese/vegetarian thin crust	¼ of 12" (4½ to 5 oz)	2 carbohydrates + 2 medium-fat meats
🧂 meat topping, thin crust	¼ of 12" (5 oz)	2 carbohydrates + 2 medium-fat meats, + 1½ fats
🧂 Pocket sandwich	1 (4½ oz)	3 carbohydrates + 1 lean meat + 1–2 fats
🧂 Pot pie	1 (7 oz)	2½ carbohydrates + 1 medium-fat meat + 3 fats
Salads (Deli-Style)		
Coleslaw	½ c	1 carbohydrate + 1½ fats
Macaroni/pasta salad	½ c	2 carbohydrates + 3 fats
🧂 Potato salad	½ c	1½ carbohydrates + 1–2 fats
Soups		
🧂 Bean, lentil, or split pea	1 cup	1 carbohydrate + 1 lean meat

Food	Serving Size	Count as
🧂 Chowder (made with milk)	1 c (8 oz)	1 carbohydrate + 1 lean meat + 1½ fats
🧂 Cream (made with water)	1 c (8 oz)	1 carbohydrate + 1 fat
🧂 Instant	6 oz prepared	1 carbohydrate
🧂 with beans or lentils	8 oz prepared	2½ carbohydrates + 1 lean meat
🧂 Miso soup	1 c	½ carbohydrate + 1 fat
🧂 Oriental noodle	1 c	2 carbohydrates + 2 fats
Rice (congee)	1 c	1 carbohydrate
🧂 Tomato (made with water)	1 c (8 oz)	1 carbohydrate
🧂 Vegetable beef, chicken noodle, or other broth-type	1 c (8 oz)	1 carbohydrate

Fast Foods List[a]

Icon Key

😊 = More than 3 g of dietary fiber per serving.

! = Extra fat, or prepared with added fat.

🧂 = 600 mg or more sodium per serving (for fast food main dishes/meals).

Food	Serving Size	Exchanges per Serving
Breakfast Sandwiches		
🧂 Egg, cheese, meat, English muffin	1 sandwich	2 carbohydrates + 2 medium-fat meats
🧂 Sausage biscuit sandwich	1 sandwich	2 carbohydrates + 2 high-fat meats + 3½ fats
Main Dishes/Entrees		
🧂😊 Burrito (beef and beans)	1 (about 8 oz)	3 carbohydrates + 3 medium-fat meats + 3 fats
🧂 Chicken breast, breaded and fried	1 (about 5 oz)	1 carbohydrate + 4 medium-fat meats
Chicken drumstick, breaded and fried	1 (about 2 oz)	2 medium-fat meats
🧂 Chicken nuggets	6 (about 3½ oz)	1 carbohydrate + 2 medium-fat meats + 1 fat
🧂 Chicken thigh, breaded and fried	1 (about 4 oz)	½ carbohydrate + 3 medium-fat meats + 1½ fats
🧂 Chicken wings, hot	6 (5 oz)	5 medium-fat meats + 1½ fats
Oriental		
🧂 Beef/chicken/shrimp with vegetables in sauce	1 c (about 5 oz)	1 carbohydrate + 1 lean meat + 1 fat
🧂 Egg roll, meat	1 (about 3 oz)	1 carbohydrate + 1 lean meat + 1 fat
Fried rice, meatless	½ c	1½ carbohydrates + 1½ fats
🧂 Meat and sweet sauce (orange chicken)	1 c	3 carbohydrates + 3 medium-fat meats + 2 fats
🧂😊 Noodles and vegetables in sauce (chow mein, lo mein)	1 c	2 carbohydrates + 1 fat
Pizza		
🧂 Cheese, pepperoni, regular crust	⅛ of 14" (about 4 oz)	2½ carbohydrates + 1 medium-fat meat + 1½ fats
🧂 Cheese/vegetarian, thin crust	¼ of 12" (about 6 oz)	2½ carbohydrates + 2 medium-fat meats + 1½ fats
Sandwiches		
🧂 Chicken sandwich, grilled	1	3 carbohydrates + 4 lean meats
🧂 Chicken sandwich, crispy	1	3½ carbohydrates + 3 medium-fat meats + 1 fat
Fish sandwich with tartar sauce	1	2½ carbohydrates + 2 medium-fat meats + 2 fats
Hamburger		
🧂 large with cheese	1	2½ carbohydrates + 4 medium-fat meats + 1 fat
regular	1	2 carbohydrates + 1 medium-fat meat + 1 fat
🧂 Hot dog with bun	1	1 carbohydrate + 1 high-fat meat + 1 fat
Submarine sandwich		
🧂 less than 6 grams fat	6" sub	3 carbohydrates + 2 lean meats
🧂 regular	6" sub	3½ carbohydrates + 2 medium-fat meats + 1 fat

[a]The choices in the Fast Foods list are not specific fast food meals or items, but are estimates based on popular foods. You can get specific nutrition information for almost every fast food or restaurant chain. Ask the restaurant or check its website for nutrition information about your favorite fast foods.

Food	Serving Size	Exchanges per Serving
Taco, hard or soft shell (meat and cheese)	1 small	1 carbohydrate + 1 medium-fat meat + 1½ fats
Salads		
Salad, main dish (grilled chcken type, no dressing or croutons)	salad	1 carbohydrate + 4 lean meats
Salad, side, no dressing or cheese	Small (about 5 oz)	1 vegetable
Sides/Appetizers		
French fries, restaurant style	Small	3 carbohydrates + 3 fats
Medium		4 carbohydrates + 4 fats
Large		5 carbohydrates + 6 fats
Nachos with cheese	Small (about 4½ oz)	2½ carbohydrates + 4 fats
Onion rings	1 serving (about 3 oz)	2½ carbohydrates + 3 fats
Desserts		
Milkshake, any flavor	12 oz	6 carbohydrates + 2 fats
Soft-serve ice cream cone	1 small	2½ carbohydrates + 1 fat

Alcohol List

In general, 1 alcohol choice (½ oz absolute alcohol) has about 100 calories.

Alcoholic Beverage	Serving Size	Count as
Beer		
light (4.2%)	12 fl. oz	1 alcohol equivalent + ½ carbohydrate
regular (4.9%)	12 fl. oz	1 alcohol equivalent + 1 carbohydrate
Distilled spirits: vodka, rum, gin, whiskey, 80 or 86 proof	1½ fl. oz	1 alcohol equivalent
Liqueur, coffee (53 proof)	1 fl. oz	1 alcohol equivalent + 1 carbohydrate
Sake	1 fl. oz	½ alcohol equivalent
Wine		
dessert (sherry)	3½ fl. oz	1 alcohol equivalent + 1 carbohydrate
dry, red or white (10%)	5 fl. oz	1 alcohol equivalent

APPENDIX E STATURE-FOR-AGE CHARTS

CDC Growth Charts: United States
Stature-for-age percentiles: Boys, 2 to 20 years

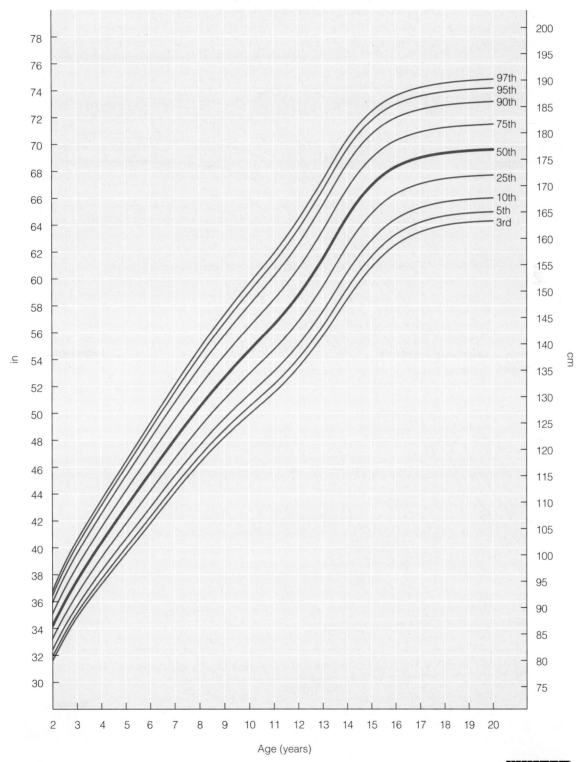

Published May 30, 2000.
Source: Developed by the National Center for Health Statistics
in collaboration with the National Center for Chronic
Disease Prevention and Health Promotion (2000).

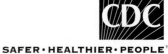

SAFER · HEALTHIER · PEOPLE™

CDC Growth Charts: United States
Stature-for-age percentiles: Girls, 2 to 20 years

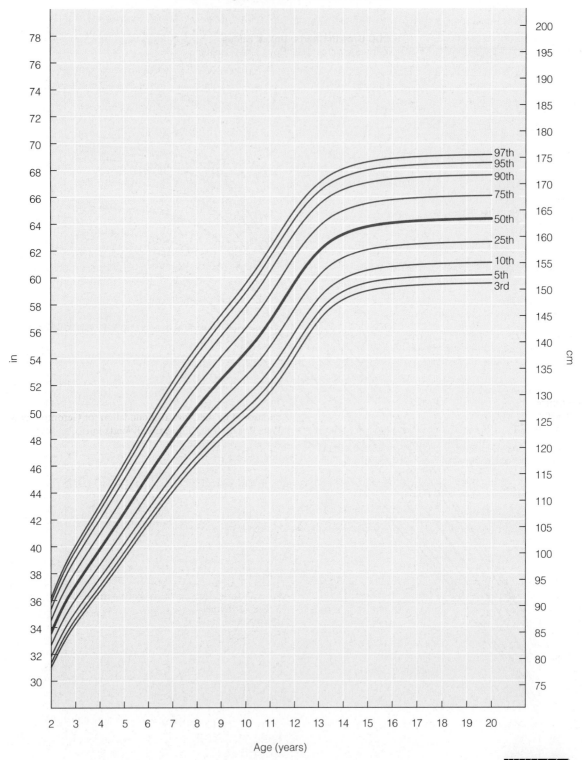

Age (years)

Published May 30, 2000.

Source: Developed by the National Center for Health Statistics
in collaboration with the National Center for Chronic
Disease Prevention and Health Promotion (2000).

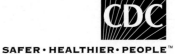

SAFER · HEALTHIER · PEOPLE™

APPENDIX F ORGANIZATIONS AND RESOURCES

Academic Journals

International Journal of Sport Nutrition and Exercise Metabolism
Human Kinetics
P.O. Box 5076
Champaign, IL 61825-5076
(800) 747-4457
www.humankinetics.com/IJSNEM

Journal of Nutrition
9650 Rockville Pike
Bethesda, MD 20814
(301) 634-7892
www.nutrition.org

Nutrition Research
Elsevier: Journals Customer Service
6277 Sea Harbor Drive
Orlando, FL 32887
(877) 839-7126
www.journals.elsevierhealth.com/periodicals/NTR

Nutrition
Elsevier: Journals Customer Service
6277 Sea Harbor Drive
Orlando, FL 32887
(877) 839-7126
www.journals.elsevierhealth.com/periodicals/NUT

Nutrition Reviews
International Life Sciences Institute
Subscription Office
P.O. Box 830430
Birmingham, AL 35283
(800) 633-4931
www.ingentaconnect.com/content/ilsi/nure

Obesity Research
North American Association for the Study of Obesity (NAASO)
8630 Fenton Street, Suite 918
Silver Spring, MD 20910
(301) 563-6526
www.obesityresearch.org

International Journal of Obesity
Journal of the International Association for the Study of Obesity
Nature Publishing Group
The Macmillan Building
4 Crinan Street
London N1 9XW
United Kingdom
www.nature.com/ijo

Journal of the American Medical Association
American Medical Association
P.O. Box 10946
Chicago, IL 60610-0946
(800) 262-2350
http://jama.ama-assn.org

New England Journal of Medicine
10 Shattuck Street
Boston, MA 02115-6094
(617) 734-9800
http://content.nejm.org/

American Journal of Clinical Nutrition
The American Journal of Clinical Nutrition
9650 Rockville Pike
Bethesda, MD 20814
(301) 634-7892
www.nutrition.org

Journal of the American Dietetic Association
Elsevier, Health Sciences Division
Subscription Customer Service
6277 Sea Harbor Drive
Orlando, FL 32887
(800) 654-2452
www.adajournal.org

Aging

Administration on Aging
U.S. Health & Human Services
200 Independence Avenue, SW
Washington, DC 20201
(877) 696-6775
www.aoa.gov

American Association of Retired Persons (AARP)
601 E. Street, NW
Washington, DC 20049
(888) 687-2277
www.aarp.org

Health and Age
Sponsored by the Novartis Foundation for Gerontology & The Web-Based Health Education Foundation
Robert Griffith MD
Executive Director
573 Vista de la Ciudad
Santa Fe, NM 87501
www.healthandage.com

National Council on the Aging
300 D Street, SW, Suite 801
Washington, DC 20024
(202) 479-1200
www.ncoa.org

International Osteoporosis Foundation
5 Rue Perdtemps
1260 Nyon
Switzerland
41 22 994 01 00
www.osteofound.org

National Institute on Aging
Building 31, Room 5C27
31 Center Drive, MSC 2292
Bethesda, MD 20892
(301) 496-1752
www.nia.nih.gov

Osteoporosis and Related Bone Diseases National Resource Center
2 AMS Circle
Bethesda, MD 20892-3676
(800) 624-BONE
www.osteo.org

American Geriatrics Society
The Empire State Building
350 Fifth Avenue, Suite 801
New York, NY 10118
(212) 308-1414
www.americangeriatrics.org

National Osteoporosis Foundation
1232 22nd Street, NW
Washington, DC 20037-1292
(202) 223-2226
www.nof.org/

Alcohol and Drug Abuse
National Institute on Drug Abuse
6001 Executive Boulevard, Room 5213
Bethesda, MD 20892-9561
(301) 443-1124
www.nida.nih.gov

National Institute on Alcohol Abuse and Alcoholism
5635 Fishers Lane, MSC 9304
Bethesda, MD 20892-9304
www.niaaa.nih.gov

Alcoholics Anonymous
Grand Central Station
P.O. Box 459
New York, NY 10163
www.alcoholics-anonymous.org

Narcotics Anonymous
P.O. Box 9999
Van Nuys, California 91409
(818) 773-9999
www.na.org

National Council on Alcoholism and Drug Dependence
20 Exchange Place, Suite 2902
New York, NY 10005
(212) 269-7797
www.ncadd.org

National Clearinghouse for Alcohol and Drug Information
11420 Rockville Pike
Rockville, MD 20852
(800) 729-6686
www.health.org

Canadian Government
Health Canada
A.L. 0900C2
Ottawa, ON
K1A 0K9
(613) 957-2991
www.hc-sc.gc.ca/english

National Institute of Nutrition
408 Queen Street, 3rd Floor
Ottawa, ON K1R 5A7
(613) 235-3355
www.nin.ca/public_html/index.html

Agricultural and Agri-Food Canada
Public Information Request Service
Sir John Carling Building
930 Carling Avenue
Ottawa, ON K1A 0C5
(613) 759-1000
www.agr.gc.ca

Bureau of Nutritional Sciences
Sir Frederick G. Banting Research Centre
Tunney's Pasture (2203A)
Ottawa, ON K1A 0L2
(613) 957-0352
www.hc-sc.gc.ca/food-aliment/ns-sc/e_nutrition.html

Canadian Food Inspection Agency
59 Camelot Drive
Ottawa, ON K1A 0Y9
(613) 225-2342
www.inspection.gc.ca/english/toce.shtml

Canadian Institute for Health Information
CIHI Ottawa
377 Dalhousie Street, Suite 200
Ottawa, ON K1N 9N8
(613) 241-7860
www.cihi.ca

Canadian Public Health Association
1565 Carling Avenue, Suite 400
Ottawa, ON K1Z 8R1
(613) 725-3769
www.cpha.ca

Canadian Nutrition and Professional Organizations
Dietitians of Canada
480 University Avenue, Suite 604
Toronto, ON M5G 1V2
(416) 596-0857
www.dietitians.ca

Canadian Diabetes Association
National Life Building
1400-522 University Avenue
Toronto, ON M5G 2R5
(800) 226-8464
www.diabetes.ca

National Eating Disorder Information Centre
CW 1-211, 200 Elizabeth Street
Toronto, ON M5G 2C4
(866) NEDIC-20
www.nedic.ca

Canadian Pediatric Society
100-2204 Walkley Road
Ottawa, ON K1G 4G8
(613) 526-9397
www.cps.ca

Canadian Dietetic Association
480 University Avenue, Suite 604
Toronto, ON M5G 1V2
(416) 596-0857
www.dietitians.ca

Disordered Eating/Eating Disorders

American Psychiatric Association
1000 Wilson Boulevard, Suite 1825
Arlington, VA 22209
(703) 907-7300
www.psych.org

Harvard Eating Disorders Center
WACC 725
15 Parkman Street
Boston, MA 02114
(617) 236-7766
www.hedc.org

National Institute of Mental Health
Office of Communications
6001 Executive Boulevard, Room 8184, MSC 9663
Bethesda, MD 20892
(866) 615-6464
www.nimh.nih.gov

National Association of Anorexia Nervosa and Associated Disorders (ANAD)
Box 7
Highland Park, IL 60035
(847) 831-3438
www.anad.org

National Eating Disorders Association
603 Stewart Street, Suite 803
Seattle, WA 98101
(206) 382-3587
www.nationaleatingdisorders.org

Eating Disorder Referral and Information Center
2923 Sandy Pointe, Suite 6
Del Mar, CA 92014
(858) 792-7463
www.edreferral.com

Anorexia Nervosa and Related Eating Disorders, Inc. (ANRED)
Email:jarinor@rio.com
www.anred.com

Overeaters Anonymous
P.O. Box 44020
Rio Rancho, NM 87174
(505) 891-2664
www.oa.org

Exercise, Physical Activity, and Sports

American College of Sports Medicine (ACSM)
P.O. Box 1440
Indianapolis, IN 46206-1440
(317) 637-9200
www.acsm.org

American Physical Therapy Association (ASNA)
1111 North Fairfax Street
Alexandria, VA 22314
(800) 999-APTA
www.apta.org

Gatorade Sports Science Institute (GSSI)
617 West Main Street
Barrington, IL 60010
(800) 616-GSSI
www.gssiweb.com

National Coalition for Promoting Physical Activity (NCPPA)
1010 Massachusetts Avenue, Suite 350
Washington, DC 20001
(202) 454-7518
www.ncppa.org

Sports, Wellness, Eating Disorder and Cardiovascular Nutritionists (SCAN)
P.O. Box 60820
Colorado Springs, CO 80960
(719) 635-6005
www.scandpg.org

President's Council on Physical Fitness and Sports
Department W
200 Independence Avenue, SW
Room 738-H
Washington, DC 20201-0004
(202) 690-9000
www.fitness.gov

American Council on Exercise (ACE)
4851 Paramount Drive
San Diego, CA 92123
(858) 279-8227
www.acefitness.org

The International Association for Fitness Professionals (IDEA)
10455 Pacific Center Court
San Diego, CA 92121
(800) 999-4332, ext. 7
www.ideafit.com

International Society of Sports Nutrition
Executive Director, Maelu Fleck
600 Pembrook Drive
Woodland Park, CO 80863
(866) 472-4650
www.sportsnutritionsociety.org

Food Safety

Food Marketing Institute
655 15th Street, NW
Washington, DC 20005
(202) 452-8444
www.fmi.org

Agency for Toxic Substances and Disease Registry (ATSDR)
ORO Washington Office
Ariel Rios Building
1200 Pennsylvania Avenue, NW
M/C 5204G
Washington, DC 20460
(888) 422-8737
www.atsdr.cdc.gov

Food Allergy and Anaphylaxis Network
11781 Lee Jackson Highway, Suite 160
Fairfax, VA 22033-3309
(800) 929-4040
www.foodallergy.org

Foodsafety.gov
www.foodsafety.gov

The USDA Food Safety and Inspection Service
Food Safety and Inspection Service
United States Department of Agriculture
Washington, DC 20250
www.fsis.usda.gov

Consumer Reports
Web Site Customer Relations Department
101 Truman Avenue
Yonkers, NY 10703
www.consumerreports.org

Center for Science in the Public Interest: Food Safety
1875 Connecticut Avenue, NW
Washington, DC 20009
(202) 332-9110
www.cspinet.org/foodsafety/index.html

Center for Food Safety and Applied Nutrition
5100 Paint Branch Parkway
College Park, MD 20740
(888) SAFEFOOD
www.cfsan.fda.gov

Food Safety Project
Dan Henroid, MS, RD, CFSP
HRIM Extension Specialist and Website Coordinator
Hotel, Restaurant and Institution Management
9e MacKay Hall
Iowa State University
Ames, IA 50011
(515) 294-3527
www.extension.iastate.edu/foodsafety

Organic Consumers Association
6101 Cliff Estate Road
Little Marais, MN 55614
(218) 226-4164
www.organicconsumers.org

Infancy and Childhood
Administration for Children and Families
370 L'Enfant Promenade, SW
Washington, DC 20447
www.acf.dhhs.gov

The American Academy of Pediatrics
141 Northwest Point Boulevard
Elk Grove Village, IL 60007
(847) 434-4000
www.aap.org

Kidnetic.com
Email:contactus@kidnetic.com
www.kidnetic.com

Kidshealth: The Nemours Foundation
12735 West Gran Bay Parkway
Jacksonville, FL 32258
(866) 390-3610
www.kidshealth.org

National Center for Education in Maternal and Child Health
Georgetown University
Box 571272
Washington, DC 20057
(202) 784-9770
www.ncemch.org

Birth Defects Research for Children, Inc.
930 Woodcock Road, Suite 225
Orlando, FL 32803
(407) 895-0802
www.birthdefects.org

USDA/ARS Children's Nutrition Research Center at Baylor College of Medicine
1100 Bates Street
Houston, TX 77030
www.kidsnutrition.org

Keep Kids Healthy.com
www.keepkidshealthy.com

International Agencies
UNICEF
3 United Nations Plaza
New York, NY 10017
(212) 326-7000
www.unicef.org

World Health Organization
Avenue Appia 20
1211 Geneva 27
Switzerland
41 22 791 21 11
www.who.int/en

The Stockholm Convention on Persistent Organic Pollutants
11-13 Chemin des Anémones
1219 Châtelaine
Geneva, Switzerland
41 22 917 8191
www.pops.int

Food and Agricultural Organization of the United Nations
Viale delle Terme di Caracalla
00100 Rome, Italy
39 06 57051
www.fao.org

International Food Information Council Foundation
1100 Connecticut Avenue, NW
Suite 430
Washington, DC 20036
(202) 296-6540

Pregnancy and Lactation
San Diego County Breastfeeding Coalition
c/o Children's Hospital and Health Center
3020 Children's Way, MC 5073
San Diego, CA 92123
(800) 371-MILK
www.breastfeeding.org

National Alliance for Breastfeeding Advocacy
Barbara Heiser, Executive Director
9684 Oak Hill Drive
Ellicott City, MD 21042-6321
OR
Marsha Walker, Executive Director
254 Conant Road
Weston, MA 02493-1756
www.naba-breastfeeding.org

American College of Obstetricians and Gynecologists
409 12th Street, SW, P.O. Box 96920
Washington, DC 20090
www.acog.org

La Leche League
1400 N. Meacham Road
Schaumburg, IL 60173
(847) 519-7730
www.lalecheleague.org

National Organization on Fetal Alcohol Syndrome
900 17th Street, NW
Suite 910
Washington, DC 20006
(800) 66 NOFAS
www.nofas.org

March of Dimes Birth Defects Foundation
1275 Mamaroneck Avenue
White Plains, NY 10605
(888) 663-4637
http://modimes.org

Professional Nutrition Organizations
Association of Departments and Programs of Nutrition (ANDP)
Dr. Carolyn M. Bednar, ANDP Chair
Dept. of Nutrition and Food Sciences
Texas Woman's University
P.O. Box 425888
Denton, TX 76204-5888
(940) 898-2658
http://andpnet.org

North American Association for the Study of Obesity (NAASO)
8630 Fenton Street, Suite 918
Silver Spring, MD 20910
(301) 563-6526
www.naaso.org

American Dental Association
211 East Chicago Avenue
Chicago, IL 60611-2678
(312) 440-2500
www.ada.org

American Heart Association
National Center
7272 Greenville Avenue
Dallas, TX 75231
(800) 242-8721
www.americanheart.org

American Dietetic Association (ADA)
120 South Riverside Plaza, Suite 2000
Chicago, IL 60606-6995
(800) 877-1600
www.eatright.org

The American Society for Nutrition (ASN)
9650 Rockville Pike
Bethesda, MD 20814
(301) 634-7892
www.nutrition.org

The Society for Nutrition Education (SNE)
7150 Winton Drive, Suite 300
Indianapolis, IN 46268
(800) 235-6690
www.sne.org

American College of Nutrition
300 S. Duncan Avenue, Suite 225
Clearwater, FL 33755
(727) 446-6086
www.amcollnutr.org

American Obesity Association
1250 24th Street, NW, Suite 300
Washington, DC 20037
(800) 98-OBESE

American Council on Health and Science
1995 Broadway
Second Floor
New York, NY 10023
(212) 362-7044
www.acsh.org

American Diabetes Association
ATTN: National Call Center
1701 North Beauregard Street
Alexandria, VA 22311
(800) 342-2383
www.diabetes.org

Institute of Food Technologies
525 W. Van Buren, Suite 1000
Chicago, IL 60607
(312) 782-8424
www.ift.org

ILSI Human Nutrition Institute
One Thomas Circle, Ninth Floor
Washington, DC 20005
(202) 659-0524
http://hni.ilsi.org

Trade Organizations
American Meat Institute
1700 North Moore Street
Suite 1600
Arlington, VA 22209
(703) 841-2400
www.meatami.com

National Dairy Council
10255 W. Higgins Road, Suite 900
Rosemont, IL 60018
(312) 240-2880
www.nationaldairycouncil.org

United Fresh Fruit and Vegetable Association
1901 Pennsylvania Ave. NW, Suite 1100
Washington, DC 20006
(202) 303-3400
www.uffva.org

U.S.A. Rice Federation
Washington, DC
4301 North Fairfax Drive, Suite 425
Arlington, VA 22203
(703) 236-2300
www.usarice.com

U.S. Government

The USDA National Organic Program
Agricultural Marketing Service
USDA-AMS-TMP-NOP
Room 4008-South Building
1400 Independence Avenue, SW
Washington, DC 20250-0020
(202) 720-3252
www.ams.usda.gov

U.S. Department of Health and Human Services
200 Independence Avenue, SW
Washington, DC 20201
(877) 696-6775
www.os.dhhs.gov

Food and Drug Administration (FDA)
5600 Fishers Lane
Rockville, MD 20857
(888) 463-6332
www.fda.gov

Environmental Protection Agency
Ariel Rios Building
1200 Pennsylvania Avenue, NW
Washington, DC 20460
(202) 272-0167
www.epa.gov

Federal Trade Commission
600 Pennsylvania Avenue, NW
Washington, DC 20580
(202) 326-2222
www.ftc.gov

Partnership for Healthy Weight Management
www.consumer.gov/weightloss

Office of Dietary Supplements
National Institutes of Health
6100 Executive Boulevard, Room 3B01, MSC 7517
Bethesda, MD 20892
(301) 435-2920
http://dietary-supplements.info.nih.gov

Nutrient Data Laboratory Homepage
Beltsville Human Nutrition Center
10300 Baltimore Avenue
Building 307-C Room 117
BARC-East
Beltsville, MD 20705
(301) 504-8157
www.nal.usda.gov/fnic/foodcomp

National Digestive Disease Clearinghouse
2 Information Way
Bethesda, MD 20892-3570
(800) 891-5389
http://digestive.niddk.nih.gov

The National Cancer Institute
NCI Public Inquiries Office
Suite 3036A
6116 Executive Boulevard, MSC 8322
Bethesda, MD 20892-8322
(800) 4-CANCER
www.cancer.gov

The National Eye Institute
31 Center Drive MSC 2510
Bethesda, MD 20892-2510
(301) 496-5248
www.nei.nih.gov

The National Heart, Lung, and Blood Institute
Building 31, Room 5A52
31 Center Drive MSC 2486
Bethesda, MD 20892
(301) 592-8573
www.nhlbi.nih.gov/index.htm

The National Institute of Diabetes and Digestive and Kidney Diseases
Office of Communications and Public Liaison
NIDDK, NIH, Building 31, Room 9A04
Center Drive, MSC 2560
Bethesda, MD 20892
(301) 496-4000
www.niddk.nih.gov

National Center for Complementary and Alternative Medicine
NCCAM Clearinghouse
P.O. Box 7923
Gaithersburg, MD 20898
(888) 644-6226
http://nccam.nih.gov

U.S. Department of Agriculture (USDA)
14th Street, SW
Washington, DC 20250
(202) 720-2791
www.usda.gov

Centers for Disease Control and Prevention (CDC)
1600 Clifton Rd
Atlanta, GA 30333
(404) 639-3311 / Public Inquiries: (800) 311-3435
www.cdc.gov

National Institutes of Health (NIH)
9000 Rockville Pike
Bethesda, MD 20892
(301) 496-4000
www.nih.gov

Food and Nutrition Information Center
Agricultural Research Service, USDA
National Agricultural Library, Room 105
10301 Baltimore Avenue
Beltsville, MD 20705-2351
(301) 504-5719
www.nal.usda.gov/fnic

National Institute of Allergy and Infectious Diseases
NIAID Office of Communications and Public Liaison
6610 Rockledge Drive, MSC 6612
Bethesda, MD 20892
(301) 496-5717
www.niaid.nih.gov

Weight and Health Management
The Vegetarian Resource Group
P.O. Box 1463, Dept. IN
Baltimore, MD 21203
(410) 366-VEGE
www.vrg.org

American Obesity Association
1250 24th Street, NW
Suite 300
Washington, DC 20037
(202) 776-7711
www.obesity.org

Anemia Lifeline
(888) 722-4407
www.anemia.com

Bottled Water Web
P.O. Box 5658
Santa Barbara, CA 93150
(805) 879-1564
www.bottledwaterweb.com

The Food and Nutrition Board
Institute of Medicine
500 Fifth Street, NW
Washington, DC 20001
(202) 334-2352
www.iom.edu/board.asp?id-3788

The Calorie Control Council
www.caloriecontrol.org

TOPS (Take Off Pounds Sensibly)
4575 South Fifth Street
P.O. Box 07360
Milwaukee, WI 53207
(800) 932-8677
www.tops.org

Shape Up America!
15009 Native Dancer Road
N. Potomac, MD 20878
(240) 631-6533
www.shapeup.org

World Hunger
Center on Hunger, Poverty, and Nutrition Policy
Tufts University
Medford, MA 02155
(617) 627-3020
www.tufts.edu/nutrition

Freedom from Hunger
1644 DaVinci Court
Davis, CA 95616
(800) 708-2555
www.freefromhunger.org

Oxfam International
1112 16th Street, NW, Suite 600
Washington, DC 20036
(202) 496-1170
www.oxfam.org

WorldWatch Institute
1776 Massachusetts Avenue, NW
Washington, DC 20036
(202) 452-1999
www.worldwatch.org

Food First
398 60th Street
Oakland, CA 94618
(510) 654-4400
www.foodfirst.org

The Hunger Project
15 East 26th Street
New York, NY 10010
(212) 251-9100
www.thp.org

U.S. Agency for International Development
Information Center
Ronald Reagan Building
Washington, DC 20523
(202) 712-0000
www.usaid.gov

ANSWERS TO REVIEW QUESTIONS

Chapter 1
1. **d.** all of the above.
2. **b.** provides enough of the energy, nutrients, and fiber to maintain a person's health.
3. **c.** Being physically active each day.
4. **b.** eating more dark green and orange vegetables.
5. **b.** vitamin A, vitamin C, sodium, iron, and calcium.
6. False. Vitamins do not provide any energy, although many vitamins are critical to the metabolic processes that assist us in generating energy from carbohydrates, fats, and proteins.
7. True.
8. True. There is some evidence that drinking alcoholic beverages in moderation is associated with cardiovascular health benefits. However, because drinking in excess can lead to significant health and social problems, the Dietary Guidelines for Americans recommend that if someone does drink alcoholic beverages, they should do so in moderation.
9. False. Although eating a variety of foods is one component of a healthful diet, it is not the only factor to ensure that one's diet is healthful. Other factors to consider include adequacy, moderation, and balance.
10. True.

Chapter 2
1. **b.** chemicals that help speed up body processes.
2. **d.** emulsifies fats.
3. **c.** hypothalamus.
4. **a.** seepage of gastric acid into the esophagus.
5. **c.** small intestine.
6. False. Cells are the smallest units of life. Atoms are the smallest units of matter in nature.
7. True.
8. True.
9. False. Vitamins and minerals are not really "digested" the same way that macronutrients are. These compounds do not have to be broken down because they are small enough to be readily absorbed by the small intestine. For example, fat-soluble vitamins, such as vitamins A, D, E, and K, are soluble in lipids and are absorbed into the intestinal cells along with the fats in our foods. Water-soluble vitamins, such as the B vitamins and vitamin C, typically undergo some type of active transport process that helps assure the vitamin is absorbed by the small intestine. Minerals are absorbed all along the small intestine, and in some cases in the large intestine as well, by a wide variety of mechanisms.
10. False. People with irritable bowel syndrome may experience constipation, diarrhea, or a combination of both.

Chapter 3
1. **b.** the potential of foods to raise blood glucose and insulin levels.
2. **d.** carbon, hydrogen, and oxygen.
3. **d.** sweetened soft drinks.
4. **a.** monosaccharides.
5. **c.** type 2 diabetes.
6. False. Although in the past this was true, recently there has been a significant increase in the incidence of type 2 diabetes among children and teens.
7. True.
8. False. A person with lactose intolerance [has a difficult] time tolerating milk and other dairy produc[ts. This] person does not have an allergy to milk, as he o[r she] does not exhibit an immune response indicative of a[n] allergy. Instead, this person does not digest lactose completely, which causes intestinal distress and symptoms such as gas, bloating, diarrhea, and nausea.
9. False. Plants store glucose as starch.
10. False. Salivary amylase breaks starches into maltose and shorter polysaccharides.

Chapter 4
1. **c.** synthesized in the liver and small intestine.
2. **b.** exercise regularly.
3. **a.** transport of dietary fat to the wall of the small intestine.
4. **d.** high-density lipoproteins.
5. **a.** monounsaturated fats.
6. True.
7. False. Fat is an important source of energy during rest and during exercise, and adipose tissue is our primary storage site for fat. We rely significantly on the fat stored in our adipose tissue to provide energy during rest and exercise.
8. False. A triglyceride is a lipid comprised of a glycerol molecule and three fatty acids. Thus, fatty acids are a component of triglycerides.
9. False. While most *trans* fatty acids result from the hydrogenation of vegetable oils by food manufacturers, a small amount of *trans* fatty acids are found in cow's milk.
10. False. A serving of food labeled *reduced fat* has at least 25% less fat than a standard serving, but may not have fewer calories than a full-fat version of the same food.

Chapter 5
1. **d.** mutual supplementation.
2. **a.** Rice, pinto beans, acorn squash, soy butter, and almond milk.
3. **b.** DNA.
4. **b.** amine group.
5. **c.** carbon, oxygen, hydrogen, and nitrogen.
6. True.
7. False. Both shape and function are lost when a protein is denatured.
8. False. Some hormones are made from lipids.
9. True.
10. False. Depending upon the type of sport, athletes may require the same or up to two times as much protein as nonactive people.

Chapter 6
1. **b.** thiamin, pantothenic acid, and biotin.
2. **d.** is destroyed by exposure to high heat.
3. **d.** nitrates.
4. **a.** vitamin A
5. **b.** vitamin K.
6. False. Neural tube defects occur during the first 4 weeks of pregnancy; this is often before a woman even

she is pregnant. Thus, the best way for a
n to protect her fetus against neural tube defects
make sure she is consuming adequate folate
ore she is pregnant.
alse. Our bodies make vitamin D by converting a
cholesterol compound in our skin to the active form of
vitamin D that we need to function. We do not absorb
vitamin D from sunlight, but when the ultraviolet rays
of the sun hit our skin, they react to eventually form
calcitriol, which is considered the primary active form
of vitamin D in our bodies.
8. True.
9. False. Pregnant women should not consume beef liver
very often, as it can lead to vitamin A toxicity and
potentially serious birth defects.
10. True.

Chapter 7
1. **c.** It is freely permeable to water but not to all
electrolytes.
2. **b.** Iron is a component of hemoglobin, myoglobin, and
certain enzymes.
3. **a.** sodium, chloride, and iodine.
4. **d.** It provides the scaffolding for cortical bone.
5. **d.** structure of bone, nerve transmission, and muscle
contraction.
6. True.
7. True.
8. True.
9. True.
10. False. The fractures that result from osteoporosis
cause an increased risk of infection and other related
illnesses that can lead to premature death.

Chapter 8
1. **d.** A healthy infant of average weight.
2. **a.** fluid outside our cells.
3. **c.** adequate hydration.
4. **c.** 7 kcal of energy.
5. **d.** All of the above are true.
6. True.
7. False. Our thirst mechanism is triggered by an
increase in the concentration of electrolytes in our
blood.
8. False. The recommendations state, "If you don't drink,
don't start. If you do drink, do so in moderation."
9. False. One "drink" of wine is equivalent to 5 oz of
wine.
10. True.

Chapter 9
1. **d.** body mass index.
2. **a.** basal metabolic rate, thermal effect of food, and
effect of physical activity.
3. **b.** take in more energy than they expend.
4. **c.** all people have a genetic set point for their body
weight.
5. **d.** disordered eating, menstrual dysfunction, and
osteoporosis.
6. False. It is the apple-shaped fat patterning, or excess
fat in the trunk region, that is known to increase a
person's risk for many chronic diseases.
7. True
8. False. People with binge-eating disorder typically do
not purge to compensate for the binge; thus, these
individuals are usually overweight or obese.

9. False. Healthful weight gain includes eating more
energy than you expend and also exercising to
maintain both aerobic fitness and to build muscle
mass.
10. True.

Chapter 10
1. **c.** 64% to 90% of your estimated maximal heart rate.
2. **a.** 1 to 3 seconds.
3. **b.** fat
4. **c.** seems to increase strength gained in resistance
exercise.
5. **b.** beverages containing carbohydrates and
electrolytes.
6. True.
7. False. A dietary fat intake of 20% to 25% is typically
recommended.
8. False. Carbohydrate loading involves altering
duration and intensity of exercise and intake of
carbohydrate such that the storage of carbohydrate is
maximized.
9. False. Sports anemia is not true anemia, but a
transient decrease in iron stores that occurs at the
start of an exercise program. This is a result of an
initial increase in plasma volume (or water in our
blood) that is not matched by an increase in
hemoglobin.
10. True.

Chapter 11
1. **b.** neural tube defects
2. **c.** iron
3. **d.** greater than that for children, adults, and pregnant
adults.
4. **b.** vitamin D.
5. **d.** all of the above.
6. False. These issues are most likely to occur in the first
trimester of pregnancy.
7. False. Honey may contain spores of the bacterium
Clostridium botulinum, which can be fatal for infants.
8. False. Toddlers are greatly influenced by their
parents' own examples of eating, and also are
influenced by the foods parents choose for them to eat.
9. True.
10. True.

Chapter 12
1. **b.** a flavor enhancer used in a variety of foods.
2. **a.** contain only organically produced ingredients,
excluding water and salt.
3. **d.** pasteurization
4. **d.** kwashiorkor
5. **a.** the nutrition transition.
6. False. Bacteria that cause food-borne illnesses
multiply rapidly at room temperature. Foods should
be refrigerated promptly to keep microbes from
multiplying.
7. True, it is easier for them to be infected (low vitamin A)
and harder for them to fight off the infection.
8. True.
9. False. Irradiation kills microbes that can cause food-
borne illness or leaves them unable to reproduce.
10. True.

GLOSSARY

A

absorption   The physiologic process by which molecules of food are taken from the GI tract into the body.

acceptable daily intake (ADI)   An estimate made by the Food and Drug Administration of the amount of a non-nutritive sweetener that someone can consume each day over a lifetime without adverse effects.

Acceptable Macronutrient Distribution Range (AMDR)   A range of intakes for a particular energy source that is associated with reduced risk of chronic disease while providing adequate intake of essential nutrients.

added sugars   Sugars and syrups that are added to food during processing or preparation.

adenosine triphosphate (ATP)   The common currency of energy for virtually all cells of the body.

adequate diet   A diet that provides enough energy, nutrients, and fiber to maintain a person's health.

Adequate Intake (AI)   A recommended average daily nutrient intake level based on observed or experimentally determined estimates of nutrient intake by a group of healthy people.

aerobic   Means "with oxygen." Term used to refer to metabolic reactions that occur only in the presence of oxygen.

aerobic exercise   Exercise that involves the repetitive movement of large muscle groups, increasing the body's use of oxygen and promoting cardiovascular health.

alcohol   A beverage made from fermented fruits, vegetables, or grains and containing the chemical ethanol.

alpha-linolenic acid   An essential fatty acid found in leafy green vegetables, flax seed oil, soy oil, fish oil, and fish products; an omega-3 fatty acid.

amenorrhea   Amenorrhea is the absence of menstruation. In females who had previously been menstruating, it is defined as the absence of menstrual periods for 3 or more months.

amino acids   Nitrogen-containing molecules that combine to form proteins.

amniotic fluid   The watery fluid contained within the innermost membrane of the sac containing the fetus. It cushions and protects the growing fetus.

anabolic   Refers to a substance that builds muscle and increases strength.

anaerobic   Means "without oxygen." Term used to refer to metabolic reactions that occur in the absence of oxygen.

anencephaly   A fatal neural tube defect in which there is partial absence of brain tissue most likely caused by failure of the neural tube to close.

anorexia nervosa   A serious, potentially life-threatening eating disorder that is characterized by self-starvation, which eventually leads to a deficiency in energy and essential nutrients that are required by the body to function normally.

antibodies   Defensive proteins of the immune system. Their production is prompted by the presence of bacteria, viruses, toxins, or allergens.

antioxidant   A compound that has the ability to prevent or repair the damage caused by oxidation.

appetite   A psychological desire to consume specific foods.

ariboflavinosis   A condition caused by riboflavin deficiency.

aseptic packaging   Sterile packaging that does not require refrigeration or preservatives while seal is maintained.

athlete   Any person trained to compete in sports.

atrophic gastritis   A condition that results in low stomach acid secretion; estimated to occur in about 10% to 30% of adults older than 50 years of age.

B

bacteria   Microorganisms that lack a true nucleus and have a chemical called peptidoglycan in their cell walls.

balanced diet   A diet that contains the combinations of foods that provide the proper proportion of nutrients.

basal metabolic rate (BMR)   The energy the body expends to maintain its fundamental physiologic functions.

beriberi   A disease caused by thiamin deficiency.

bile   Fluid produced by the liver and stored in the gallbladder that emulsifies fats in the small intestine.

binge drinking   The consumption of five or more alcoholic drinks on one occasion.

binge-eating   Consumption of a large amount of food in a short period of time, usually accompanied by a feeling of loss of self-control.

binge-eating disorder   A disorder characterized by binge-eating an average of twice a week or more, typically without compensatory purging.

bioavailability   The degree to which our bodies can absorb and use any given nutrient.

biologic age   Physiologic age as determined by health and functional status; often estimated by scored questionnaires.

biopesticides   Primarily insecticides, these chemicals use natural methods to reduce damage to crops.

blood volume   The amount of fluid in blood.

body composition   The ratio of a person's body fat to lean body mass.

body image   A person's perception of his or her body's appearance and functioning.

body mass index (BMI)   A measurement representing the ratio of a person's body weight to his or her height.

bone density   The degree of compactness of bone tissue, reflecting the strength of the bones. *Peak bone density* is the point at which a bone is strongest.

brush border   Term that describes the microvilli of the small intestine's lining, which tremendously increase its absorptive capacity.

buffers   Proteins that help maintain proper acid–base balance by attaching to, or releasing, hydrogen ions as conditions change in the body.

bulimia nervosa   A serious eating disorder characterized by recurrent episodes of binge-eating and recurrent inappropriate compensatory behaviors in order to prevent weight gain, such as self-induced vomiting, fasting, excessive exercise, or misuse of laxatives, diuretics, enemas, or other medications.

C

cancer   A group of diseases characterized by cells that reproduce spontaneously and independently and may invade other tissues and organs.

carbohydrate   One of the three macronutrients, a compound made up of carbon, hydrogen, and oxygen. It is derived from plants and provides energy. Carbohydrate is the primary fuel source for our bodies, particularly for the brain and for physical exercise.

carbohydrate loading   Also known as glycogen loading. A process that involves altering training and carbohydrate intake so that muscle glycogen storage is maximized.

carcinogens   Cancer-causing agents, such as certain pesticides, industrial chemicals, and pollutants.

cardiovascular disease   A general term that refers to abnormal conditions involving dysfunction of the heart and blood vessels; cardiovascular disease can result in heart attack or stroke.

carotenoids   Fat-soluble plant pigments that the body stores in the liver and adipose tissues. The body is able to convert certain carotenoids to vitamin A.

celiac disease   A genetic disorder characterized by an inability to absorb a protein called gluten. This causes an inflammatory immune response that damages the lining of the small intestine.

cell   The smallest unit of matter that exhibits the properties of living things, such as growth, reproduction, and the taking in of nutrients.

cell differentiation   The process by which immature, undifferentiated cells develop into highly specialized functional cells of discrete organs and tissues.

cell membrane   The boundary of an animal cell that separates its internal cytoplasm, nucleus, and other structures from the external environment.

chronologic age   Age as defined by calendar years, from date of birth.

chylomicron   A lipoprotein produced in the mucosal cell of the intestine; transports dietary fat out of the intestinal tract.

chyme   Semifluid mass consisting of partially digested food, water, and gastric juices.

cirrhosis   End-stage liver disease characterized by significant abnormalities in liver structure and function; may lead to complete liver failure.

coenzyme   A compound that combines with an inactive enzyme to form an active enzyme.

colic   Unconsolable infant crying of unknown origin that lasts for hours at a time.

collagen   A protein found in all connective tissues in our bodies.

colostrum   The first fluid made and secreted by the breasts from late in pregnancy to about a week after birth. It is rich in immune factors and protein.

complementary proteins   Two or more foods that together contain all nine essential amino acids necessary for a complete protein. It is not necessary to eat complementary proteins at the same meal.

complete proteins   Foods that contain all nine essential amino acids.

complex carbohydrate   A nutrient compound consisting of long chains of glucose molecules, such as starch, glycogen, and fiber.

conception (also called *fertilization*)   The uniting of an ovum (egg) and sperm to create a fertilized egg.

constipation   Condition characterized by the absence of bowel movements for a period of time that is significantly longer than normal for the individual. When a bowel movement does occur, stools are usually small, hard, and difficult to pass.

cool-down   Activities done after an exercise session is completed. Should be gradual and allow your body to slowly recover from exercise.

cortical bone (compact bone)   A dense bone tissue that makes up the outer surface of all bones as well as the entirety of most small bones of the body.

creatine phosphate (CP)   A high-energy compound that can be broken down for energy and used to regenerate ATP.

cretinism   A form of mental retardation that occurs in individuals whose mothers experienced iodine deficiency during pregnancy.

cross contamination   Contamination of one food by another via the transfer of microorganisms through physical contact.

cytoplasm   The liquid within an animal cell.

D

danger zone   Range of temperature (about 40°F to 135°F [4°C to 57°C]) at which many microorganisms capable of causing human disease thrive.

dehydration   Depletion of body fluid that results when fluid excretion exceeds fluid intake.

desiccants   Chemicals that prevent foods from absorbing moisture from the air.

diabetes   A chronic disease in which the body can no longer regulate glucose.

diarrhea   Condition characterized by the frequent passage of loose, watery stools.

dietary fiber   The type of fiber that occurs naturally in foods.

Dietary Guidelines for Americans   A set of principles developed by the U.S. Department of Agriculture and the U.S. Department of Health and Human Services to assist Americans in designing a healthful diet and lifestyle.

Dietary Reference Intakes (DRIs)   A set of nutritional reference values for the United States and Canada that apply to healthy people.

digestion   The process by which foods are broken down into their component molecules, both mechanically and chemically.

disaccharide   A carbohydrate compound consisting of two sugar molecules joined together.

discretionary calories   A term used in the MyPyramid food guidance system that represents the extra amount of energy you can consume after you have met all of your essential needs by consuming the most nutrient-dense foods that are low fat or fat free and that have no added sugars.

disordered eating   Disordered eating is a general term used to describe a variety of abnormal or atypical eating behaviors that are used to keep or maintain a lower body weight.

diuretic   A substance that increases fluid loss via the urine. Common diuretics include alcohol and some prescription medications for high blood pressure and other disorders.

DNA   A molecule present in the nucleus of all body cells that directs the assembly of amino acids into body proteins.

docosahexaenoic acid (DHA)   A type of omega-3 fatty acid that can be made in the body from alpha-linolenic acid and found in our diet primarily in marine plants and animals; together with EPA, it appears to reduce our risk of a heart attack.

drink   The amount of an alcoholic beverage that provides approximately ½ fl. oz of pure ethanol.

E

eating disorder An eating disorder is a clinically diagnosed psychiatric disorder characterized by severe disturbances in body image and eating behaviors.

edema A disorder in which fluids build up in the tissue spaces of the body, causing fluid imbalances and a swollen appearance.

eicosapentaenoic acid (EPA) A type of omega-3 fatty acid that can be made in the body from alpha-linolenic acid and found in our diet primarily in marine plants and animals.

electrolyte A substance that dissociates in solution into positively and negatively charged ions and is thus capable of carrying an electric current.

elimination The process by which the undigested portions of food and waste products are removed from the body.

embryo Human growth and developmental stage lasting from the third week to the end of the eighth week after fertilization.

emulsifiers Chemicals that improve texture and smoothness in foods; stabilize oil–water mixtures.

energy cost of physical activity The energy expended on body movement and muscular work above basal levels.

energy expenditure The energy the body expends to maintain its basic functions and to perform all levels of movement and activity.

energy intake The amount of food a person eats; in other words, it is the number of kilocalories consumed.

enteric nerves The nerves of the GI tract.

enzymes Chemicals, usually proteins, that act on other chemicals to speed up body processes.

ergogenic aids Substances used to improve exercise and athletic performance.

esophagus Muscular tube of the GI tract connecting the back of the mouth to the stomach.

essential amino acids Amino acids not produced by the body that must be obtained from food.

essential fatty acids (EFA) Fatty acids that must be consumed in the diet because they cannot be made by our bodies. The two essential fatty acids are linoleic acid and alpha-linolenic acid.

Estimated Average Requirement (EAR) The average daily nutrient intake level estimated to meet the requirement of half of the healthy individuals in a particular life stage and gender group.

Estimated Energy Requirement (EER) The average dietary energy intake that is predicted to maintain energy balance in a healthy adult.

evaporative cooling Another term for sweating, which is the primary way in which we dissipate heat.

exercise A subcategory of leisure-time physical activity; any activity that is purposeful, planned, and structured.

F

famine A widespread and severe food shortage that causes starvation and death in a large portion of a population in a region.

fats An important energy source for our bodies at rest and during low-intensity exercise.

fat-soluble vitamins Vitamins that are not soluble in water but soluble in fat. These include vitamins A, D, E, and K.

fatty acids Long chains of carbon atoms bound to each other as well as to hydrogen atoms.

female athlete triad A serious syndrome that consists of three medical disorders seen in some female athletes: disordered eating, amenorrhea, and osteoporosis.

fetal alcohol spectrum disorders (FASD) An umbrella term describing the range of effects that can occur in the child of a woman who drinks during her pregnancy. Fetal alcohol syndrome (FAS), alcohol-related neurodevelopmental disorder (ARND), and alcohol-related birth defects (ARBD) are components of FASD.

fetal alcohol syndrome (FAS) Cluster of birth defects in the offspring of a mother who consumed alcohol during pregnancy, including facial deformities, impaired growth, and a spectrum of mild to severe cognitive, emotional, and physical problems.

fetus Human growth and developmental stage lasting from the beginning of the ninth week after conception to birth.

fiber The nondigestible carbohydrate parts of plants that form the support structures of leaves, stems, and seeds.

fiber-rich carbohydrates A group of foods containing either simple or complex carbohydrates that are rich in dietary fiber. These foods, which include most fruits, vegetables, and whole grains, are typically fresh or only moderately processed.

FIT principle The principle used to achieve an appropriate overload for physical training. Stands for frequency, intensity, and time of activity.

flavoring agents Obtained from either natural or synthetic sources; they allow manufacturers to maintain a consistent flavor from batch to batch.

fluid A substance composed of molecules that move past one another freely. Fluids are characterized by their ability to conform to the shape of whatever container holds them.

fluorosis A condition marked by staining and pitting of the teeth; caused by an abnormally high intake of fluoride.

food The plants and animals we consume.

food additive A substance or mixture of substances intentionally put into food to enhance its appearance, safety, palatability, and quality.

food allergy An inflammatory reaction caused by an immune system hypersensitivity to a protein component of a food.

food-borne illness An illness transmitted through food or water either by an infectious agent, a poisonous substance, or a protein that causes an immune reaction.

food insecurity Situation in which one or more factors limit an individual's access to a safe and adequate nutrient-rich food supply.

food intolerance A cluster of GI symptoms that occur following consumption of a particular food but are not caused by an immune system response.

food preservatives Chemicals that help prevent microbial spoilage and enzymatic deterioration.

food security A situation in which a person has daily access to a supply of safe foods with enough energy and sufficiently rich nutrient quality to promote a healthy, active life.

free radical A highly unstable atom with an unpaired electron in its outermost shell.

frequency Refers to the number of activity sessions per week you perform.

fructose The sweetest natural sugar; a monosaccharide that occurs in fruits and vegetables. Also called *levulose*, or *fruit sugar*.

functional fiber   The nondigestible forms of carbohydrate that are extracted from plants or manufactured in the laboratory and have known health benefits.

fungi   Plantlike spore-forming organisms that can grow either as single cells or multicellular colonies.

G

galactose   A monosaccharide that joins with glucose to create lactose, one of the three most common disaccharides.

gallbladder   A sack of tissue beneath the liver that stores bile and secretes it into the small intestine.

gastric juice   Acidic liquid secreted within the stomach that contains hydrochloric acid, pepsin, and other chemicals.

gastroesophageal reflux disease (GERD)   A painful type of heartburn that occurs more than twice per week.

gastrointestinal (GI) tract   A long, muscular tube consisting of several organs: the mouth, esophagus, stomach, small intestine, and large intestine.

gene   Segment of DNA that carries the instructions for assembling available amino acids into a unique protein.

Generally Recognized as Safe (GRAS) list   Established by Congress to identify substances used in foods that are generally recognized as safe based on a history of long-term use or on the consensus of qualified research experts.

genetic modification/genetically modified organisms (GMOs)   Terms used to signify that the organism has been created through manipulation of the genetic material.

gestational diabetes   Insufficient insulin production or insulin resistance that results in consistently high blood glucose levels, specifically during pregnancy; condition typically resolves after birth occurs.

giardiasis   A diarrheal illness caused by the intestinal parasite *Giardia intestinalis* (or *Giardia lamblia*).

glucagon   Hormone secreted by the alpha cells of the pancreas in response to decreased blood levels of glucose. Causes breakdown of liver stores of glycogen into glucose.

gluconeogenesis   The generation of glucose from the breakdown of proteins into amino acids.

glucose   The most abundant sugar molecule: a monosaccharide generally found in combination with other sugars. The preferred source of energy for the brain and an important source of energy for all cells.

glycemic index   Rating of the potential of foods to raise blood glucose and insulin levels.

glycemic load   The amount of carbohydrate contained in a particular food, multiplied by its glycemic index.

glycerol   An alcohol composed of three carbon atoms; it is the backbone of a triglyceride molecule.

glycogen   A polysaccharide stored in animals; the storage form of glucose in animals.

glycolysis   The breakdown of glucose; yields two ATP molecules and two pyruvic acid molecules for each molecule of glucose.

goiter   Enlargement of the thyroid gland; can be caused by iodine toxicity or deficiency.

grazing   Consistently eating small meals throughout the day; done by many athletes to meet their high-energy demands.

H

healthful diet   A diet that provides the proper combination of energy and nutrients and is adequate, moderate, balanced, and varied.

heartburn   The painful sensation that occurs over the sternum when hydrochloric acid backs up into the lower esophagus.

heat cramps   Muscle spasms that occur several hours after strenuous exercise; most often occur when sweat losses and fluid intakes are high, urine volume is low, and sodium intake is inadequate.

heat exhaustion   A heat illness that is characterized by excessive sweating, weakness, nausea, dizziness, headache, and difficulty concentrating. Unchecked heat exhaustion can lead to heatstroke.

heat stroke   A potentially fatal response to high temperature characterized by failure of the body's heat-regulating mechanisms. Symptoms include rapid pulse, reduced sweating, hot, dry skin, high temperature, headache, weakness, and sudden loss of consciousness. Commonly called *sunstroke*.

heat syncope   Dizziness that occurs when people stand for too long in the heat or when they stop suddenly after a race or stand suddenly from a lying position; results from blood pooling in the lower extremities.

helminth   Multicellular microscopic worm.

heme   The iron-containing molecule found in hemoglobin.

heme iron   Iron that is part of hemoglobin and myoglobin; found only in animal-based foods.

hemoglobin   The oxygen-carrying protein found in our red blood cells; almost two-thirds of all the iron in our bodies is found in hemoglobin.

hepatitis   Inflammation of the liver; can be caused by a virus or toxic agent such as alcohol.

high-density lipoprotein (HDL)   Small, dense lipoprotein with a very low cholesterol content and a high protein content.

homocysteine   An amino acid that requires adequate levels of folate, vitamin B_6, and vitamin B_{12} for its metabolism. High levels of homocysteine in the blood are associated with an increased risk for vascular diseases such as cardiovascular disease.

hormone   Chemical messenger that is secreted into the bloodstream by one of the many glands of the body.

humectants   Chemicals that help retain moisture in foods, keeping them soft and pliable.

hunger   A physical sensation that drives us to eat.

hydrogenation   The process of adding hydrogen to unsaturated fatty acids, making them more saturated and therefore more solid at room temperature.

hypoglycemia   A condition marked by blood glucose levels that are below normal fasting levels.

hypothalamus   A region of the forebrain where visceral sensations such as hunger and thirst are regulated.

I

incomplete proteins   Foods that do not contain all of the essential amino acids in sufficient amounts to support growth and health.

insoluble fibers   Fibers that do not dissolve in water.

insulin   Hormone secreted by the beta cells of the pancreas in response to increased blood levels of glucose. Facilitates uptake of glucose by body cells.

intensity   Refers to the amount of effort expended during the activity, or how difficult the activity is to perform.

invisible fats   Fats that are hidden in foods, such as the fats found in baked goods, regular-fat dairy products, marbling in meat, and fried foods.

ion   Any electrically charged particle.

iron-deficiency anemia Disorder in which the production of healthy red blood cells decreases and hemoglobin levels are inadequate to fully oxygenate the body's cells and tissues.

irradiation A sterilization process in which food is exposed to gamma rays or high-energy electron beams to kill microorganisms. Irradiation does not impart any radiation to the food being treated.

irritable bowel syndrome (IBS) A bowel disorder that interferes with normal functions of the colon. IBS causes abdominal cramps, bloating, and constipation or diarrhea.

K

ketoacidosis A condition in which excessive ketones are present in the blood, causing the blood to become very acidic, which alters basic body functions and damages tissues. Untreated ketoacidosis can be fatal. This condition is found in individuals with untreated diabetes mellitus.

ketones Substances produced during the breakdown of fat when carbohydrate intake is insufficient to meet energy needs. Provide an alternative energy source for the brain when glucose levels are low.

ketosis The process by which the breakdown of fat during fasting states results in the production of ketones.

kwashiorkor A form of malnutrition that is typically seen in toddlers who are weaned because of the birth of a subsequent child. Denied breast milk, they are fed a cereal diet that provides adequate energy but inadequate protein.

L

lactic acid A compound that results when pyruvic acid is metabolized.

lactose Also called *milk sugar;* a disaccharide consisting of one glucose molecule and one galactose molecule. Found in milk, including human breast milk.

lactose intolerance A disorder in which the body does not produce sufficient lactase enzyme and therefore cannot digest foods that contain lactose, such as cow's milk.

large intestine Final organ of the GI tract consisting of the cecum, colon, rectum, and anal canal, and in which most water is absorbed and feces are formed.

leptin A hormone that is produced by body fat that acts to reduce food intake, and it causes a decrease in body weight and body fat.

life expectancy The expected number of years remaining in one's life; typically stated from the time of birth: children born in the United States in 2003 could expect to live, on average, 77.6 years.

life span The highest age reached by any member of a species; currently, the human life span is 122 years.

limiting amino acid The essential amino acid that is missing or in the smallest supply in the amino acid pool and is thus responsible for slowing or halting protein synthesis.

linoleic acid An essential fatty acid found in vegetable and nut oils; also known as omega-6 fatty acid.

lipids A diverse group of organic substances that are insoluble in water; lipids include triglycerides, phospholipids, and sterols.

lipoprotein A spherical compound in which fat clusters in the center and phospholipids and proteins form the outside.

liver The largest organ of the GI tract and one of the most important organs of the body. Its functions include production of bile and processing of nutrient-rich blood from the small intestine.

low birth weight A weight of less than 5.5 lb at birth.

low-density lipoprotein (LDL) Molecule resulting when a VLDL releases its triglyceride load. Higher cholesterol and protein content makes LDLs somewhat more dense than VLDLs.

low-intensity activities Activities that cause very mild increases in breathing, sweating, and heart rate.

M

macronutrients Nutrients that our bodies need in relatively large amounts to support normal function and health. Carbohydrates, fats, and proteins are macronutrients.

major minerals Minerals we need to consume in amounts of at least 100 mg per day and of which the total amount in our bodies is at least 5 g.

maltose A disaccharide consisting of two molecules of glucose. Does not generally occur independently in foods but results as a by-product of digestion. Also called *malt sugar.*

marasmus A form of malnutrition seen in children and resulting from grossly inadequate intakes of protein, carbohydrates, fats, and micronutrients.

maximal heart rate The rate at which your heart beats during maximal-intensity exercise.

megadosing Taking a dose of a nutrient that is ten or more times greater than the recommended amount.

metabolic water The water formed as a by-product of our body's metabolic reactions.

metabolism The sum of all the chemical and physical processes by which the body breaks down and builds up molecules.

micronutrients Nutrients needed in relatively small amounts to support normal health and body functions. Vitamins and minerals are micronutrients.

minerals Micronutrients that do not contain carbon, are not broken down during digestion and absorption, and are not destroyed by heat or light. Minerals assist in the regulation of many body processes and are classified as major minerals or trace minerals.

moderate-intensity activities Activities that cause noticeable increases in breathing, sweating, and heart rate.

moderation Eating the right amounts of foods to maintain a healthy weight and to optimize our bodies' functioning.

monosaccharide The simplest of carbohydrates: consists of one sugar molecule; the most common form is glucose.

monounsaturated fatty acids (MUFA) Fatty acids that have two carbons in the chain bound to each other with one double bond; these types of fatty acids are generally liquid at room temperature.

morbid obesity A condition in which a person's body weight exceeds 100% of normal, putting him or her at very high risk for serious health consequences.

morning sickness Varying degrees of nausea and vomiting associated with pregnancy, most commonly in the first trimester.

multifactorial disease Any disease that may be attributable to one or more of a variety of causes.

mutual supplementation The process of combining two or more incomplete protein sources to make a complete protein.

myoglobin An iron-containing protein similar to hemoglobin, except that it is found in muscle cells.

MyPyramid   A revised pyramid-based food guidance system developed by the USDA and based on the 2005 Dietary Guidelines for Americans and the Dietary Reference Intakes from the National Academy of Sciences.

N

neural tube   Embryonic tissue that forms a tube, which eventually becomes the brain and spinal cord.

night blindness   A vitamin A–deficiency disorder that results in the loss of the ability to see in dim light.

nitrites   Chemicals used in meat curing to develop and stabilize the pink color associated with cured meat, also functions as an antibacterial agent.

noncommunicable diseases   Diseases that are not infectious but are largely determined by genetics and lifestyle. Chronic diseases are typically noncommunicable.

nonessential amino acids   Amino acids that can be manufactured by the body in sufficient quantities and therefore do not need to be consumed regularly in our diet.

non-heme iron   The form of iron that is not a part of hemoglobin or myoglobin; found in animal- and plant-based foods.

non-nutritive sweeteners   Also called *alternative sweeteners;* manufactured sweeteners that provide little or no energy.

nutrient deficiency   Malnutrition defined by a poor-quality diet that may or may not be adequate in energy. One or more nutrient-deficiency diseases may occur.

nutrient density   The relative amount of nutrients per amount of energy (number of calories).

nutrients   Chemicals found in foods that are critical to human growth and function.

nutrition   The scientific study of food and how food nourishes the body and influences health.

Nutrition Facts Panel   The label on a food package that contains the nutrition information required by the FDA.

nutrition transition   A shift in dietary pattern toward greater food security, greater variety of foods, and more foods with high energy density because of added fat and sugar. It is accompanied by access to motorized transportation, sedentary occupations, and economic growth.

nutritive sweeteners   Sweeteners such as sucrose, fructose, honey, and brown sugar that contribute calories (or energy).

O

obesity   Having an excess body fat that adversely affects health, resulting in a person having a weight for a given height that is substantially greater than an accepted standard.

organ   A body structure composed of two or more tissues and performing a specific function, for example, the esophagus.

organism   A complete and independent living being.

osteoblasts   Cells that prompt the formation of new bone matrix by laying down the collagen-containing component of bone that is then mineralized.

osteoclasts   Cells that break down the surface of bones by secreting enzymes and acids that dig grooves into the bone matrix.

osteomalacia   Vitamin D–deficiency disease in adults, in which bones become weak and prone to fractures.

osteoporosis   A disease characterized by low bone mass and deterioration of bone tissue, leading to increased bone fragility and fracture risk.

ounce-equivalent (or oz-equivalent)   A term used to define a serving size that is 1 ounce, or equivalent to an ounce, for the grains section and the meats and beans section of MyPyramid.

overload principle   Placing an extra physical demand on your body in order to improve your fitness level.

overnutrition   Malnutrition defined by an absolute excess of energy leading to overweight. Diet may be high-quality or poor-quality.

overweight   Having a moderate amount of excess body fat, resulting in a person having a weight for a given height that is greater than an accepted standard but is not considered obese.

ovulation   The release of an ovum (egg) from a woman's ovary.

P

pancreas   Gland located behind the stomach that secretes digestive enzymes.

pancreatic amylase   An enzyme secreted by the pancreas into the small intestine that digests any remaining starch into maltose.

pasteurization   A form of sterilization using high temperatures for short periods of time.

pellagra   A disease that results from severe niacin deficiency.

pepsin   An enzyme in the stomach that begins the breakdown of proteins into shorter polypeptide chains and single amino acids.

peptic ulcer   Area of the GI tract that has been eroded away by the acidic gastric juice of the stomach. The two main causes of peptic ulcers are an *H. pylori* infection or use of nonsteroidal anti-inflammatory drugs.

peptide bonds   Unique types of chemical bonds in which the amine group of one amino acid binds to the acid group of another in order to manufacture dipeptides and all larger peptide molecules.

percent daily values (%DV)   Information on a Nutrition Facts Panel that tells you how much a serving of food contributes to your overall intake of nutrients listed on the label. The information is based on an energy intake of 2,000 kcal per day.

peristalsis   Waves of squeezing and pushing contractions that move food in one direction through the length of the GI tract.

persistent organic pollutants (POPs)   Chemicals released into the environment as a result of industry, agriculture, or improper waste disposal; automobile emissions also are considered POPs.

pesticides   Chemicals used either in the field or in storage to decrease destruction by predators or disease.

pH   Stands for percentage of hydrogen. It is a measure of the acidity—or level of hydrogen—of any solution, including human blood.

phospholipids   A type of lipid in which a fatty acid is combined with another compound that contains phosphate; unlike other lipids, phospholipids are soluble in water.

photosynthesis   Process by which plants use sunlight to fuel a chemical reaction that combines carbon and water into glucose, which is then stored in their cells.

physical activity   Any movement produced by muscles that increases energy expenditure; includes occupational, household, leisure-time, and transportation activities.

Physical Activity Pyramid   A pyramid similar to the previous USDA Food Guide Pyramid that makes recommendations for the type and amount of activity that should be done weekly to increase physical activity levels.

physical fitness The ability to carry out daily tasks with vigor and alertness, without undue fatigue, and with ample energy to enjoy leisure-time pursuits and meet unforeseen emergencies.

phytochemicals Chemicals found in plants (*phyto-* is from the Greek word for "plant"), such as pigments and other substances, that may reduce our risk for diseases such as cancer and heart disease.

pica An abnormal craving to eat something not fit for food, such as clay, paint, and so forth.

placebo effect Improved performance based on the belief that a product is beneficial although the product has been proved to have no physiologic benefits.

placenta A pregnancy-specific organ formed from both maternal and embryonic tissues. It is responsible for oxygen, nutrient, and waste exchange between mother and fetus.

polypharmacy Concurrent use of three or more medications.

polysaccharide A complex carbohydrate consisting of long chains of glucose.

polyunsaturated fatty acids (PUFA) Fatty acids that have more than one double bond in the chain; these types of fatty acids are generally liquid at room temperature.

prion A protein that misfolds and becomes infectious; prions are not living cellular organisms or viruses.

proof A measure of the alcohol content of a liquid. For example, 100-proof liquor is 50% alcohol by volume, whereas 80-proof liquor is 40% alcohol by volume.

proteases Enzymes that continue the breakdown of polypeptides in the small intestine.

proteins Large, complex molecules made up of amino acids and found as essential components of all living cells.

provitamin An inactive form of a vitamin that the body can convert to an active form. An example is beta-carotene.

puberty The period in life in which secondary sexual characteristics develop and people are biologically capable of reproducing.

purging An attempt to rid the body of unwanted food by vomiting or other compensatory means, such as excessive exercise, fasting, or laxative abuse.

pyruvic acid The primary end product of glycolysis.

Q

quackery The promotion of an unproven remedy, such as a supplement or other product or service, usually by someone unlicensed and untrained.

R

recombinant bovine growth hormone (rBGH) A genetically engineered hormone injected into dairy cows to enhance their milk output.

Recommended Dietary Allowance (RDA) The average daily nutrient intake level that meets the nutrient requirements of 97% to 98% of healthy individuals in a particular life stage and gender group.

remodeling The two-step process by which bone tissue is recycled; includes the breakdown of existing bone and the formation of new bone.

residues Chemicals that remain in the foods we eat despite cleaning and processing.

resistance training Exercise in which our muscles act against resistance.

retina The delicate, light-sensitive membrane lining the inner eyeball and connected to the optic nerve. It contains retinal.

rickets Vitamin D–deficiency disease in children. Symptoms include deformities of the skeleton such as bowed legs and knocked knees.

S

saliva A mixture of water, mucus, enzymes, and other chemicals that moistens the mouth and food, binds food particles together, and begins the digestion of carbohydrates.

salivary amylase An enzyme in saliva that breaks starch into smaller particles and eventually into the disaccharide maltose.

salivary glands Group of glands found under and behind the tongue and beneath the jaw that release saliva continually as well as in response to the thought, sight, smell, or presence of food.

satiation State of satisfaction, especially with food intake; fullness.

saturated fatty acids (SFA) Fatty acids that have no carbons joined together with a double bond; these types of fatty acids are generally solid at room temperature.

set-point theory A theory that suggests that the body raises or lowers energy expenditure in response to increased and decreased food intake and physical activity. This action serves to maintain an individual's body weight within a narrow range.

simple carbohydrate Commonly called *sugar*; a monosaccharide or disaccharide such as glucose.

small intestine The largest portion of the GI tract where most digestion and absorption take place.

soluble fibers Fibers that dissolve in water.

solvent A substance that is capable of mixing with and breaking apart compounds. Water is an excellent solvent.

sphincter A tight ring of muscle separating organs of the GI tract that opens in response to nerve signals indicating that food is ready to pass into the next section.

spina bifida Embryonic neural tube defect that occurs when the spinal vertebrae fail to completely enclose the spinal cord, allowing it to protrude.

spontaneous abortion (also called *miscarriage*) Natural termination of a pregnancy and expulsion of fetus and pregnancy tissues because of a genetic, developmental, or physiological abnormality that is so severe that the pregnancy cannot be maintained.

stabilizer A chemical that helps maintain smooth texture and uniform color and flavor in some foods.

starch A polysaccharide stored in plants; the storage form of glucose in plants.

steroid Man-made derivatives of testosterone, the male sex hormone.

sterols A type of lipid found in foods and the body that has a ring structure; cholesterol is the most common sterol that occurs in our diets.

stomach J-shaped organ where food is partially digested, churned, and stored until released into the small intestine.

stretching Exercise in which muscles are gently lengthened using slow, controlled movements.

stunting Low height for age.

sucrose   A disaccharide composed of one glucose molecule and one fructose molecule. Sweeter than lactose or maltose.

sudden infant death syndrome (SIDS)   The sudden death of a previously healthy infant; the most common cause of death in infants more than 1 month of age.

sulfites   A mold inhibitor that is very effective in controlling growth in grapes and wine.

sustainable agriculture   Techniques of food production that preserve the environment indefinitely.

system   A group of organs that work together to perform a unique function, for example, the gastrointestinal system.

T

teratogen   Any substance that can cause a birth defect.

texturizer   A chemical used to improve the texture of various foods.

thermic effect of food   The energy expended as a result of processing food consumed.

thickening agents   Natural or chemically modified carbohydrates that absorb some of the water present in food, making the food thicker.

thirst mechanism   A cluster of nerve cells in the hypothalamus that stimulate our desire to drink fluids in response to an increase in the concentration of salt in our blood or a decrease in blood pressure and blood volume.

thrifty gene theory   A theory that suggests that some people possess a gene (or genes) that causes them to be energetically thrifty, resulting in them expending less energy at rest and during physical activity.

time of activity   How long each exercise session lasts, not including warm-up and cool-down periods.

tissue   A sheet or other grouping of like cells that performs like functions, for example, muscle tissue.

Tolerable Upper Intake Level (UL)   The highest average daily nutrient intake level likely to pose no risk of adverse health effects to almost all individuals in a particular life stage and gender group.

total fiber   The sum of dietary fiber and functional fiber.

toxin   Any harmful substance; in microbiology, a chemical produced by a microorganism that harms tissues or causes harmful immune responses.

trabecular bone (spongy bone)   A porous bone tissue that is found within the ends of the long bones, and inside the spinal vertebrae, flat bones (breastbone, ribs, and most bones of the skull), and bones of the pelvis.

trace minerals   Minerals we need to consume in amounts less than 100 mg per day and of which the total amount in our bodies is less than 5 g.

transport proteins   Protein molecules that help to transport substances throughout the body and across cell membranes.

triglyceride   A molecule consisting of three fatty acids attached to a three-carbon glycerol backbone.

trimester   Any one of three stages of pregnancy, each lasting 13 to 14 weeks.

tumor   Any newly formed mass of undifferentiated cells.

type 1 diabetes   Disorder in which the body cannot produce enough insulin.

type 2 diabetes   Progressive disorder in which body cells become less responsive to insulin or the body does not produce enough insulin.

U

ultra-trace minerals   Minerals we need to consume in amounts less than 1 mg/kg body weight per day.

umbilical cord   The cord containing arteries and veins that connects the baby (from the navel) to the mother via the placenta.

undernutrition   Malnutrition defined by an absolute lack of adequate energy leading to underweight.

underweight   Having too little body fat to maintain health, causing a person to have a weight for a given height that is below an acceptably defined standard.

V

variety   Eating a lot of different foods each day.

vegetarianism   The practice of restricting the diet to food substances of plant origin, including vegetables, fruits, grains, and nuts.

very-low-density lipoprotein (VLDL)   Large lipoprotein made up mostly of triglyceride. Functions primarily to transport triglycerides from their source to the body's cells, including to adipose tissues for storage.

vigorous-intensity activities   Activities that produce significant increases in breathing, sweating, and heart rate; talking is difficult when exercising at a vigorous intensity.

viruses   A group of infectious agents that are much smaller than bacteria, lack independent metabolism, and are incapable of growth or reproduction outside of living cells.

viscous   Term referring to a gel-like consistency; viscous fibers form a gel when dissolved in water.

visible fats   Fat we can see in our foods or see added to foods, such as butter, margarine, cream, shortening, salad dressings, chicken skin, and untrimmed fat on meat.

vitamins   Micronutrients that contain carbon and assist us in regulating the processes of our bodies. They are classified as water soluble or fat soluble.

W

warm-up   Also called preliminary exercise; includes activities that prepare you for an exercise session, including stretching, calisthenics, and movements specific to the exercise you are about to engage in.

wasting   Very low weight for height.

water intoxication   Dilution of body fluid. It results when water intake or retention is excessive, and can lead to hyponatremia.

water-soluble vitamins   Vitamins that are soluble in water. These include vitamin C and the B vitamins.

wellness   A multidimensional, lifelong process that includes physical, emotional, and spiritual health.

INDEX

Page numbers in *italics* refer to figures and tables.

CREDITS

Photo Credits

Chapter 1

Opening photo: Masterfile; **p. 3:** Lew Robertson/Picture Arts/Corbis; **p. 7:** Tom Stewart/Corbis; **p. 8:** FoodPix/PictureArts Corporation/Jupiter Images; **p. 9 top:** Andy Crawford/Dorling Kindersley; **p. 9 bottom:** Jean Luc Morales/Getty Images; **p. 10 top:** Jon Riley/Getty Images; **p. 10 bottom:** Paul Poplis/Foodpix/Jupiter Images; **p. 11:** Photodisc/Getty; **p. 13 left:** Duomo/Corbis; **p. 13 right:** Alex Mares-Manton/Asia Images/Getty Images; **p. 15:** Jon Feingersh/Getty Images; **p. 16:** David Sacks/Getty Images; **p. 17:** Adams Picture Library t/a apl/Alamy; **p. 18 top:** Alexander Walter/Taxi/Getty Images; **p. 18 bottom:** Andrew Whittuck/Dorling Kindersley; **p. 21:** Steve Terrill/Corbis; **fig. 1.7:** PLG, Pearson Science; **fig. 1.8:** Kristin Piljay; **p. 24 top:** Chris Collins/Corbis; **fig. 1.9a-b:** PLG, Pearson Science; **p. 26:** PLG, Pearson Science; **p. 29:** Ned Frisk Photography/Corbis; **p. 30:** LA/Tevy Battini/Phototake NYC; **p. 35:** Kristin Piljay, Pearson Science.

Chapter 2

Opening photo: Andreas Schlegel/fStop/Getty Images; **p. 43:** Howard Kingsnorth/Getty Images; **p. 44:** George Doyle & Claran Griffin/Stockbyte/Getty; **p. 45:** Jonelle Weaver/Taxi/Getty Images; **fig. 2.10 left:** Dr. Richard Kessel & Dr. Gene Shih/Visuals Unlimited; **fig. 2.10 right:** Dr. David M. Philips/Visuals Unlimited; **p. 51:** Tim Hawley/Foodpix/Jupiter Images; **p. 53 top:** SPL/Photo Researchers; **p. 53 bottom:** Trysker/Shutterstock; **p. 54:** PLG, Pearson Science; **p. 56:** Peter Southwick/Stock Boston; **fig. 2.14:** Dr. E. Walker/SPL/Photo Researchers; **p. 59 top:** David Murray and Jules Selmes/Dorling Kindersley; **p. 59 bottom:** Cordelia Molloy/Photo Researchers; **p. 60 top:** Gerald Zanetti/Foodpix/Jupiter Images; **p. 60 bottom:** Rubberball/Getty Images; **p. 61:** Peter Adams/Taxi/Getty Images; **p. 62:** Pramod Mistry/Lonely Planet Images.

Chapter 3

Opening photo: Colin Anderson/Blend Images/Jupiter Images; **p. 69:** Michael Newman/PhotoEdit; **p. 70 left:** Foodcollection/Getty Images; **p. 70 right:** Envision/Corbis; **p. 71 top:** Robert J. Bennett/AGE Fotostock; **p. 71 bottom:** Kristin Piljay; **p. 73:** Rob Lewine/Bettmann/Corbis; **p. 74:** Jeff Greenburg/PhotoEdit; **p. 75:** Stockbyte/Getty Images; **p. 76:** Dorling Kindersley; **p. 79 top:** Steve Shott/Dorling Kindersley; **p. 79 bottom:** Ryan McVay/Getty Images; **p. 81:** Joe Raedle/Getty Images; **p. 82:** Kristin Piljay; **p. 85:** Dorling Kindersley; **fig. 3.12 top:** Eduard Andras/iStockphoto; **fig. 3.12 upper middle:** DarjaVorontsova/Shutterstock; **fig. 3.12 lower middle:** Jurga Rubinovaite/iStockphoto; **fig. 3.12 bottom:** Julie Masson Deshaies/iStockphoto; **p. 86 bottom:** Dorling Kindersley; **p. 88 top:** Photodisc/Getty Images; **p. 88 bottom:** AGE Fotostock; **fig. 3.13 all:** Creative Digital Visions; **fig. 3.14a:** Rebecca Ellis/iStockphoto; **fig. 3.14b:** Ben Beltman/iStockphoto; **p. 92:** Trysker/Shutterstock; **fig. 3.16:** Roche Diagnostics Corporation; **p. 94:** Getty Images.

Chapter 4

Opening photo: Masterfile; **p. 100:** Dorling Kindersley; **p. 102 top:** J.Garcia/Corbis; **p. 102 bottom:** David Murray/Dorling Kindersley; **p. 103:** AP Wide World Photos; **p. 105 top:** Michael Newman/PhotoEdit; **p. 105 bottom:** Maximilian Weinzierl/Alamy; **fig. 4.6:** Myrleen Ferguson Caféé/PhotoEdit; **p. 107:** Andersen Floss/Photodisc/Getty Images; **p. 108 top:** Doug Pensinger/Getty Im-

ages; **p. 108 bottom:** Odd Andersen/Getty Images; **p. 109 top:** Gerald Zanetti/Foodpix/Jupiter Images; **p. 109 bottom:** Kip Peticolas/Fundamental Photographs, NYC; **p. 111:** Michael Newman/Photo Edit; **p. 112:** Rubberball/Getty; **p. 113:** Jeff Greenberg/AGE Fotostock; **p. 114 bottom:** Spencer Platt/Getty Images; **fig. 4.9:** foodfolio/Alamy; **p. 118:** James Leynse/Bettmann/Corbis; **p. 119:** Trysker/Shutterstock; **fig. 4.12a:** Ed Reschke/Visuals Unlimited; **fig. 4.12b:** William Ober/Visuals Unlimited; **p. 124 top:** AP Wide World Photos; **p. 124 bottom:** George Doyle & Claran Griffin/Stockbyte/Getty; **p. 126:** Eric Meacher/Dorling Kindersley.

Chapter 5

Opening photo: Masterfile; **p. 131:** Duomo/Corbis; **p. 133 top:** Foodfolio/Jupiter Images; **fig. 5.3a:** Ed Reschke/Peter Arnold; **fig. 5.3b:** Andrew Syred/Photo Researchers; **fig. 5.4:** Creative Digital Visions; **fig. 5.6:** Visuals Unlimited; **p. 139:** Ian O'Leary/Dorling Kindersley; **p. 140:** AP Wide World Photos; **p. 141:** Rubberball/Getty Images; **p. 142:** Chris Hondros/Getty Images; **p. 143 top:** Ryan McVay/Getty Images; **p. 143 bottom:** Ranald MacKechnie/Dorling Kindersley; **p. 146:** Trysker/Shutterstock; **p. 149:** StockFood/Getty Images; **p. 150:** Jennifer Levy/FoodPix/Jupiter Images; **p. 152 top:** Stockbyte/Getty Images; **p. 152 bottom:** Dorling Kindersley.

Chapter 6

Opening photo: Creatas Images/Jupiter Images; **fig. 6.1 all:** Shutterstock; **p. 159:** www.blende11.de/Getty Images; **p. 161:** Dorling Kindersley; **p. 162:** Ian O'Leary/Dorling Kindersley; **fig. 6.3 top:** Ross Durant/Foodpix/Jupiter Images; **fig. 6.3 bottom:** Steve Cohen/Foodpix/Jupiter Images; **p. 164:** Peter Turnley/Bettmann/Corbis; **fig. 6.4 top:** Inmagine/Inspirestock/Jupiter Images; **fig. 6.4 bottom:** Barry Gregg/Corbis; **fig. 6.5:** Biophoto Associates/Photo Researchers; **fig. 6.8 top:** Corbis Premium RF/Alamy; **fig. 6.8 bottom:** Darja Vorontsova/Shutterstock; **p. 167 top:** Philip Dowell/Dorling Kindersley; **p. 167 bottom:** Dorling Kindersley; **p. 168 top:** Dorling Kindersley; **p. 168 bottom:** Bill Aron/PhotoEdit; **p. 169:** Cordelia Molloy/Photo Researchers; **p. 170:** Nancy R. Cohen/Getty Images; **fig. 6.9 top:** Suzannah Skelton/iStockphoto; **fig. 6.9 bottom:** Craig Veltri/iStockphoto; **p. 171:** Deborah Davis/Getty Images; **p. 172:** Steve Gorton/ Dorling Kindersley; **p. 173 top:** Dorling Kindersley; **fig. 6.10 both:** Barry Gregg/Corbis; **p. 174:** Photodisc/Getty Images: **fig. 6.12 top:** PLG/Pearson Science; **fig. 6.12 bottom:** Suzannah Skelton/iStockphoto; **fig. 6.13 top:** Ross Durant/Foodpix/Jupiter Images; **fig. 6.13 bottom:** Barry Gregg/Corbis; **fig. 6.14 top:** Jupiter Images/Brand X/Alamy; **fig. 6.14 bottom:** Craig Veltri/iStockphoto; **fig. 6.15:** Lester V. Bergman/Corbis; **fig. 6.16 top:** Spauln/Shutterstock; **fig. 6.16 bottom:** Spauln/iStockphoto; **p. 179:** Robert Fiocca/Picture Arts/Corbis; **fig. 6.17 top:** Gretchen Halverson/iStockphoto; **fig. 6.17 bottom:** PLG/Pearson Science; **fig. 6.18 top:** Ross Durant/Foodpix/Jupiter Images; **fig. 6.18 bottom:** Inmagine/Inspirestock/Jupiter Images; **p. 181 top:** Food Features/Alamy; **p. 181 middle:** David Murray/Dorling Kindersley; **p. 181 bottom:** Corbis; **p. 182 top:** Rubberball/Getty Images; **p. 182 bottom:** Trysker/Shutterstock; **p. 184:** Guy Ryecart and David Jordan/The Ivy Press Limited/Dorling Kindersley; **p. 186:** Eric Risberg/AP Photo; **p. 187:** Dorling Kindersley; **fig. 6.20 top to bottom:** Southern Illinois University/Photo Researchers; Lew Robertson/Foodpix/Jupiter Images; Image Source

Pink/Getty Images; Pixtal/AGE Fotostock; Carol and Mike Werner/ Phototake USA.

Chapter 7
Opening photo: David Buffington/Blend Images/Getty images; **fig. 7.1 broccoli:** PM Images/Photodisc/Getty Images; **fig. 7.1 all others:** Shutterstock; **p. 197:** Polka Dot Images/Jupiter Images; **p. 200:** Masterfile; **p. 202:** Michael Pohuski/Jupiter Images; **fig. 7.3 top:** Barry Gregg/Corbis; **fig. 7.3 bottom:** Spauln/iStockphoto; **p. 204 top:** Foodcollection/Getty Images; **p. 204 bottom:** Shaun Egan/Getty Images; **fig. 7.4 top:** Barry Gregg/Corbis; **fig. 7.4 bottom:** marco testa/iStockphoto; **p. 205:** George Doyle & Claran Griffin/Stockbyte/Getty Images; **p. 206 top:** Monique le Luhandre/ Dorling Kindersley; **p. 206 bottom:** Dorling Kindersley; **fig. 7.5 top:** Rudi Tapper/iStockphoto; **fig. 7.5 bottom:** Nigel Paul Monckton/ Shutterstock; **fig. 7.6:** Alison Wright/Corbis; **p. 208:** Kristin Piljay; **fig. 7.7 top:** Stephen Rees/iStockphoto; **fig. 7.7 bottom:** Brian Hagiwara/Foodpix/Jupiter Images; **p. 209:** Dorling Kindersley; **p. 211:** Burke/Triolo Productions/Foodpix/Jupiter Images; **fig. 7.10 top:** Laitr Keiows/Shutterstock; **fig. 7.10 bottom:** Suzannah Skelton/iStockphoto; **p. 213:** Isabelle Rozenbaum & Frederic Cirou/Getty Images; **fig. 7.11 both:** Dorling Kindersley; **p. 214:** Ian O'Leary/Dorling Kindersley; **p. 215:** Kristin Piljay; **fig. 7.12 top:** Morgan Lane Photography/Shutterstock; **fig. 7.12 bottom:** Kelly Cline/iStockphoto; **p. 218:** Dave King/Dorling Kindersley; **fig. 7.15 top:** Bill Varie/Workbook Stock/Jupiter Images; **fig. 7.15 bottom:** Barry Gregg/Corbis; **p. 221 top:** Catherine Ledner/Getty Images; **p. 221 bottom:** Spencer Jones/Photodisc/Getty Images; **fig. 7.17 top:** Greg Nicholas/iStockphoto; **fig. 7.17 bottom:** Suzannah Skelton/iStockphoto; **fig. 7.18:** National Institute of Dental Research; **fig. 7.19:** Michael Klein/Peter Arnold; **p. 223 top left:** Trysker/Shutterstock; **p. 223 bottom right:** Larry Williams/ Bettmann/Corbis; **fig. 7.20:** Yoav Levy/Phototake NYC; **p. 224:** Spencer Platt/Getty Images; **p. 225 top:** Duomo/Bettmann/Corbis; **p. 225 bottom:** Ned Frisk Photography/Corbis.

Chapter 8
Opening photo: Image Source/Getty images; **p. 233:** Arthur Tilley/Getty Images; **p. 235:** Theo Allots/Corbis; **fig. 8.3:** Yong Hian Lim/iStockphoto; **p. 237:** Randy Sidman-Moore/Masterfile; **p. 238:** Stockbyte/Getty Images; **p. 239:** Eyewire Collection/ Photodisc/Getty Images; **p. 240:** Network Productions/The Image Works; **p. 243 left:** Trysker/Shutterstock; **p. 243 right:** Corbis; **p. 245:** Ned Frisk Photography/Corbis; **fig. 8.6:** Kristin Piljay; **p. 247:** Corbis; **p. 248:** Michael Newman/PhotoEdit; **p. 250:** David Young-Wolff/PhotoEdit; **fig. 8.7a:** CNRI/Science Photo Library; **fig. 8.7b:** Martin M. Rotker/Photo Researchers; **p. 252 top:** Paul Conklin/Photo Edit; **p. 252 bottom:** Stockbyte/Getty Images; **p. 253:** Trysker/Shutterstock; **fig. 8.8:** George Steinmetz Photography.

Chapter 9
Opening photo: Manchan/Photographer's Choice/Getty Images; **p. 259:** Photodisc/Getty Images; **fig. 9.2:** PhotoEdit; **fig. 9.3:** Custom Medical Stock Photo; **fig. 9.4:** Phototake NYC; **fig. 9.5:** Life Measurement, Inc; **fig. 9.7:** Kristin Piljay; **p. 263:** Dorling Kindersley; **fig. 9.8a:** Stockbyte/Getty Images; **fig. 9.8b:** M. L. Harris/ Getty Images; **fig. 9.8c:** LWA/Sharie Kennedy/Getty Images; **p. 265:** Xavier Bonghi/Image Bank/Getty Images; **p. 268:** Mark Douet/Getty Images; **p. 270:** Bruce Dale/Getty Images; **fig. 9.11:** Creative Digital Visions; **p. 274:** Image Source/Jupiter Images; **p. 276:** David Young-Wolff/PhotoEdit; **p. 279:** Lew Robertson/ Corbis; **p. 280:** BananaStock/Jupiter Images; **p. 281 top:**

Photodisc/Getty Images; **p. 281 bottom:** Trysker/Shutterstock; **p. 284:** Ariel Skelley/Corbis; **p. 285:** LIU Jin/APF/Corbis; **p. 286 top:** Sheri Giblin/Foodpix/Jupiter Images; **p. 286 bottom:** Food Alan King/Alamy; **p. 287 top:** Stockbyte/Getty Images; **p. 287 bottom:** Trysker/Shutterstock; **fig. 9.16:** Laura Murray; **fig. 9.17:** Karl Prouse/Catwalking/Getty Images; **p. 291:** Blake Little/Getty Images; **fig. 9.18:** Express Newspapers/Getty Images; **fig. 9.20:** Baumgartner Olivia/Corbis; **p. 294:** Rel Loopers/Photolibrary; **p. 296:** Rubberball/Getty Images.

Chapter 10
Opening photo: Sheer Photo/Photodisc/Getty Images; **p. 302:** Caleb Kennal/PNI/Aurora & Quanta Productions; **p. 305:** Photodisc/Getty Images; **p. 306:** AP Wide World Photos; **fig. 10.3 top:** BananaStock/Jupiter Images; **fig. 10.3 middle:** Alan Jakubek/ Corbis; **fig. 10.3 bottom:** Comstock Images/Jupiter Images; **p. 308:** Will & Deni McIntyre/Photo Researchers; **p. 310:** Marc Romanelli/ Getty Images; **p. 311:** George Doyle & Claran Griffin/Stockbyte/ Getty Images; **p. 318:** Stephen Oliver/Dorling Kindersley; **fig. 10.8:** Laura Murray; **p. 319:** Photodisc/Getty Images; **p. 320:** Scott T. Smith/Corbis; **fig. 10.9 top:** Lily Valde/Pixland/Jupiter Images; **fig. 10.9 bottom:** Dominic Burke/Alamy; **p. 323:** Dave King/ Dorling Kindersley; **p. 324:** David Young-Wolff/Getty Images; **p. 326 top:** Stockbyte/Getty Images; **p. 326 bottom:** Trysker/ Shutterstock; **p. 328:** Altrendo/Getty Images; **p. 329:** Derek Hall/ Dorling Kindersley.

Chapter 11
Opening photo: Blend Images/Veer; **p. 334:** David Phillips/The Population Council/Photo Researchers; **fig. 11.1 top:** Lennart Nilsson/Albert Bonniers Forlag AB; **fig. 11.1 upper middle:** Lennart Nilsson/Albert Bonniers Forlag AB; **fig. 11.1 lower middle:** Neil Bromhall/Photo Researchers; **fig. 11.1 bottom:** Tom Galliher/ Corbis; **p. 338:** Ian O'Leary/Getty Images; **p. 339:** Dave King/ Dorling Kindersley; **fig. 11.3:** Biophoto Associates/Science Source/ Photo Researchers; **p. 341:** Carl Tremblay/StockFood Creative/ Getty Images; **p. 342:** Allana Wesley White/Corbis; **p. 344 top:** George Doyle & Claran Griffin/Stockbyte/Getty Images; **p. 344 bottom:** Jim Craigmyle/Corbis; **p. 346:** Phanie/Photo Researchers; **p. 347:** Rick Gomez/AGE Fotostock; **fig. 11.4:** Dr. Pamela R. Erickson; **p. 352:** Corbis; **p. 354:** Anne Flinn Powell/Index Stock Imagery; **p. 356 top:** Michael Newman/PhotoEdit; **p. 356 bottom:** Dave King/Dorling Kindersley; **fig. 11.5:** Laura Dwight; **p. 357:** Roger Phillips/Dorling Kindersley; **p. 359 top:** Laura Murray; **p. 359 bottom:** Vince Streano/Corbis; **p. 361:** Bob Daemmrich/ The Image Works; **p. 362:** Gary Buss/Getty Images; **p. 364:** Tom Stewart/Corbis; **p. 368:** Tom & Dee Ann McCarthy/Corbis; **p. 369:** Richard Koek/Getty Images; **p. 370:** Raymond Gehman/Corbis; **p. 371:** Don Smetzer/Getty Images; **p. 373:** Deborah Jaffe/ Foodpix/Jupiter Images; **p. 374 top:** Donna Day/Getty Images; **p. 374 bottom:** Ryan McVay/Getty Images; **p. 376:** Ned Frisk Photography/Corbis; **p. 377:** Andreas Pollok/Getty Images; **p. 378:** Karen Pruess/The Image Works.

Chapter 12
Opening photo: Masterfile; **fig. 12.1:** Barry Dowsett/Photo Researchers; **fig. 12.2:** Andrew Syred/Photo Researchers; **fig. 12.3:** Matt Meadows/Peter Arnold; **fig. 12.4:** Neil Fletcher/Dorling Kindersley; **p. 390:** Vanessa Davies/Dorling Kindersley; **p. 391:** Digital Vision/Getty Images; **p. 396:** Alan Richardson/Foodpix/Jupiter Images; **p. 398:** Stockbyte/Getty Images; **p. 399 top:** Owen Franken/Corbis; **p. 399 bottom:** Hulton Archive Photos/Getty Images; **p. 400:** Digital Vision/Getty Images; **fig. 12.9:** Lon C. Diehl/

PhotoEdit; **p. 402:** Martin Bond/Peter Arnold; **p. 403 top:** Corbis; **p. 403 bottom:** Travis Amos; **fig. 12.12 left:** Carl Walsh/Aurora; **fig. 12.12 right:** Brian Hagiwara/Foodpix/Jupiter Images; **p. 406 top:** Corbis; **p. 406 bottom:** Judith Miller/Dorling Kindersley/ Woolley and Wallis; **p. 407:** Ned Frisk Photography/Corbis; **p. 411:** Reuters/Corbis; **fig. 12.15:** Getty Images; **p. 413:** Trysker/ Shutterstock Images; **fig. 12.16:** Alexandra Avakian/Corbis; **fig. 12.17:** AP Wide World Photos.

Figure and Text Credits

Fig. 1.8 From Salge Blake, J. *Nutrition and You,* Fig. 2.8. © 2008. Reprinted by permission of Pearson Education. **Fig. 1.14** Flow chart based on Bauman, R. *Microbiology,* Figure 1.13 © 2003 Benjamin Cummings. Used by permission of Pearson Education. **p. 190** © 2006 Produce for Better Health Foundation. Fruits & Veggies— More Matters and the Fruits & Veggies—More Matters Logo are registered trademarks and servicemarks of Produce for Better Health Foundation. All rights reserved. **Fig. 6.6b** From Germann, W. and Stanfield, C. *Principles of Human Physiology,* Fig. 2.9. Copyright © 2001 Benjamin Cummings. **Fig. 6.1** Eyeball from Marieb, *Human Anatomy and Physiology,* 5e, Fig. 16.7. © 2003. Reprinted by permission of Pearson Education. **Figure 7.9** Hemoglobin and myoglobin illustrations, Irving Geis. Rights owned by Howard Hughes Medical Institute. Not to be reproduced without permission. **p. 294** National Institute of Mental Health. 2007. Eating Disorders. P. 10. **Fig. 7.13** From Germann, W. and Stanfield, C. *Principles of Human Physiology,* Fig. 20.14. Copyright © 2001 Benjamin Cummings. **Fig. 7.14** From Germann, W. and Stanfield, C. *Principles of Human Physiology,* Fig. 20.14. Copyright © 2001 Benjamin Cummings. **Fig 10.5** From *Biology: Exploring Life* by Neil Campbell, Brad Williamson, and Robin Heyden. © 2003 by Pearson Education, Inc. Publishing as Prentice Hall. **Fig. 11.1** Adapted from Germann, W. and Stanfield, C. *Principles of Human Physiology,* 2/e, Fig. 22.20a. Copyright © 2001 Benjamin Cummings. Reprinted by permission of Pearson Education, Inc. **Fig. 11.3** Adapted from Germann, W. and Stanfield, C. *Principles of Human Physiology,* 2/e, Fig. 22.22. Copyright © 2001 Benjamin Cummings. Reprinted by permission of Pearson Education, Inc. **Fig. 11.4** Adapted from Germann, W. and Stanfield, C. *Principles of Human Physiology,* 2/e, Fig. 22.25a. Copyright © 2001 Benjamin Cummings. Reprinted by permission of Pearson Education, Inc.

DIETARY REFERENCE INTAKES: RDA, AI*, (AMDR)

	Macronutrients					
Life-Stage Group	Carbohydrate— Total Digestible (g/d)	Total Fiber (g/d)	Total Fat (g/d)	n-6 polyunsaturated fatty acids (linoleic acid) (g/d)	n-3 polyunsaturated fatty acids (α-linolenic acid) (g/d)	Protein and Amino Acids (g/d) [a]
Infants						
0–6 mo	60* (ND[b])[c]	ND	31*	4.4* (ND)	0.5* (ND)	9.1* (ND)
7–12 mo	95* (ND)	ND	30*	4.6* (ND)	0.5* (ND)	13.5 (ND)
Children						
1–3 y	130 (45–65)	19*	(30–40)	7* (5–10)	0.7* (0.6–1.2)	13 (5–20)
4–8 y	130 (45–65)	25*	(25–35)	10* (5–10)	0.9* (0.6–1.2)	19 (10–30)
Males						
9–13 y	130 (45–65)	31*	(25–35)	12* (5–10)	1.2* (0.6–1.2)	34 (10–30)
14–18 y	130 (45–65)	38*	(25–35)	16* (5–10)	1.6* (0.6–1.2)	52 (10–30)
19–30 y	130 (45–65)	38*	(20–35)	17* (5–10)	1.6* (0.6–1.2)	56 (10–35)
31–50 y	130 (45–65)	38*	(20–35)	17* (5–10)	1.6* (0.6–1.2)	56 (10–35)
51–70 y	130 (45–65)	30*	(20–35)	14* (5–10)	1.6* (0.6–1.2)	56 (10–35)
>70 y	130 (45–65)	30*	(20–35)	14* (5–10)	1.6* (0.6–1.2)	56 (10–35)
Females						
9–13 y	130 (45–65)	26*	(25–35)	10* (5–10)	1.0* (0.6–1.2)	34 (10–30)
14–18 y	130 (45–65)	26*	(25–35)	11* (5–10)	1.1* (0.6–1.2)	46 (10–30)
19–30 y	130 (45–65)	25*	(20–35)	12* (5–10)	1.1* (0.6–1.2)	46 (10–35)
31–50 y	130 (45–65)	25*	(20–35)	12* (5–10)	1.1* (0.6–1.2)	46 (10–35)
51–70 y	130 (45–65)	21*	(20–35)	11* (5–10)	1.1* (0.6–1.2)	46 (10–35)
>70 y	130 (45–65)	21*	(20–35)	11* (5–10)	1.1* (0.6–1.2)	46 (10–35)
Pregnancy						
≤18 y	175 (45–65)	28*	(20–35)	13* (5–10)	1.4* (0.6–1.2)	71 (10–35)
19–30 y	175 (45–65)	28*	(20–35)	13* (5–10)	1.4* (0.6–1.2)	71 (10–35)
31–50 y	(45–65)	28*	(20–35)	13* (5–10)	1.4* (0.6–1.2)	71 (10–35)
Lactation						
≤18 y	210 (45–65)	29*	(20–35)	13* (5–10)	1.3* (0.6–1.2)	71 (10–35)
19–30 y	210 (45–65)	29*	(20–35)	13* (5–10)	1.3* (0.6–1.2)	71 (10–35)
31–50 y	210 (45–65)	29*	(20–35)	13* (5–10)	1.3* (0.6–1.2)	71 (10–35)

Source: Reprinted with permission from "Dietary Reference Intakes for Energy, Carbohydrates, Fiber, Fat, Fatty Acids, Cholesterol, Protein, and Amino Acids (Macronutrients)," © 2005 by the National Academy of Sciences, courtesy of the National Academies Press, Washington, DC.

Note: This table is adapted from the DRI reports, see www.nap.edu. It lists Recommended Dietary Allowances (RDAs), with Adequate Intakes (AIs) indicated by an asterisk (*), and Acceptable Macronutrient Distribution Range (AMDR) data provided in parentheses. RDAs and AIs may both be used as goals for individual intake. RDAs are set to meet the needs of almost all (97% to 98%) individuals in a group. For healthy breastfed infants, the AI is the mean intake. The AI for other life stage and gender groups is believed to cover the needs of all individuals in the group, but lack of data prevent being able to specify with confidence the percentage of individuals covered by this intake.

[a] Based on 1.5 g/kg/day for infants, 1.1 g/kg/day for 1–3 y, 0.95 g/kg/day for 4–13 y, 0.85 g/kg/day for 14–18 y, 0.8 g/kg/day for adults, and 1.1 g/kg/day for pregnant (using pre-pregnancy weight) and lactating women.

[b] ND = Not determinable due to lack of data of adverse effects in this age group and concern with regard to lack of ability to handle excess amounts. Source of intake should be from food only to prevent high levels of intake.

[c] Data in parentheses are Acceptable Macronutrient Distribution Range (AMDR). This is the range of intake for a particular energy source that is associated with reduced risk of chronic disease while providing intakes of essential nutrients. If an individual consumes in excess of the AMDR, there is a potential of increasing the risk of chronic diseases and/or insufficient intakes of essential nutrients.